Register Now for Online Access to Your Book!

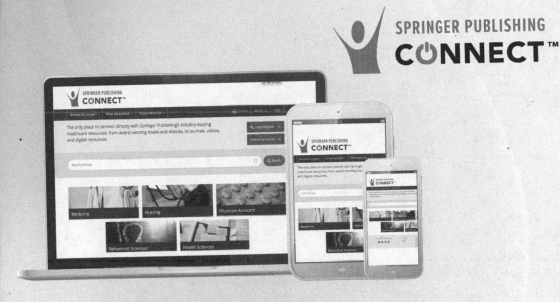

SPRINGER PUBLISHING CONNECT™

Your print purchase of *Tumor Board Review, Third Edition*, **includes online access to the contents of your book**—increasing accessibility, portability, and searchability!

Access today at:
http://connect.springerpub.com/content/book/978-0-8261-4598-7
or scan the QR code at the right with your smartphone. Log in or register, then click "Redeem a voucher" and use the code below.

5VMV25U4

Scan here for quick access.

Having trouble redeeming a voucher code?
Go to https://connect.springerpub.com/redeeming-voucher-code

If you are experiencing problems accessing the digital component of this product, please contact our customer service department at cs@springerpub.com

The online access with your print purchase is available at the publisher's discretion and may be removed at any time without notice.

Publisher's Note: New and used products purchased from third-party sellers are not guaranteed for quality, authenticity, or access to any included digital components.

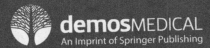

demosMEDICAL
An Imprint of Springer Publishing

View all our products at springerpub.com/demosmedical

Tumor Board Review

Tumor Board Review

Evidence-Based Case Reviews and Questions

Third Edition

Editors

Francis P. Worden, MD
Professor of Medicine
Director of the Hematology/Oncology Fellowship Program
University of Michigan Medical School
Ann Arbor, Michigan

Martha P. Mims, MD, PhD
Professor
Chief of Hematology-Oncology
Baylor College of Medicine
Houston, Texas

Helen K. Chew, MD
Professor of Medicine
Director of the Clinical Breast Cancer Program
University of California Davis
Davis, California

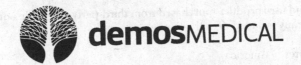

demosMEDICAL

Springer Publishing Company, LLC
11 West 42nd Street, New York, NY 10036
www.springerpub.com
connect.springerpub.com/

Acquisitions Editor: David D'Addona
Compositor: Exeter Premedia Services Private Limited

ISBN: 978-0-8261-4597-0
ebook ISBN: 978-0-8261-4598-7
DOI: 10.1891/9780826145987

Printed by BnT

Medicine is an ever-changing science. Research and clinical experience are continually expanding our
knowledge, in particular our understanding of proper treatment and drug therapy. The authors, editors,
and publisher have made every effort to ensure that all information in this book is in accordance with the
state of knowledge at the time of production of the book. Nevertheless, the authors, editors, and publisher
are not responsible for any errors or omissions or for any consequence from application of the information in this book and make no warranty, expressed or implied, with respect to the content of this publication. Every reader should examine carefully the package inserts accompanying each drug and should
carefully check whether the dosage schedules therein or the contraindications stated by the manufacturer
differ from the statements made in this book. Such examination is particularly important with drugs that
are either rarely used or have been newly released on the market.

Library of Congress Cataloging-in-Publication Data

Names: Worden, Francis P., editor. | Mims, Martha Pritchett, editor. |
  Chew, Helen K., editor.
Title: Tumor board review : evidence-based case reviews and questions /
  editors, Francis P. Worden, Martha Pritchett Mims, Helen K. Chew.
Description: Third edition. | New York, NY : Springer Publishing Company,
  [2023] | Includes bibliographical references and index.
Identifiers: LCCN 2022019636 (print) | LCCN 2022019637 (ebook) | ISBN
  9780826145970 (paperback) | ISBN 9780826145987 (ebook)
Subjects: MESH: Neoplasms | Evidence-Based Medicine | Practice Guideline |
  Case Reports
Classification: LCC RC254 (print) | LCC RC254 (ebook) | NLM QZ 200 | DDC
  616.99/4--dc23/eng/20220624
LC record available at https://lccn.loc.gov/2022019636
LC ebook record available at https://lccn.loc.gov/2022019637

Contents

Contributors *xv*
Preface *xxi*

1. Head and Neck Cancer **1**
   Irene Tsung, Samuel B. Reynolds, and Paul L. Swiecicki

   Introduction 1
   Case Summaries 1
   Case 1.1: Locally Advanced Cancer of the Oropharynx 1
   Case 1.2: Locally Advanced Nasopharyngeal Cancer 4
   Case 1.3: Metastatic Adenoid Cystic Carcinoma 7
   Case 1.4: Metastatic Squamous Cell Carcinoma 9
   Review Questions 12
   Answers and Rationales 15
   References 16

2. Thyroid Cancer **19**
   Kamya Sankar and Francis P. Worden

   Introduction 19
   Case Summaries 21
   Case 2.1: Locally Advanced Anaplastic Thyroid Cancer 21
   Case 2.2: Metastatic Medullary Thyroid Cancer 22
   Case 2.3: Metastatic Radioactive Iodine Refractory Differentiated Thyroid Cancer 24
   Review Questions 29
   Answers and Rationales 31
   References 32

3. Non-Small Cell Lung Cancer **35**
   Natalie Chen, Cyrus A. Iqbal, Omayra Gonzalez-Pagan, Meera Patel, Daniel Wang, and Quillan Huang

   Introduction 35
   Case Summaries 36
   Case 3.1: Early-Stage Resectable Lung Cancer 36
   Case 3.2: Locally Advanced Unresectable Lung Cancer 38
   Case 3.3: Metastatic Lung Cancer Without Driver Mutations 40
   Case 3.4: Metastatic Lung Adenocarcinoma With a Targetable Driver Mutation 43
   Case 3.5: Metastatic Non-Small Cell Lung Cancer in the Second Line 45
   Review Questions 47
   Answers and Rationales 49
   References 50

4. Small Cell Lung Cancer   53
  Ebaa Al-Obeidi and Karen Kelly

  Introduction   53
  Case Summaries   53
  Case 4.1: Newly Diagnosed Extensive-Stage Small Cell Lung Cancer   53
  Case 4.2: Relapsed Small Cell Lung Cancer   56
  Case 4.3: Limited-Stage Small Cell Lung Cancer and the Role of Prophylactic Cranial
        Irradiation Versus MRI Brain Surveillance   57
  Review Questions   61
  Answers and Rationales   64
  References   65

5. Hormone Receptor-Positive Breast Cancer   67
  *Katherine Sanchez, Jennifer Collins, Sudha Yarlagadda, Jingxin Sun, Sarah Premji,
  Maryam Nemati Shafaee, and Julie Nangia*

  Introduction   67
  Case Summaries   67
  Case 5.1: Early-Stage Breast Cancer   67
  Case 5.2: Early-Stage Hormone-Positive Breast Cancer   71
  Case 5.3: Locally Advanced Breast Cancer   73
  Case 5.4: Stage IV Breast Cancer   75
  Case 5.5: Recurrent Stage IV Breast Cancer   78
  Review Questions   81
  Answers and Rationales   83
  References   84

6. Triple-Negative Breast Cancer   87
  Richard Benjamin Young and Helen K. Chew

  Introduction   87
  Case Summaries   87
  Case 6.1: Localized Triple-Negative Breast Cancer   87
  Case 6.2: Locally Advanced Triple-Negative Breast Cancer   89
  Case 6.3: Metastatic Triple-Negative Breast Cancer   92
  Review Questions   96
  Answers and Rationales   98
  References   98

7. Esophageal Cancer   101
  Kamya Sankar, Charles B. Nguyen, and Bryan J. Schneider

  Introduction   101
  Case Summaries   103
  Case 7.1: Locally Advanced, Resectable Esophageal Adenocarcinoma   103
  Case 7.2: Locally Advanced Esophageal Squamous Cell Carcinoma   106
  Case 7.3: Locally Advanced Cervical Esophageal Squamous Cell Carcinoma   106
  Case 7.4: Metastatic Esophageal Adenocarcinoma   107
  Case 7.5: Human Epidermal Growth Factor Receptor 2-Positive Metastatic Esophageal
        Cancer   110
  Review Questions   112
  Answers and Rationales   115
  References   116

8. Gastric Cancer *119*
    Karen Riggins and Huili Zhu

    Introduction *119*
    Case Summaries *119*
    Case 8.1: Resectable Gastric Cancer *119*
    Case 8.2: Unresectable Locally Advanced Gastric Cancer *123*
    Case 8.3: Metastatic Gastric Adenocarcinoma *125*
    Review Questions *131*
    Answers and Rationales *134*
    References *135*

9. Pancreatic Cancer *139*
    Huili Zhu, Zachary Phillip Yeung, Benjamin Musher, and Shalini Makawita

    Introduction *139*
    Case Summaries *139*
    Case 9.1: Resectable Pancreatic Cancer *139*
    Case 9.2: Borderline Resectable Pancreatic Cancer *143*
    Case 9.3: Locally Advanced Pancreatic Cancer *145*
    Case 9.4: Metastatic Pancreatic Cancer *146*
    Review Questions *149*
    Answers and Rationales *151*
    References *152*

10. Neuroendocrine Cancer *155*
    Tannaz Armaghany and Zachary Phillip Yeung

    Introduction *155*
    Case Summaries *156*
    Case 10.1: Gastric Neuroendocrine Neoplasm *156*
    Case 10.2: Pancreatic Neuroendocrine Neoplasm *159*
    Case 10.3: Midgut Neuroendocrine Tumor and Carcinoid Syndrome *165*
    Case 10.4: Poorly Differentiated Neuroendocrine Carcinoma *170*
    Review Questions *173*
    Answers and Rationales *176*
    References *177*

11. Hepatobiliary Cancer *181*
    Brian Pham and Edward J. Kim

    Introduction *181*
    Case Summaries *181*
    Case 11.1: Metastatic Hepatocellular Carcinoma *181*
    Case 11.2: Locally Advanced Cholangiocarcinoma *184*
    Case 11.3: Metastatic Cholangiocarcinoma *186*
    Review Questions *188*
    Answers and Rationales *190*
    References *190*

12. Colorectal Cancer *193*
    Brian Pham and Edward J. Kim

    Introduction *193*
    Case Summaries *194*

Case 12.1: Locally Advanced Colon Adenocarcinoma 194
Case 12.2: Locally Advanced Rectal Cancer 196
Case 12.3: Unresectable Metastatic Colon Adenocarcinoma 197
Review Questions 200
Answers and Rationales 203
References 204

13. Anal Cancer 207
Arathi Mohan and John C. Krauss

Introduction 207
Case Summaries 208
Case 13.1: Locally Advanced Anal Cancer 208
Case 13.2: Very Early-Stage Anal Cancer Requiring Surgery Alone 210
Case 13.3: Metastatic Anal Cancer 211
Review Questions 212
Answers and Rationales 214
References 214

14. Prostate Cancer 217
Monica Tamil, Nagaishwarya Moka, Aihua Edward Yen, and Arpit Rao

Introduction 217
Case Summaries 217
Case 14.1: Localized Prostate Cancer 217
Case 14.2: Biochemically Recurrent Prostate Cancer 220
Case 14.3: Metastatic Hormone-Sensitive Prostate Cancer 222
Review Questions 225
Answers and Rationales 228
References 229

15. Testicular Cancer 231
Thomas C. Westbrook, Eric B. Schwartz, and Zachery R. Reichert

Introduction 231
Case Summaries 231
Case 15.1: Localized Testicular Cancer—Seminoma 231
Case 15.2: Advanced Testicular Cancer—Seminoma 233
Case 15.3: Locally Advanced Nonseminoma Testicular Cancer 236
Case 15.4: Metastatic Nonseminoma Testicular Cancer 237
Review Questions 240
Answers and Rationales 243
References 244

16. Renal Cancer 245
Eric Granowicz and Mamta Parikh

Introduction 245
Case Summaries 245
Case 16.1: Early-Stage Renal Cell Carcinoma 245
Case 16.2: Metastatic Renal Cell Carcinoma 248
Case 16.3: Oligometastatic Disease 251
Review Questions 253

Answers and Rationales *256*
References *257*

17. Bladder Cancer *259*
    Eric Granowicz and Mamta Parikh

    Introduction *259*
    Case Summaries *259*
    Case 17.1: Muscle-Invasive Bladder Cancer in a Surgical Candidate *259*
    Case 17.2: Muscle-Invasive Bladder Cancer in a Nonsurgical Candidate *262*
    Case 17.3: Metastatic Bladder Cancer *263*
    Case 17.4: Platinum-Refractory Metastatic Bladder Cancer *265*
    Review Questions *267*
    Answers and Rationales *270*
    References *271*

18. Cervical Cancer *273*
    Alli M. Straubhar and Jean H. Siedel

    Introduction *273*
    Case Summaries *274*
    Case 18.1: Early Cervical Cancer *274*
    Case 18.2: Locally Advanced Cervical Cancer *277*
    Case 18.3: Distant Metastatic and Recurrent Cervical Cancer *278*
    Review Questions *281*
    Answers and Rationales *284*
    References *285*

19. Uterine Cancer *289*
    Claire Hoppenot

    Introduction *289*
    Case Summaries *289*
    Case 19.1: Type 1 Endometrial Cancer *289*
    Case 19.2: Advanced Type 2 Endometrial Cancer *292*
    Case 19.3: Leiomyosarcoma *294*
    Review Questions *298*
    Answers and Rationales *300*
    References *300*

20. Ovarian Cancer *303*
    Katelyn Tondo-Steele and Jean H. Siedel

    Introduction *303*
    Case Summaries *304*
    Case 20.1: Early Ovarian Cancer *304*
    Case 20.2: Borderline Ovarian Tumor *306*
    Case 20.3: Primary Treatment: Neoadjuvant Treatment Versus Primary Cytoreductive
        Surgery *308*
    Case 20.4: Recurrent Ovarian Cancer *310*
    Case 20.5: Malignant Germ Cell Tumor *311*
    Review Questions *313*
    Answers and Rationales *316*
    References *318*

21. Melanoma *321*
    Vincent T. Ma, Luke T. Fraley, and Leslie A. Fecher

    Introduction *321*
    Case Summaries *322*
    Case 21.1: Stage I to II Disease *322*
    Case 21.2: Locally Advanced Stage III With Positive Sentinel Node *324*
    Case 21.3: Metastatic *BRAF* V600 Mutation-Positive Disease *327*
    Case 21.4: Merkel Cell Carcinoma *329*
    Review Questions *332*
    Answers and Rationales *335*
    References *336*

22. Bone Sarcoma *339*
    James Liu and Janai R. Carr-Ascher

    Introduction *339*
    Case Summaries *339*
    Case 22.1: Osteosarcoma *339*
    Case 22.2: Ewing Sarcoma *341*
    Case 22.3: Chondrosarcoma *343*
    Review Questions *345*
    Answers and Rationales *347*
    References *348*

23. Soft-Tissue Sarcoma *349*
    James Liu and Janai R. Carr-Ascher

    Introduction *349*
    Case Summaries *349*
    Case 23.1: Localized Soft-Tissue Sarcoma *349*
    Case 23.2: Metastatic Soft-Tissue Sarcoma *351*
    Case 23.3: Rhabdomyosarcoma *352*
    Case 23.4: Gastrointestinal Stromal Tumor *353*
    Review Questions *355*
    Answers and Rationales *357*
    References *358*

24. Primary Brain Tumors *361*
    Akaolisa S. Eziokwu and Jacob Mandel

    Introduction *361*
    Case Summaries *361*
    Case 24.1: Glioblastoma, *IDH* Wildtype *361*
    Case 24.2: Astrocytoma, *IDH* Mutant *366*
    Case 24.3: Oligodendroglioma, *IDH* Mutant, 1p/19q Co-Deleted *371*
    Review Questions *376*
    Answers and Rationales *378*
    References *379*

25. Cancer of Unknown Primary *381*
    Marcus Geer, Jennifer Girard, and Francis P. Worden

    Introduction *381*
    Case Summaries *384*

Case 25.1: Squamous Cell Carcinoma of the Head and Neck *384*
Case 25.2: Poorly Differentiated Carcinoma of Unknown Primary *387*
Case 25.3: Neuroendocrine Cancer of Unknown Primary *390*
Case 25.4: Adenocarcinoma of Unknown Primary *394*
Review Questions *398*
Answers and Rationales *401*
References *402*

26. Hodgkin Lymphoma *405*
    Radhika Takiar, Lisa P. Chu, and Tycel J. Phillips

    Introduction *405*
    Case Summaries *405*
    Case 26.1: Early-Stage, Favorable Risk Hodgkin Lymphoma *405*
    Case 26.2: Early-Stage, Unfavorable Risk Hodgkin Lymphoma *408*
    Case 26.3: Advanced-Stage Hodgkin Lymphoma *410*
    Review Questions *413*
    Answers and Rationales *415*
    References *415*

27. Non-Hodgkin Lymphoma *417*
    Alejandro Marinos, Colbert A. Parker, Akiva Diamond, and Sravanti P. Teegavarapu

    Introduction *417*
    Case Summaries *420*
    Case 27.1: Mantle Cell Lymphoma *420*
    Case 27.2: Follicular Lymphoma *422*
    Case 27.3: Diffuse Large B-Cell Lymphoma *424*
    Case 27.4: Peripheral T-Cell Lymphoma *428*
    Case 27.5: Burkitt Lymphoma *431*
    Review Questions *434*
    Answers and Rationales *437*
    References *438*

28. Multiple Myeloma and Plasma Cell Neoplasms *441*
    Christopher T. Su, Jason C. Chen, and Matthew J. Pianko

    Introduction *441*
    Case Summaries *441*
    Case 28.1: Precursor Disease (Monoclonal Gammopathy of Undetermined Significance,
       Smoldering Multiple Myeloma) *441*
    Case 28.2: Newly Diagnosed, Transplant-Eligible Multiple Myeloma *446*
    Case 28.3: Newly Diagnosed, Transplant-Ineligible Multiple Myeloma *448*
    Case 28.4: Relapsed/Refractory Multiple Myeloma *449*
    Case 28.5: Amyloid Light Chain Amyloidosis *451*
    Review Questions *453*
    Answers and Rationales *456*
    References *458*

29. Acute Lymphoblastic Leukemia *461*
    Colbert A. Parker, Cyrus A. Iqbal, and Martha P. Mims

    Introduction *461*
    Case Summaries *462*

Case 29.1: Adolescent and Young Adult Acute Lymphoblastic Leukemia *462*
Case 29.2: Philadelphia Chromosome-Positive Acute Lymphoblastic Leukemia *465*
Case 29.3: Pre-B Cell Acute Lymphoblastic Leukemia *467*
Case 29.4: T-Cell Acute Lymphoblastic Leukemia *469*
Review Questions *471*
Answers and Rationales *474*
References *475*

30. Acute Myelogenous Leukemia *477*
    Elizabeth F. Eisenmenger, Maria Siddiqui, and Gustavo Rivero

    Introduction *477*
    Case Summaries *477*
    Case 30.1: Acute Promyelocytic Leukemia *477*
    Case 30.2: Acute Myeloid Leukemia With Favorable Risk in Younger Adults
       (18 to 60 Years Old) *482*
    Case 30.3: Acute Myeloid Leukemia With Intermediate Risk/Unfavorable Risk in
       Younger Adults *483*
    Case 30.4: Acute Myeloid Leukemia in the Older Adult (Age Older Than
       60 Years) *484*
    Review Questions *487*
    Answers and Rationales *490*
    References *491*

31. Chronic Myeloid Leukemia *493*
    Tamer Othman and Brian A. Jonas

    Introduction *493*
    Case Summaries *493*
    Case 31.1: Newly Diagnosed Chronic Myeloid Leukemia *493*
    Case 31.2: Chronic Myeloid Leukemia With a *T315I* Mutation *498*
    Case 31.3: Chronic Myeloid Leukemia With Lymphoid Blast Crisis *500*
    Review Questions *503*
    Answers and Rationales *506*
    References *507*

32. Chronic Lymphocytic Leukemia *511*
    Tamer Othman and Brian A. Jonas

    Introduction *511*
    Case Summaries *511*
    Case 32.1: Newly Diagnosed Chronic Lymphocytic Leukemia *511*
    Case 32.2: Chronic Lymphocytic Leukemia Requiring Treatment *514*
    Case 32.3: Chronic Lymphocytic Leukemia Undergoing Richter's Transformation *517*
    Review Questions *519*
    Answers and Rationales *522*
    References *523*

33. Myelodysplastic Syndrome *527*
    Tamer Othman and Brian A. Jonas

    Introduction *527*

Case Summaries 527
Case 33.1: Myelodysplastic Syndrome With Excess Blasts-1 527
Case 33.2: Myelodysplastic Syndrome With Ring Sideroblasts 533
Case 33.3: Myelodysplastic Syndrome With Isolated Del(5q) 536
Review Questions 537
Answers and Rationales 540
References 541

Index 545

Contributors

Ebaa Al-Obeidi, MD   Fellow, Department of Internal Medicine, Division of Hematology/Oncology, University of California Davis Comprehensive Cancer Center, Sacramento, California

Tannaz Armaghany, MD   Assistant Professor, Section of Hematology/Oncology, Department of Medicine, Dan L Duncan Comprehensive Cancer Center, Baylor College of Medicine, Houston, Texas

Janai R. Carr-Ascher, MD, PhD   Assistant Professor, Department of Internal Medicine, Division of Hematology/Oncology, University of California Davis Comprehensive Cancer Center, Sacramento, California

Jason C. Chen, MD   Clinical Assistant Professor, Department of Internal Medicine, University of Michigan, Ann Arbor, Michigan

Natalie Chen, MD, PhD   Hematology/Oncology Fellow, Department of Medicine, Baylor College of Medicine, Houston, Texas

Helen K. Chew, MD   Professor of Medicine, Department of Internal Medicine, Division of Hematology/Oncology, University of California Davis Comprehensive Cancer Center, Sacramento, California

Lisa P. Chu, MD   Fellow, Department of Internal Medicine, Division of Hematology/Oncology, University of Michigan, Ann Arbor, Michigan

Jennifer Collins, MD   Hematology/Oncology Fellow, Baylor College of Medicine, Houston, Texas

Akiva Diamond, MD   Assistant Professor, Section of Hematology/Oncology, Department of Medicine, Dan L Duncan Comprehensive Cancer Center, Baylor College of Medicine, Houston, Texas

Elizabeth F. Eisenmenger, MD   Hematology/Oncology Fellow, Department of Medicine, Baylor College of Medicine, Houston, Texas

Akaolisa S. Eziokwu, MD, MS   Hematology/Oncology Fellow, Department of Medicine, Baylor College of Medicine, Houston, Texas

Leslie A. Fecher, MD   Clinical Professor of Medicine and Dermatology, Department of Internal Medicine, Division of Hematology and Oncology, Rogel Cancer Center, University of Michigan, Ann Arbor, Michigan

Luke T. Fraley, MD Hematology/Oncology Fellow, Department of Internal Medicine, University of Michigan Medical School, Ann Arbor, Michigan

Marcus Geer, MD Hematology/Oncology Fellow, Department of Internal Medicine, University of Michigan, Ann Arbor, Michigan

Jennifer Girard, MD Assistant Professor, Division of Hematology/Oncology, Department of Internal Medicine, University of Michigan, Ann Arbor, Michigan

Omayra Gonzalez-Pagan, MD, PhD Hematology/Oncology Fellow, Department of Medicine, Baylor College of Medicine, Houston, Texas

Eric Granowicz, MD Fellow, Department of Internal Medicine, Division of Hematology/Oncology, University of California Davis Comprehensive Cancer Center, Sacramento, California

Claire Hoppenot, MD Assistant Professor, Division of Gynecologic Oncology, Department of Obstetrics and Gynecology, Baylor College of Medicine, Dan L Duncan Comprehensive Cancer Center, Houston, Texas

Quillan Huang, MD Assistant Professor, Section of Hematology/Oncology, Department of Medicine, Dan L Duncan Comprehensive Cancer Center, Baylor College of Medicine, Houston, Texas

Cyrus A. Iqbal, MD Hematology/Oncology Fellow, Department of Medicine, Baylor College of Medicine, Houston, Texas

Brian A. Jonas, MD, PhD, FACP Associate Professor of Medicine, Department of Internal Medicine, Division of Hematology/Oncology, University of California Davis Comprehensive Cancer Center, Sacramento, California

Karen Kelly, MD Professor of Medicine, Associate Director for Clinical Research, Jennifer Rene Harmon Tegley and Elizabeth Erica Harmon Endowed Chair in Cancer Clinical Research; Department of Internal Medicine, Division of Hematology/Oncology, University of California Davis Comprehensive Cancer Center, Sacramento, California

Edward J. Kim, MD, PhD Associate Professor of Medicine, Department of Internal Medicine, Division of Hematology/Oncology, University of California Davis Comprehensive Cancer Center, Sacramento, California

John C. Krauss, MD Associate Professor, Department of Internal Medicine, Division of Hematology/Oncology, University of Michigan, Ann Arbor, Michigan

James Liu, MD Fellow, Department of Internal Medicine, Division of Hematology/Oncology, University of California Davis Comprehensive Cancer Center, Sacramento, California

Vincent T. Ma, MD Assistant Professor, Department of Internal Medicine, University of Wisconsin, Madison, Wisconsin

Shalini Makawita, MD, MSc Assistant Professor, Section of Hematology/Oncology, Department of Medicine, Dan L Duncan Comprehensive Cancer Center, Baylor College of Medicine, Houston, Texas

Jacob Mandel, MD Assistant Professor, Neurology and Neurosurgery, Dan L Duncan Comprehensive Cancer Center, Baylor College of Medicine, Houston, Texas

Alejandro Marinos, MD Hematology/Oncology Fellow, Department of Medicine, Baylor College of Medicine, Houston, Texas

Martha P. Mims, MD, PhD Professor and Chief, Section of Hematology/Oncology, Department of Medicine, Dan L Duncan Comprehensive Cancer Center, Baylor College of Medicine, Houston, Texas

Arathi Mohan, MD Fellow, Department of Internal Medicine, Division of Hematology/Oncology, University of Michigan, Ann Arbor, Michigan

Nagaishwarya Moka, MD Hematology/Oncology Fellow, Department of Medicine, Baylor College of Medicine, Houston, Texas

Benjamin Musher, MD Associate Professor, Barry S. Smith Endowed Professorship in Pancreatic Malignancies, Section of Hematology/Oncology, Department of Medicine, Dan L Duncan Comprehensive Cancer Center, Baylor College of Medicine, Houston, Texas

Julie Nangia, MD Associate Professor, Section of Hematology/Oncology, Department of Medicine, Dan L Duncan Comprehensive Cancer Center, Baylor College of Medicine, Houston, Texas

Charles B. Nguyen, MD Fellow, Department of Internal Medicine, Division of Hematology/Oncology, University of Michigan, Ann Arbor, Michigan

Tamer Othman, MD Fellow, Department of Internal Medicine, Division of Hematology/Oncology, University of California Davis Comprehensive Cancer Center, Sacramento, California

Mamta Parikh, MD, MS Assistant Professor of Medicine, Department of Internal Medicine, Division of Hematology/Oncology, University of California Davis Comprehensive Cancer Center, Sacramento, California

Colbert A. Parker, MD Hematology/Oncology Fellow, Department of Medicine, Baylor College of Medicine, Houston, Texas

Meera Patel, MD, MHS Assistant Professor, Section of Hematology/Oncology, Department of Medicine, Dan L Duncan Comprehensive Cancer Center, Baylor College of Medicine, Houston, Texas

Brian Pham, MD Fellow, Department of Internal Medicine, Division of Hematology/Oncology, University of California Davis Comprehensive Cancer Center, Sacramento, California

Tycel J. Phillips, MD Maria Reinhardt Decesare Research Professor of Blood Cancers and Bone Marrow Transplantation, Associate Professor, Division of Hematology, Department of Internal Medicine, University of Michigan, Ann Arbor, Michigan

Matthew J. Pianko, MD Clinical Assistant Professor, Department of Internal Medicine, Division of Hematology/Oncology, University of Michigan, Ann Arbor, Michigan

Sarah Premji, MD Internal Medicine Resident, Baylor College of Medicine, Houston, Texas

Arpit Rao, MD   Associate Professor, Section of Hematology/Oncology, Department of Medicine, Dan L Duncan Comprehensive Cancer Center, Baylor College of Medicine, Houston, Texas

Zachery R. Reichert, MD   Assistant Professor of Medical Oncology, Department of Internal Medicine, University of Michigan, Ann Arbor, Michigan

Samuel B. Reynolds, MD   Hematology/Oncology Fellow, Division of Hematology/Oncology, Department of Internal Medicine, University of Michigan, Ann Arbor, Michigan

Karen Riggins, MD, PhD   Section of Hematology/Oncology, Dan L Duncan Comprehensive Cancer Center, Baylor College of Medicine, Houston, Texas

Gustavo Rivero, MD   Associate Professor, Section of Hematology/Oncology, Department of Medicine, Dan L Duncan Comprehensive Cancer Center, Baylor College of Medicine, Houston, Texas

Katherine Sanchez, MD   Hematology/Oncology Fellow, Baylor College of Medicine, Houston, Texas

Kamya Sankar, MD   Hematology/Oncology Fellow, Division of Hematology/Oncology, Department of Internal Medicine, University of Michigan, Ann Arbor, Michigan

Bryan J. Schneider, MD   Professor, Division of Medical Oncology, University of Michigan, Ann Arbor, Michigan

Eric B. Schwartz, MD   Fellow, Division of Hematology/Oncology, University of Michigan, Ann Arbor, Michigan

Maryam Nemati Shafaee, MD, MPH   Assistant Professor, Section of Hematology/Oncology, Department of Medicine, Dan L Duncan Comprehensive Cancer Center, Baylor College of Medicine, Houston, Texas

Maria Siddiqui, MD   Hematology/Oncology Fellow, Department of Medicine, Baylor College of Medicine, Houston, Texas

Jean H. Siedel, DO, MS   Assistant Professor, Division of Gynecologic Oncology, Department of Obstetrics and Gynecology, University of Michigan, Ann Arbor, Michigan

Alli M. Straubhar, MD   Division of Gynecologic Oncology, Department of Obstetrics and Gynecology, University of Michigan, Ann Arbor, Michigan

Christopher T. Su, MD, MPH   Clinical Fellow, Division of Hematology/Oncology, Department of Internal Medicine, University of Michigan, Ann Arbor, Michigan

Jingxin Sun, MD   Hematology/Oncology Fellow, Baylor College of Medicine, Houston, Texas

Paul L. Swiecicki, MD   Clinical Associate Professor, Division of Hematology/Oncology, Department of Internal Medicine, University of Michigan, Ann Arbor, Michigan

Radhika Takiar, MD   Fellow, Department of Internal Medicine, Division of Hematology/Oncology, University of Michigan, Ann Arbor, Michigan

Monica Tamil, MD Hematology/Oncology Fellow, Department of Medicine, Baylor College of Medicine, Houston, Texas

Sravanti P. Teegavarapu, MD Assistant Professor, Section of Hematology/Oncology, Department of Medicine, Dan L Duncan Comprehensive Cancer Center, Baylor College of Medicine, Houston, Texas

Katelyn Tondo-Steele, DO Fellow, Division of Gynecologic Oncology, Department of Obstetrics and Gynecology, University of Michigan, Ann Arbor, Michigan

Irene Tsung, MD Hematology/Oncology Fellow, Division of Hematology/Oncology, Department of Internal Medicine, University of Michigan, Ann Arbor, Michigan

Daniel Wang, MD Assistant Professor, Section of Hematology/Oncology, Department of Medicine, Dan L Duncan Comprehensive Cancer Center, Baylor College of Medicine, Houston, Texas

Thomas C. Westbrook, MD Fellow, Division of Hematology/Oncology, University of Michigan, Ann Arbor, Michigan

Francis P. Worden, MD Professor, Division of Medical Oncology, University of Michigan, Ann Arbor, Michigan

Sudha Yarlagadda, MD Hematology/Oncology Fellow, Baylor College of Medicine, Houston, Texas

Aihua Edward Yen, MD Assistant Professor, Section of Hematology/Oncology, Department of Medicine, Dan L Duncan Comprehensive Cancer Center, Baylor College of Medicine, Houston, Texas

Zachary Phillip Yeung, MD Hematology/Oncology Fellow, Section of Hematology/Oncology, Department of Medicine, Dan L Duncan Comprehensive Cancer Center, Baylor College of Medicine, Houston, Texas

Richard Benjamin Young, MD Fellow, Department of Internal Medicine, Division of Hematology/Oncology, University of California Davis Comprehensive Cancer Center, Sacramento, California

Huili Zhu, MD Hematology/Oncology Fellow, Section of Hematology/Oncology, Department of Medicine, Dan L Duncan Comprehensive Cancer Center, Baylor College of Medicine, Houston, Texas

Preface

As the field of medical oncology evolves, we have developed a new format for the third edition of this textbook, now titled: *Tumor Board Review: Evidence-Based Case Reviews and Questions*. Here we include recent advances in the diagnosis and treatment of the most common malignancies encountered by oncology providers. The text includes recently published clinical studies and updated cancer guidelines. Further, we discuss the importance of genetic mutations in the selection of anticancer drugs (e.g., *BRAF* mutations in melanoma) based on Phase III clinical trials in both solid tumors and hematologic malignancies. The content of this third edition represents our best effort to incorporate and highlight the most recent clinically relevant data in our field. We continue to use a case-based format, but each oncologic disease type is now presented in a tumor board format, with a brief synopsis of a patient case followed by a discussion of the imaging and molecular and/or genomic sequencing required for a correct diagnosis. We finish each chapter with a dialogue on staging and treatment including chemotherapy, immunotherapy, and targeted agent regimens. Finally, we close with pertinent information related to follow-up and survivorship. Up to 10 board-style questions are also included at the end of each chapter to help enhance the reader's knowledge base. The third edition continues to represent a joint effort among oncology faculty and subspecialty fellows based at the Baylor College of Medicine (Houston, Texas), the University of Michigan Medical School (Ann Arbor, Michigan), and the University of California Davis Medical Center (Sacramento, California). All three institutions are the homes of National Cancer Institute (NCI) designated cancer centers: the Dan L Duncan Comprehensive Cancer Center, the Rogel Cancer Center, and the UC Davis Comprehensive Cancer Center. Contributors to the third edition were selected based on their interest and expertise in the relevant cancers. The editors gratefully acknowledge the contributions of our trainee and faculty authors, as well as the support staff who assisted in the preparation of each chapter. We also thank the editorial staff of Springer Publishing Company/Demos Medical Publishing, particularly David D'Addona, senior editor, and Hannah Grace Greco, assistant editor. In closing, we dedicate this book to our fellows and faculty. This book would not have been possible without their steadfast devotion and immeasurable service to each of our respective institutions.

Francis P. Worden
Martha P. Mims
Helen K. Chew

CHAPTER 1

Head and Neck Cancer

Irene Tsung, Samuel B. Reynolds, and Paul L. Swiecicki

INTRODUCTION

In the United States, head and neck malignancies have accounted for an estimated 3% of all new cancer diagnoses (54,010 new cases) and 2% of cancer-related deaths in the year 2021.[1] The majority of these cancers originate from the squamous cells that line the mucosal surface of the head and neck (oral cavity, pharynx, larynx). In addition to these squamous cell carcinomas (SCCs), head and neck cancers can less commonly develop in the sinuses, nasal cavity, or salivary glands.

The strongest risk factors for head and neck cancer are alcohol and tobacco use, although the incidence of human papilloma virus (HPV)-associated oropharyngeal cancer is notably increasing.[2,3] Infection with Epstein-Barr virus (EBV) is also a risk factor for the development of nasopharyngeal and salivary gland cancers.[4,5]

Due to the diverse anatomic structures that comprise the head and neck, the presenting symptoms, staging, prognosis, and treatment vary greatly depending on the site of origin of the malignancy. Management, accordingly, requires a multidisciplinary approach that may include surgery, radiation, and/or systemic therapy with cytotoxic chemotherapy, targeted therapy, or immunotherapy. The cancer itself as well as its treatments can be associated with significant long-term morbidity that includes anatomic defects, speech impairment, dysphagia, or chronic pain.

CASE SUMMARIES

Case 1.1: Locally Advanced Cancer of the Oropharynx

A 58-year-old male presents for an evaluation for persistent swelling in his right neck that has worsened over the past 3 months. He is otherwise healthy, is a lifetime nonsmoker, drinks alcohol occasionally, and denies a history of marijuana use or use of other recreational drugs. During this period of neck swelling, the patient was treated with a course of antibiotics for an upper respiratory tract infection, after which his swelling became less pronounced. Two weeks later, the swelling returned but was attributed to a dental procedure. Upon return to his dentist 3 weeks later, the patient noted a palpable, fixed mass in his right neck that was mildly tender to palpation. He also reported a persistent mild sore throat but denied fever, cough, or dysphagia. Clinical evaluation by his dentist confirmed the presence of a 1 cm x 1 cm right neck mass at level IIA, prompting referral to a head and neck surgeon for further evaluation. His physical examination revealed a palpable mass on the right base of the tongue that does not cross the midline but extends into the glossotonsillar sulcus. The remainder of his physical exam was normal with no additional palpable neck masses.

How Is a Diagnosis Established?

- Evaluation occurs under anesthesia by direct laryngoscopy or pan-endoscopy and with tumor fine needle aspiration (FNA) biopsy.

Patient's Diagnosis

- *Examination of the larynx under anesthesia identifies a mass at the base of the tongue.*
- *FNA Biopsy: non-keratinizing SCC of the base of the tongue. Note that non-keratinizing tumors are often virus-associated (specifically with HPV); keratinizing tumors are more likely to be caused by tobacco and alcohol exposure.*

What Further Molecular or Genomic Testing Is Required?

- Whole body PET/CT is used to evaluate the extent of local regional disease and to rule out distant metastases. Note that only 10% of patients with SCCs of the head and neck will present with distant metastases at the time of diagnosis.
- All newly diagnosed oropharyngeal primary malignancies must undergo testing for HPV, as 60% to 70% of all new primaries of the oropharynx are attributable to the virus.[6]
- p16, detectable by immunohistochemistry (IHC), is predominantly used as a surrogate biomarker for HPV as it closely correlates with HPV status by HPV E6/E7 mRNA oncogene expression.[7]
- FNA biopsy provides sufficient pathological tissue for HPV testing.[8]
- HPV is a prognostic but not a predictive biomarker.

Whole Body PET/CT Results

- *PET/CT: A 5-cm intensely fluorodeoxyglucose (FDG) avid mass centered at the right base of the tongue/lingular tonsil with a standardized uptake value (SUV) of 3.5, consistent with malignancy, is noted. A large centrally necrotic right level 2A/3 cervical chain with an SUV of 2.5, consistent with metastatic disease, is also present. Mild FDG uptake within several non-enlarged left cervical chain nodes is appreciated but is nonspecific.*

Patient's Molecular and Genomic Testing

- *IHC Staining on tissue biopsy was positive for p16.*

How Is This Tumor Staged?

- The American Joint Committee on Cancer (AJCC) eighth edition staging system is used to stage cancers of the head and neck and employs clinical examination, CT, and PET imaging. Table 1.1 summarizes this staging system.
- Oropharyngeal tumors measuring greater than 4 cm in diameter, as seen in this patient, or those with extension into the epiglottis are considered T3.
- Absence of disease beyond the neck indicates M0 disease.

Patient's Clinical Stage

- *T3, N1, M0, p16+ (stage II)*

What Are Appropriate Treatment Options?

- Concomitant chemoradiotherapy with cisplatin 100 mg/m² IV delivered every 21 days during radiation is considered a standard of care for patients with locally advanced head and neck cancers.[9]

Table 1.1 AJCC Eighth Edition Staging for Cancers of the Oral Cavity

Stage	Tumor	Nodes	Metastases
Stage 0	Tis	N0	M0
Stage I	T1	N0	M0
Stage II	T2	N0	M0
Stage III	T1, T2	N1	M0
	T3	N0, N1	M0
Stage IVA	T1	N2	M0
	T2	N2	M0
	T3	N2	M0
	T4a	N0, N1, N2	M0
Stage IVB	Any T	N3	M0
	T4b	Any N	M0
Stage IVC	Any T	Any N	M1

AJCC, American Joint Committee on Cancer.

Source: Data from Amin MB, Edge SB, Greene FL, et al., eds. *AJCC Cancer Staging Manual.* 8th ed. Springer Nature; 2017.

- Concomitant cetuximab with radiation is inferior to concomitant cisplatin and radiation, as documented by RTOG 1016.[10]
- Induction chemotherapy with docetaxel (Taxotere), cisplatin (Platinol), and 5-fluorouracil (TPF) prior to treatment with cisplatin and radiation may be considered for patients with large bulky disease for symptomatic cytoreduction and to possibly decrease the risk of developing distant metastases. Induction chemotherapy, however, provides no improvement in overall survival and poses the risks of increased toxicity and potential delay in definitive therapy.
- Tumors approaching the midline, as in the case of this patient, are at risk of contralateral metastases and should be managed with bilateral neck radiation. Furthermore, the patient's PET scan highlighted mild uptake in the contralateral neck. Since radiation will be administered bilaterally, there is no need to biopsy these lymph nodes (LNs).

Recommended Treatment Plan for This Patient
- *Cisplatin 100 mg/m² IV every 21 days with radiation to a total dose of 70 Gy*

What Are the Toxicities Associated With Chemoradiotherapy?

- Radiation can lead to long-term swallowing dysfunction and associated risk for chronic aspiration, xerostomia, changes to skin pigmentation, and an increased risk of carotid artery plaque formation.
- Cisplatin may be associated with nausea, vomiting, permanent hearing loss, peripheral neuropathy, renal failure, and infusion reactions. Adequate intravenous hydration administered with magnesium sulfate, mannitol, and antiemetics must be delivered concomitantly with cisplatin to minimize such outcomes. Dosage reductions are also required to help alleviate toxic side effects and to ensure that patients receive a minimum of 200 mg/m² of cisplatin during radiation, as doses of less than 200 mg/m² provide no added benefit to radiotherapy.[11]

What Are Other Treatment Considerations?

Treatment De-Escalation

- Because HPV-related head and neck cancers garner an improved prognosis over HPV-negative disease, there is movement to improve long-term toxicity without compromising survival.
- Until formal confirmatory data is available from larger studies defining the safety and long-term survival benefits of de-intensification regimens, these therapeutic strategies remain experimental and should not be adopted into practice outside of clinical trials.

What Is Required for This Patient's Follow-Up and Survivorship?

- A PET/CT should be performed at 12 weeks following definitive chemoradiation for assessment of treatment response and to identify any residual tumor. A negative PET at this time-point predicts improved overall survival at 2 years.
  - Early PET/CT scans before 12 weeks are associated with significant false-positive rates and should not be performed.
  - If a PET/CT at 3 months post-treatment is negative, there is no data to support substantial benefit for further routine imaging in an asymptomatic patient with negative clinical exams.
- The patient should have clinical histories, physical examinations, and flexible laryngoscopies every 3 months for the first 2 years following completion of treatment, extending every 6 months for years 3 to 5, and yearly after 5 years.

General Surveillance Recommendations

- All patients should receive education on the signs and symptoms of locally recurrent disease (that is, palpable neck masses, change in voice, sore throat) and distant metastases (that is, back pain, dyspnea, cough, hemoptysis).
- Patients should be examined and treated for lymphedema and/or fibrosis of the neck and for swelling of the jaw to evaluate for osteonecrosis. Referrals to occupational therapy, physical therapy, and oral surgery should be made as indicated.
- All patients who undergo neck irradiation should be screened for hypothyroidism and supplemented appropriately with thyroid-stimulating hormone (TSH) monitoring every 6 to 12 months.
- Patients should be evaluated for late and long-term effects. Carotid artery ultrasonography, for example, should be performed 5 years following radiotherapy to evaluate for radiation-induced carotid artery stenosis. Additional late effects include chronic fatigue, depression, anxiety, and thoughts of suicide.

Case 1.2: Locally Advanced Nasopharyngeal Cancer

A 54-year-old male with a history of alcohol and tobacco use and whose family was stationed in southeast Asia for military duty for the majority of his childhood presents with a painless mass on the left side of his neck. He also notes intermittent nose bleeds with difficulty swallowing. Examination confirms a 2 × 1.5 cm left-sided neck mass at the level IIb LNs; the observable nares revealed normal inferior turbinates bilaterally. Cranial nerve exam is unremarkable and visual fields are intact.

How Is a Diagnosis Established?

- Evaluation occurs under anesthesia by direct imaging with assessment of the maxillary sinuses with tumor FNA biopsy for tissue diagnosis.

- Functional MRI of the head and neck will provide a higher resolution as compared to CT to evaluate the skull base and parapharyngeal spaces. Whole body PET/CT should also be performed to identify the extent of local regional and distant metastatic disease, if present.[12]
- Note, again, that only 10% of patients with head and neck SCCs have distant metastases at the time of original diagnosis.

Patient's Diagnosis

- *The patient was referred to an otolaryngology clinic, where on direct imaging physicians visualized an exophytic mass in the fossa of Rosenmüller.*
- *FNA Biopsy of parapharyngeal mass: Well-differentiated non-keratinizing SCC of the posterior pharynx.*
- *MRI Neck—soft tissues and brain: A 2.5 × 1.5 cm mass is visualized in the posterior pharynx with thickening of the posterior nasal septum, although without invasion into the nasal septum, oropharynx retropharyngeal, nor prevertebral spaces; involvement of pterygoid muscles and skull base extension are also absent. No retropharyngeal lymphadenopathy is present but an enlarged, 1.5-cm left-sided anterior cervical LN is visualized at level IIB.*
- *PET/CT: An approximately 2.5-cm FDG-avid mass is visualized in the retropharynx with an SUV of 3.0. An enlarged level IIB LN, 1.5 cm, with FDG-avid uptake is also appreciated. No evidence of retropharyngeal LN uptake is seen.*

What Are the Histological Subclassifications for This Diagnosis?

The World Health Organization (WHO) classifies nasopharyngeal carcinoma into three types as follows:

1. Type I: Keratinizing SCC
2. Type II: Non-keratinizing SCC
3. Type III: Undifferentiated carcinoma

Also note that a new subtype in basaloid SCC is also now recognized by the WHO, and, while rare, it exhibits aggressive clinical behavior.[13,14]

What Further Molecular or Genomic Testing Is Recommended?

- Tumor EBV testing should be conducted through in situ hybridization for EBV-coded RNA (EBER).[15]

Patient's Molecular and Genomic Testing

- *A biopsy of the patient's FDG-avid cervical LN was obtained and was confirmed as a non-keratinizing SCC. EBER by fluorescent in situ hybridization (FISH) was positive.*

How Is This Tumor Staged?

- The AJCC eighth edition staging system, which is summarized in the text that follows, is used to stage cancers of the head and neck, and employs clinical examination, endoscopy, CT, and PET imaging (Table 1.2).[16]
- Tumors confined to the nasopharynx are staged as T1.
- Extension into the parapharyngeal space or soft tissues (pterygoid and/or prevertebral musculature) are considered T2 and infiltration of the skull base and/or cervical vertebrae are designated as T3.
- The FDG-avid left-sided cervical LN at level IIB in this patient is suggestive of malignancy. Any unilateral metastatic cervical LN that is 6 cm or less is considered N1 while those greater than 6 cm are N3. Bilateral cervical LN metastases that are 6 cm or less are designated as N2.
- Disease beyond the head and neck is indicative of M1 disease.

Table 1.2   AJCC Eighth Edition Staging for Cancers of the Nasopharynx

Stage	Tumor	Nodes	Metastases
Stage 0	Tis	N0	M0
Stage I	T1	N0	M0
Stage II	T0, T1	N1	M0
	T2	N0, N1	
Stage III	T0, T1, T2	N2	M0
	T3	N0, N1, N2	M0
Stage IVA	T4	N0, N1, N2	M0
	Any T	N3	M0
Stage IVB	Any T	Any N	M1

AJCC, American Joint Committee on Cancer.

Source: Data from Amin MB, Edge SB, Greene FL, et al, eds. *AJCC Cancer Staging Manual.* 8th ed. Springer Nature; 2017.

Patient's Clinical Stage
- *Stage II EBV+ nasopharyngeal carcinoma (T2, N1, M0)*

What Are Appropriate Treatment Options?
- The best approach in patients with regionally advanced disease is concurrent chemoradiation with either neoadjuvant or adjuvant chemotherapy.
- Concurrent chemoradiotherapy consists of cisplatin 100 mg/m² delivered every 21 days during radiation.
- Neoadjuvant/adjuvant therapy generally involves 3 cycles of cisplatin and 5-fluorouracil (5-FU).[17,18]

What Are Other Treatment Considerations?
- Intensity modulated radiotherapy (IMRT) is the mainstay of treatment for local, non-metastatic nasopharyngeal carcinoma and is recommended as monotherapy for stage I (T1N0M0) disease.

Recommended Treatment Plan for This Patient
- *Cisplatin 100 mg/m² IV every 21 days with IMRT to a total dose of 70 Gy, followed by 3 cycles of adjuvant cisplatin with 5-FU*

What Are the Toxicities Associated With Chemoradiotherapy?
- Please see the section on toxicities under the section on locally advanced cancer of the oropharynx.

What Is Required for This Patient's Follow-Up and Survivorship?
- *A PET/CT is recommended at 12 weeks after definitive chemoradiation to assess treatment response. Similar to the previous discussion, imaging prior to 12 weeks has the potential for false-positive results.*
- *Additionally, clinical history and physical examinations with rhinolaryngoscopy are generally recommended at least every 3 months for the first year following completion of primary therapy every 6 months for the second year, 8 months for years 3 to 5, and annually thereafter.*

- *TSH monitoring every 6 to 12 months should be performed in the setting of any neck irradiation, as in this patient.*

General Surveillance Recommendations[19-21]

- All patients should be educated on the symptoms of locally recurrent disease (that is, palpable neck masses, change in voice, sore throat) and distant metastases (that is, back pain, dyspnea, cough).
- At office visits, providers should examine and treat patients for local effects of therapy as they arise, including jaw swelling and/or osteonecrosis, fibrosis of the neck, and/or speech deficits. Referrals to occupational, speech, and physical therapy should be made as indicated.
- Again, screen all patients who undergo neck radiotherapy with TSH every 6 to 12 months and supplement thyroid hormone as indicated.
- Evaluate patients for late and long-term effects, including chronic fatigue, depression, anxiety, and thoughts of suicide. Also perform carotid ultrasonography every 5 years following radiotherapy to evaluate for radiation-induced carotid artery stenosis. Additional late effects include chronic fatigue, depression, anxiety, and thoughts of suicide.

Case 1.3: Metastatic Adenoid Cystic Carcinoma

A 70-year-old woman presents for evaluation of right facial swelling, which her friend recently noticed, as well as a mild right facial droop. She notes that the swelling has gradually worsened over the past year, but as she had no pain or other significant symptoms, she did not seek medical attention until now. She is otherwise healthy and does not smoke or drink alcohol; there is no family history of cancer. Physical exam was notable for a 2-cm fixed, painless lump in the preauricular region and a mild droop at the corner of her right lip when smiling; cervical lymphadenopathy was not appreciated and the remainder of her physical exam was unremarkable.

How Is a Diagnosis Established?

- Tissue diagnosis with FNA. Consider image-guided (ultrasound [US] or CT) FNA depending on tumor location and accessibility.
- Imaging with head and neck CT +/- MRI with contrast to assess the extent of disease (local, bony, or perineural invasion; LN metastases). Adenoid cystic carcinoma (ACC) is characterized by an infiltrative growth pattern and can have perineural spread.
- CT of the chest is used to evaluate for distant metastases.

Patient's Diagnosis
- *US-guided FNA biopsy of the right parotid lesion: ACC with MYB-NFIB fusion. MYB-NFIB and MYBL1-NFIB rearrangements by FISH are seen in most ACC cases and can be a useful confirmatory test.[22]*
- *CT and MRI of the head and neck demonstrated a localized right-sided parotid tumor without evidence of local invasion, perineural spread, or lymphadenopathy.*
- *CT of the chest was unremarkable.*

What Is the Appropriate Treatment for Localized Disease?

- Surgical consultation for complete tumor resection. ACC is considered a high-grade malignant tumor, which is often treated with total parotidectomy.
- If there is clinical concern for facial nerve involvement, resection of the involved portion of the facial nerve can be considered.

- Management of the clinically negative neck is controversial, but for tumors with high risk for occult nodal disease (high-grade tumor, large tumor, or facial nerve involvement), elective neck dissection can be considered.[23]

Patient's Diagnosis

- *Surgical pathology confirmed a 2.2-cm lesion separated from the normal parotid gland by a thin fibrous capsule consisting of ductal and myoepithelial cells in a cribriform pattern and some areas of solid pattern. No capsular or perineural invasion is present. pT2 N0 M0, stage group II based on AJCC Union for International Cancer Control (UICC) eighth edition TNM staging.*

Is Adjuvant Therapy Indicated?

- Adjuvant radiation should be offered to all patients with resected ACC as it has been shown to improve locoregional control.[24–26]
- *Routine adjuvant systemic therapy is not indicated in this case.*[23]

What Is the Recommended Follow-Up?

- Despite locoregional control with surgical resection and adjuvant radiation therapy, many patients eventually experience distant recurrence of disease which can occur as late as 10 to 30 years after the initial diagnosis and treatment, making routine monitoring essential.[27]
- History and physical at least every 3 months in year 1, every 6 months in year 2, every 8 months in years 3 to 5, and yearly after year 5.
- There is no consensus on the guidelines for frequency or modality of routine post-treatment imaging.

Patient's Diagnosis

- *In year 6 of follow-up, the patient noticed recurrent right-sided facial swelling. On physical exam, several cervical LNs are enlarged.*
- *CT imaging of the head, neck, and chest revealed a right parotid lesion, multiple enlarged cervical LNs, and bilateral lung nodules. Whole body PET/CT scan demonstrated FDG-avid lesions in the right parotid gland, cervical LNs, lung nodules, and liver.*
- *Biopsy of a liver lesion was consistent with ACC.*

What Are the Treatment Options for Metastatic Disease?

- For patients with ACC with slow disease progression who are minimally symptomatic, observation can be considered.
- For patients with more indolent disease and limited number of metastases (5), local ablative treatment such as surgery for metastasectomy or stereotactic body radiation therapy can be considered to delay local disease progression.[23]
- Patients may be candidates for systemic therapy if the metastases are symptomatic or if their growth has the potential to compromise organ function.
- Other indications for systemic therapy are if patients are not candidates for palliative local therapy or if their metastatic lesions are more rapidly growing (greater than 20% over 6 months).[23]
- Options for systemic therapy include:
  - Clinical trial if available
  - A multitargeted tyrosine kinase inhibitor (TKI) such as lenvatinib or sorafenib[28–31]
  - Cytotoxic chemotherapy if rapid tumor debulking is needed

Case 1.4: Metastatic Squamous Cell Carcinoma

A 61-year-old man with a 50 pack-year smoking history presents with a persistent sore throat over the past year despite treatment with antibiotics and various allergy medications. CT of the head and neck demonstrated a 2.8-cm mass at the right pyriform sinus with multiple surrounding enlarged LNs. Biopsy of the mass and cervical LNs revealed a moderately to poorly differentiated SCC (T3 N2 M0, stage IVA) of the hypopharynx. He completed definitive concurrent chemoradiation (carboplatin + paclitaxel) but had a local recurrence 3 months later. He was then treated with salvage total laryngectomy, partial pharyngectomy, and bilateral selective neck dissection. Surveillance CT scans 1 year later showed new lung nodules and mediastinal lymphadenopathy which were FDG avid on PET scan. Biopsy of a lung nodule confirmed metastatic SCC.

What Further Molecular or Genomic Testing Is Required?

- For unresectable recurrent or metastatic SCC of the head and neck (HNSCC), tumor programmed death-ligand 1 (PD-L1) combined positive score (CPS) should be obtained.

How Is This Tumor Staged?

- Staging varies depending on the primary tumor site (oral cavity, nasopharynx, oropharynx, hypopharynx, larynx, etc.).
- Regardless of stage, a patient is treated similarly with systemic therapy if there are distant metastases or if there is recurrent disease that is not amenable to definitive treatment with surgery and/or radiation.

What Are Treatment Considerations?

- Platinum-refractory disease (recurrence within 6 months of receiving a platinum agent for locally advanced disease)
- Eastern Cooperative Oncology Group (ECOG) performance status
- PD-L1 CPS score (0 or 1 or greater)
- Bulk of disease and any need for rapid cytoreduction
- Medical comorbidities (which may guide whether patient is a candidate for immunotherapy or combination chemotherapy + immunotherapy)

Patient's Diagnosis

- *He does not have platinum-refractory disease since his metastatic recurrence was greater than 6 months from last receipt of platinum-based chemotherapy (given during initial chemoradiation).*
- *His ECOG performance status (PS) is 1 and tumor PD-L1 CPS score is 15.*
- *He has noticed progressive worsening of his neck swelling from lymphadenopathy and feels short of breath with exertion.*
- *There are no medical contraindications for immunotherapy.*

What Are Available First-Line Treatment Options for Unresectable Recurrent or Metastatic Head and Neck Squamous Cell Carcinoma? (Figure 1.1)

- Platinum-refractory disease
  - Immunotherapy (checkpoint inhibitors of PD-1)

- Pembrolizumab

  In KEYNOTE-040, a Phase III, open-label, randomized study, patients with platinum-refractory recurrent or metastatic (R/M) HNSCC received either single-agent pembrolizumab or investigator's choice of methotrexate, docetaxel, or cetuximab. Pembrolizumab showed statistically significant improved median overall survival (OS; 8.4 vs. 6.9 months; hazard ratio [HR] 0.80, 95% confidence interval [CI] 0.65–0.98, P = 0.02), response rates, and duration of response.[32]

- Nivolumab

  In an open-label, randomized, Phase III trial (CheckMate 141), single-agent nivolumab was compared to the investigator's choice of methotrexate, docetaxel, or cetuximab in patients with platinum-refractory R/M disease and demonstrated significantly improved median OS (7.5 vs. 5.1 months; HR 0.70, 97.73% CI 0.51–0.96, P = 0.01) and overall response rates (ORR; 13.3% vs. 5.8%) in patients treated with nivolumab.[33]

- Non-platinum-refractory disease
  - Pembrolizumab +/- chemotherapy (platinum + 5-FU)

    The KEYNOTE-048 trial evaluated pembrolizumab with or without chemotherapy as first-line treatment for R/M HNSCC. Pembrolizumab in combination with platinum and 5-FU improved OS compared with cetuximab with platinum and 5-FU (13 vs. 10.7 months). In patients with PD-L1 CPS score 1, single-agent pembrolizumab improved OS compared to cetuximab + chemotherapy (12.3 vs. 10.3 months).[34]

  - Consider addition of chemotherapy for patients with rapidly progressive disease who may benefit from more rapid tumor debulking regardless of PD-L1 CPS score.

  - Cetuximab + chemotherapy (platinum + 5-FU)

    For patients who are not immunotherapy candidates, cetuximab + platinum + 5-FU can be considered as first-line treatment. In the Phase III EXTREME trial, platinum + 5-FU was compared with platinum + 5-FU + cetuximab. The addition of cetuximab showed improvement in median OS (10.1 vs. 7.4 months) compared to chemotherapy alone.[35]

Patient's Case

- *Platinum + 5-FU + pembrolizumab was chosen for treatment as he does not have platinum-refractory disease and has a positive PD-L1 CPS score. He is becoming symptomatic with bulky lymphadenopathy, so chemotherapy + immunotherapy will provide more rapid tumor debulking and symptom relief.*

What Are Second-Line Treatment Options?

- Optimal second-line therapy upon progression is unclear.
- Consider clinical trials if available.
- For patients who progressed after receiving immunotherapy, reasonable treatment options include single-agent chemotherapy or targeted therapy such as cetuximab, methotrexate, or docetaxel (Figure 1.1).[36–38]

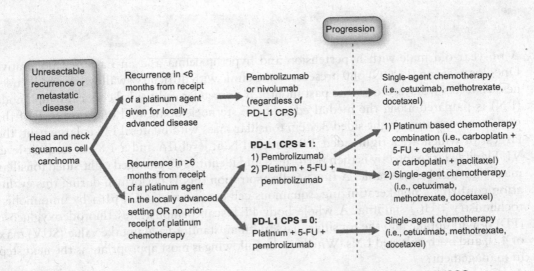

Figure 1.1 Systemic therapy treatment paradigms in unresectable recurrent or metastatic HNSCC

CPS, combined positive score; 5-FU, 5-fluorouracil; HNSCC, head and neck squamous cell carcinoma; PD-L1, programmed death-ligand 1.

1. A 66-year-old male with hypertension and hyperlipidemia and an Eastern Cooperative Oncology Group (ECOG) of 0 presents to the clinic with difficulty swallowing and hoarseness that has worsened over the past month. A nontender right-sided cervical lymph node (LN) is palpated along the medial edge of the sternocleidomastoid on exam. CT of the neck demonstrates a right-sided 3.5-cm tonsillar mass with bilateral LN enlargement, the largest of which are a right-sided 2.0-cm left LN at level IIA and a 1.8-cm node at level VI. Flexible laryngoscopy is then performed and identifies an enlarged right-sided tonsillar mass that will be resectable. A fine needle aspiration (FNA) performed during this evaluation confirms a non-keratinizing, squamous cell carcinoma (SCC), p16+ by immunohistochemistry (IHC) staining. A whole body PET scan demonstrates fluorodeoxyglucose (FDG)-avid uptake into the tonsillar mass, with an standardized uptake value (SUV) max of 4.0, and both enlarged LNs. Which of the following is most appropriate as the next step in management?
   A. Concurrent cetuximab and radiation
   B. Induction docetaxel, cisplatin, and 5-fluorouracil (TPF) followed by concurrent cetuximab and radiation
   C. Concurrent chemoradiation with cisplatin-radiotherapy (RT)
   D. Radiation alone

2. A 55-year-old male with a 35 pack-year cigarette smoking history and daily alcohol use presents to the hospital with dysphonia and decreased oral intake over the past 3 months. He is found on exam to have a palpable mass deep into his oral cavity on the left side of his tongue, confirmed on subsequent CT imaging as a 5.5-cm mass on the base of the tongue (BOT); an accompanying level IIB lymph node (LN) is also visualized. Fluorodeoxyglucose (FDG)-avidity in both lesions is highlighted by PET scan, which demonstrates no evidence of metastatic disease. A biopsy of the BOT lesion confirms a keratinizing squamous cell carcinoma (SCC), p16-negative by immunohistochemistry (IHC). The patient successfully undergoes primary tumor resection with bilateral neck dissections and adjuvant chemoradiation with cisplatin 100 mg/m² and unilateral neck radiation with 70 Gy total. A PET/CT is performed at 2 months after completion of concurrent chemoradiation and demonstrates diffuse FDG-avid uptake in the left neck surgical bed. What is the most appropriate next step in management?
   A. Concurrent chemoradiation with weekly cisplatin
   B. Repeat PET/CT 12 weeks post-therapy
   C. Modified left radical neck dissection
   D. Clinical surveillance alone

3. A 58-year-old male with a past medical history of hypertension, hyperlipidemia, and a 40 pack-year smoking history presents to your clinic with a 3-month history of progressive dysphagia and right-sided submandibular swelling. He also notes occasional pain with mastication. Physical examination of the visible nares and oropharynx is normal but a firm 1.5-cm nodule is palpated beneath the right lateral mandible. MRI of the brain, head, and neck demonstrated a 3.0-cm posterior pharyngeal mass with invasion into the right medial pterygoid muscle. PET/CT then confirms an fluorodeoxyglucose (FDG)-avid 3.0-cm invasive parapharyngeal mass with accompanying uptake into right level IIA (1.5 cm) and retropharyngeal lymph nodes (LNs). Fine needle aspiration (FNA) biopsy of the

primary tumor confirms a non-keratinizing nasopharyngeal squamous cell carcinoma (SCC). What is the most appropriate next step in therapy?

A. Surgery with adjuvant radiotherapy
B. Radiation to the mass and bilateral neck alone
C. Concurrent chemoradiation with cisplatin followed by observation with PET/CT at 12 weeks
D. Concurrent chemoradiation with cisplatin followed by 3 cycles of adjuvant cisplatin/5-fluorouracil (5-FU)

4. A 78-year-old male with a past medical history of type 2 diabetes complicated by chronic kidney disease (CKD) with nephrotic-range proteinuria as well as presbycusis presents to your clinic with recurrent epistaxis and deep, burning pains in his right neck, which have worsened over the last 6 months. The patient is otherwise able to ambulate, drive, and carry out all activities of daily living independently. An MRI of the brain and neck demonstrates a 2.5 x 3 cm nasopharyngeal mass with extension anteriorly into the nasal septum and posteriorly into the right medial pterygoid wing. Whole-body PET/CT highlights an fluorodeoxyglucose (FDG)-avid mass in the nasopharynx, although imaging is partially obscured by intracranial glucose uptake. Fine needle aspiration (FNA) biopsy by flexible rhinolaryngoscopy confirms a keratinizing nasopharyngeal squamous cell carcinoma (SCC). What is the most appropriate course in management?

A. Concurrent chemoradiation with cisplatin followed by 3 cycles of adjuvant cisplatin/5-fluorouracil (5-FU)
B. Concurrent chemoradiation with carboplatin followed by 3 cycles of adjuvant carboplatin/5-FU
C. Cisplatin with gemcitabine
D. Cisplatin with 5-FU

5. A healthy 83-year-old man presents with a small painless lump on the hard palate. Fine needle aspiration (FNA) of the lesion reveals adenoid cystic carcinoma (ACC). Imaging does not show evidence of distant metastases. What is the recommended treatment?

A. Surgical resection alone
B. Surgical resection followed by adjuvant radiation
C. Surgical resection followed by adjuvant chemotherapy + radiation
D. Observation
E. Systemic therapy with lenvatinib

6. A 67-year-old woman with a previous diagnosis of localized parotid adenoid cystic carcinoma (ACC) who underwent complete resection and adjuvant radiation 8 years ago presents for routine follow-up. She has been having a mild cough for the past 3 months. Chest imaging reveals two lung nodules (less than 2 cm) in the right upper lobe (RUL) which were not present on imaging 1 year ago. PET/CT scan was negative. Image-guided biopsy of a lung nodule revealed ACC. She is otherwise healthy. What is the recommended treatment?

A. Chemotherapy
B. Lenvatinib
C. Surgical resection of the lung nodules
D. Hospice

7. A 55-year-old previously healthy woman presents for a second opinion on treatment for biopsy proven recurrent laryngeal squamous cell carcinoma (SCC). Re-staging scans show

several lung nodules. Her tumor programmed death-ligand 1 (PD-L1) combined positive score (CPS) score is 0. She reports she completed definitive concurrent chemoradiation with cisplatin about 4 months ago. She is currently asymptomatic with Eastern Cooperative Oncology Group (ECOG) performance status (PS) 1. What is the next best treatment option?

A. Platinum + 5-fluorouracil (5-FU) + pembrolizumab
B. Platinum + 5-FU
C. Ipilimumab and nivolumab
D. Pembrolizumab
E. Hospice

8. An 80-year-old man with past medical history (PMH) of coronary artery disease, type 2 diabetes, chronic obstructive pulmonary disease (COPD), and a 60 pack-year smoking history presents for evaluation of newly diagnosed metastatic pharyngeal squamous cell carcinoma (SCC). Biopsy of a distant metastasis showed a programmed death-ligand 1 (PD-L1) combined positive score (CPS) score of 1. He has baseline dyspnea on exertion and severe peripheral neuropathy but is asymptomatic from his cancer. What is the recommended treatment?

A. Pembrolizumab
B. Pembrolizumab + platinum + 5-fluorouracil (5-FU)
C. Nivolumab
D. Platinum + 5-FU
E. Cetuximab

ANSWERS AND RATIONALES

1. **C. Concurrent chemoradiation with cisplatin-RT.** This patient has a clinical T2, N2, M0, p16+ (stage II) SCC of the oropharynx and should be treated with concurrent chemoradiation with cisplatin-RT as first-line therapy. While both concurrent cetuximab-radiation and induction TPF followed by cetuximab-radiation are options, they are inferior to cisplatin-RT but may be considered for cisplatin-ineligible patients. Radiation alone should not be pursued in this patient with stage II disease.

2. **B. Repeat PET/CT 12 weeks post-therapy.** Although a negative PET/CT at 12 weeks following receipt of definitive chemoradiation is predictive of improved overall 2-year survival, early studies (as in this case) are associated with false positives and should be avoided. The diffuse FDG-avid uptake described here is likely reactive from the patient's recent surgery and subsequent treatment effect from adjuvant radiotherapy.

3. **D. Concurrent chemoradiation with cisplatin followed by 3 cycles of adjuvant cisplatin/5-fluorouracil (5-FU).** This patient has T2N1M0, or stage II, nasopharyngeal carcinoma and should receive concurrent chemoradiation followed by adjuvant chemotherapy. Please note that surgery does not have a role at this stage and radiation alone is reserved for localized disease, generally stage I or IIA. Omitting adjuvant therapy (C) would also be inappropriate as adjuvant therapy has been shown to improve overall survival in this setting.

4. **B. Concurrent chemoradiation with carboplatin followed by 3 cycles of adjuvant carboplatin/5-FU.** For this patient with T3N0M0 (stage III) nasopharyngeal carcinoma, concurrent chemoradiation followed by adjuvant therapy may be administered. The standard in care, traditionally, has been option A, but, given this patient's extensive medical comorbidities, he would not be a cisplatin candidate and a carboplatin-based regimen in B is more appropriate. Options C and D are both therapies for metastatic disease and are not indicated in this patient with localized nasopharyngeal carcinoma.

5. **B. Surgical resection followed by adjuvant radiation.** This patient should be referred for a surgical evaluation for complete resection of the tumor given it is localized. All ACC should have adjuvant radiation as it has been shown to improve locoregional control. Adjuvant chemotherapy has not shown to provide any additional benefit. Observation is incorrect as these tumors can be locally invasive and metastasize to distant locations over time. Systemic therapy is not indicated at this time as he has only localized disease.

6. **C. Surgical resection of the lung nodules.** This patient has oligo-metastatic ACC with only two lung lesions. She is minimally symptomatic. The next best step is evaluation for metastasectomy (or stereotactic radiation). Systemic chemotherapy can be reserved for rapidly growing disease with symptoms and need for tumor debulking. Tyrosine kinase inhibitor (TKI), such as lenvatinib, can be reserved for slower growing disease which is not amenable to local ablative therapy with surgery or radiation.

7. **D. Pembrolizumab.** This patient has platinum-refractory disease as she has disease progression within 6 months of receiving cisplatin for locally advanced disease. Approved therapies for platinum-refractory recurrent or metastatic (R/M) head and neck squamous cell carcinoma (HNSCC) include pembrolizumab and nivolumab. Platinum-based chemotherapy regimens are not recommended since she progressed on these agents. Hospice is not recommended at this time given she is otherwise healthy and asymptomatic.

8. **A. Pembrolizumab.** For patients with nonplatinum-refractory disease and PD-L1 CPS score of 1, pembrolizumab or pembrolizumab + chemotherapy are available treatment options. As this patient does not need rapid tumor debulking and has medical comorbidities which may be worsened with platinum-based chemotherapy, pembrolizumab alone should be chosen. Nivolumab is approved for platinum-refractory disease. This patient does not have contraindications for immunotherapy and has severe peripheral neuropathy, so platinum + 5-FU is less favored. Cetuximab can be given as second-line therapy.

REFERENCES

1. Siegel RL, Miller KD, Fuchs HE, et al. Cancer statistics 2021. *CA Cancer J Clin.* 2021;71:7–33. doi:10.3322/caac.21654

2. Hashim D, Genden E, Posner M, et al. Head and neck cancer prevention: from primary prevention to impact of clinicians on reducing burden. *Ann Oncol.* 2019;30:744–756. doi:10.1093/annonc/mdz084

3. Chaturvedi AK, Engels EA, Pfeiffer RM, et al. Human papillomavirus and rising oropharyngeal cancer incidence in the United States. *J Clin Oncol.* 2011;29:4294–4301. doi:10.1200/JCO.2011.36.4596

4. Tsao SW, Tsang CM, Lo KW. Epstein-Barr virus infection and nasopharyngeal carcinoma. *Philos Trans R Soc Lond B Biol Sci.* 2017;372:20160270. doi:10.1098/rstb.2016.0270

5. Mozaffari HR, Ramezani M, Janbakhsh A, Sadeghi M. Malignant salivary gland tumors and Epstein-Barr virus (EBV) infection: a systematic review and meta-analysis. *Asian Pac J Cancer Prev.* 2017;18:1201–1206. doi:10.22034/APJCP.2017.18.5.1201

6. Chaturvedi AK, Engels EA, Anderson WF, Gillison ML. Incidence trends for human papillomavirus-related and -unrelated oral squamous cell carcinomas in the United States. *J Clin Oncol.* 2008;26:612–619. doi:10.1200/JCO.2007.14.1713

7. Jordan RC, Lingen MW, Perez-Ordonez B, et al. Validation of methods for oropharyngeal cancer HPV status determination in US cooperative group trials. *Am J Surg Pathol.* 2012;36:945–954. doi:10.1097/PAS.0b013e318253a2d1

8. Snow AN, Laudadio J. Human papillomavirus detection in head and neck squamous cell carcinomas. *Adv Anat Pathol.* 2010;17:394–403. doi:10.1097/PAP.0b013e3181f895c1

9. Gillison M, Trotti A, Harris J, et al. Radiotherapy plus cetuximab or cisplatin in human papillomavirus positive oropharyngeal cancer (RTOG 1016): a randomised, multicentre, non-inferiority trial [published correction appears in *Lancet.* 2020;395(10226):784]. *Lancet.* 2019;393(10166):40–50. doi:10.1016/S0140-6736(18)32779-X

10. Mehanna H, Robinson M, Hartley A, et al. Radiotherapy plus cisplatin or cetuximab in low-risk human papillomavirus-positive oropharyngeal cancer (De-ESCALaTE HPV): an open-lable randomised controlled phase 3 trial. *Lancet.* 2019;393(10166):51–60. doi:10.1016/S0140-6736(18)32752-1

11. Nguyen-Tan PF, Zhang Q, Ang KK, et al. Randomized phase III trial to test accelerated versus standard fractionation in combination with concurrent cisplatin for head and neck carcinomas in the Radiation Therapy Oncology Group 0129 trial: long-term report of efficacy and toxicity. *J Clin Oncol.* 2014;32:3858–3866. doi:10.1200/JCO.2014.55.3925

12. Chua MLK, Wee JTS, Hui EP, Chan ATC. Nasopharyngeal carcinoma. *Lancet.* 2016;387(10022):1012–1024. doi:10.1016/S0140-6736(15)00055-0

13. Barnes L, Eveson JW, Reichart P, Sidransky D, eds. *World Health Organization Classification of Tumors: Pathology and Genetics of Head and Neck Tumours.* Lyon: IARC Press, 2005.

14. Müller E, Beleites E. The basaloid squamous cell carcinoma of the nasopharynx. *Rhinology.* 2000;38(4):208–211. https://www.rhinologyjournal.com/Rhinology_issues/65.pdf

15. Kimura H, Ito Y, Suzuki R, Nishiyama Y. Measuring Epstein-Barr virus (EBV) load: the significance and application for each EBV-associated disease. *Rev Med Virol.* 2008;18(5):305–319. doi:10.1002/rmv.582

16. Kang M, Zhou P, Li G, et al. Validation of the 8th edition of the UICC/AJCC staging system for nasopharyngeal carcinoma treated with intensity-modulated radiotherapy. *Oncotarget.* 2017;8(41):70586–70594. doi:10.18632/oncotarget.19829

17. Gillison M, Trotti A, Harris J, et al. Radiotherapy plus cetuximab or cisplatin in human papillomavirus positive oropharyngeal cancer (RTOG 1016). *Lancet.* 2019;393(10166):40-50. doi:10.1016/S0140-6736(18)32779-X

18. Lee AWM, Tung SY, Ng WT, et al. A multicenter, phase 3, randomized trial of concurrent chemoradiotherapy plus adjuvant chemotherapy versus radiotherapy alone in patients with regionally advanced nasopharyngeal carcinoma: 10-year outcomes for efficacy and toxicity. *Cancer.* 2017;123(21):4147–4157. doi:10.1002/cncr.30850

19. Bossi P, Chan AT, Licitra L, et al. Nasopharyngeal carcinoma: ESMO-EURACAN clinical practice guidelines for diagnosis, treatment and follow-up. *Ann Oncol.* 2021;32(4):452–465. doi:10.1016/j.annonc.2020.12.007

20. Lee A, Chow J, Lee NY. Treatment deescalation strategies for nasopharyngeal cancer: a review. *JAMA Oncol.* 2021;7(3):445-453. doi:10.1001/jamaoncol.2020.6154

21. Wang X, Wang Y, Jiang S, et al. Safety and effectiveness of de-escalated radiation dose in T1-3 nasopharyngeal carcinoma: a propensity matched analysis. *J Cancer.* 2019;10(21):5057-5064. doi:10.7150/jca.33303

22. Togashi Y, Dobashi A, Sakata S, et al. *MYB* and *MYBL1* in adenoid cystic carcinoma: diversity in the mode of genomic rearrangement and transcripts. *Mod Pathol.* 2018;31:934-946. doi:10.1038/s41379-018-0008-8

23. Geiger JL, Ismaila N, Beadle B, et al. Management of salivary gland malignancy: ASCO guideline. *J Clin Oncol.* 2021;39:1909-1941. doi:10.1200/JCO.21.00449

24. Chen Y, Zheng ZQ, Chen FP, et al. Role of postoperative radiotherapy in nonmetastatic head and neck adenoid cystic carcinoma. *J Natl Compr Canc Netw.* 2020;18:1476-1484. doi:10.6004/jnccn.2020.7593

25. Bjørndal K, Krogdahl A, Therkildsen MH, et al. Salivary adenoid cystic carcinoma in Denmark 1990-2005: outcome and independent prognostic factors including the benefit of radiotherapy. Results of the Danish Head and Neck Cancer Group (DAHANCA). *Oral Oncol.* 2015;51:1138-1142. doi:10.1016/j.oraloncology.2015.10.002

26. Mendenhall WM, Morris CG, Amdur RJ, et al. Radiotherapy alone or combined with surgery for adenoid cystic carcinoma of the head and neck. *Head Neck.* 2004;26:154-162. doi:10.1002/hed.10380

27. Gao M, Hao Y, Huang MX, et al. Clinicopathological study of distant metastases of salivary adenoid cystic carcinoma. *Int J Oral Maxillofac Surg.* 2013;42:923-928. doi:10.1016/j.ijom.2013.04.006

28. Locati LD, Perrone F, Cortelazzi B, et al. A phase II study of sorafenib in recurrent and/or metastatic salivary gland carcinomas: translational analyses and clinical impact. *Eur J Cancer.* 2016;69:158-165. doi:10.1016/j.ejca.2016.09.022

29. Thomson DJ, Silva P, Denton K, et al. Phase II trial of sorafenib in advanced salivary adenoid cystic carcinoma of the head and neck. *Head Neck.* 2015;37:182-187. doi:10.1002/hed.23577

30. Tchekmedyian V, Sherman EJ, Dunn L, et al. Phase II study of lenvatinib in patients with progressive, recurrent or metastatic adenoid cystic carcinoma. *J Clin Oncol.* 2019;37:1529-1537. doi:10.1200/JCO.18.01859

31. Locati LD, Galbiati D, Calareso G, et al. Patients with adenoid cystic carcinomas of the salivary glands treated with lenvatinib: activity and quality of life. *Cancer.* 2020;126:1888-1894. doi:10.1002/cncr.32754

32. Cohen EEW, Soulières D, Le Tourneau C, et al. Pembrolizumab versus methotrexate, docetaxel, or cetuximab for recurrent or metastatic head-and-neck squamous cell carcinoma (KEYNOTE-040): a randomised, open-label, phase 3 study. *Lancet.* 2019;393:156-167. doi:10.1016/S0140-6736(18)31999-8

33. Ferris RL, Blumenschein G, Fayette J, et al. Nivolumab for recurrent squamous-cell carcinoma of the head and neck. *N Engl J Med.* 2016;375:1856-1867. doi:10.1056/NEJMoa1602252

34. Burtness B, Harrington KJ, Greil R, et al. Pembrolizumab alone or with chemotherapy versus cetuximab with chemotherapy for recurrent or metastatic squamous cell carcinoma of the head and neck (KEYNOTE-048): a randomised, open-label, phase 3 study. *Lancet.* 2019;394:1915-1928. doi:10.1016/S0140-6736(19)32591-7

35. Vermorken JB, Mesia R, Rivera F, et al. Platinum-based chemotherapy plus cetuximab in head and neck cancer. *N Engl J Med.* 2008;359:1116-1127. doi:10.1056/NEJMoa0802656

36. Vermorken JB, Trigo J, Hitt R, et al. Open-label, uncontrolled, multicenter phase II study to evaluate the efficacy and toxicity of cetuximab as single agent in patients with recurrent and/or metastatic squamous cell carcinoma of the head and neck who failed to respond to platinum-based therapy. *J Clin Oncol.* 2007;25:2171-2177. doi:10.1200/JCO.2006.06.7447

37. Stewart JS, Cohen EE, Licitra L, et al. Phase III study of gefitinib compared with intravenous methotrexate for recurrent squamous cell carcinoma of the head and neck. *J Clin Oncol.* 2009;27:1864-1871. doi:10.1200/JCO.2008.17.0530

38. Guardiola E, Peyrade F, Chaigneau L, et al. Results of a randomised phase II study comparing docetaxel with methotrexate in patients with recurrent head and neck cancer. *Eur J Cancer.* 2004;40:2071-2076. doi:10.1016/j.ejca.2004.05.019

CHAPTER 2

Thyroid Cancer

Kamya Sankar and Francis P. Worden

INTRODUCTION

Epidemiology, risk factors, and natural history. The incidence of thyroid cancer has tripled from 1975 to 2012 and has since plateaued. During the year 2021, it was estimated that approximately 44,280 cases of thyroid cancers would be diagnosed.[1] The median age of diagnosis for all thyroid cancers is 49 years. The 5-year survival rate, which varies based on stage and the specific type of thyroid cancer, is almost 100% for localized papillary, follicular, and medullary thyroid cancer, and 31% for localized anaplastic thyroid cancer. The 5-year overall survival (OS) rate for regional papillary thyroid cancer is greater than 90% for regional papillary, follicular, and medullary thyroid cancer, and 10% for regional anaplastic thyroid cancer. The 5-year OS rate for metastatic thyroid cancer is 76% for papillary, 64% for follicular, 38% for medullary, and 3% for anaplastic.[2]

The three main histology categories of thyroid cancer are differentiated (that is, papillary, follicular, and Hürthle cell), medullary, and anaplastic. Radiation exposure to the thyroid during childhood is the most defined environmental risk factor for thyroid cancer. Other risk factors include a family history of thyroid cancer or a thyroid cancer syndrome (that is, multiple endocrine neoplasia [MEN] 2 syndrome, familial polyposis, Werner syndrome) and iodine deficiency.

Differentiated Thyroid Cancer

Papillary thyroid cancer. Papillary thyroid cancer accounts for ~80% of all thyroid cancers and may present as an incidental imaging finding or as an enlarged symptomatic thyroid nodule. Papillary thyroid cancers predominate in the fourth and fifth decades of life, with a female predominance of 2.5:1.[1] A diagnosis of papillary thyroid cancer is made by fine needle aspiration (FNA). Most patients with papillary thyroid cancer do not die of their disease.[3] Poor prognostic features include age older than 55 years,[4] presence of distant metastases, and/or local invasion into airways, vessels, or surrounding tissue. The median survival may range by site of metastasis, and can range from a 10-year OS of 30% to 50%[5] in those with pulmonary metastases alone as compared to median survival of approximately 1 year in those with brain metastases.[5]

Follicular thyroid cancer. Follicular thyroid cancer accounts for ~5% to 8% of thyroid cancers. The peak incidence is in the fifth or sixth decades of life, with a female predominance. An FNA is not adequate for diagnosis of follicular cancer as growth beyond the tumor capsule cannot be assessed with FNA; therefore, an excisional biopsy or lobectomy is required for diagnosis. More than 75% of follicular thyroid carcinomas have either a *PAX8* or *RAS* mutation. Given that follicular carcinoma typically occurs later in life, it is generally associated with a more aggressive clinical course, higher incidence of distant metastases, and higher mortality as compared to papillary thyroid cancer.

Hürthle cell carcinoma. Hürthle cell carcinomas comprise 3% of all thyroid cancers and often manifest as thyroid nodules, as in other thyroid cancers. As with follicular carcinoma, an FNA is inadequate to establish a diagnosis, therefore requiring an excisional biopsy or lobectomy for pathological analysis. The tumor is comprised of at least 75% Hürthle cells which are large eosinophilic thyroglobulin-producing cells, designated as "oncocytes." A significant percentage of Hürthle cell carcinomas demonstrate the *RET/PTC gene rearrangement.* Hürthle cell carcinoma is a more aggressive disease with higher mortality than either papillary or follicular carcinoma, perhaps related to the tumor's poor ability to take up radioactive iodine (RAI). The 10-year disease-free survival has been quoted to be ~41% as compared to 75% in follicular carcinoma.[6]

Treatment overview of differentiated thyroid cancer. Surgical excision is the primary modality of treatment for patients with differentiated thyroid cancer (DTC). The type of procedure (that is, thyroid lobectomy, total thyroidectomy) is dependent on the size of the tumor, extrathyroidal extension, and presence of metastasis. Radioactive iodine ablation (RIA) to ablate residual normal thyroid tissue is administered in patients who are high risk and selected intermediate-risk patients based on specific tumor characteristics which portend higher risk for recurrence or persistent disease.[7] Further, thyroid hormone replacement is required to prevent hypothyroidism and for reducing the risk of thyroid-stimulating hormone (TSH) stimulated tumor growth. Surveillance typically involves physical exam, TSH and thyroglobulin measurement at 6 and 12 months, then annually if disease-free, as well as periodic neck ultrasound. Between 4% and 5% of DTCs are RAI refractory. RAI-refractory disease is defined as lack of RAI uptake within one target lesion, progression following treatment dose of RAI, or cumulative RAI treatment of greater than 600 mCI.[8] Treatment for RAI-refractory disease can include watchful waiting for stable or slowly progressive asymptomatic disease, local therapies such as surgery or radiation for isolated growing distant metastases, or systemic therapy (that is, with tyrosine kinase inhibitors [TKIs]) for progressive symptomatic disease.

Medullary thyroid cancer. Medullary thyroid carcinoma constitutes approximately 4% of all thyroid cancers. It occurs most frequently in the fourth or fifth decades of life and in equal frequency among men and women. Medullary thyroid carcinoma is a type of neuroendocrine tumor which arises from the parafollicular C cell of the thyroid gland and produces calcitonin. Calcitonin levels are characteristically elevated at the time of diagnosis. Somatic mutations in the *RET* proto-oncogene occurs in greater than 70% of medullary thyroid carcinomas. The rest are accounted for by inherited germ-line mutations as part of cancer predisposition syndromes including MEN 2A or 2B, or familial medullary thyroid cancer (FMTC). MEN 2A is associated with medullary thyroid carcinoma, parathyroid hyperplasia, and pheochromocytoma. MEN 2B is associated with medullary thyroid carcinoma, pheochromocytoma, marfanoid features, and neuroganglioneuromas. Because most medullary thyroid carcinomas have identifiable mutations, they are usually amenable for treatment with targeted TKIs. Medullary thyroid cancer has a worse prognosis than either papillary or follicular thyroid cancer. Poor prognostic features include older age, presence of distant metastases, larger tumor, and number of positive regional lymph nodes (LNs).

Anaplastic thyroid cancer. Anaplastic thyroid carcinoma is the least common thyroid cancer (~2% of thyroid cancers) and is the most aggressive solid tumor, characterized by heterogenous histology. It is an undifferentiated carcinoma arising from the thyroid follicular epithelium. It typically presents as an enlarging neck mass with local symptoms and tends to present in the seventh or eighth decades of life with a female predominance. FNA establishes the diagnosis. Molecular testing should be performed to identify mutations which are associated with anaplastic thyroid carcinoma, which include *BRAF, TSC1, TSC2, ALK, NTRK,* and *RET,* as presence of some of these mutations may have therapeutic implications. Anaplastic thyroid carcinoma is extremely aggressive with a disease-specific mortality of almost 100% and a median survival ranging from 3 to 12 months.[9]

CASE SUMMARIES

Case 2.1: Locally Advanced Anaplastic Thyroid Cancer

Mr. J.S. is a 66-year-old man who presented to his primary care physician with voice hoarseness. He was sent to an otolaryngologist who performed a flexible laryngoscopy, which revealed sluggish vocal cord on the right side. A CT scan of the neck demonstrated a bulky heterogenous enhancing mass involving the right thyroid lobe, inseparable from the upper thoracic esophagus and right paravertebral soft tissue with infiltration of the right lateral distal cervical and upper thoracic trachea, with evidence of leftward tracheal deviation. A fluorodeoxyglucose (FDG)-PET scan revealed an FDG-avid large thyroid mass, without evidence of distant metastases. An FNA of the thyroid mass revealed high-grade follicular thyroid carcinoma with significant necrosis, favoring a more aggressive anaplastic histology.

What Is the Initial Evaluation and Management of Anaplastic Thyroid Carcinoma?

- Anaplastic thyroid carcinoma is an aggressive solid tumor malignancy with median survival of less than 1 year. Around 90% of cases present with locoregionally advanced or metastatic disease.
- In a patient with newly diagnosed anaplastic thyroid carcinoma, a multidisciplinary team should be consulted for evaluation of resectability.
- Molecular testing with next-generation sequencing (NGS) should be performed to test for actionable mutations (including *BRAF, NTRK, ALK, RET*), microsatellite instability (MSI), and tumor mutational burden.
- The prognosis and goals of treatment including risks and benefits should be discussed with the patient. The patient's comorbidities and physical fitness with the Eastern Cooperative Oncology Group (ECOG) performance status should be assessed prior to consideration of therapies.

Case Update
- *The patient's molecular testing identified a BRAF V600E mutation, microsatellite stable, and tumor mutational burden of five mutations/megabase.*

What Is the Management for Locoregionally Advanced Anaplastic Thyroid Carcinoma?

- In patients with good performance status with resectable disease, total thyroidectomy with therapeutic LN dissection is performed. If an R0 or R1 resection is achieved, adjuvant external beam radiotherapy or intensity-modulated radiation therapy is administered postoperatively. If an R2 resection is achieved, concurrent chemoradiotherapy may be considered with radiosensitizing agents such as paclitaxel, docetaxel, doxorubicin, cisplatin, or combination agents such as carboplatin/paclitaxel or docetaxel/doxorubicin.[9]
- In patients with locoregionally advanced unresectable disease, external beam radiotherapy or intensity-modulated radiation therapy with or without concurrent chemotherapy is administered.

What Is the Management for Locoregionally Advanced, Unresectable, or Metastatic Anaplastic Thyroid Carcinoma?

- Patients with targetable mutations:

- ○ Between 20% and 50% of patients with anaplastic thyroid cancer harbor the *BRAF* V600E mutation. In patients with *BRAF* V600E-mutant anaplastic thyroid carcinoma, combination of dabrafenib and trametinib is approved.
  - ▪ In a Phase II study, patients with *BRAF* V600E-mutant malignancies received dabrafenib in combination with trametinib. In this study, the overall response rate (ORR) was 61% in 23 patients with anaplastic thyroid carcinoma.[10]
- ○ Other targeted therapies may be considered including larotrectinib and entrectinib for *NTRK* gene fusion-positive tumors,[11,12] and pralsetinib or selpercatinib for *RET* fusion-positive patients.[13,14]
- Patients without targetable mutations:
  - ○ There are no randomized trials to support prolongation of survival or quality of life in patients with anaplastic thyroid carcinoma with systemic cytotoxic chemotherapy. However, tumor regression can be induced, and anecdotal nonrandomized study evidence supports use of cytotoxic chemotherapies in select patients. Palliation of symptomatic and/or imminently life-threatening lesions should be given high priority for systemic therapy.
    - ▪ Taxanes (paclitaxel, docetaxel) may be administered alone or in combination with carboplatin. Anthracyclines (doxorubicin) may be administered in combination with cisplatin or taxane.[15]
  - ○ Pembrolizumab may be considered in patients with tumor mutational burden [Equation]10 mutations/megabase.

Case Update

- *Mr. J.S.'s tumor was considered to be locoregionally advanced and unresectable. He underwent radiotherapy alone (7000 Gy) followed by systemic therapy with combination dabrafenib and trametinib, achieving a partial response and symptomatic improvement.*

Case 2.2: Metastatic Medullary Thyroid Cancer

Ms. D.P. is a 58-year-old woman who presented initially with diarrhea and unintentional 60-lb weight loss. A CT scan of her abdomen and pelvis discovered diffuse bony metastasis in her spine as well as necrotic iliac LNs. A left iliac bone biopsy demonstrated neuroendocrine tumor, most consistent with medullary thyroid carcinoma. Her serum calcitonin was greater than 40,000 pg/mL. She then underwent FNA of a left thyroid nodule which confirmed medullary thyroid carcinoma.

What Is the Initial Evaluation for a Patient Diagnosed With Medullary Thyroid Carcinoma?

- Serum measurements of carcinoembryonic antigen (CEA) and calcitonin should be performed.
- Genetic testing to identify germline *RET* mutation should be performed.
- If germline *RET* mutation is identified, screening for hyperparathyroidism and/or pheochromocytoma should be performed. Patient should be referred for genetic counseling
- *RET* somatic genotyping may be performed in patients who are germline wild-type or if germline status is unknown.

Case Update

- *Patient underwent genetic testing which did not identify any inheritable mutations. The tumor was sent for NGS and was identified to harbor an RET exon 16 single nucleotide substitution.*

What Are the Primary Treatment Options for Medullary Thyroid Cancer?

- The primary treatment for medullary thyroid cancer in local or locally advanced disease is surgical resection. There is a limited role for external beam radiotherapy.
- Since medullary thyroid cancer is a neuroendocrine tumor of the thyroid parafollicular cells, it is not responsive to either radioiodine or TSH suppression.
- For patients who are not candidates for surgery or radiotherapy and/or have metastatic disease, systemic therapy can be offered.

When Should Systemic Therapy Be Considered?

- For patients with asymptomatic distant metastatic disease without radiographic evidence of progression, disease monitoring is generally accepted, given the lack of data regarding the alteration of outcome if patients are initiated on early systemic therapy.[7]
- Patients with symptomatic disease and/or evidence of radiographic progression by Response Evaluation Criteria in Solid Tumors (RECIST) should be considered for systemic therapy options.

What Are the Systemic Therapy Options for Medullary Thyroid Cancer?

- TKIs are the standard approach to treating metastatic medullary thyroid cancer. *RET* mutations account for the majority (greater than 70%) of medullary thyroid cancers. The multikinase TKIs and selective *RET* inhibitors which have been approved for medullary thyroid cancer are described in the text that follows. Currently, there is no data regarding the optimal sequencing of multikinase and targeted TKIs in patients with medullary thyroid cancer.
- Multikinase inhibitors:
  - *Vandetanib.* Vandetanib is a multikinase inhibitor which targets *RET, VEGFR,* and *EGFR.* In a Phase III randomized double-blind study, vandetanib 300 mg/day was compared to placebo in patients with unresectable locally advanced or metastatic medullary thyroid cancer. The primary endpoint, progression-free survival (PFS), was significantly prolonged in the vandetanib group (hazard ratio [HR] 0.35, 95% confidence interval [CI] 0.24 to 0.53, P less than 0.0001).[16] The ORR was 37% in the vandetanib group. OS data were immature at data cutoff (HR 0.89, 95% CI 0.48 to 1.65). The most common adverse events included diarrhea, rash, nausea, hypertension, and headache. Based on these data, vandetanib was the first drug to be approved by the U.S. Food and Drug Administration (FDA) for progressive or symptomatic medullary thyroid cancer in 2011.
  - *Cabozantinib.* Cabozantinib is a multikinase inhibitor which targets *RET, VEGFR2,* and *MET.* In a Phase III randomized controlled study, patients with locally advanced or metastatic medullary thyroid cancer with documented progression were randomized to receive cabozantinib 140 mg/day or placebo.[17] The median PFS was noted to be prolonged in the cabozantinib group (11.2 vs. 4.0 months, HR 0.28, 95% CI 0.19 to 0.40, P less than 0.0001). The ORR with cabozantinib was 28% with a median duration of response of 14.6 months. There was no significant difference in OS despite lack of crossover in this trial, most likely due to presence of other active agents such as vandetanib. Common toxicities included diarrhea, palmar-plantar erythrodysesthesia, decreased weight, nausea, and fatigue. Cabozantinib can be associated with fistula formation or perforations of the GI tract. Cabozantinib was approved in 2012 for progressive metastatic medullary thyroid cancer.
- Selective *RET* inhibitors:
  - *Selpercatinib.* Selpercatinib is a potent selective *RET* inhibitor which was evaluated in a Phase I to II study.[14] In patients with *RET*-mutated medullary thyroid cancer who had

previously received vandetanib, cabozantinib, or both, the response rate was 69%, and 1-year PFS was 82%. In treatment-naive patients with *RET*-mutated medullary thyroid cancer, the response rate was 73% and 1-year PFS was 92%. The most common side effects were hypertension, increased liver function tests, hyponatremia, and diarrhea. Selpercatinib was approved in 2020 for patients with advanced or metastatic medullary thyroid cancer who require systemic therapy.

○ *Pralsetinib.* Pralsetinib is another highly potent selective *RET* inhibitor which was studied in a Phase I to II study. In patients with *RET*-mutant medullary thyroid cancer who had previously received cabozantinib, vandetanib, or both, the response rate was 71%. The ORR was 89% in treatment-naive patients with *RET*-mutant medullary thyroid cancer.[13] Pralsetinib was generally well tolerated with common side effects reported to be hypertension, neutropenia, lymphopenia, and anemia. Although most adverse events are limited, tumor lysis syndrome has been reported, prompting the FDA to issue a black box warning. Pralsetinib was approved in 2020 for patients with *RET*-mutated medullary thyroid cancer who require systemic therapy.

What Are Other Options for Patients Who Progress on the Approved Tyrosine Kinase Inhibitors?

- While not approved by the FDA, other small molecule multikinase inhibitors (for example, sorafenib, sunitinib, lenvatinib, or pazopanib) can be considered if patients progress on preferred frontline therapies.
- Dacarbazine-based chemotherapy may be considered.
- If tumor mutational burden has been assessed, pembrolizumab can be an option for patients with tumors where tumor mutational burden is [Equation]10 mutations/ megabase.

What Are Some Other Considerations to Offer Best Supportive Care for Patients With Metastatic Medullary Thyroid Cancer?

- External beam radiotherapy or intensity-modulated radiation therapy to the thyroid may be considered for patients with local symptoms but should *never* be administered in the adjuvant setting. Palliative resection, ablation, or other regional treatments may be considered.
- Patients with bone metastases should receive intravenous bisphosphonate or denosumab.
- As with other advanced malignancies, best supportive care for symptomatic comfort and integration with the palliative care team should be provided.

Case Update

- *Patient was initiated on selpercatinib. She was additionally started on denosumab for presence of bone metastases. She required a 25% dose reduction of selpercatinib due to elevated liver function tests, but otherwise tolerated therapy well. She initially had a partial response on radiographic imaging and remains on selpercatinib with stable disease.*

Case 2.3: Metastatic Radioactive Iodine Refractory Differentiated Thyroid Cancer

Mr. D.O. is a 57-year-old man who initially presented to his primary care physician with a mass in his left neck, which was confirmed on ultrasound. He underwent a total thyroidectomy with compartmental dissection, and pathology revealed a 4-cm tumor with large vessel involvement, consistent with unifocal columnar cell variant of papillary thyroid carcinoma. Surgical margins were positive, and he had two out of three cervical LNs positive for papillary thyroid carcinoma. He was subsequently treated with RAI therapy, and a post-therapy ablation scan showed no evidence of metastatic papillary thyroid cancer. Six months later, he developed lower extremity numbness on the right side. A CT scan revealed thoracic adenopathy, multiple pulmonary nodules, and osseous lesions involving the ribs, as well as T12, L2, and L4 vertebral bodies. Biopsy of a pulmonary nodule confirmed recurrent metastatic papillary thyroid carcinoma. He had no abnormal RAI uptake on his thyroid scan, making his disease compatible with non-iodine avid metastatic disease. He first underwent palliative radiation to the spine.

What Is the Stage of His Recurrent Thyroid Cancer?

- This is a 55-year-old man who after local therapy for a papillary thyroid carcinoma has developed metastatic disease involving the LNs, lungs, and spine within 1 year. Given the metastatic spread of the cancer and the patient's age, this thyroid cancer is prognostically classified as stage IVB based on the American Joint Committee on Cancer/Union for International Cancer Control (AJCC/UICC) eighth edition staging manual (Tables 2.1 and 2.2). If this patient had been younger than 55 years, he would have been classified as having stage II disease.
- Most patients with papillary thyroid cancer do not die of their disease.
- Prognostic features include age at diagnosis (greater than 55 years), size of tumor and gross invasion of adjacent structures, and the presence of distant metastases.

What Further Testing Would You Recommend for Recurrent or Metastatic Radioactive Iodine-Refractory Differentiated Thyroid Cancer?

- NGS should be performed on patients with recurrent or metastatic, RAI-refractory DTC. NGS allows for identification of genomic alterations that are targets of directed TKI therapy.

Table 2.1   Staging for Differentiated Thyroid Cancer Based on the Eighth Edition of AJCC Staging System

AJCC Stage	Age at Diagnosis	Description
Stage I	≤55 y old	Tumor of any size without distant metastasis (any T, any N, M0)
	>55 y old	Tumors ≤4 cm that are confined to the thyroid without LN or distant metastasis (T1–T2, N0, M0)
Stage II	≤55 y old	Tumor of any size with distant metastasis present (any T, any N, M1)
	>55 y old	Tumors >4 cm and confined to the thyroid (T3a, any N) or with gross extra-thyroidal extension into the strap muscles (T3b, any N), or tumors <4 cm with metastasis to regional LNs (T1-T2, N1). No distant metastasis (M0)
Stage III	>55 y old	Tumors of any size with gross extra-thyroidal extension into subcutaneous tissue, larynx, trachea, esophagus, recurrent laryngeal nerve without distant metastasis (T4a, any N, M0)
Stage IV	>55 y old	Tumors of any size with gross extra-thyroidal extension into prevertebral fascia, encasing major vessels (T4b, any N, M0), or presence of distant metastasis (any T, any N, M1)

AJCC, American Joint Committee on Cancer; LN, lymph node.

Source: Data from Amin MB, Edge SB, Greene FL, et al., eds. *AJCC Cancer Staging Manual.* 8th ed. Springer Nature; 2017.

Table 2.2   AJCC Prognostic Stage Groups for Differentiated and Anaplastic Thyroid Cancer

Stage	T	N	M
Differentiated Thyroid Cancer Age <55 years			
I	Any	Any	0
II	Any	Any	M1
Differentiated Thyroid Cancer Age >55 years			
I	T1	N0	M0
	T2	N0	M0
II	T1	N1	M0
	T2	N1	M0
	T3a/3b	Any	M0
III	T4a	Any	M0
IVA	T4b	Any	M0
IVB	Any	Any	M1
Anaplastic			
IVA	T1-3a	N0	M0
IVB	T1-3a	N1	M0
	T3b	Any	M0
	T4	Any	M0
IVC	Any	Any	M1

AJCC, American Joint Committee on Cancer; M, metastasis; N, node; T, tumor.

Source: Data from Amin MB, Edge SB, Greene FL, et al., eds. *AJCC Cancer Staging Manual.* 8th ed. Springer Nature; 2017.

What Are the Frontline Options for Treatment of Metastatic Radioactive Iodine-Refractory Differentiated Thyroid Cancer?

- TKIs are now the first-line therapy for RAI-refractory metastatic DTC. NGS testing guides the choice of TKI. Patients whose tumors harbor potentially targetable mutations may be candidates for directed TKI. Those without targetable mutations are candidates for multikinase TKIs.
- **Multikinase inhibitors.** The two currently approved TKIs for RAI-refractory metastatic DTC (regardless of mutational status) are sorafenib and lenvantinib.
  - *Sorafenib.* Sorafenib is a multi-target TKI which targets *VEGFR1-3*, *RET*, *PDGFR-B*, and *RAF* including *BRAF* V600E. Sorafenib was evaluated in a randomized controlled Phase III trial where patients with RAI-refractory locally advanced or metastatic thyroid cancer who had progressed within the last 14 months were randomized to sorafenib or placebo. The median PFS was significantly longer in the sorafenib group (10.8 vs. 5.8 months, HR 0.59, 95% CI 0.45 to 0.76; *P* less than 0.0001).[18] The ORR was 12.2% in the sorafenib group. There was no significant difference in OS between the groups. The most common toxicities in the sorafenib group were hand–foot syndrome, diarrhea, and alopecia. Based on these data, sorafenib was approved for patients with metastatic thyroid cancer after progression on RAI therapy.

- *Lenvatinib*. Lenvatinib is a TKI which targets the following pathways: *VEGFR* 1-3, *PDGFR*-alpha, *RET, KIT,* and *FGFR* 1-4. Lenvatinib was evaluated in a randomized Phase III clinical trial which evaluated lenvatinib 24 mg versus placebo in patients with progressive metastatic RAI-refractory DTC. The median PFS was 18.3 versus 3.6 months (P less than 0.001) and response rate was 64.8% versus 1.5% (P less than 0.001).[19] The most common adverse effects in the lenvatinib group occurring in 97.3% of patients included hypertension, proteinuria, and arterial and venous thromboembolic events. Based on this study, lenvatinib was also approved for patients who had progressive DTC following RAI therapy.

- **Targeted therapies.** The most common genetic alteration in DTC is a mutation of the *BRAF* gene, found in ~45% of patients with papillary thyroid cancer. Other mutations which have been identified include *RET, NTRK,* and *ALK.*
  - **BRAF-*inhibitors*.** Vemurafenib and dabrafenib have each been studied separately in patients with metastatic *BRAF*-mutated RAI-refractory DTC in the frontline setting and after progression on multikinase inhibitors. In a nonrandomized Phase II study evaluating vemurafenib 960 mg twice daily in patients with *BRAF* V600E-positive RAI-refractory metastatic or unresectable papillary thyroid cancer, patients who were treatment-naive had a response rate of 38.5%, and median PFS of 18.2 months. In contrast, patients who had previously received treatment with a multikinase inhibitor achieved a response rate of 27.3% and median PFS of 8.9 months.[20] Dabrafenib was evaluated in a Phase I study of patients with *BRAF* V600E-positive metastatic DTC, where partial response was achieved in 29% of patients, with a median PFS of 11.3 months.[21] Dabrafenib has also been studied in combination with trametinib, a *MEK* inhibitor. In a Phase II randomized study, patients with *BRAF*-mutated RAI-refractory DTC were randomized to dabrafenib alone or dabrafenib plus trametinib. There was no significant difference in the primary outcomes between the arms (objective response rate 50% vs. 54% [P = 0.78] and median PFS 11.4 vs. 15.1 months [P = 0.27]).[22] Though *BRAF* inhibitors are still under evaluation in RAI-refractory metastatic DTC and OS data are not yet mature, *BRAF* inhibitors may be considered in a select population both as first- or second-line therapy.
  - **RET *inhibitors*.** *RET* alterations are less commonly found in DTC (less than 10% of DTC) as compared to medullary thyroid cancer. Selpercatinib and pralsetinib are both highly selective and potent *RET* inhibitors which have been evaluated in thyroid cancer. In a Phase I to II study evaluating efficacy of selpercatinib in *RET*-altered thyroid cancers, in 19 patients with previously treated *RET* fusion-positive nonmedullary thyroid cancer, selpercatinib 160 mg twice daily resulted in a 79% objective response rate, with 64% of patients progression-free at 1 year (median PFS not reached).[14] Similarly, pralsetinib was evaluated in a Phase I to II study, which included nine patients with previously treated *RET*-fusion positive, nonmedullary thyroid cancer who were treated with pralsetinib 400 mg once daily.[13] This resulted in an ORR of 89% and a 1-year PFS rate of 81% (median PFS not reached). Toxicities to consider for selpercatinib include edema, elevated liver function tests and hyponatremia. Adverse effects of pralsetinib may include anemia, elevated liver function tests, hypertension, and pneumonitis. Based on these data, both selpercatinib and pralsetinib were approved by the FDA for patients with RAI-refractory metastatic DTC.
  - **NTRK *inhibitors*.** Rearrangements of the *NTRK* gene have been identified in many solid malignancies including papillary thyroid cancer. From a pooled efficacy analysis of three clinical trials, five of 55 patients included had *TRK* fusion-positive thyroid cancer and were treated with larotrectinib, with an ORR of 79%.[11] In another pooled analysis, treatment with larotrectinib in *NTRK* fusion-positive DTC resulted in an ORR of 90% with a 12-month PFS rate of 81%.[11] Similarly, in a pooled efficacy

analysis of three clinical trials which evaluated entrectinib in previously treated patients with *NTRK* fusion-positive advanced malignancies, five of 54 patients had thyroid cancer. The objective response rate in the entire study population was 57% with a median PFS of 11.2 months.[12] Based on these data, both entrectinib and larotrectinib have tissue-agnostic approval for advanced malignancies with *NTRK* fusion who have progressed after prior lines of therapy. Therefore, both are options for patients with RAI-refractory metastatic or unresectable DTC.

What Are the Second-Line Therapy Options for Treatment of Metastatic Radioactive Iodine-Refractory Differentiated Thyroid Cancer?

- In patients who have progressive symptom disease after treatment with lenvantinib or sorafenib, cabozantinib is approved. This is based on a randomized Phase III trial which compared cabozantinib to placebo in patients who had received previous *VEGFR*-targeted therapy. The median PFS was significantly higher in the cabozantinib group.[23]
- Other small molecule kinase inhibitors such as axitinib, everolimus, pazopanib, sunitinib, and vandetanib can also be considered.
- Pembrolizumab may be considered for patients with tumor mutational burden-high (TMB-H; [Equation]10 mutations/megabase) tumors.
- For patients who harbor *BRAF* mutations, vemurafenib or dabrafenib may be used.
- Patients who progress on upfront selective TKI therapy may be treated with sorafenib or lenvantinib.

Case Update

- *The patient was initiated on lenvantinib 24 mg daily and required subsequent dose reductions for hypertension and fatigue. NGS was performed and revealed a BRAF mutation. He was then started on dabrafenib 150 mg daily.*

REVIEW QUESTIONS

1. A 34-year-old female is diagnosed with papillary thyroid cancer. Staging CT of the neck and chest reveals a 2-cm primary thyroid tumor and multiple less than 2-mm bilateral pulmonary nodules. Her stage is:
   A. II
   B. III
   C. IVA
   D. IVB

2. A 54-year-old female with metastatic radioactive iodine (RAI)-refractory differentiated thyroid cancer (DTC) has asymptomatic disease and is on observation. Her most recent set of scans demonstrate doubling in size of metastatic lesions in the pulmonary right lower lobe (RLL) nodule, mediastinal lymph nodes (LNs), and sacrum. Next-generation sequencing (NGS) at diagnosis did not reveal any targetable mutations. What are your treatment options?
   A. Observation
   B. Sorafenib
   C. Lenvatinib
   D. All of the above could be options

3. A 60-year-old man with a history of medullary thyroid cancer presents with low back pain. On CT scan, he is found to have osseous lytic lesions involving the L2, L3, and L4 vertebral bodies with soft tissue extension and neural foraminal narrowing. There is no evidence of spinal cord compression. Further imaging reveals a suspicious right thyroid nodule, right supraclavicular, and mediastinal lymphadenopathy along with bilateral pulmonary nodules measuring up to 2 cm. A biopsy of the right supraclavicular lymph node (LN) reveals medullary thyroid carcinoma. Next-generation sequencing (NGS) reveals *RET* mutation. What do you recommend for treatment?
   A. Sorafenib
   B. Sunitinib
   C. Lenvatinib
   D. Pralsetinib

4. A 72-year-old man presents with anaplastic thyroid cancer. He was treated with combination therapy including surgery, chemotherapy, and radiation. His most recent CT scans show progressive disease in the liver and lung. The patient has no other comorbidities but has an Eastern Cooperative Oncology Group (ECOG) performance status of 3 due to ongoing fatigue. He additionally has had significant weight loss of 30 lbs over the last 2 months. Laboratory examination is within normal parameters. What do you recommend?
   A. Hospice
   B. Sorafenib
   C. Gemcitabine
   D. Cabozantinib

5. A 46-year-old female presents with stage II papillary thyroid carcinoma and undergoes total thyroidectomy followed by radioactive iodine ablation (RIA). What additional treatment is indicated?
   A. Chemotherapy
   B. Adjuvant external beam radiation to the neck
   C. Thyroid-stimulating hormone (TSH) suppression
   D. Observation

6. A 68-year-old man presents with metastatic radioactive iodine (RAI)-refractory follicular thyroid carcinoma involving lymph nodes (LNs), lung, and bone. He has no targetable mutations on next-generation sequencing (NGS) panel. He was initially treated with lenvatinib with partial response and tolerated this treatment well for approximately 1 year. His most recent CT of the chest, abdomen, and pelvis demonstrates increase in size of retroperitoneal and mediastinal LNs as well as doubling in size of osseous lesions in the right femur and sacrum. He has an Eastern Cooperative Oncology Group (ECOG) performance status of 1. What are your next steps in management?
   A. Pralsetinib
   B. Dabrafenib
   C. Cabozantinib
   D. Vandetinib

7. A 49-year-old woman presents to discuss management of newly diagnosed thyroid cancer. She has a 3-cm papillary thyroid carcinoma, with extra-thyroidal extension, without any lymph node (LN) involvement or distant metastases. Which is an indication to perform a total thyroidectomy?
   A. Extra-thyroid extension
   B. Size of tumor
   C. Papillary histology
   D. Age of patient

8. A 55-year-old woman is status post partial thyroidectomy for papillary thyroid cancer. Pathology reveals a unifocal 0.8-cm tumor with no extra-thyroid extension. Preoperative imaging showed no involvement of lymph nodes (LNs) or distant metastasis. The postoperative unstimulated thyroglobulin level is less than 1 ng/mL and no detectable anti-thyroglobulin antibodies are seen. What adjuvant therapy do you offer?
   A. Radioactive iodine (RAI)
   B. Observation
   C. External beam radiotherapy
   D. Lenvatinib

9. Which of the following tumor markers can aid in both diagnosis and surveillance after treatment for medullary thyroid cancer?
   A. CA-125
   B. Calcium
   C. Calcitonin
   D. Thyroglobulin

10. A 48-year-old female presents for preoperative clearance prior to surgery for recently diagnosed medullary thyroid cancer. Calcitonin level was 550 pg/mL. Imaging did not show distant metastases. Which of the following should be evaluated for prior to surgery?
    A. Diabetes insipidus
    B. Syndrome of inappropriate antidiuretic hormone (SIADH)
    C. Parathyroid hyperplasia
    D. Pheochromocytoma

ANSWERS AND RATIONALES

1. **A. II.** According to the American Joint Committee on Cancer (AJCC) eighth edition thyroid cancer staging manual, there are two stages for papillary thyroid carcinoma in patients younger than 55 years of age. Stage II disease is defined as patients younger than 55 who have presence of M1 disease (regardless of tumor size and/or lymph node [LN] status).

2. **D. All of the above could be options.** For patients with RAI-refractory DTC, watchful waiting is a reasonable treatment option in patients with stable asymptomatic disease. For patients with symptomatic progressive disease, systemic therapy is indicated with multi-kinase inhibitor. Sorafenib and lenvatinib are both approved in the frontline setting for patients with metastatic RAI-refractory DTC.

3. **D. Pralsetinib.** For patients with metastatic medullary thyroid cancer, mutations in *RET* are identified in greater than 70% of cases. Frontline therapy options include pralsetinib and selpercatinib, which are both highly potent selective *RET* inhibitors. To date, there are no randomized controlled trials directly comparing these two agents in the frontline setting; therefore, either may be used after discussion of toxicity profiles with the patient.

4. **A. Hospice.** Anaplastic thyroid carcinoma is the most aggressive solid tumor malignancy with median survival of less than 12 months. In a patient who has already had aggressive trimodal therapy, now with declining performance status and significant weight loss, goals of treatment and prognosis must be discussed with the patient. Hospice referral is most appropriate in this situation.

5. **C. Thyroid-stimulating hormone (TSH) suppression.** In patients with DTC following RIA, TSH suppression has been shown to prolong survival. In addition, ultrasound and thyroglobulin monitoring are indicated.

6. **C. Cabozantinib.** In patients with metastatic RAI-refractory differentiated thyroid cancer (DTC) who have previously progressed on lenvatinib or sorafenib, cabozantinib was shown to prolong median progression-free survival (PFS) as compared to supportive care in a randomized Phase II study. Pralsetinib and dabrafenib are not indicated given that this patient's NGS panel did not show a targetable mutation. Vandetinib could be considered; however, use of cabozantinib in the second-line setting has a higher level of evidence.

7. **A. Extra-thyroid extension.** The indications for consideration of total thyroidectomy include extra-thyroid extension, poorly differentiated histology, cervical LN involvement, tumor greater than 4 cm, and known distant metastases. Total thyroidectomy is also considered for bilateral nodularity and history of radiation exposure to the neck.

8. **B. Observation.** Patients are considered for adjuvant RAI therapy based on their risk for relapse. Those who meet all criteria for low-risk disease do not require adjuvant RAI and can be placed on surveillance. These criteria for low-risk disease include classic papillary cancer, tumor less than 2 cm, unifocal or multifocal (all are less than 1 cm), intra-thyroidal disease, postoperative unstimulated thyroglobulin less than 1 ng/mL, and no detectable anti-thyroglobulin antibodies.

9. **C. Calcitonin.** Medullary thyroid carcinomas secrete calcitonin and other peptides. Calcitonin levels are often elevated at time of diagnosis and can be used to aid surveillance after treatment.

10. D. Pheochromocytoma. Medullary thyroid carcinoma is associated with familial syndromes multiple endocrine neoplasia (MEN) 2A and MEN 2B. Pheochromocytomas can co-occur with medullary thyroid carcinoma in patients who have MEN 2A or 2B disease and should be screened for prior to surgery. Patients who have pheochromocytoma will require alpha blockade prior to surgery.

REFERENCES

1. Siegel RL, Miller KD, Fuchs HE, Jemal A. Cancer statistics, 2021. *CA Cancer J Clin*. 2021;71(1):7–33. doi:10.3322/caac.21654
2. American Cancer Society. Thyroid cancer survival rates, by type and stage. Updated March 1, 2022. https://www.cancer.org/cancer/thyroid-cancer/detection-diagnosis-staging/survival-rates.html
3. Mazzaferri EL, Jhiang SM. Long-term impact of initial surgical and medical therapy on papillary and follicular thyroid cancer. *Am J Med*. 1994;97(5):418–428. doi:10.1016/0002-9343(94)90321-2
4. Tuttle RM, Haugen B, Perrier ND. Updated American Joint Committee on Cancer/tumor-node-metastasis staging system for differentiated and anaplastic thyroid cancer (eighth edition): what changed and why? *Thyroid*. 2017;27(6):751–756. doi:10.1089/thy.2017.0102
5. Casara D, Rubello D, Saladini G, et al. Different features of pulmonary metastases in differentiated thyroid cancer: natural history and multivariate statistical analysis of prognostic variables. *J Nucl Med*. 1993;34(10):1626–1631. https://jnm.snmjournals.org/content/34/10/1626
6. Kushchayeva Y, Duh Q-Y, Kebebew E, D'Avanzo A, Clark OH. Comparison of clinical characteristics at diagnosis and during follow-up in 118 patients with Hurthle cell or follicular thyroid cancer. *Am J Surg*. 2008;195(4):457–462. doi:10.1016/j.amjsurg.2007.06.001
7. Haugen BR, Alexander EK, Bible KC, et al. 2015 American Thyroid Association management guidelines for adult patients with thyroid nodules and differentiated thyroid cancer: the American Thyroid Association guidelines task force on thyroid nodules and differentiated thyroid cancer. *Thyroid*. 2016;26(1):1–133. doi:10.1089/thy.2015.0020
8. Naoum GE, Morkos M, Kim B, Arafat W. Novel targeted therapies and immunotherapy for advanced thyroid cancers. *Mol Cancer*. 2018;17(1):51. doi:10.1186/s12943-018-0786-0
9. Smallridge RC, Copland JA. Anaplastic thyroid carcinoma: pathogenesis and emerging therapies. *Clin Oncol (R Coll Radiol)*. 2010;22(6):486–497. doi:10.1016/j.clon.2010.03.013
10. Subbiah V, Kreitman RJ, Wainberg ZA, et al. Dabrafenib and trametinib treatment in patients with locally advanced or metastatic *BRAF* V600-mutant anaplastic thyroid cancer. *J Clin Oncol*. 2018;36(1):7–13. doi:10.1200/JCO.2017.73.6785
11. Drilon A, Laetsch TW, Kummar S, et al. Efficacy of larotrectinib in TRK fusion-positive cancers in adults and children. *N Engl J Med*. 2018;378(8):731–739. doi:10.1056/NEJMoa1714448
12. Doebele RC, Drilon A, Paz-Ares L, et al. Entrectinib in patients with advanced or metastatic *NTRK* fusion-positive solid tumours: integrated analysis of three phase 1-2 trials. *Lancet Oncol*. 2020;21(2):271–282. doi:10.1016/S1470-2045(19)30691-6
13. Subbiah V, Hu MI, Wirth LJ, et al. Pralsetinib for patients with advanced or metastatic RET-altered thyroid cancer (ARROW): a multi-cohort, open-label, registrational, phase 1/2 study. *Lancet Diabetes Endocrinol*. 2021;9(8):491–501. doi:10.1016/S2213-8587(21)00120-0
14. Wirth LJ, Sherman E, Robinson B, et al. Efficacy of selpercatinib in RET-altered thyroid cancers. *N Engl J Med*. 2020;383(9):825–835. doi:10.1056/NEJMoa2005651
15. Smallridge RC, Ain KB, Asa SL, et al. American Thyroid Association guidelines for management of patients with anaplastic thyroid cancer. *Thyroid*. 2012;22(11):1104–1139. doi:doi: 10.1089/thy.2012.0302
16. Wells Jr SA, Robinson BG, Gagel RF, et al. Vandetanib in patients with locally advanced or metastatic medullary thyroid cancer: a randomized, double-blind phase III trial. *J Clin Oncol*. 2012;30(2):134–141. doi:10.1200/JCO.2011.35.5040
17. Elisei R, Schlumberger MJ, Müller SP, et al. Cabozantinib in progressive medullary thyroid cancer. *J Clin Oncol*. 2013;31(29):3639–3646. doi:10.1200/JCO.2012.48.4659
18. Brose MS, Nutting CM, Jarzab B, et al. Sorafenib in radioactive iodine-refractory, locally advanced or metastatic differentiated thyroid cancer: a randomised, double-blind, phase 3 trial. *Lancet*. 2014;384(9940):319–328. doi:10.1016/S0140-6736(14)60421-9
19. Schlumberger M, Tahara M, Wirth LJ, et al. Lenvatinib versus placebo in radioiodine-refractory thyroid cancer. *N Engl J Med*. 2015;372(7):621–630. doi:10.1056/NEJMoa1406470
20. Brose MS, Cabanillas ME, Cohen EE, et al. Vemurafenib in patients with *BRAF*(V600E)-positive metastatic or unresectable papillary thyroid cancer refractory to radioactive iodine: a non-randomised, multicentre, open-label, phase 2 trial. *Lancet Oncol*. 2016;17(9):1272–1282. doi:10.1016/S1470-2045(16)30166-8

21. Falchook GS, Millward M, Hong D, et al. *BRAF* inhibitor dabrafenib in patients with metastatic *BRAF*-mutant thyroid cancer. *Thyroid.* 2015;25(1):71–77. doi:10.1089/thy.2014.0123

22. Shah MH, Wei L, Wirth LJ, et al. Results of randomized phase II trial of dabrafenib versus dabrafenib plus trametinib in *BRAF*-mutated papillary thyroid carcinoma. *J Clin Oncol.* 2017;35(15 suppl):6022. doi:10.1200/JCO.2017.35.15_suppl.6022

23. Brose MS, Robinson B, Sherman SI, et al. Cabozantinib for radioiodine-refractory differentiated thyroid cancer (COSMIC-311): a randomised, double-blind, placebo-controlled, phase 3 trial. *Lancet Oncol.* 2021;22(8):1126–1138. doi:10.1016/S1470-2045(21)00332-6

CHAPTER 3

Non-Small Cell Lung Cancer

Natalie Chen, Cyrus A. Iqbal, Omayra Gonzalez-Pagan, Meera Patel, Daniel Wang, and Quillan Huang

INTRODUCTION

Non-small cell lung cancer (NSCLC) encompasses a heterogeneous array of malignancies of the lungs. In the year 2021, there were nearly 235,000 new cases of lung cancer diagnosed in the United States, making it the second most common malignancy in both male and female patients (behind prostate and breast cancer, respectively). Lung cancer is also overwhelmingly the most lethal malignancy in the United States, with over 130,000 deaths estimated annually.[1] While major advances in systemic therapy have emerged in recent years, including targeted therapies and expanding roles of immunotherapy, the 5-year overall survival for all stages combined is still estimated to be approximately 20%.[1] While tobacco use represents the most prevalent and important risk factor, some 15,000 to 20,000 deaths annually occur in nonsmokers. This highlights the importance of environmental exposures, such as to asbestos, arsenic, and radon. Prior radiation exposure also represents an important risk factor, particularly at a younger age (such as in Hodgkin lymphoma patients).

Tumor histology (for example, squamous vs. nonsquamous, namely adenocarcinoma), resectability, the presence of molecular targets ("driver mutations"), programmed death-ligand 1 (PD-L1) expression (in terms of tumor proportion score [TPS], rather than combined positive score [CPS] as used elsewhere), and a patient's own performance status and baseline state of health are just some of many important factors which guide the management of the patient with NSCLC.

In general, an algorithmic or decision-tree model can neatly guide oncologists and enable optimal management of patients with clearly complex diseases. For example, a proposed model for the management of NSCLC could be approximated by the following series of hierarchical questions:

- Is the cancer resectable? If so, does the patient require adjuvant therapy and what is the role of epidermal growth factor receptor (*EGFR*) mutation analysis and immunotherapy?
- If unresectable, has the cancer metastasized? If not, what are the options for concurrent chemoRT (based on histology) and what is the role for and data underlying immunotherapy maintenance?
- If the cancer has metastasized, which, if any, of the known targetable driver mutations, including mutations in the genes encoding *EGFR* (for example, exon 19 deletion, L858R, or exon 20 insertion), *ALK* rearrangement, *KRAS* (for example, newly G12C), *ROS1* rearrangement, *BRAF* V600E, *NTRK1/2/3* gene fusion, *METex14* skipping, and *RET* rearrangement are present?
- In metastatic disease *without* driver mutations, what is the PD-L1 expression and how does this guide implementation of immunotherapy, with or without chemotherapy (based on histology)?

The cases that follow in this chapter aim to explore each of these branches and clinical scenarios and provide concise but robust discussions regarding the evidence underlying these key clinical decisions.

CASE SUMMARIES

Case 3.1: Early-Stage Resectable Lung Cancer

A 68-year-old male presents after having a low dose screening CT of the chest. He notes a persistent nonproductive cough for the last month. He is a current 1 pack per day smoker with a 30 pack-year smoking history. He is otherwise healthy. On physical exam, lungs were clear to auscultation bilaterally and no palpable lymphadenopathy. He was found to have a 5.6-cm left upper lobe (LUL) lung mass and no enlarged lymph nodes (LNs) on screening CT of the chest.

How Is a Diagnosis Established?

- Complete staging with CT scan of the chest and upper abdomen (including the adrenal glands) with contrast, fluorodeoxyglucose (FDG) PET/CT scan to evaluate for mediastinal involvement and distant metastasis, and MRI brain scan with and without contrast is used to evaluate for intracranial metastasis.
- Tissue biopsy is needed for diagnosis by either percutaneous interventional radiology (IR) guided biopsy of the mass or endobrachial ultrasound (EBUS) with fine needle aspiration (FNA) of the mass and LNs. Assessing the safety of biopsy to minimize complications and feasibility to access the lesion percutaneously or via EBUS should be discussed with the pulmonologist and interventional radiologist.

Patient's Diagnosis

- *Initial screening CT of the chest for smokers showed a 5.6-cm LUL mass with no lymphadenopathy.*
- *FDG PET/CT scan: Hypermetabolic 5.6-cm LUL mass with an standardized uptake value (SUV) of 16.5. Mediastinal and hilar LNs with no increased FDG uptake. No evidence of extrathoracic FDG-avid disease.*
- *MRI brain with and without contrast showed no intracranial metastases.*
- *Percutaneous IR-guided biopsy of the lung mass revealed adenocarcinoma. Immunohistochemistry (IHC) was positive for thyroid transcription factor (TTF)-1 and Napsin A, consistent with lung primary.*

How Is This Tumor Staged?

- Staging was determined according to the American Joint Committee on Cancer (AJCC) eighth edition staging system for NSCLC.
- Tumor is staged based on clinical exam; CT of the chest, abdomen, and pelvis with contrast; and FDG PET/CT scan.
- Pathological mediastinal staging should be strongly considered for primary tumors >1 cm.
- MRI brain should be considered for stage IB or higher tumors.

Patient's Clinical Stage

- *T3: tumor size of 5.6 cm; N0: given no LN involvement; M0: since no distant metastases identified, which correlates with stage IIB.*

- *Pathology after lobectomy and mediastinal LN dissection was consistent with previous biopsy. Mediastinal LNs were negative for malignancy. Surgical margins were negative. Pathological staging was pT3N0.*

What Further Molecular or Genomic Testing Is Required?

- After surgical resection, all newly diagnosed stage IB to IIIA NSCLC patients should have their tumor tested for *EGFR* mutations and PD-L1 with VENTANA (SP263) assay postoperatively for adjuvant therapy selection.[2,3]

Patient's Molecular and Genomic Testing

- *Patient's tumor PD-L1 was less than 1%; however, it was positive for EGFR exon 19 deletion.*

What Are Appropriate Treatment Options?

- If the tumor clinically appears resectable, pulmonary function tests (PFTs) need to be evaluated for the likelihood of adequate cardiopulmonary reserve postoperatively. The forced expiratory volume in 1 second (FEV_1) of 1.5L for lobectomy or 2L for pneumonectomy or values greater than 80% predicted are considered adequate PFTs, which are necessary for moving forward with surgical resection.
- Adjuvant cisplatin and pemetrexed (75 mg/m^2 and 500 mg/m^2) can be given per the Trial to Reduce Cardiovascular Events With Aranesp Therapy (TREAT) study as standard of care for stage IIB of greater (tumors 4 cm or greater or with LN involvement) or high-risk factors for stage IB disease or greater, which includes poorly differentiated tumors, vascular invasion, wedge resection, visceral pleural involvement, or unknown LN status.[4]
- The IMpower010 Phase III trial demonstrated disease-free survival benefit in resected stage II to IIIA NSCLC patients treated with adjuvant atezolizumab (1200 mg every 21 days for 16 cycles or 1 year) after adjuvant platinum-based chemotherapy compared to best supportive care. Of note, the subgroup of patients with a PD-L1 of 1% or more showed the most significant benefit.[3] Adjuvant atezolizumab is not recommended for patients with driver mutations such as EGFR.
- The randomized, Phase III ADAURA trial demonstrated significant disease-free survival benefit for 3 years of adjuvant osimertinib following standard of care platinum-based chemotherapy in resected stage IB to III patients harboring an exon 19del or exon 21 L858R mutation in *EGFR*.[2] Based on this data, the U.S. Food and Drug Administration (FDA) has approved the use of adjuvant osimertinib in resected stage IB to III NSCLC.

Recommended Patient Treatment Plan

- *PFTs for this patient showed an FEV_1 of 1.9L and diffusing capacity (DLCO) of 85%, adequate for a lobectomy.*
- *Surgical resection with lobectomy → cisplatin + pemetrexed for 4 cycles → 3 years of osimertinib.*

What Are the Toxicities Associated With Treatment?

- Cisplatin: peripheral neuropathy, nausea and vomiting, nephrotoxicity, anemia, leukopenia, thrombocytopenia, ototoxicity
- Pemetrexed: fatigue, skin rash, nausea and vomiting, diarrhea, anemia, neutropenia
- Atezolizumab: immune-mediated pneumonitis, colitis, hepatitis, endocrinopathies, dermatologic reaction, and nephritis
- Osimertinib: anemia, leukopenia, lymphocytopenia, neutropenia, thrombocytopenia, nail disease, skin rash, diarrhea, nausea, stomatitis, vomiting, prolonged QT interval

What Are Other Treatment Considerations?

What Is Required for This Patient's Follow-Up and Survivorship?

- Once patients with stage I to II disease treated with surgery with or without adjuvant chemotherapy complete treatment, the patient will be on surveillance and need to present to the oncology clinic for history and physical (H&P) and CT of the chest ± contrast every 6 months for 2 to 3 years, then H&P and a low dose non–contrast-enhanced CT of the chest annually.
- Smoking cessation with counseling and pharmacotherapy should be discussed at every visit if the patient remains an active smoker.
- Patient would need age-appropriate screening for other cancers as well as annual influenza vaccination, herpes zoster vaccination, and pneumococcal vaccination with revaccination as appropriate.

Case 3.2: Locally Advanced Unresectable Lung Cancer

A 60-year-old man with a 25 pack-year smoking history and emphysema presented to the ED with one episode of hemoptysis. Physical exam was notable for decreased breath sounds in the right lower lobe (RLL) and no palpable lymphadenopathy. CT of the chest with contrast showed 2.3 × 2.0 cm soft tissue mass in medial RLL with prominent right hilar LNs.

How Is a Diagnosis Established?

- Imaging and biopsy are required. Refer to Case 3.1 for details.

Patient's Diagnosis

- Patient had CT of the chest and FDG PET/CT demonstrating an FDG avid 2.4-cm mass in the RLL of the lung with an SUV 12.5 and subcarinal LN adjacent to the right mainstem bronchus measuring 1.2 cm with an SUV of 7.5 and no extrathoracic disease. MRI brain was negative for intracranial metastasis.
- EBUS–TBNA (endobronchial ultrasound transbronchial needle aspiration) confirmed the diagnosis of adenocarcinoma of the lung involving subcarinal LN, station VII. IHC positive for TTF-1 and Napsin A.

How Is This Tumor Staged?

- Staging is determined according to the AJCC eighth edition staging system for lung cancer with imaging and biopsies. Refer to Case 3.1 for details.
- T1c: Tumors greater than 2 cm but 3 cm or less. N2; ipsilateral mediastinal or subcarinal LNs.
  - Note: Ipsilateral hilar/lobar LN (stations 10 to 14) are N1, ipsilateral mediastinal LNs (single-digit stations) are N2, and contralateral mediastinal LNs are N3.

Patient's Clinical Stage

- T1cN2M0 (stage IIIA)

Patient's Pathological Stage After Neoadjuvant Chemotherapy

- ypT1cN0M0 (stage IA3)

What Further Molecular or Genomic Testing Is Required?

- All newly diagnosed stage IB to III NSCLC patients should be tested for *EGFR* mutations and PD-L1. Refer to Case 3.1 for details.

Patient's Molecular and Genomic Testing
- *Patient's tumor PD-L1 was less than 1% and negative for EGFR mutations.*

What Are Appropriate Treatment Options?

- All stage III NSCLC patients should be discussed with the multidisciplinary teams to determine the best treatment plan.
- Determination of resectability, type of resection, and adequate cardiopulmonary reserve should be performed by cardiothoracic surgeons. For medically operable disease, oncological resection is the preferred curative local therapy. See Case 3.1 for values of adequate PFTs needed for surgery.
- Disease involving the mediastinal LNs are typically medically inoperable.
- The role of surgery in patients with stage IIIA (N2) disease remains controversial[5] and decisions should be determined after multidisciplinary discussion involving medical oncologists, radiation oncologists, pulmonologists, and cardiothoracic surgeons who are experienced in managing lung cancers.
- National Comprehensive Cancer Network (NCCN) Member Institutions made the following recommendations regarding their approach to patients with N2 disease:[6]
  - Consider surgery in patients with single station N2 LN involved, and non-bulky disease with LNs less than 3 cm.
  - Use EBUS in the initial evaluation of the mediastinum.
  - Consider neoadjuvant therapy.
  - Consider adjuvant radiotherapy (RT) for positive residual N2 disease.
- While active smokers have increased risks of postoperative complications, surgery should not be denied to patients who actively smoke. Smoking cessation counseling should be provided.
- For cases that are medically inoperable including stage IIIB and IIIC, definitive concurrent chemoradiation followed by consolidation immunotherapy with durvalumab is recommended. Durvalumab significantly prolonged both progression-free survival and overall survival among patients with stage III, unresectable NSCLC who did not have disease progression after concurrent chemoradiation compared to placebo in the PACIFIC trial.[7] Patients were enrolled regardless of their PD-L1 expression status. FDA approved durvalumab after concurrent chemoradiation regardless of PD-L1 expression.
- Concurrent chemoradiation therapy is recommended for patients with inoperable stage II and stage III NSCLC. Sequential chemotherapy and radiation therapy or radiation therapy alone can be used for patients who are too frail to tolerate concurrent therapy, in which case accelerated radiation therapy may be beneficial.[8]
- In resectable Stage IB to IIIA NSCLC, the recent CheckMate 816 study found the use of neoadjuvant nivolumab + platinum doublet for 3 cycles had up to 24% of patients with a pathological complete response at the time of surgery. Additionally, the event-free survival was 31.6 months with the addition of immunotherapy to a platinum doublet versus 20.8 months with a platinum doublet alone. The overall survival data is not yet available. In resectable Stage IB to IIIA NSCLC, neoadjuvant nivolumab plus platinum doublet is another option to consider.

Recommended Patient Treatment Plan
- *Case was discussed at tumor board and patient's lung cancer was deemed borderline resectable. Recommendations were made to proceed with cisplatin, pemetrexed, and nivolumab followed by reassessment for surgical resection.[9]*
- *PFTs showed FEV$_1$ of 1.9L with a DLCO of 91% predicted.*
- *Cisplatin, pemetrexed, and nivolumab is used for 3 cycles.*

- *FDG PET/CT done after completion of neoadjuvant therapy showed size reduction in the lower lobe lung mass (now 2.2 cm) and resolution of the subcarinal LN hypermetabolism consistent with treatment response.*
- *Cardiothoracic surgical re-evaluation determined patient would be a candidate for RLL lobectomy with mediastinal LN dissection.*
- *Surgical pathology showed 2.3-cm adenocarcinoma with positive margin and negative LNs (pT1cpN0pM0, stage IA3).*
- *Adjuvant radiation was completed for an R1 resection with a positive margin.*
- *Smoking cessation counseling was provided throughout treatment and patient successfully quit smoking.*

What Are the Toxicities Associated With Chemoradiotherapy?

Radiation therapy damages cell DNA leading to tissue damages in the acute, subacute, and late phase.
- Acute (occur during treatment period and resolve within 1 to 2 weeks after completion): mucositis, esophagitis, and dermatitis
- Subacute (occur 4 weeks to 3 months after treatment completion): pneumonitis
- Late (6 months or longer after treatment completion): fibrosis, fistula, and secondary cancers

The addition of chemotherapy results in increased severity of the toxicities induced by radiation alone.[10]

What Are Other Treatment Considerations?

What Is Required for This Patient's Follow-Up and Survivorship?
- H&P and CT of the chest ± contrast every 3 to 6 months for 3 years, then H&P and CT of the chest ± contrast every 6 months for 2 years, then H&P and a low-dose non–contrast-enhanced CT of the chest annually. If the patient has residual or new radiographic abnormalities, more frequent imaging may be required.
- See Case 3.1 for other survivorship recommendations.

Case 3.3: Metastatic Lung Cancer Without Driver Mutations

A 58-year-old male presents for an evaluation for persistent cough for 3 months. He also reports a 15-pound weight loss during that time. He currently smokes 1 pack per day with a 30 pack-year smoking history. He denies any significant past medical history or use of recreational drugs. He denies occupational exposures. Given his smoking history, a low dose CT of the chest was done which showed a 3.8-cm right upper lobe (RUL) mass, spiculated appearance with a contralateral pulmonary nodule suspicious for metastasis.

How Is a Diagnosis Established?
- Complete staging with MRI brain with contrast and FDG PET/CT scan to confirm distant disease is recommended.
- For patients with clinically suspected metastatic lung cancer, pathological confirmation of metastatic lesion is generally preferred over the suspected primary lesion to confirm the highest stage of disease.
- Distant metastatic sites can by categorized into intrathoracic (M1a: pleura, contralateral lung, and/or pericardium) and extrathoracic disease (M1 b/c: commonly liver, adrenal gland, brain, and bone).
- Based on the site of distant disease, a multidisciplinary discussion should occur to decide on the least invasive biopsy with the highest yield.

- Due to the importance of molecular testing, a core biopsy is preferred over an FNA. Additionally, due to the acid decalcifying solutions used on bone biopsies, a soft tissue lesion may be reasonable to consider.

Patient's Diagnosis

- *MRI brain: negative for intracranial metastasis*
- *FDG PET/CT: abnormal increased FDG metabolism seen in RUL mass with a maximum SUV of 12.5 corresponding to the spiculated mass noted in recent CT. Abnormal increased FDG metabolism noted in nodule in left lower lobe (LLL) with a maximum SUV of 4.5 highly consistent with metastatic disease. Extensive metastatic disease involving the liver (right lobe greater than the left).*
- *A percutaneous image-guided biopsy of the liver was recommended as it was least invasive and would confer the highest stage. The pathology confirms the diagnosis of adenocarcinoma with IHC strongly positive for TTF1 and Napsin A were strongly positive. p63, p40 and CK5/6 were negative.*
- *There can be overlap in the immunophenotype, so in those cases a diagnosis of adenocarcinoma is favored versus squamous cell carcinoma (SCC) based on morphology.*
- *The 2015 World Health Organization (WHO) classification defines adenocarcinoma as carcinoma with an acinar/tubular structure or mucin production with immunohistochemical positivity for TTF-1 (NKX2-1) and/or Napsin A. SCC is diagnosed as a solid carcinoma without keratinization or intercellular bridges with immunohistochemical positivity for p40, CK5/6, and TP63 (p63).[11,12]*

What Further Molecular or Genomic Testing Is Required?

- All newly diagnosed metastatic lung adenocarcinoma must undergo molecular testing, when possible, for *EGFR, ALK, KRAS, ROS1, BRAF, NTRK1/2/3, METex14* skipping, and *RET*. Most commonly this is now done via commercially available next-generation sequencing panels that include all actionable biomarkers. This is in contrast to SCC lung cancer, in which it would be done most likely only in nonsmoker patients, because targetable driver genetic alterations are mostly identified in adenocarcinoma.[12]
- PD-L1 is tested in all types of NSCLC. There are many methods for analyzing PD-L1 expression based on the assay, but they generally rely on measuring expression on tumor cells (for example, TPS), immune cells (IC), or both (for example, CPS).
  - TPS looks at tumor cells only, dividing the number of tumor cells showing partial or complete membrane staining divided by total tumor cell count in the area used to evaluate.[13]
  - CPS is evaluated based on the number of PD-L1–positive cells including tumor, lymphocytes, and macrophages, in relation to total tumor cells, and hence allows the capture of tumor and immune cells in a single read.
- PD-L1–negative tumors are defined as TPS less than 1%, low PD-L1 expression is defined as greater than 1%, and high PD-L1 expression is defined as greater than 50%.[13,14] At this time, PD-L1 expression in NSCLC refers primarily to PD-L1 expression on the tumor cells (that is, TPS or tumor proportion score), unlike in other tumor types.

Patient's Molecular and Genomic Testing

- *PD-L1 TPS is 6%. No biologically relevant molecular targets are present.*

How Is This Tumor Staged?

- T2a: tumor greater than 3 cm but less than 4 cm in greatest dimension
- N3: metastasis in contralateral mediastinal, contralateral hilar, ipsilateral, contralateral scalene, or supraclavicular LN(s)

- M1
  - M1a: separate tumor nodule(s) in a contralateral lobe; tumor with pleural or pericardial nodules or malignant pleural or pericardial effusion
  - M1b: single extrathoracic metastasis in a single organ (including involvement of a single nonregional node)
  - M1c: multiple extrathoracic metastasis in a single organ or multiple organs

Patient's Clinical Stage
- T2a, N3, M1c (Stage IV)

What Are Appropriate Treatment Options?

- Adenocarcinoma
  - No or unknown PD-L1 expression (less than 1%)
    - Pembrolizumab/carboplatin or cisplatin/pemetrexed
      - KEYNOTE-189 median overal survival rate (OS) was 22.0 months in the pembrolizumab-combination group versus 10.7 months in the placebo-combination group.[15,16]
    - Nivolumab plus ipilimumab ± 2 cycles of chemotherapy (pemetrexed/carboplatin or cisplatin)
      - CheckMate-227 showed OS benefit in the nivolumab plus ipilimumab alone cohort over chemotherapy for patients with no PD-L1 expression.[17]
      - CheckMate-9LA showed improved median OS with nivolumab plus ipilimumab and 2 cycles of platinum doublet over standard chemotherapy (PD-L1 less than 1%: 17.7 vs. 9.8 months, PD-L1 greater than 1%: 15.8 vs. 10.9 months).[18]
    - Atezolizumab/carboplatin/paclitaxel/bevacizumab
      - IMpower150 showed statistically significant improvements in OS with atezolizumab versus placebo in combination with chemotherapy and bevacizumab (19.0 vs. 14.9 months).[19,20]
  - Low PD-L1 expression (1% to 49%)
    - Generally prefer chemo-immunotherapy as previously noted but can consider single agent immunotherapy (pembrolizumab from KEYNOTE-042) in cases where chemotherapy may not be tolerated.
  - High PD-L1 expression (greater than 50%)
    - Pembrolizumab monotherapy
      - KEYNOTE-024 showed a median OS of 30 months with pembrolizumab versus 14.2 months with chemotherapy.[21]
    - Atezolizumab monotherapy
      - IMpower110 showed improved OS with atezolizumab compared to chemotherapy (20 vs. 13 months).[22]
    - Cemiplimab monotherapy
      - EMPOWER-Lung 1 showed cemiplimab had improved median OS (not reached vs. 14.2 months).[23]
- SCC
  - No or unknown PD-L1 expression (less than 1%)
    - Pembrolizumab/paclitaxel/carboplatin
      - KEYNOTE-407 showed pembrolizumab plus chemotherapy exhibited improved OS median compared to chemotherapy alone (17.1 vs. 11.6 months).[24]
    - Nivolumab plus ipilimumab with 2 cycles of chemotherapy (paclitaxel/carboplatin).
      - CheckMate-227 showed OS benefit in the nivolumab plus ipilimumab alone cohort over chemotherapy for patients with no PD-L1 expression.[17]

- CheckMate-9LA showed improved median OS with nivolumab plus ipilimumab and 2 cycles of platinum doublet over standard chemotherapy (PD-L1 less than 1%: 17.7 vs. 9.8 months, PD-L1 greater than 1%: 15.8 vs. 10.9 months).[18]
  - o Low PD-L1 expression (1% to 49%)
    - Generally prefer chemo-immunotherapy as previously noted but can consider single agent immunotherapy (pembrolizumab from KEYNOTE-042) in cases where chemotherapy may not be tolerated.
  - o High PD-L1 expression (greater than 50%)
    - Pembrolizumab monotherapy
      - KEYNOTE-024 showed a median OS of 30 months with pembrolizumab versus 14.2 months with chemotherapy.[21]
    - Atezolizumab monotherapy
      - IMpower110 showed improved OS with atezolizumab compared to chemotherapy (20 vs. 13 months).[22]
    - Cemiplimab monotherapy
      - EMPOWER-Lung 1 showed cemiplimab had improved median OS (not reached vs. 14.2 months).[23]

Recommended Patient Treatment Plan

- *Pembrolizumab/carboplatin/pemetrexed as per KEYNOTE-189.*

What Are the Toxicities Associated With Immunotherapy?

- Anti–CTLA-4 antibodies (ipilimumab, tremelimumab), PD-1 (pembrolizumab, nivolumab, cemiplimab), and PD-L1 (atezolizumab) try to overcome the tumor-suppression of T-cell function, which can cause a spectrum of inflammatory side effects, or irAEs.[25]
- Dermatologic toxicity is the most common irAE reported with CTLA-4 or PD-1/PD-L1 blockade (presentation is diverse), GI toxicity (colitis, hepatitis), endocrinopathies (hypothyroidsm or hyperthyroidism, thyroiditis, hypophysitis, primary adrenal insufficiency, insulin-dependent diabetes mellitus), or pulmonary toxicity (pneumonitis). Other rare toxicities include neurological, renal, ocular, or cardiovascular.[25]

Should the Patient Receive Maintenance Therapy?

- Pemetrexed maintenance had been the standard for metastatic lung adenocarcinoma.[26]
- Patient receiving nivolumab showed a median progression-free survival (PFS) of 24.7 months with continuous treatment versus 9.4 months with 1-year fixed-duration treatment.[27]
- 35 cycles/2 years of pembrolizumab showed a significant increase in OS (median 16.9 vs. 8.2 months among those with PD-L1 greater than 50% and 11.8 vs. 8.4 months among those with PD-L1 TPS greater than 1%) in comparison with docetaxel.[28]
- Re-challenging with immune checkpoint inhibitors has also been shown to be effective; five in 11 patients (45%) achieved partial response (PR) or stable disease (SD).[28,29]

Recommended Patient Maintenance Treatment Plan

- *Pemetrexed/pembrolizumab for 35 cycles*

Case 3.4: Metastatic Lung Adenocarcinoma With a Targetable Driver Mutation

A 58-year-old East Asian woman (A.B.) with no prior medical history and, of note, no smoking history presented for evaluation for a subacute cough and generalized fatigue. Physical exam was notable for regular heart rate and rhythm, adequate air movement without crackles or wheezing, and no palpable adenopathy. After initial lack of response to antibiotics and as-needed bronchodilator therapy, she received plain radiographs of her chest with a suspicious RUL mass-like lesion. This was followed up by a CT scan of the chest which revealed a 5.6 ×3.4 cm mass in the RUL as well as enlarged hilar and supraclavicular LNs bilaterally.

How Is a Diagnosis Established?

- Although this patient is relatively asymptomatic and has no tobacco use history, the presence of an RUL lung mass and enlarged locoregional LNs is concerning for malignancy.
- Full staging imaging should be performed, with options (as aforementioned, since Case 3.3 is metastatic disease without a driver mutation) including PET/CT or contrast-enhanced CT scans of the chest and abdomen with or without bone scintigraphy.
- Brain imaging using MRI should be performed to evaluate for intracranial metastatic lesions.
- Biopsy should subsequently be performed on the most easily accessible lesion, with preference given to biopsy of a metastatic site as this could establish both diagnosis and stage. For molecular testing, a soft tissue site (not bone) is preferred, as bone decalcification will make the sample unsuitable for molecular testing.

Patient's Diagnosis

- *FDG PET/CT is performed, disclosing the previously noted intensely FDG-avid RUL lung mass as well as FDG-avid hilar and supraclavicular LNs. Additionally, the right adrenal gland is noted to harbor a 3.2-cm FDG-avid lesion, and the liver is noted to harbor a 2.6-cm FDG-avid lesion. Both the adrenal and hepatic lesions are suspicious for metastases.*
- *MRI of the brain is performed, and is negative for intracranial metastatic lesions.*
- *Percutaneous biopsy of the adrenal lesion reveals findings consistent with metastatic lung adenocarcinoma.*

How Is This Tumor Staged?

- The AJCC eighth edition staging system tumor, lymph node, metastasis (TNM) system is used to stage NSCLC.
- T3 disease is defined as a tumor greater than 5 cm but 7 cm or less in greatest dimension or directly invading any of the following: parietal pleura, chest wall (including superior sulcus tumors), phrenic nerve, parietal pericardium, or separate tumor nodule(s) in the same lobe as the primary.
- N3 disease is defined as metastasis in contralateral mediastinal, contralateral hilar, ipsilateral or contralateral scalene, or supraclavicular LN(s).
- M1c disease is defined as multiple extrathoracic metastases in a single organ or in multiple organs.
  - Note: A malignant pleural effusion is classified as M1a disease and thus should be treated as stage IV disease.

Patient's Clinical Stage

- *T3N3M1c (stage IVB)*

What Further Molecular or Genomic Testing Is Required? Should Treatment Be Initiated Immediately?

- The next step is to obtain next-generation sequencing (NGS) to disclose the presence of actionable biomarkers such as driver mutations and high PD-L1 expression levels. Several commercial labs (for example, Foundation, Tempus) perform this testing as a bundle.
- Note that it is appropriate to await NGS results before treating, as outcomes with targeted therapy are superior to systemic chemo-immunotherapy and this patient is relatively asymptomatic.

Furthermore, as discussed in the text that follows, there can be an increased risk of toxicity, specifically pneumonitis, if anti-PD-L1 agents are given prior to *EGFR* tyrosine kinase inhibitors (TKIs), such as if pembrolizumab were to be administered prior to osimertinib.

Patient's Next-Generation Sequencing Results
- *Positive for EGFR L858R point mutation (exon 21). PD-L1 TPS is 60%.*

What Are Appropriate Treatment Options?

- Synthesizing the available information, this patient has stage IVB *EGFR*-mutated lung adenocarcinoma, specifically with an exon 21 L858R mutation.
- *EGFR* mutations are the most common targetable driver mutations in lung adenocarcinomas, which are comprised predominantly (approximately 90% of cases) by the L858R mutation in exon 21 and the exon 19 deletion.
- *EGFR* TKIs are used to target these mutations (exon 19 deletions and exon 21 L858R); the preferred *EGFR* TKI is osimertinib, a third generation *EGFR* TKI notable for superior ORR and PFS when compared to second and first generation *EGFR* TKIs as well as having good CNS penetration.[30]
- Note: Driver mutation status always trumps PD-L1 expression status when deciding on frontline therapy. *EGFR* mutations are known to upregulate PD-L1 expression, but these patients are insensitive to PD-1/PD-L1 monotherapy.[31]
- Note: For patients who present with symptomatic disease, it may not be feasible to wait 2 to 4 weeks for molecular testing results. In such patients, it is reasonable to start with upfront chemotherapy (for example, carboplatin plus pemetrexed). Immunotherapy should generally be avoided in these situations, since if a patient receives immunotherapy they are at risk for pneumonitis should they subsequently receive osimertinib.[32]

Recommended Patient Treatment Plan
- *Osimertinib 80 mg PO daily*

What Are the Toxicities Associated With Treatment?

- Common (~30% of patients) adverse effects include cutaneous rash, cytopenias (particularly neutropenia), GI toxicities (nausea, vomiting, and diarrhea), and paronychia.
- Cardiac monitoring with left ventricular ejection fraction (LVEF) assessment and periodic QTc monitoring are recommended.

Other Considerations

- For patients harboring a targetable driver mutation with small/asymptomatic brain metastases, consideration should be given for avoidance of up-front whole-brain radiotherapy (WBRT) as many newer-generation targeted therapies have excellent CNS penetration, thus sparing the patient the toxicities of WBRT.
- Table 3.1 characterizes preferred targeted therapies associated with the various targetable driver mutations found in metastatic lung adenocarcinoma.

Case 3.5: Metastatic Non-Small Cell Lung Cancer in the Second Line

The patient received 4 cycles of pembrolizumab/carboplatin/pemetrexed which were well tolerated. Re-staging CT CAP showed response to therapy. He then started maintenance with pemetrexed/pembrolizumab; however, he was noted to have oligometastatic progression of disease as evidenced by a new L4 lesion; RUL mass and liver lesion were smaller in size. Multidisciplinary

Table 3.1 Frontline Targetable Alterations in Metastatic Lung Adenocarcinoma

Target	Details	Drug	CNS Pen?	ORR	mPFS
EGFR, classic	Ex 19 del, ex 21 L858R	osimertinib	Yes	~ 80%	18 months
EGFR, rare point mutations	S768I, L861Q, G719X	afatinib	Yes	60–100%	12–14 months
ALK	rearrangement	alectinib, brigatinib, lorlatinib	Yes	80–85%	26 months
ROS1	rearrangement	entrectinib, crizotinib	Yes (entrec)	~ 70%	16–20 months
BRAF	V600E	dabrafenib/ trametinib	Limited	~ 60%	9–10 months
NTRK	fusion	larotrectinib, entrectinib	Yes	60–80%	12+ months
MET	Exon 14 skip	capmatinib, tepotinib	Yes	70%	12 months
RET	rearrangement	selpercatinib, pralsetinib	Yes	60–80%	12+ months

CNS, central nervous system; mPFS, modified progression-free survival; ORR, objective response rate.

tumor board discussion recommended palliative radiation to the L4 lesion for symptomatic control and continuation of pembrolizumab.

The patient was able to tolerate well 6 months of maintenance therapy with stable disease. However, re-staging scans showed disseminated osseous metastasis and new adrenal mass. Also, an increase in size and number of bilateral pulmonary nodules was noted.

What Are Appropriate Second-Line Treatment Options?

- If feasible, repeat tissue and/or liquid biopsy should be performed upon progression to evaluate for targetable resistance mechanisms.
- For patients without actionable genomic alterations, the treatment is generally sequential use of single-agent chemotherapy. As examples:
  - Docetaxel was shown to be superior to alternative chemotherapy (vinorelbine or ifosfamide) in the TAX 320 study. Of note, prior paclitaxel did not impact the likelihood of response to docetaxel.[33,34]
  - Ramucirumab plus docetaxel improves survival as second-line treatment based on the REVEL study which showed an improved OS from 10.5 months from 9.1 months compared to single agent docetaxel.[35]
  - Single agent gemcitabine is also used as salvage chemotherapy in advanced NSCLC with the main goal to achieve symptom relief.[36] The overall response rate is 18.5%, with a median overall survival of 38 weeks.[37]
  - Single agent abraxane is another option for second-line treatment which is generally well tolerated; the overall response rate is 35.3%, OS is 9 months.[36,37]

1. A 65-year-old male with a 60 pack-year smoking history presents to his physician with worsening cough. CT scan of the thorax reveals a spiculated left upper lobe (LUL) mass, extensive hilar and mediastinal lymphadenopathy, as well as bilateral adrenal masses. Biopsy of the left adrenal mass reveals adenocarcinoma which is CK7+, CK20-, thyroid transcription factor 1-positive (TTF1+) consistent with adenocarcinoma of lung primary. MRI of the brain is negative for intracranial metastases. The patient has an Eastern Cooperative Oncology Group (ECOG) performance status of 0, and aside from his cough he is relatively asymptomatic. Which of the following is true about further molecular testing for this patient?
   A. Testing for molecular driver mutations is important in this patient despite his smoking history, as targetable drivers can occur regardless of tobacco history
   B. Given that he has adenocarcinoma and not squamous cell carcinoma (SCC), he is unlikely to have a targetable driver mutation
   C. Given his extensive smoking history, his programmed death-ligand 1 (PD-L1) expression status outweighs the importance of molecular testing for driver mutations
   D. Given his extensive smoking history, National Comprehensive Cancer Network (NCCN) guidelines recommend only testing for PD-L1 expression status as well as single-gene mutation testing for epidermal growth factor receptor (*EGFR*) and anaplastic lymphoma kinase (*ALK*) mutations

2. A 52-year-old woman with no smoking history presents with a dry cough. CT scan of the chest reveals a 2.4-cm left upper lobe (LUL) mass, but no other sites of disease. PET scan and endobronchial ultrasound (EBUS)-guided sampling of mediastinal lymph nodes (LNs) confirm lack of nodal involvement, and the patient undergoes a lobectomy. Her final pathological stage is pT1cN0 = stage IAC, and she is not felt to have any adverse features such as lymphovascular invasion. She is referred to you for consideration of adjuvant therapy. She has an excellent performance status with no relevant comorbidities. What do you recommend?
   A. 4 cycles of cisplatin/pemetrexed, along with molecular testing for consideration of adjuvant targeted or immune therapy
   B. 4 cycles of carboplatin/paclitaxel, along with molecular testing for consideration of adjuvant targeted or immune therapy
   C. Molecular testing for consideration of adjuvant targeted therapy alone
   D. Programmed death-ligand 1 (PD-L1) expression testing for consideration of adjuvant immunotherapy alone
   E. Observation alone

3. A 69-year-old man with a 30 pack-year smoking history presents with hemoptysis and weight loss. Imaging reveals a 5.1-cm left hilar mass. Endobronchial ultrasound (EBUS)-guided biopsy reveals squamous cell carcinoma (SCC), but all sampled mediastinal nodes are negative. The patient undergoes a left upper lobectomy, with pathology confirming hilar but no mediastinal lymph node (LN) involvement. Molecular testing is performed, revealing programmed death-ligand 1 (PD-L1) tumor proportion score (TPS) of 10%. The patient is referred for consideration of adjuvant therapy. His Eastern Cooperative Oncology Group (ECOG) performance status is 1, but otherwise he has no relevant comorbidities. Which of the following do you recommend?
   A. Observation alone
   B. 4 cycles of cisplatin/docetaxel alone

    C. 4 cycles of cisplatin/gemcitabine, followed by atezolizumab

    D. 4 cycles of carboplatin/paclitaxel, followed by bevacizumab

    E. Either C or D, followed by postoperative radiotherapy (PORT)

4. A 55-year-old woman with no smoking history presents to you with a new diagnosis of metastatic lung adenocarcinoma. PET/CT reveals bilateral pulmonary nodules, extensive bilateral mediastinal lymphadenopathy, bilateral adrenal lesions, and extensive bony involvement. MRI of the brain demonstrates two to three 3-mm lesions suspicious for metastatic involvement; the patient does not have any focal neurological symptoms. She has a good performance status and is relatively asymptomatic. You review her biopsy result which shows adenocarcinoma consistent with lung origin, thyroid transcription factor 1-positive (TTF1+), programmed death-ligand 1 (PD-L1) tumor proportion score (TPS) 70%. What do you recommend?

    A. Initiate therapy with pembrolizumab

    B. Initiate therapy with carboplatin, pemetrexed, pembrolizumab

    C. Continue to hold therapy while ordering molecular testing

    D. Refer for whole brain radiotherapy while ordering molecular testing

5. A 58-year-old man with a 30 pack-year smoking history is reviewed at your tumor board with a new diagnosis of lung adenocarcinoma. His staging PET scan reveals a right lower lobe (RLL) primary tumor as well as hilar, subcarinal, and bilateral paratracheal lymphadenopathy. He has no additional disease in his body, and his MRI of the brain is negative for metastatic disease. Aside from his tobacco use, he has no relevant comorbidities. The pathologist reveals that his programmed death-ligand 1 (PD-L1) tumor proportion score (TPS) is 1%. Which of the following do you recommend?

    A. Neoadjuvant chemoradiation with intent to proceed to surgery if he has a response

    B. Definitive chemoradiation followed by durvalumab consolidation

    C. Definitive chemoradiation alone, given the relatively low PD-L1 expression

    D. Radiation alone, followed by chemotherapy and durvalumab consolidation

6. A 72-year-old woman is referred to you with a new diagnosis of metastatic lung adenocarcinoma. You perform molecular testing which reveals an activating insertion mutation in exon 20 of the epidermal growth factor receptor (*EGFR*) gene. Her programmed death-ligand 1 (PD-L1) tumor proportion score (TPS) is 40%. She has a good performance status without relevant comorbidities. Which of the following do you recommend?

    A. Carboplatin/pemetrexed/pembrolizumab

    B. Pembrolizumab

    C. Osimertinib

    D. Mobocertinib

    E. Amivantamab

ANSWERS AND RATIONALES

1. **A. Testing for molecular driver mutations is important in this patient despite his smoking history, as targetable drivers can occur regardless of tobacco history.** Testing for molecular driver mutations using a broad-based next-generation sequencing (NGS) panel is recommended for all patients with metastatic lung adenocarcinoma regardless of smoking history. Although patients with pure SCC of the lung have a much lower incidence of targetable driver mutations, broad molecular testing should still be considered. PD-L1 expression status is important as well for all patients, although when making front-line treatment decisions the presence of a targetable driver almost always trumps high PD-L1 expression status. The only driver mutations currently approved in the second-line settings are *KRAS* G12C (sotorasib) and *EGFR* exon 20 insertion mutations (mobocertinib and amivantamab).

2. **E. Observation alone.** For stage IA cancers treated with definitive surgery, there is currently no role for adjuvant systemic therapy of any kind. For stage IB and up tumors with a sensitizing epidermal growth factor receptor (*EGFR*) mutation (exon 19 del or exon 21 L858R), the Phase III ADAURA trial demonstrated a significant PFS benefit (hazard ratio [HR] 0.21) with the addition of osimertinib to standard treatment. For stage II to III resected tumors (either 4 cm or node-positive), the standard of care has long been cisplatin-based chemotherapy based on the LACE meta-analysis which demonstrated a 5-year survival benefit of 5.4%. Recently, the IMpower010 Phase III study also demonstrated a PFS benefit for the addition of atezolizumab for stage II to III resected tumors with a PD-L1 tumor proportion score (TPS) of at least 1%, resulting in the approval of atezolizumab for this population.

3. **C. 4 cycles of cisplatin/gemcitabine, followed by atezolizumab.** Given the patient's tumor and nodal stage, he qualifies for adjuvant cisplatin-based chemotherapy. He also qualifies for adjuvant atezolizumab based on his PD-L1 TPS of at least 1%. Although carboplatin can be considered for patients who are cisplatin-ineligible, it cannot be considered as standard of care given the lack of level 1 evidence for benefit of carboplatin in the adjuvant setting (this is in contrast to the metastatic setting, where the toxicities of cisplatin generally outweigh any marginal efficacy benefit it might have). All cisplatin doublets are generally considered acceptable; vinorelbine, docetaxel, or gemcitabine can be considered in squamous patients, while pemetrexed is reserved for adenocarcinomas. There is no role for bevacizumab in the adjuvant setting. PORT is reserved for patients with positive resection margins; its use for those with N2 disease found at surgery has been called into question following the negative LUNG-ART trial.

4. **C. Continue to hold therapy while ordering molecular testing.** In a patient with a high likelihood of an actionable driver mutation, it is critical to wait for full molecular profiling before deciding on therapy. Patients with epidermal growth factor receptor (*EGFR*) mutations can have high PD-L1 expression levels, but despite this generally do not respond well to immunotherapy. Furthermore, if a patient is started on immunotherapy and subsequently is found to have an *EGFR* mutation and is switched to osimertinib, that patient will be at high risk for pneumonitis. Given her small and asymptomatic brain lesions, it is reasonable to wait for driver mutation status, as many small molecule tyrosine kinase inhibitors (TKIs) penetrate the blood-brain barrier well.

5. **B. Definitive chemoradiation followed by durvalumab consolidation.** In patients with mediastinal lymph node involvement, the vast majority should be treated with definitive chemoradiation followed by 1 year of durvalumab consolidation if there is no frank

progression of disease after chemoradiation. The benefit for durvalumab was shown in the Phase 3 PACIFIC trial, which now has 5-year follow-up confirming an approximately 10% absolute benefit in overall survival. Rarely, patients can be considered for surgery preceded by neoadjuvant therapy if they are in excellent shape, have single-station mediastinal node involvement, and do not require a lobectomy; however, there is no universal standard of care and these discussions are often institution-dependent. Durvalumab is approved by the U.S. Food and Drug Administration (FDA) for all patients regardless of PD-L1 expression status, although of note certain subsets (PD-L1–negative, driver-mutation–positive) derived less benefit on unpowered subset analyses.

6. **A. Carboplatin/pemetrexed/pembrolizumab.** Although the U.S. Food and Drug Administration (FDA) recently granted accelerated approval to amivantamab (a bispecific *EGFR*-MET antibody) and mobocertinib (a small-molecule inhibitor of *EGFR* specific for exon 20 insertions), neither therapy is approved in the front-line setting. Pembrolizumab monotherapy would not be the standard of care for a PD-L1 expression level less than 50%. Thus, the standard of care remains combination chemotherapy and immunotherapy based on KEYNOTE-189, with the possibility of using either amivantamab or mobocertinib in the second-line setting. Osimertinib has limited activity against exon 20 insertion mutations and is not FDA-approved for this setting.

REFERENCES

1. Siegel RL, Miller KD, Jemal A. Cancer statistics. *CA Cancer J Clin.* 2021;71(1):7–33. doi:10.3322/caac.21708
2. Wu YL, Tsuboi M, He J, et al. Osimertinib in resected EGFR-mutated non-small-cell lung cancer. *N Engl J Med.* 2020;383(18):1711–1723. doi:10.1056/NEJMoa2027071
3. Felip E, Altorki N, Zhou C, et al. Adjuvant atezolizumab after adjuvant chemotherapy in resected stage IB-IIIA non-small-cell lung cancer (IMpower010): a randomised, multicentre, open-label, phase 3 trial. *Lancet.* 2021;398(10308):1344–1357. doi:10.1016/S0140-6736(21)02098-5
4. Kreuter M, Vansteenkiste J, Fischer JR, et al. Randomized phase 2 trial on refinement of early-stage NSCLC adjuvant chemotherapy with cisplatin and pemetrexed versus cisplatin and vinorelbine: the TREAT study. *Ann Oncol.* 2013;24(4): 986–992. doi:10.1093/annonc/mds578
5. Martins RG, D'Amico TA, Loo BW, et al. The management of patients with stage IIIA non-small cell lung cancer with N2 mediastinal node involvement. *J Natl Compr Canc Netw.* 2012;10(5):599–613. doi:10.6004/jnccn.2012.0062
6. National Comprehensive Cancer Network. *Non-small cell lung cancer (Version 1.2022).* https://www.nccn.org/professionals/physician_gls/pdf/nscl.pdf
7. Antonia SJ, Villegas A, Daniel D, et al. Overall survival with durvalumab after chemoradiotherapy in stage III NSCLC. *N Engl J Med.* 2018;379(24):2342–2350.
8. Baumann M, Herrmann T, Koch R, et al. Final results of the randomized phase III CHARTWEL-trial (ARO 97-1) comparing hyperfractionated-accelerated versus conventionally fractionated radiotherapy in non-small cell lung cancer (NSCLC). *Radiother Oncol.* 2011;100(1):76–85.
9. Forde PM, Spicer J, Lu S, et al. Neoadjuvant nivolumab plus chemotherapy in resectable lung cancer. *N Engl J Med.* 2022;386(21):1973–1985. doi:10.1056/NEJMoa2202170
10. Yazbeck VY, Villaruz L, Haley M, Socinski MA. Management of normal tissue toxicity associated with chemoradiation (primary skin, esophagus, and lung). *Cancer J.* 2013;19(3):231–237.
11. Inamura K. Lung cancer: Understanding its molecular pathology and the 2015 WHO classification. *Front Oncol.* 2017;7:93.
12. Inamura K. Update on immunohistochemistry for the diagnosis of lung cancer. *Cancers (Basel).* 2018;10(3):72. doi:10.3390/cancers10030072.
13. Lantuejoul S, Damotte D, Hofman V, Adam J. Programmed death ligand 1 immunohistochemistry in non-small cell lung carcinoma. *J Thorac Dis.* 2019;11(Suppl 1):S89–S101. doi:10.21037/jtd.2018.12.103
14. Lantuejoul S, Sound-Tsao M, Cooper WA, et al. PD-L1 Testing for lung cancer in 2019: perspective from the IASLC pathology committee. *J Thoracic Oncol.* 2020;15(4):499–519. doi:10.1016/j.jtho.2019.12.107
15. Gandhi L, Rodríguez-Abreu D, Gadgeel S, et al. Pembrolizumab plus chemotherapy in metastatic non-small-cell lung cancer. *N Engl J Med.* 2018;378(22):2078–2092. doi:10.1056/NEJMoa1801005

16. Gadgeel S, Rodríguez-Abreu D, Speranza G, et al. Updated analysis from KEYNOTE-189: pembrolizumab or placebo plus pemetrexed and platinum for previously untreated metastatic nonsquamous non-small-cell lung cancer. *J Clin Oncol.* 2020;38(14):1505–1517. doi:10.1200/JCO.19.03136

17. Hellmann MD, Paz-Ares L, Bernabe Caro R, et al. Nivolumab plus ipilimumab in advanced non-small-cell lung cancer. *N Engl J Med.* 2019;381(21):2020–2031. doi:10.1056/NEJMoa1910231

18. Deng H, Zhou C. From CheckMate 227 to CheckMate 9LA: rethinking the status of chemotherapy in the immunotherapy era-chemo-free or chemo-reform? *Transl Lung Cancer Res.* 2021;10(4):1924–1927. doi:10.21037/tlcr-21-179

19. Socinski MA, Jotte RM, Cappuzzo F, et al. Atezolizumab for first-line treatment of metastatic nonsquamous NSCLC. *N Engl J Med.* 2018;378(24):2288–2301. doi:10.1056/NEJMoa1716948

20. Socinski MA, Nishio M, Jotte RM, et al. IMpower150 final overall survival analyses for atezolizumab plus bevacizumab and chemotherapy in first-line metastatic nonsquamous NSCLC. *J Thoracic Oncol.* 2021;16(11):1909–1924. doi:10.1016/j.jtho.2021.07.009

21. Reck M, Rodríguez-Abreu D, Robinson A, et al. Updated analysis of KEYNOTE-024: pembrolizumab versus platinum-based chemotherapy for advanced non–small-cell lung cancer with PD-L1 tumor proportion score of 50% or greater. *J Clinical Oncol.* 2019;37(7):537–546. doi:10.1200/JCO.18.00149

22. Herbst RS, Giaccone G, de Marinis F, et al. Atezolizumab for first-line treatment of PD-L1-selected patients with NSCLC. *N Engl J Med.* 2020;383(14):1328–1339. doi:10.1056/NEJMoa1917346

23. Sezer A, Kilickap S, Gümüş M, et al. Cemiplimab monotherapy for first-line treatment of advanced non-small-cell lung cancer with PD-L1 of at least 50%: a multicentre, open-label, global, phase 3, randomised, controlled trial. *Lancet.* 2021;397(10274):592–604. doi:10.1016/S0140-6736(21)00228-2

24. Paz-Ares L, Vicente D, Tafreshi A, et al. A randomized, placebo-controlled trial of pembrolizumab plus chemotherapy in patients with metastatic squamous NSCLC: protocol-specified final analysis of KEYNOTE-407. *J Thorac Oncol.* 2020;15(10):1657–1669. doi:10.1016/j.jtho.2020.06.015

25. Kennedy LB, Salama AKS. A review of cancer immunotherapy toxicity. *CA Cancer J Clin.* 2020;70(2):86–104. doi:10.3322/caac.21596

26. Garon EB, Kim JS, Govindan R. Pemetrexed maintenance with or without pembrolizumab in non-squamous non-small cell lung cancer: a cross-trial comparison of KEYNOTE-189 versus PARAMOUNT, PRONOUNCE, and JVBL. *Lung Cancer.* 2021;151:25–29. doi:10.1016/j.lungcan.2020.11.018

27. Waterhouse DM, Garon EB, Chandler J, et al. Continuous versus 1-year fixed-duration nivolumab in previously treated advanced non-small-cell lung cancer: CheckMate 153. *J Clin Oncol.* 2020;38(33):3863–3873. doi:10.1200/JCO.20.00131

28. Herbst RS, Garon EB, Kim D-W, et al. Five year survival update from KEYNOTE-010: pembrolizumab versus docetaxel for previously treated, programmed death-ligand 1-positive advanced NSCLC. *J Thorac Oncol.* 2021;16(10):1718–1732. doi:10.1016/j.jtho.2021.05.001

29. Niki M, Nakaya A, Kurata T, et al. Immune checkpoint inhibitor re-challenge in patients with advanced non-small cell lung cancer. *Oncotarget.* 2018;9(64):32298–32304. doi:10.18632/oncotarget.25949

30. Soria JC, Ohe Y, Vansteenkiste J, et al. Osimertinib in untreated EGFR-mutated advanced non-small-cell lung cancer. *N Engl J Med.* 2018;378(2):113–125. doi:10.1056/NEJMoa1713137

31. Chen N, Fang W, Zhan J, et al. Upregulation of PD-L1 by EGFR activation mediates the immune escape in EGFR-driven NSCLC: implication for optional immune targeted therapy for NSCLC patients with EGFR mutation. *J Thorac Oncol.* 2015;10(6):910–923. doi:10.1097/JTO.0000000000000500

32. Schoenfeld AJ, Arbour KC, Rizvi H, et al. Severe immune-related adverse events are common with sequential PD-(L)1 blockade and osimertinib. *Ann Oncol.* 2019;30(5):839–844. doi:10.1093/annonc/mdz077

33. Wong W, Sun P, Mu Z, Liu J, Yu C, Liu A. Efficacy and safety of nab-paclitaxel as second-line chemotherapy for locally advanced and metastatic non-small cell lung cancer. *Anticancer Res.* 2017;37(8):4687–4691. doi:10.21873/anticanres.11873

34. Fossella FV, DeVore R, Kerr RN, et al. Randomized phase III trial of docetaxel versus vinorelbine or ifosfamide in patients with advanced non-small-cell lung cancer previously treated with platinum-containing chemotherapy regimens. the TAX 320 non-small cell lung cancer study group [published correction appears in *J Clin Oncol.* 2004 January 1;22(1):209]. *J Clin Oncol.* 2000;18(12):2354–2362. doi:10.1200/JCO.2000.18.12.2354

35. Garon EB, Ciuleanu TE, Arrieta O, et al. Ramucirumab plus docetaxel versus placebo plus docetaxel for second-line treatment of stage IV non-small-cell lung cancer after disease progression on platinum-based therapy (REVEL): a multicentre, double-blind, randomised phase 3 trial. *Lancet.* 2014. 384(9944):665–673. doi:10.1016/S0140-6736(14)60845-X

36. Gridelli C, Perrone F, Gallo C, et al. Single-agent gemcitabine as second-line treatment in patients with advanced non small cell lung cancer (NSCLC): a phase II trial. *Anticancer Res.* 1999;19(5C):4535–4538.

37. Cho K-H, Song Y-B, Choi I-S, et al. A phase II study of single-agent gemcitabine as a second-line treatment in advanced non small cell lung cancer. *Jpn J Clin Oncol.* 2006;36(1):50–54. doi:10.1093/jjco/hyi213

CHAPTER 4

Small Cell Lung Cancer

Ebaa Al-Obeidi and Karen Kelly

INTRODUCTION

Lung cancer is the leading cause of cancer deaths for men and women worldwide. In the United States small cell lung cancer (SCLC) accounts for approximately 13% or 30,000 new cases of lung cancer each year.[1,2] It is strongly associated with tobacco smoke with 98% of patients having a smoking history. Not surprisingly, chronic obstructive lung disease is a common comorbidity. Under the microscope, small round blue cells with scant cytoplasm, crush artifact, and a high proliferation rate are observed. The molecular hallmarks of SCLC are inactivation of tumor suppressor genes *RB* and *TP53*.

SCLC has a propensity for early metastases with two-thirds of patients diagnosed with metastatic disease that translates into a poor prognosis. Sites of metastasis are similar to non-small cell lung cancer (NSCLC) and include lymph nodes (LNs), as well as contralateral lung, brain, bone, liver, and adrenal glands. SCLC is also called a high-grade neuroendocrine carcinoma and is associated with multiple paraneoplastic syndromes. Its characteristic rapid doubling time makes it sensitive to chemotherapy. Hence, chemotherapy is the cornerstone of treatment for all patients with SCLC. A platinum-containing doublet, either cisplatin or carboplatin in combination with etoposide, has been the standard of care for decades. Recently, the addition of programmed death-ligand 1 (PD-L1) inhibitors atezolizumab or durvalumab to chemotherapy followed by maintenance immunotherapy improved survival for patients with extensive-stage disease and is considered the treatment of choice.[3-6] Patients with limited stage disease receive thoracic radiotherapy concurrently with chemotherapy and have a small chance to be cured. The addition of immune checkpoint inhibitors to this multimodality regimen is being evaluated. Systemic treatment options for patients who progress or relapse are limited. Two chemotherapy agents, topotecan and lurbinectedin, are approved. Patients are encouraged to participate in clinical trials to improve quality of life and survival.

CASE SUMMARIES

Case 4.1: Newly Diagnosed Extensive-Stage Small Cell Lung Cancer

A 60-year-old woman with a 23 pack-year tobacco use history presented with dyspnea on ambulation and chest heaviness. She was treated empirically with antibiotics for presumed upper respiratory infection. Over the next 2 months her symptoms progressed. She presented to the hospital for progressive dyspnea, hemoptysis, night sweats, anorexia, and a 50-pound unintentional weight loss. Chest x-ray and CT of the chest/upper abdomen showed complete collapse of the right hemithorax due to obstruction of the right mainstem bronchus by a 10-cm mass, extensive mediastinal lymphadenopathy, and suspicious vertebral metastasis at T8 and T11. Bronchoscopy-guided lung biopsy was performed and demonstrated SCLC. MRI of the brain showed no metastatic disease. PET scan showed bone metastases in T8, T11, L2, and the left ischium.

What Is the Clinical Presentation of Small Cell Lung Cancer?

- The clinical presentation of SCLC predominantly includes cough and dyspnea due to the central location of the tumor. Constitutional symptoms of anorexia, weight loss, and weakness frequently accompany respiratory symptoms.
- Superior vena cava (SVC) syndrome occurs in 10% of patients due to SVC obstruction by the tumor itself, thrombi, or lymphadenopathy.[7]
- SCLC is characterized by its ability to metastasize early, resulting in 60% to 70% of patients having metastases in the brain, bone, bone marrow, liver, or adrenal gland at the time of diagnosis.[8]
- Paraneoplastic syndromes can contribute to the presenting symptoms of SCLC such as the syndrome of inappropriate diuretic hormone (SIADH) with resulting euvolemic hypotonic hyponatremia and Cushing's syndrome with hypercortisolism leading to hypertension, hyperglycemia, hypokalemia, muscle wasting, and central obesity. SCLC is the most common malignancy associated with neurological paraneoplastic disorders,[9] which include cerebellar degeneration, retinopathy, and Lambert-Eaton myasthenic syndrome which classically presents with weakness in the lower extremities and is improved with exertion and repeated testing. These neurological manifestations are thought to result from autoantibodies that cross-react with both SCLC cells and the central nervous system or neuromuscular junction.[9]
- Most patients with SCLC are current or former smokers but a small percentage of patients are never smokers.

How Is a Diagnosis Established?

- A diagnosis can be obtained through endobronchial or transbronchial biopsy, CT or ultrasound (US)-guided biopsies, and/or pleural fluid cytology.
- Fine needle aspirates (FNAs) have been the most frequently used procurement method, but with the increasing role for immunotherapy as well as the recent subclassification of SCLC, core biopsies are preferred.

How Is This Tumor Staged?

- In practice, the Veterans Administration (VA) two-stage system is typically used. It divides SCLC into limited-stage disease—localized to one hemithorax and regional LN involvement that can be irradiated in a single radiotherapy field—and extensive-stage disease that includes tumor spread outside of those sites. Cytology-positive pericardial or pleural effusions are considered extensive stage.
- The American Joint Committee on Cancer (AJCC) tumor, lymph node, metastasis (TNM) staging system used for NSCLC has been validated in SCLC. It is recommended that this staging system be used alone or in conjunction with the VA staging system. TNM staging is particularly helpful in identifying the rare patient with resectable disease.
- Due to its ability to metastasize, a full imaging workup is required for staging. This includes a CT of the chest and upper abdomen with contrast and brain imaging via MRI (preferably) or CT with contrast. A PET scan should be considered to prove limited stage disease. Patients with potentially resectable disease and normal mediastinal LNs on imaging (that is, clinical stage I to IIA) require a mediastinoscopy due to the propensity to have microscopic disease that would make them ineligible for a surgical resection. For

extensive-stage patients with a suspicion of bone metastases, a PET scan or bone scan may be indicated.

The Patient's Stage
This patient has extensive-stage SCLC

What Is the Role for Molecular Biomarker Analysis in Treatment Selection for Small Cell Lung Cancer?

- Molecular biomarker testing does not play a role in treatment selection for SCLC.
- Although not frequently tested, *RB1* and *TP53* mutations are the molecular hallmarks of SCLC.[8]

What Is the First-Line Treatment for Extensive-Stage Small Cell Lung Cancer?

- Platinum-based chemotherapy with a PD-L1 inhibitor is the standard of care for first-line treatment of extensive-stage disease. This is based on two trials: IMpower-133 evaluated the addition of atezolizumab, and CASPIAN evaluated the addition of durvalumab. Both agents improved overall survival (OS) when given with platinum agent and etoposide followed by maintenance immunotherapy (see Table 4.1[3,4]).
- Radiation to the chest may be an option for those with a disease response to initial therapy but who still have residual disease confined to the chest. A Phase III study of thoracic radiotherapy in patients with extensive-stage SCLC (ES-SCLC) who had persistent thoracic disease did not meet the primary endpoint of improved OS at 1 year, but a significant difference was observed at 2 years.[10] The role of thoracic radiotherapy in the modern treatment era is unclear and is currently under study.
- The role for prophylactic cranial irradiation versus MRI surveillance is under evaluation and is discussed further in Case 4.3.
- Smoking cessation should be emphasized as it is associated with improved survival, less recurrence, and lower toxicity during radiation therapy such as radiation pneumonitis and infection.[11]

What Are the Toxicities Associated With the Treatment?

- Hematologic toxicity is higher with carboplatin, and nonhematologic toxicity such as nephrotoxicity, neuropathy, and ototoxicity is higher with cisplatin. GI side effects are common with both. In the United States, carboplatin is preferred over cisplatin due to toxicity.
- The most common immunotherapy-related toxicities reported in IMpower-133 and CASPIAN were rash and thyroid disease. Other important checkpoint-inhibitor related toxicities to be aware of include pneumonitis, colitis, hepatitis, and nephritis.
- Tumor lysis syndrome (TLS) is a rare but possible event in SCLC after starting chemotherapy, particularly in patients with bulky disease, preexisting renal dysfunction, elevated lactate dehydrogenase (LDH), or hyperuricemia. Such patients should be started on TLS prophylaxis with frequent lab monitoring at the outset of therapy.

The Patient's Treatment
The patient was started on carboplatin area under the curve (AUC) 5 on day 1 with etoposide 100 mg/m² on days 1 through 3 and atezolizumab 1200 mg on day 1, every 21 days.

What Surveillance Is Recommended?

- In SCLC, relapse is unfortunately typical and expected despite the disease's responsiveness to therapy.

- Re-staging scans with CT of the chest and abdomen, and MRI of the brain, should be performed every 6 weeks (every 2 cycles) for the first 3 months, then every 9 weeks (every 3 cycles) thereafter during maintenance therapy until disease progression.[3,4]

What Is the Prognosis of Extensive-Stage Small Cell Lung Cancer?

- The median survival is 12 to 13 months (Table 4.1[5,6]). Five-year survival data with the addition of PD-L1 inhibitors is premature. Surveillance, Epidemiology, and End Results (SEER) data from 2011 to 2017 reported less than 7% of these patients survived beyond 5 years.[12]

Case 4.2: Relapsed Small Cell Lung Cancer

A 64-year-old woman who is a former smoker with no significant medical history presented with hemoptysis. A CT scan revealed an 8-cm left upper lobe (LUL) lung mass, a moderate pleural effusion, and enlarged LNs in the chest and abdomen. Her lung biopsy showed SCLC. A staging MRI of the brain was negative for metastases. She was diagnosed with ES-SCLC. Carboplatin, etoposide, and atezolizumab were initiated. After 4 cycles, imaging showed partial response and she continued maintenance atezolizumab. Ten months later, her surveillance imaging showed liver lesions. A liver biopsy confirmed small cell carcinoma.

How Frequently Does Small Cell Lung Cancer Relapse?

- Although SCLC is highly responsive to chemotherapy with or without radiotherapy, most patients will relapse within 2 years despite treatment.[8]

How Is Refractory Disease and Relapse Defined?

- Refractory disease is defined as the lack of initial response.
- Resistant relapse is defined as a disease-free interval of less than 3 months from the last day of initial therapy.
- Sensitive relapse is defined as a disease-free interval of greater than 3 months from the last day of initial therapy.
- Response to second-line treatments is associated with the time to relapse: the shorter the disease-free interval, the poorer the response to second-line therapies.

What Are the Treatment Options for Refractory and Relapsed Extensive-Stage Small Cell Lung Cancer?

- If the progression or relapse occurs within 6 months from the last dose of platinum-based doublet plus an anti-PDL-1 inhibitor, the FDA-approved subsequent therapy options are:
  - Topotecan (intravenous or oral) or lurbinectedin. A clinical trial should always be considered.
  - We have no data on the efficacy of these agents in the era of first-line immunotherapy, but the median survival is approximately 5 to 5.7 months.
  - Common adverse events with topotecan are grade 3 to 4 neutropenia, thrombocytopenia, and anemia. Lurbinectedin has less hematologic toxicity and a higher incidence of transaminitis. Both cause GI side effects.
  - Currently there is no consensus regarding whether to continue immunotherapy in patients who were on maintenance immunotherapy at the time of relapse.

- If the relapse occurs greater than 6 months from the last dose of platinum-based doublet plus an anti-PD-L1 inhibitor, the options are:
  - Re-induction with platinum-based doublet therapy if performance status allows. If the patient did not receive immunotherapy with their original induction regimen, it is reasonable to add an immune checkpoint inhibitor (atezolizumab or durvalumab) to the regimen as is recommended in the first-line setting.
  - If the patient is not a candidate for platinum-based doublet therapy, then topotecan, lurbinectedin, or a clinical trial are alternatives.
  - Median OS with any of these treatments is 10 to 12 months.
- For patients with brain metastases at relapse, brain radiation is recommended (whole brain radiation is the standard of care but stereotactic radiosurgery may be considered in selected patients).
- Patients with an Eastern Cooperative Oncology Group (ECOG) performance status of 2 were included in the clinical trials, but consideration for an initial dose reduction or the addition of growth factor support is appropriate for these patients.
- For patients with poor performance status (ECOG 3 to 4) symptom management should be offered including palliative radiation therapy.

The Patient's Treatment

The patient was deemed to have a sensitive relapse, and because greater than 6 months had passed since her last dose of platinum-based doublet therapy, she was treated again with carboplatin and etoposide.

What Is the Duration of Treatment for Relapsed Disease?

- Expert opinion suggests continuation of treatment until disease progression or unacceptable toxicity.

What Response Assessment Is Recommended?

- Evaluation for response to subsequent systemic therapy should occur every 2 to 3 cycles with a contrast-enhanced CT of the chest/abdomen/pelvis and MRI of the brain (if appropriate) to assess all sites of known disease.

Is There Subsequent Therapy If Patients Are Found to Have Recurrent Relapse or Ongoing Progression?

- If the patient has a good performance status, a clinical trial is preferred. Otherwise, treatment options include agents that have shown modest clinical benefit including topotecan (if not already given), lurbinectedin (if not already given), paclitaxel, docetaxel, irinotecan, temozolomide, CAV (cyclophosphamide, doxorubicin, vincristine), oral etoposide, and gemcitabine.

Case 4.3: Limited-Stage Small Cell Lung Cancer and the Role of Prophylactic Cranial Irradiation Versus MRI Brain Surveillance

A 60-year-old woman with a 15 pack-year smoking history presented with left-sided chest pain and was found to have a 6-cm tumor in the LUL with extension to the suprahilar, hilar, and mediastinal regions. Bronchoscopy with biopsy of the mediastinum diagnosed small cell carcinoma.

She underwent staging with a CT of the chest, abdomen, and pelvis with contrast; MRI of the brain with contrast; and PET scan which demonstrated that the tumor burden was limited to the left hemithorax and regional nodes only. A brain MRI was negative. In consultation with radiation oncology, it was confirmed that her entire disease burden could be encompassed in a single tolerable radiation field. Her disease was classified as T3N2M0 (clinical stage IIIb) or limited-stage small cell lung cancer (LS-SCLC).

How Is the Staging of Limited-Stage Small Cell Lung Cancer Different From Extensive-Stage Small Cell Lung Cancer?

- Staging for LS-SCLC is as described in Case 4.1. The important difference between staging for LS-SCLC versus ES-SCLC is the requirement for a PET scan to rule out distant metastases whereas it is optional for patients found to have ES-SCLC on CT scans because it will not change management. A minority of patients with LS-SCLC will have no evidence of hilar or mediastinal LN involvement or metastatic disease that is clinical stage I or IIA disease (N0). For these patients, mediastinal staging is required.

How Is Limited-Stage Small Cell Lung Cancer Treated?

- For patients with clinical stage I to IIA, surgery followed by adjuvant chemotherapy with cisplatin plus etoposide is the standard of care. If the patient has N1 disease at resection, radiation can be considered with chemotherapy or after chemotherapy. If the patient is found to have N2 disease at resection, radiation is recommended either concurrently or sequentially with chemotherapy.
- For patients with clinical stage II to III, concurrent chemotherapy and radiation is the standard of care.
  - Four cycles of cisplatin plus etoposide is first line. If cisplatin is contraindicated (for example, due to renal disease, congestive heart failure [CHF], neuropathy, or hearing loss) then carboplatin can be substituted.
  - Radiation must be started with cycle 1 or cycle 2 of chemotherapy.[13] Several fractionation schedules are used for LS-SCLC, including 60 to 70 Gy in 2 Gy fractions over 6 weeks (a "conventional" fractionation schedule) or 45 Gy in 1.5 Gy fractions twice daily over 3 weeks (an "accelerated" hyperfractionated schedule). The CONVERT trial demonstrated that both approaches have similar outcomes with no statistically significant difference in OS, progression-free survival (PFS), or radiation toxicity such as esophagitis or pneumonitis (Table 4.1[14]).
  - Toxicities associated with cisplatin-etoposide include hematologic (primarily neutropenia), GI (nausea/vomiting), and alopecia. Renal toxicity, neurotoxicity, and ototoxicity from cisplatin should also be monitored.
  - Concurrent administration of radiation is associated with more radiation-related toxicity including myelosuppression, esophagitis, and pneumonitis.
- There is no role for maintenance systemic therapy.
- CT surveillance every 3 months for the first 2 years then every 6 months for year 3, then annually, is recommended.
- The intent of treatment of LS-SCLC is curative, but only a small subset of patients achieves this goal.

The Patient's Treatment
The patient was started on cisplatin 80 mg/m² on day 1 with etoposide 100 mg/m² on days 1 to 3 every 21 days for 4 cycles. Concurrently she received radiation to the left lung and mediastinum. Follow-up scans showed an 80% partial response.

What Is the Prognosis for Limited-Stage Small Cell Lung Cancer?

- Response rates to chemoradiotherapy range from 70% to 90% with a median OS of 25 to 30 months and 5-year OS rates of 31% to 34%.[14]

What Is the Role of Prophylactic Cranial Irradiation Versus MRI Brain Surveillance in Small Cell Lung Cancer?

- The brain is one of the first sites of relapse in SCLC. Due to the morbidity and cognitive decline associated with brain metastases, the role of prophylactic cranial irradiation (PCI) has been studied. Prophylactic cranial irradiation (PCI) consistently demonstrated a decrease in the occurrence of brain metastases but with an increase in neurocognitive toxicity. A drawback of these studies is that they were performed before MRI was available. Studies are underway to determine which patients benefit most from PCI versus MRI surveillance.
- In patients with LS-SCLC, PCI is currently the standard of care. In addition to a decrease in the incidence of brain metastases, a survival benefit was seen among patients with LS-SCLC who have a complete or significant partial response to chemoradiotherapy and received PCI (5.4% increase in survival at 3 years).[15,16]
- In patients with ES-SCLC, there is conflicting data on the survival benefit of PCI. One study found an increase in 1-year survival of 13.8% but did not include baseline brain imaging or MRI surveillance.[17] In contrast, another study with a similar trial design but with the inclusion of baseline brain imaging and surveillance imaging found no difference in survival between patients who received PCI and those who underwent MRI surveillance.[18] It did show a statistically significant decrease in the incidence of brain metastases by 26% at 1 year among patients who underwent PCI.
- Clinical trial enrollment in the study of PCI plus MRI surveillance versus MRI surveillance alone is an available option for patients with both limited stage and extensive-stage disease to definitively answer this question.[19]

The Patient's Course
The patient discussed PCI with radiation oncology and preferred not to proceed and instead opted for MRI surveillance. Four months after completing concurrent chemoradiation, she was found to have a new 1-cm brain metastasis in the cerebellum and underwent gamma knife stereotactic radiosurgery.

Table 4.1 Recent Trials in Small Cell Lung Cancer

| | EXTENSIVE-STAGE SCLC | | | | LIMITED-STAGE SCLC | | |
	IMpower-133 (Horn et al., *NEJM* 2018)[3] (Liu et al., *JCO* 2021)[5]		CASPIAN (Paz-Ares et al., *Lancet* 2019)[4] (Goldman et al., *Lancet Onc* 2021)[6]		CONVERT (Faivre-Finn et al., *Lancet Oncology* 2017)[14]		
	Atezolizumab Group (N = 201)	Placebo Group (N = 202)	Durvalumab Group (N = 268)	Placebo Group (N = 269)		Once-Daily Chemoradiotherapy (N = 273)	Twice-Daily Chemoradiotherapy (N = 274)
OVERALL SURVIVAL							
HR	0.76 (95% CI, 0.60 to 0.95; P = 0.0154)		0.71 (95% CI, 0.60 to 0.86; P = 0.0003)		HR	1.18 (95% CI, 0.95 to 1.45; P = 0.14)	
Median (mos)	12.3	10.3	12.9	10.5	Median (mos)	25	30
12 mos	51.9%	39.0%	52.8%	39.3%	2 yrs	51%	56%
18 mos	34.0%	21.0%	32.0%	24.8%	5 yrs	31%	34%
PROGRESSION-FREE SURVIVAL							
HR	0.77 (95% CI, 0.62 to 0.96; P = 0.02)		0.80 (95% CI, 0.66 to 0.96; P value not reported)		HR	1.12 (95% CI, 0.92 to 1.38; P = 0.26)	
Median (mos)	5.2	4.3	5.1	5.4	Median (mos)	14.3	15.4
12 mos	12.6%	5.4%	17.9%	5.3%			
RESPONSE							
ORR	60.2%	64.4%	68%	58%	ORR	Not reported	Not reported
DoR (mos)	4.2	3.9	5.1	5.1	DoR (mos)	Not reported	Not reported

CI, confidence interval; DoR, duration of response, mos (months); HR, hazard ratio; ORR, objective response rate; SCLC, small cell lung cancer.

1. A 70-year-old woman with chronic kidney disease (CKD), neuropathy from type 2 diabetes, and active tobacco use is found to have extensive-stage (ES) small cell lung cancer (SCLC). Which therapy should she start?
   A. Cisplatin + etoposide
   B. Carboplatin + etoposide
   C. Carboplatin + etoposide + atezolizumab
   D. Cisplatin + etoposide + durvalumab

2. A 65-year-old former smoker presents with dyspnea on exertion and weight loss. He also reports developing progressive hoarseness and edema of the face, neck, and upper extremities. He denies stridor, syncope, or confusion. A CT of the chest with contrast shows extrinsic compression of the superior vena cava (SVC) by a right lung mass. CT of the abdomen shows a left adrenal gland mass suspicious for metastatic disease and MRI of the brain is negative. Biopsy of the lung mass identifies small cell carcinoma. What is the best next step?
   A. Start platinum-based doublet with concurrent chest radiation and prophylactic cranial irradiation (PCI)
   B. Start chest radiation for SVC syndrome along with platinum-based doublet chemotherapy and atezolizumab or durvalumab
   C. Start platinum-based doublet chemotherapy and atezolizumab or durvalumab
   D. Obtain PET scan to complete staging

3. A 49-year-old man with a 40 pack-year smoking history presents with worsening lower extremity weakness, fatigue, dry mouth, and constipation. Imaging did not show spinal cord compression or brain metastases but did identify a right upper lobe (RUL) lung lesion that is biopsied and demonstrates small cell lung cancer (SCLC). Which paraneoplastic syndrome is NOT associated with SCLC?
   A. Hypercalcemia
   B. Syndrome of inappropriate antidiuretic hormone (SIADH)
   C. Cushing's syndrome
   D. Lambert-Eaton syndrome
   E. Myasthenia gravis

4. A 66-year-old woman with a 30 pack-year smoking history presents with extensive-stage small cell lung cancer (ES-SCLC) and is treated with carboplatin + etoposide + atezolizumab. She undergoes 4 cycles followed by atezolizumab maintenance. Nine months later she is found to have new metastatic disease in the brain and liver. Her Eastern Cooperative Oncology Group (ECOG) performance status is 2. What systemic therapy would you offer her?
   A. Lurbinectedin
   B. Topotecan
   C. Carboplatin + etoposide
   D. Switch to durvalumab maintenance

5. A 75-year-old-man with extensive-stage small cell lung cancer (ES-SCLC) completes 4 cycles of carboplatin + etoposide + durvalumab. He continues durvalumab maintenance. Ten months since starting therapy, he calls your clinic to report several days of diarrhea

with four to six episodes per day. He has had no fevers, recent travel, or change in diet and his *Clostridium difficile* stool test is negative. What is the best next step?
A. Refer to the primary care provider (PCP) for gastritis workup
B. Start empiric antibiotics
C. Hold durvalumab
D. Hold durvalumab and start high-dose steroids
E. Switch to lurbinectedin

6. A 62-year-old woman with limited-stage small cell lung cancer (LS-SCLC) has completed 4 cycles of concurrent chemo-radiation with cisplatin + etoposide. Her response assessment scans unfortunately show metastatic disease to the liver. Her Eastern Cooperative Oncology Group (ECOG) performance status is 2. What therapy would you offer her?
A. Topotecan
B. Irinotecan
C. Lurbinectedin
D. Re-induction with platinum-based doublet therapy
E. A or C

7. A 60-year-old former smoker of 45 pack-years presents with a cough. A chest x-ray identifies a mass in the right lung. CT of the chest confirms a 3-cm right middle lobe mass with ipsilateral hilar and mediastinal lymph node (LN) involvement but no left chest involvement or effusions. CT of the abdomen and MRI of the brain are negative for metastases. Her disease is classified as stage IIIA (T1cN2M0). What is the best next step?
A. PET scan to confirm limited-stage disease
B. Mediastinal staging to confirm limited-stage disease
C. Start chemotherapy alone for limited-stage disease
D. Start concurrent chemo-radiation for limited-stage disease

8. A 55-year-old woman with a 40 pack-year smoking history is diagnosed with limited-stage small cell lung cancer (LS-SCLC). She is being started on cisplatin and etoposide. When is the best time to add thoracic radiation and to perform response assessment scans?
A. Add radiation after cycle 4 of chemotherapy and do response scans at that time
B. Add radiation only if residual disease after 4 cycles of chemotherapy and do response scans at that time
C. Start radiation concurrently with chemotherapy and obtain response scans after 4 cycles
D. Start radiation after cycle 1 of chemotherapy and do response scans after every 2 cycles

9. A 52-year-old man with a 20 pack-year smoking history comes to see you after undergoing a bronchoscopy-guided lung biopsy of a 3.5-cm lung tumor in the right chest that shows small cell carcinoma. Staging shows metastases to the ipsilateral mediastinal lymph nodes (LNs), no disease in the contralateral chest, and no distant metastases, and his MRI of the brain is negative. He has normal kidney function and no preexisting neuropathy or hearing issues. What is the best treatment to offer?
A. Lobectomy then adjuvant chemotherapy
B. Sequential chemotherapy with cisplatin + etoposide followed by chest radiation and prophylactic cranial irradiation (PCI)
C. Concurrent chemo-radiation with cisplatin + etoposide and chest radiation administered in daily fractions; no brain radiation due to negative MRI of the brain
D. Concurrent chemo-radiation with carboplatin + etoposide and chest radiation administered in twice daily fractions and PCI
E. Concurrent chemo-radiation with cisplatin + etoposide and chest radiation administered in once OR twice daily fractions followed by PCI

10. A 60-year-old woman with a 25 pack-year smoking history is found to have a 1.2-cm left upper lobe (LUL) lung mass and biopsy shows small cell lung cancer (SCLC). CT scan of the chest shows no contralateral chest metastases. CT of the abdomen and MRI of the brain show no metastatic disease. She undergoes a PET/CT which confirms no other evidence of disease. Mediastinoscopy is performed and all lymph nodes (LNs) examined are negative for cancer. She is deemed to have T1bN0 (stage IA2) limited-stage small cell lung cancer (LS-SCLC). A lobectomy with mediastinal LN dissection is performed and she is found to have N2 disease. What adjuvant treatment should be offered?

A. Radiation alone
B. Chemotherapy alone
C. Chemo-radiation
D. Chemo-radiation followed by prophylactic cranial irradiation (PCI)
E. Observation

ANSWERS AND RATIONALES

1. **C. Carboplatin + etoposide + atezolizumab.** The standard of care for ES-SCLC is platinum-based doublet chemotherapy with the addition of a checkpoint inhibitor—either atezolizumab as in IMpower-133[3,5] or durvalumab as in CASPIAN.[4,6] A meta-analysis showed that for SCLC carboplatin is equivalent to cisplatin for both overall survival (OS) and progression-free survival (PFS).[20] Their toxicity profile differs with more hematologic toxicity seen with carboplatin and nonhematologic toxicity (for example, nephrotoxicity, neuropathy, and ototoxicity) with cisplatin. Given this patient's preexisting kidney disease and neuropathy, a carboplatin-based regimen would be a better option.

2. **C. Start platinum-based doublet chemotherapy and atezolizumab or durvalumab.** This patient has SVC syndrome due to extensive-stage small cell lung cancer (ES-SCLC). His symptoms from the SVC syndrome are moderate and non-life threatening; therefore, the best next step is to treat the underlying SCLC with chemotherapy + anti-programmed death-ligand 1 (PD-L1) agent. In cases of life-threatening symptoms from SVC syndrome such as stridor, respiratory failure, or central nervous system (CNS) symptoms like syncope or confusion, the treatment is endovenous recanalization (if thrombus is present) and SVC stenting. Immediate radiation therapy (RT) is no longer recommended as the response to chemotherapy alone is usually rapid.

3. **A. Hypercalcemia.** Hypercalcemia is found in association with squamous cell lung cancer due to production of the protein parathyroid hormone-related peptide (PTHrP) but is not associated with SCLC. This patient is presenting with Lambert-Eaton myasthenic syndrome, which is one of the most diagnosed paraneoplastic syndromes associated with SCLC.[9] Patients typically demonstrate progressively worsening lower extremity weakness, diminished or absent reflexes, fatigue, and autonomic symptoms like dry mouth and constipation. Myasthenia gravis is also a paraneoplastic syndrome associated with SCLC and thymoma, and symptoms are similar to Lambert-Eaton myasthenic syndrome. SIADH is the most common paraneoplastic syndrome associated with SCLC.

4. **C. Carboplatin + etoposide.** For relapse or progression that occur greater than 6 months from the last dose of platinum-based doublet, re-induction with platinum-based doublet therapy is recommended if performance status allows. If the patient is not a candidate for platinum-based doublet therapy, then topotecan, lurbinectedin, or a clinical trial are alternatives. Patients with brain metastasis should also receive brain radiation.

5. **D. Hold durvalumab and start high-dose steroids.** This patient is presenting with immune-mediated colitis due to durvalumab and should receive high-dose steroids (for example, prednisone/methylprednisolone 1 to 2 mg/kg/day for at least 2 weeks followed by a taper over 6 weeks once symptoms improve). This patient's presentation is consistent with a grade 2 colitis so the durvalumab should be held while the patient receives steroids and could be resumed when symptoms improve to a grade 1. Patients who experience a grade 4 colitis (that is, a colitis that is associated with life-threatening consequences and requires urgent intervention) should have their checkpoint inhibitor permanently discontinued.

6. **E. A or C.** For patients who have progressive disease or relapse within 6 months from the last dose of platinum-based doublet therapy, topotecan (intravenous [IV] or by mouth [PO]), lurbinectedin, or a clinical trial are recommended.

7. **A. PET scan to confirm limited-stage disease.** A PET scan is recommended to prove limited-stage disease prior to starting therapy. Mediastinal staging is only indicated for clinical stage I to IIA as those patients are candidates for surgical resection if no mediastinal metastases are found.

8. **C. Start radiation concurrently with chemotherapy and obtain response scans after 4 cycles.** The standard of care for LS-SCLC is concurrent chemo-radiation. Response assessment by CT of the chest/abdomen/pelvis with contrast should occur after completion of therapy, which is 4 cycles (there is no maintenance systemic therapy). In contrast, for extensive-stage small cell lung cancer (ES-SCLC) thoracic radiation is optional for patients with residual disease confined to the chest, and response assessment by CT of the chest/abdomen/pelvis + MRI of the brain (if applicable) should occur after every 2 cycles for the first 3 months, then after every 3 cycles during maintenance therapy.

9. **E. Concurrent chemo-radiation with cisplatin + etoposide and chest radiation administered in once OR twice daily fractions followed by PCI.** This patient has limited-stage disease (stage IIIA: T2aN2M0), for which cisplatin + etoposide is preferred over carboplatin + etoposide for patients with normal kidney function (whereas for extensive stage either platinum agent is acceptable). Based on the CONVERT trial, there was no significant difference in outcomes for chest radiotherapy with once-daily compared to twice-daily fractions and both are acceptable.[14] PCI is the standard of care for limited-stage disease.

10. **D. Chemo-radiation followed by prophylactic cranial irradiation (PCI).** Early-stage presentation of SCLC is rare; thus, PET scan is recommended for further staging of apparent LS-SCLC to rule out distant metastases. Mediastinoscopy is necessary for clinical stage I to IIA to confirm early stage and candidacy for surgical resection. Surgery followed by adjuvant cisplatin + etoposide is the standard of care for stage I to IIA disease (T1-T2, N0). If the patient is N0 at resection, adjuvant chemotherapy alone is offered. If the patient is N1 at resection, chemo-radiation can be offered (sequential or concurrent). If the patient is N2 at resection (like this patient, who was upstaged after finding positive LNs), chemo-radiation is recommended (sequential or concurrent). PCI is the standard of care for all LS-SCLC. Treatment for limited-stage small cell lung cancer (LS-SCLC) is curative intent, but only a small subset of patients achieves this goal.

REFERENCES

1. Govindan R, Page N, Morgensztern D, et al. Changing epidemiology of small-cell lung cancer in the United States over the last 30 years: analysis of the surveillance, epidemiologic, and end results database. *J Clin Oncol.* 2006;24(28):4539–4544. doi:10.1200/JCO.2005.04.4859

2. Siegel RL, Miller KD, Fuchs HE, Jemal A. Cancer statistics, 2022. *CA Cancer J Clin.* 2022;72(1):7–33. doi:10.3322/CAAC.21708

3. Horn L, Mansfield AS, Szczęsna A, et al. First-line atezolizumab plus chemotherapy in extensive-stage small-cell lung cancer. *N Engl J Med.* 2018;379(23):2220–2229. doi:10.1056/NEJMOA1809064

4. Paz-Ares L, Dvorkin M, Chen Y, et al. Durvalumab plus platinum-etoposide versus platinum-etoposide in first-line treatment of extensive-stage small-cell lung cancer (CASPIAN): a randomised, controlled, open-label, phase 3 trial. *Lancet (London, England).* 2019;394(10212):1929–1939. doi:10.1016/S0140-6736(19)32222-6

5. Liu SV, Reck M, Mansfield AS, et al. Updated overall survival and PD-L1 subgroup analysis of patients with extensive-stage small-cell lung cancer treated with atezolizumab, carboplatin, and etoposide (IMpower133). *J Clin Oncol.* 2021;39(6):619–630. doi:10.1200/JCO.20.01055

6. Goldman JW, Dvorkin M, Chen Y, et al. Durvalumab, with or without tremelimumab, plus platinum–etoposide versus platinum–etoposide alone in first-line treatment of extensive-stage small-cell lung cancer (CASPIAN): updated results from a randomised, controlled, open-label, phase 3 trial. *Lancet Oncol.* 2021;22(1):51–65. doi:10.1016/S1470-2045(20)30539-8

7. Lepper PM, Ott SR, Hoppe H, et al. Superior vena cava syndrome in thoracic malignancies. *Respir Care.* 2011;56(5):653–666. doi:10.4187/RESPCARE.00947

8. Rudin CM, Brambilla E, Faivre-Finn C, Sage J. Small-cell lung cancer. *Nat Rev Dis Prim.* 2021;7:3. doi:10.1038/S41572-020-00235-0

9. Soomro Z, Youssef M, Yust-Katz S, Jalali A, Patel AJ, Mandel J. Paraneoplastic syndromes in small cell lung cancer. *J Thorac Dis.* 2020;12(10):6253. doi:10.21037/JTD.2020.03.88

10. Slotman BJ, van Tinteren H, Praag JO, et al. Use of thoracic radiotherapy for extensive stage small-cell lung cancer: a phase 3 randomised controlled trial. *Lancet.* 2015;385(9962):36–42. doi:10.1016/S0140-6736(14)61085-0

11. Andreas S, Rittmeyer A, Hinterthaner M, Huber RM. Smoking cessation in lung cancer—achievable and effective. *Dtsch Arztebl Int.* 2013;110(43):719–724. doi:10.3238/arztebl.2013.0719

12. Surveillance, Epidemiology, and End Results Program. Cancer stat facts: lung and bronchus cancer. National Cancer Institute. Accessed January 26, 2022. https://seer.cancer.gov/statfacts/html/lungb.html

13. Takada M, Fukuoka M, Kawahara M, et al. Phase III study of concurrent versus sequential thoracic radiotherapy in combination with cisplatin and etoposide for limited-stage small-cell lung cancer: results of the Japan Clinical Oncology Group Study 9104. *J Clin Oncol.* 2002;20(14):3054–3060, doi:10.1200/JCO.2002.12.071

14. Faivre-Finn C, Snee M, Ashcroft L, et al. Concurrent once-daily versus twice-daily chemoradiotherapy in patients with limited-stage small-cell lung cancer (CONVERT): an open-label, phase 3, randomised, superiority trial. *Lancet Oncol.* 2017;18(8):1116–1125. doi:10.1016/S1470-2045(17)30318-2

15. Aupérin A, Arriagada R, Pignon JP, et al. Prophylactic cranial irradiation for patients with small-cell lung cancer in complete remission. *N Engl J Med.* 1999;341(7):476–484. doi:10.1056/NEJM199908123410703

16. Meert AP, Paesmans M, Berghmans T, et al. Prophylactic cranial irradiation in small cell lung cancer: a systematic review of the literature with meta-analysis. *BMC Cancer* 2001;1:5. doi:10.1186/1471-2407-1-5

17. Slotman B, Faivre-Finn C, Kramer G, et al. Prophylactic cranial irradiation in extensive small-cell lung cancer. *N Engl J Med.* 2007;357(7):664–672, doi:10.1056/NEJMOA071780

18. Takahashi T, Yamanaka T, Seto T, et al. Prophylactic cranial irradiation versus observation in patients with extensive-disease small-cell lung cancer: a multicentre, randomised, open-label, phase 3 trial. *Lancet Oncol.* 2017;18(5):663–671. doi:10.1016/S1470-2045(17)30230-9

19. SWOG S1827 (MAVERICK) testing whether the use of brain scans alone instead of brain scans plus preventive brain radiation affects lifespan in patients with small cell lung cancer. ClinicalTrials.gov Identifier: NCT04155034. Updated December 7, 2021. https://clinicaltrials.gov/ct2/show/NCT04155034

20. Rossi A, Di Maio M, Chiodini P, et al. Carboplatin- or cisplatin-based chemotherapy in first-line treatment of small-cell lung cancer: the COCIS meta-analysis of individual patient data. *J Clin Oncol.* 2012;30(14):1692–1698. doi:10.1200/JCO.2011.40.4905

CHAPTER 5

Hormone Receptor-Positive Breast Cancer

Katherine Sanchez, Jennifer Collins, Sudha Yarlagadda, Jingxin Sun, Sarah Premji, Maryam Nemati Shafaee, and Julie Nangia

INTRODUCTION

Breast cancer (BC) is the most common cancer in women. In fact, one in eight women will be diagnosed with BC in their lifetime. The majority (70%) of BCs are hormone receptor-positive (HR+), expressing estrogen receptors (ERs) and/or progesterone receptors (PRs). HR+ BC has been the prototype for chemo-sparing therapies in oncology, and endocrine therapies (ETs) which were approved decades ago have remained the backbone of therapy. The mainstay of treating HR+ BCs are anti-estrogen therapies: selective ER modulators, aromatase inhibitors (AIs), and/or selective ER degraders. Studying the mechanisms of resistance in HR+ BC has led to the development of new classes of therapies targeting the downstream molecules of the ER, cyclin-dependent kinase (CDK) 4/6 inhibitors, and other pathways such as PI3K, AKT, and mTOR inhibitors. These next-generation therapies are currently used in the metastatic setting where they improve quality of life, enhance overall survival (OS), and delay initiation of chemotherapy. Use of these combination therapies are also being studied in early-stage disease in patients with disease features associated with high risk for relapse. Ongoing research evaluating potential biomarkers and mechanisms of resistance is anticipated to continue to improve outcomes for patients with HR+ metastatic BC. While BC patients have multiple treatment options that provide favorable outcomes, there are many nuances to treatment in both the neoadjuvant, adjuvant, and the metastatic settings. We have selected five HR+ BC cases to demonstrate how therapy can be personalized.

CASE SUMMARIES

Case 5.1: Early-Stage Breast Cancer

A 46-year-old Caucasian, premenopausal woman presents to an oncologist after being diagnosed with right-sided BC. The mass was found on a screening mammogram. Mammogram and ultrasound showed a 3.1-cm spiculated mass associated with calcifications at 3 o'clock, 6 cm from the nipple. A 0.7-cm axillary lymph node (LN) was biopsied and revealed to be negative for metastatic BC. The biopsy also revealed invasive ductal carcinoma (IDC). The patient is coming to the clinic for an initial visit with oncology.

How Is a Diagnosis Established?

Screening
- Most BCs are diagnosed because of an abnormal finding on screening mammogram.
- Screening guidelines are based on an individual's BC risk. Though guidelines vary, for a woman with average risk annual screening mammograms are recommended starting at age 40 to 50. While there is some debate about screening those over 70 years of age, mammograms should be continued if a woman is in good health and has a life expectancy of more than 5 to 7 years.

Workup
- Breast core biopsies should be considered for all palpable masses and any mass suspicious on imaging.
- Early-stage (stage I or II) disease does not require further imaging for staging. Stage III disease or patients with biopsy proven or clinically suspicious LNs should have a staging CT scan in combination with a bone scan or whole body PET.
- If someone with early-stage BC has clinical concern for metastatic disease, such as bone pain or weight loss, imaging should be performed.
- Genetic testing should be considered if patients meet criteria

What Are the Subtypes of Breast Cancer?

- BC can be divided into different subtypes based on histology, predictive markers, and molecular features. All BCs arise from the terminal duct lobular units.
- The two main histological subtypes are ductal and lobular carcinoma:
  ○ IDC is more common, accounting for ~80% of invasive cancer. It presents clinically with a mass and most commonly metastasizes through the lymphatics and blood.
  ○ Invasive lobular cancer (ILC) accounts for ~20% of invasive cancer. These cancers are nearly always HR+ and respond to ET. They clinically present in a later stage, often without a mass, and metastasize to visceral organs.
- There are three predictive biomarkers performed routinely to make treatment choices (ER, PR, and human epidermal growth factor receptor 2 [HER2]).
  ○ The ER is expressed on both carcinoma in situ and invasive cells. It is an immuno-histochemistry (IHC) test and is scored with the Allred scale. This scale combines intensity of staining and a proportion of tumor cells positive (total score 1 to 8), which is calculated by adding the proportion score of 1 to 5 (% of cells positive) + intensity score of 1 to 3 (weak, moderate, strong). Even patients with 1% of ER staining have been shown to benefit from ET.
  ○ The PR is expressed on both in situ and invasive cells. This IHC test is also scored on the Allred scale (score 1 to 2 negative, 3 to 10 positive). This biomarker commonly decreases and can become negative with ET.
  ○ HER2 is an oncogene which can be amplified and overexpressed in a subset of BCs. HER2 testing is performed with combination testing of IHC and fluorescent in situ hybridization (FISH). The IHC tests HER2 receptor, and low or high (IHC 1+ or 3+) expression has been clinically validated to correspond to the level of gene amplification. If the IHC testing is equivocal (IHC 2+), FISH testing is required to predict response to HER2-directed therapies.
- There are four molecular subtypes currently recognized, though this will likely change.
  1. Luminal A is a low-grade tumor with high estrogen receptor-positive (ER+), high progesterone receptor-positive (PR+), and HER2- expression.
  2. Luminal B is a moderate- to high-grade tumor with moderate to high ER+, moderate to low PR+, and HER2 +/- expression.
  3. HER2+ is a moderate- to high-grade tumor with negative low ER+, negative low PR+, and high HER2 expression.

4. Triple-negative breast cancer (TNBC) is a high-grade cancer with negative expression of ER, PR, and HER2 predictive biomarkers. This subtype will likely be further categorized beyond being negative for other markers as the clinical use multi-omics expands (Figure 5.1).

Patient's Diagnosis

- *Breast core biopsy showed IDC, grade 2. Biomarker analysis resulted in ER+ (8/8, 100%), PR+ (7/8, 95%), and HER2-negative (IHC2+, reflex FISH-negative, HER2 ratio 1.9), Ki-67 17% (High greater than 20%).*

What Other Biomarkers Are Important in Hormone Receptor-Positive Breast Cancer?

- Ki-67 is a proliferation marker classified in many tumor types. In BC, Ki-67 can clinically distinguish molecular subtypes (Ki-67 luminal A less than luminal B, TNBC usually high Ki-67) and is predictive of relapse and progression-free survival (PFS).[1,2]

How Is Breast Cancer Staged?

- The American Joint Committee on Cancer (AJCC) eighth edition staging system is used to stage BCs. This is a tumor, lymph node, metastasis (TNM) staging system. There is also a predictive staging system which also includes predictive biomarkers.[3]
  - Stage 0 is preinvasive cancer of both histologies (ductal carcinoma in situ [DCIS] and lobular carcinoma in situ) of any size. This can't involve any LNs, skin, or metastasizes.
  - Stage 1 is a small tumor (less than 2 cm) with negative axillary LNs (micro metastasis is permitted). The 5-year relative survival is 100%.
  - Stage 2 BCs are moderately sized (less than 5 cm with negative LNs or 5 cm or greater with movable axillary LNs).
  - Stage 3 BCs are larger (5 cm or greater) and/or have matted LNs or other non-local LNs (internal mammary). The 5-year relative survival is 72%.
  - Stage 4 cancers are metastatic. The 5-year relative survival is ~22%.

Patient's Clinical Stage

- *By the AJCC eighth edition staging system, the patient has T2N0 or stage.*
- *The patient denied bone pain or weight loss. Staging was not performed with early-stage disease.*

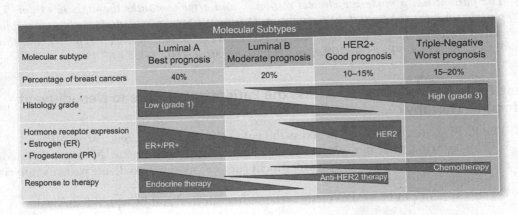

	Molecular Subtypes			
Molecular subtype	Luminal A Best prognosis	Luminal B Moderate prognosis	HER2+ Good prognosis	Triple-Negative Worst prognosis
Percentage of breast cancers	40%	20%	10–15%	15–20%
Histology grade	Low (grade 1)			High (grade 3)
Hormone receptor expression • Estrogen (ER) • Progesterone (PR)	ER+/PR+		HER2	
Response to therapy	Endocrine therapy		Anti-HER2 therapy	Chemotherapy

Figure 5.1 Four recognized molecular subtypes of breast cancer

What Treatment Should You Offer a Premenopausal Woman With Early-Stage Breast Cancer?

- Neoadjuvant chemotherapy (NAC) should be considered for patients with locally advanced cancer and/or large tumors. However, it is recognized that ER+ BCs respond poorly to NAC.[4]
- It is debated whether BC outcomes in premenopausal women are improved by the NAC or by the ovarian suppression caused by chemotherapy.
- Neoadjuvant endocrine therapy (NET) can be used to both facilitate down-staging of the tumor and increase rates of breast-conserving surgery. Additionally, the treatment response of ET can be assessed by comparing biomarkers in biopsy and surgery specimens.
- The preoperative endocrine prognostic index (PEPI) score compares clinical features (tumor size, nodal status) and biomarkers (Ki-67 and ER) between biopsy and post-NET treatment at surgery. This scoring system allows for a prediction of relapse risk and can highlight patients for escalated therapy, who's cancer had a poor response to NET.
- In postmenopausal females, NET is associated with similar response rates to NAC for breast-conserving surgery.[5]
- Despite ER+ BC being the most common subtype, there are few clinical guidelines for NET, including which ET agent to use and optimal duration of use. Randomized controlled trials have shown that AIs are an NET more effective than tamoxifen.[6] A meta-analysis supports a clinical guideline for AIs greater than 6 months.[7]
- While data is limited for NET in premenopausal women, it is a feasible neoadjuvant treatment for women with small tumors and negative LNs, in which you would omit NAC.
- One main benefit of NET with ovarian suppression in this population is to measure clinical response and Ki-67 in vivo. Escalated therapy may be selected for those "high risk" patients who don't have a significant drop in Ki-67 or reduction in size of their tumor (Table 5.1).

Patient's Treatment

- *The patient is seen by surgery who recommends partial mastectomy (lumpectomy). She is small breasted and NET should be considered as it can lead to improved cosmesis of the lumpectomy.*
- *After discussion with the surgery team and the patient, NET with letrozole 2.5 mg daily and ovarian suppression with goserelin 3.6 mg subcutaneously (SQ) monthly (q3 month dosing isn't as effective in suppressing ovarian function as q28 days in BC) is started.*
- *The patient has a moderate clinical response, and after 6 months the mass is ~1 cm. The patient undergoes a partial mastectomy and sentinel LN biopsy. Pathology showed residual disease with the largest area of invasive cancer 0.6 cm. Biomarkers were repeated and show ER+ (7/8, 80%), PR+ (3/8, 20%), and HER2-negative (IHC 1+), Ki-67 1%.*

What Tools Are Available to Access the Patient's Response to Neoadjuvant Endocrine Therapy?

- The PEPI score can be used to access the patient's risk for recurrence after NET.
  - This scoring system ranks pathological T stage, pathological N stage, ER score (Allred), and Ki-67 on the posttreatment surgical specimen to divide patients into risk groups.
  - This system can be used to predict relapse-free survival and BC-specific survival.

Table 5.1 Classes of Endocrine Therapy

Classes of Endocrine Therapy	Endocrine Agents	Mechanism of Action	Common Adverse Events
Selective estrogen receptor modulators (SERM)	Tamoxifen	– Competes with estrogen for binding of the ER – Partial estrogen agonist on other organs (uterus, bone)	– Hot flashes – Vaginal dryness – Low libido – ~1% chance per year of ovarian cancer – ~1% increase in risk for DVT in first 2 years
Aromatase inhibitors (AI)	Nonsteroidal AIs: Anastrozole – Letrozole Steroidal AI: – Exemestane	Inhibits aromatase, the enzyme that converts androgens to estrogen	– Vaginal dryness – Hot flashes – Joint pains – Fatigue – 2- to 4-fold increase in osteoporosis
Selective estrogen receptor degrader (SERD)	Fulvestrant	– Competes with estrogen for binding of the ER – Inactivated and leads to destruction of ER	– Mild menopause symptoms – Pain at the injection sites
Chemotherapy** **Not endocrine therapy, but affects hormone production	Multiple chemotherapy agents	Suppress ovaries and decrease levels of estrogen and progesterone	– Nausea/vomiting – Neutropenia – Alopecia – Fatigue

DVT, deep vein thrombosis; ER, estrogen receptor.

Patient's Preoperative Endocrine Prognostic Index Score

- *The patient's score is low because the posttreatment residual disease was small, LNs were negative for metastasis, the ER was highly expressed, and the Ki-67 score dropped in response to treatment. The patient had a favorable response to NET (PEPI score 0). Favorable response to NET is reassuring for continuation of adjuvant ET alone. If the PEPI score had been high, this patient may benefit from escalated therapy such as chemotherapy.*

What Treatment Should the Patient Receive After Surgery?

- Per National Comprehensive Cancer Network (NCCN) guidelines, if the patient has high-risk disease (positive LNs, high Ki-67, or grade 3 histology), adjuvant chemotherapy could be considered.
- A gene panel (21-gene oncotype) can be used to determine if the patient would benefit from adjuvant chemotherapy.[8] This test is performed on the diagnosis biopsy and will not be affected by any NET.

Case 5.2: Early-Stage Hormone-Positive Breast Cancer

A 58-year-old postmenopausal female was diagnosed with a small 0.4-cm left-sided BC 2 months ago. Pathology revealed IDC, grade 1/3, ER+ 8/8, PR+ 7/8, HER2- (IHC 1+), and Ki-67 of 10%.

She saw breast surgery, underwent a lumpectomy, and has been referred for radiation therapy. She presents for her initial visit with a breast oncologist to discuss adjuvant therapy to prevent recurrence of BC.

Invasive Ductal Carcinoma

- IDC is the most common histology of BC, compromising 80% of BCs. IDC often starts as DCIS when contained in the terminal milk duct lobular unit. When it invades beyond the basement membrane, it is considered malignant.[9]

Staging and Prognosis of Early Breast Cancer?

- Small tumors without LN involvement or distant metastasis have excellent prognosis.
- Other factors that affect prognosis include the expression of hormone receptors. The presence of hormone receptors are indicative of more differentiated tumors that may respond to ET.
- Low-grade tumors and low Ki-67 (less than 20%) also predict a luminal A molecular subtype, which carries a better prognosis and responds better to ET.

Treatment of Early-Stage Breast Cancer?

- Most early-stage (T1-2, N0) HR+ BCs are treated initially with upfront surgery and then radiation for curative intent. Most patients with early-stage BC undergo breast-conserving surgery with lumpectomy, but some patients may have mastectomy depending on tumor size, surgical margins, genetic risks, and patient preference. Radiation to the whole breast or partial breast typically follows, which decreases the risk of local recurrence.[10]

What Treatment Is Given After Surgery in Patients With Early-Stage Hormone Receptor-Positive Breast Cancer?

- Patients with early-stage HR+ BC should be offered adjuvant ET, which lowers the risk of distance recurrence and/or a second cancer. Patients should be offered 5 to 10 years of adjuvant ET based on high-risk disease and age. Anti-estrogen therapy should include 5 to 10 years of tamoxifen or 5 to 10 years of an AI (anastrozole, exemestane, or letrozole).[6] Both SERMs and AI have been shown to reduce the risk of contralateral BC. In premenopausal females, AI must be combined with OS.
- In patients who have very small tumors (0.5 cm or smaller), adjuvant ET is optional but may be prescribed for chemoprevention of a second cancer.
- Tamoxifen is better tolerated as it has fewer menopause side effects and less arthritis. Studies which have evaluated tamoxifen versus AI have shown that with better tolerance, adherence to tamoxifen is better.[11,12]

Patient's Adjuvant Treatment Recommendations
- *This patient is offered adjuvant ET with tamoxifen. If well tolerated, tamoxifen should be recommended for 5 years in this patient with stage 1 BC.*

Are There Adverse Effects Associated With Selective Estrogen Receptor Modulators? And What Are the Adverse Effects With Aromatase Inhibitors?

- All ETs can cause menopause symptoms including hot flashes, vaginal dryness, night sweats, and sexual dysfunction.

- Tamoxifen has two rare side effects that patients should be counseled about. First, tamoxifen carries an increased risk of venous thromboembolic events. Second, there is an increased risk of endometrial cancer, and all women should be referred to gynecology if they experience abnormal uterine bleeding.
- AIs have the unique side effects of increased risk of osteoporosis. Arthritis is a common side effect.[13]

When Do You Choose Between Selective Estrogen Receptor Modulators and Aromatase Inhibitors?

- Tamoxifen acts as a selective modulator to the ER; it blocks estrogen in the breast and acts as an agonist in other tissues (bone and uterus). It is effective in both pre- and post-menopausal women.
- In recent years, AIs have been recommended more often following their U.S. Food and Drug Administration (FDA) approval, which showed a slight advantage at 5 years in post-menopausal females. While these studies showed slight clinical benefit, they have more side effects and adherence is worse. One strategy in high-risk patients, who may benefit from 10 years of therapy, is to switch from AI to tamoxifen after 5 years, which was shown to be equally effective as 10 years of AI.
- Tamoxifen should be recommended when patients can't tolerate the side effects of AIs or have low-risk disease (because in this setting ET is primarily for chemoprevention of a second cancer). Another possible benefit of tamoxifen is a slight advantage in prevention of contralateral BC.[14]
- A recent meta-analysis, published in 2021, concluded that AI and tamoxifen had equal OS, and suggested that tamoxifen is being underutilized. This meta-analysis included four Phase III multi-center, international, randomized clinical trials comparing third-generation AIs with tamoxifen in postmenopausal females with advanced HR+ BC. They showed that AIs were associated with increased PFS, although there was no change in OS.[15]

Recommended Treatment Plan for This Patient
- *This patient is postmenopausal and has stage 1 BC. In this setting, adjuvant ET with tamoxifen was recommended.*

Case 5.3: Locally Advanced Breast Cancer

A 37-year-old healthy female presents for evaluation of a growing palpable right breast mass. Two months ago she noticed a firm nodule in her right breast while showering. She denies nipple discharge, skin changes, or any changes in her menstruation cycle. She denies any nodules or changes in the left breast. Her family history is notable for endometrial cancer in maternal grandmother, diagnosed in her seventies. She has one son and one daughter, ages 12 and 10. She breastfed both children for at least 6 months. Physical examination is remarkable for a right breast mass in the upper outer quadrant measuring 5 x 4 cm associated with palpable LNs in the right axilla. Right breast mammogram identified a solid mass of 5.5 cm x 4.5 cm at 10 o'clock about 3 cm away from the nipple.

How Is This Diagnosis Established: Patient's Workup and Staging
- *Patient underwent ultrasound guided biopsy of the right breast mass and axillary LNs. Pathology confirmed IDC, grade 3/3, ER+ (6/8), PR- (0/8), HER2- (IHC 0), and Ki-67 75%.*
- *Bilateral breast MRI is negative for multifocal disease or contralateral disease but shows bulky axillary lymphadenopathy suspicious for metastasis.*

- With positive LNs staging, imaging was ordered. CT of the chest, abdomen, and pelvis did not reveal any distant metastasis.
- Patient is clinical stage IIIA (cT3N2M0).

What Further Molecular or Genomic Testing Is Recommended?

- Genetic testing should be offered to:
  - all women diagnosed with metastatic BC, any BC patient age 45 or younger, those diagnosed with TNBC, an unknown family history, relative with a known inherited mutation associated with BC, Ashkenazi Jewish ancestry, prior diagnosis of ovarian cancer, lobular cancer with a personal history of gastric cancer, one or more relatives with high-risk history (BC less than age 50, ovarian cancer, male BC, pancreatic cancer, metastatic prostate cancer); and
  - women ages 45 to 50 who have bilateral BC or a second BC.

Patient's Genetic Testing Recommendation

- Given the patient's young age at the time of diagnosis and family history of endometrial cancer, she was referred for genetic testing. She was found to have pathogenic BRCA-1 mutation.

Patient's Treatment Course

- The patient was treated with neoadjuvant weekly paclitaxel for 12 doses followed by 4 doses of dose dense doxorubicin and cyclophosphamide. She underwent bilateral mastectomy with right axillary dissection. Pathology showed residual disease (11 mm), IDC, ER+, PR-, HER2-, and four positive LNs, which equated to a residual cancer burden score (RCB) of III. Patient now comes for consultation of adjuvant therapy for pathological stage IIIA (pT1N2).

What Adjuvant Therapy Should Be Offered to High-Risk Patients?

- Up to 30% of patients with high-risk clinical and/or pathological features may experience early distant recurrence.
- The MonarchE trial led to the approval of abemacilib, a CDK 4/6 inhibitor, combined with ET for the adjuvant treatment of HR+, HER2-, node-positive, and high-grade early-stage BC. High-risk patients were defined as four or more +LN or 1 to 3 +LN AND greater than 5 cm, histological grade 3, or Ki-67 greater than 20%. This Phase III, randomized, multicenter trial (n = 5637) showed that when daily abemaciclib for 2 years was added to at least 5 years of ET there was a clinically meaningful benefit in invasive disease-free survival (IDFS; hazard ratio [HR] = 0.71, 95% confidence interval [CI] 0.58-0.87; nominal $P < 0.001$) and in distant relapse-free survival (DRFS; HR = 0.69, 95% CI 0.55-0.86; nominal P less than 0.001). The 2-year IDFS rates were 91.3% in abemacicib + ET and 86.1% in ET alone, with an absolute improvement of 5.2% at primary outcome. Abemaciclib + ET also significantly reduced the risk of developing an invasive disease event in the Ki-67-high population by 36% (HR = 0.64, 95% CI 0.48 to 0.87; two-sided $P = 0.0042$). In this trial there was a higher incidence of grade 3 adverse events (AEs) and serious AEs in the abemacicib + ET group (50% vs. 16% and 15% vs. 9%, respectively). The most frequent AEs were diarrhea, neutropenia, and fatigue in the abemacicib arm.[16]

What Adjuvant Therapy Should Be Offered to Patients With a Germline *BRCA* Mutation?

- Patients with germline *BRCA1* or *BRCA2* mutations have deficiencies in homologous DNA repair. Patients with a *BRCA1* pathogenic variant have a particular predisposition to TNBC, and patients with a *BRCA2* pathogenic variant are predisposed to HR+ BCs.

- Olaparib is a poly adenosine diphosphate-ribose polymerase (PARP) inhibitor. PARP inhibitors exploit the DNA repair deficiency caused by the *BRCA1/2* mutation, leading to cancer cell death.
- The OlympiAD trial led to the FDA approval of olaparib for patients with metastatic BC who carry a germline *BRCA* mutation in 2018.[17]
- The OlympiA trial led to the FDA approval of adjuvant olaparib for high-risk patients with *BRCA1* or *BRCA2* mutated early-stage BC following NAC or adjuvant chemotherapy. In this Phase III, double-blind, randomized trial (n = 1836, including six men) patients received olaparib (300 mg twice daily) for 1 year. Olaparib has led to an 8.8% improvement in the 3-year IDFS (olaparib 85.9%, placebo 77.1%, 95% CI 4.5 to 13.0). The 3-year distant disease free survival in olaparib group was 87.5% compared to 80.4% in the placebo group (7.7% improvement, 95% CI 3.0 to 11.1, HR 0.57, 99.5% CI 0.39 to 0.83, *P* less than 0.001). The olaparib arm also had increased OS (92% in olaparib, 88.3% in placebo, 95% CI 0.3 to 7.1, HR 0.68, 99% CI 0.44 to 1.05, *P* = 0.02). Notable AEs were anemia (8.7%), decreased neutrophil count (4.8%), decreased white-cell count (3.0%), fatigue (1.8%), and lymphopenia (1.2%). In addition, combination of olaparib and ET was found to be safe and well tolerated.[18]

Conclusions

- Per the OlympiA trial, patients with high-risk disease who harbor a germline *BRCA1* or *BCRA2* mutation should be offered adjuvant olaparib for 1 year following chemotherapy and local management of their BC.
- Per the MonarchE trial, patient with high-risk HR+ early-stage BC should be offered adjuvant abemacicib (for 2 years) + ET (for 5 years total).
- At this time there is not enough safety and efficacy data for combination of abemacicib and olaparib. If a patient has a *BRCA* mutation, the greatest evidence would support giving adjuvant olaparib versus abemaciclib.

Case 5.4: Stage IV Breast Cancer

A 57-year-old Caucasian female presented to an urgent care center for evaluation of lower back pain which started 6 months ago. She is otherwise healthy, a nonsmoker, drinks alcohol occasionally, works as a schoolteacher, and lives with her husband. She had one daughter when she was 38 years old. She has not seen a primary care provider (PCP) in over 10 years and has not kept up with her routine cancer screenings. She is adopted and has no knowledge of her family history. Physical exam was normal except for tenderness on palpation along her lower back; breast exam and LN examination were deferred. She was given a prescription for nonsteroidal anti-inflammatory drugs (NSAIDs) and her doctor ordered routine lab work and x-rays of her lower back.

On review of the x-rays, multiple osteoblastic lesions were seen in the lumbar/sacral area and right iliac crest. Basic labs were within normal limits apart from mildly elevated alkaline phosphatase and calcium. Her physician called her with the results, and she reported her back pain was worsening and she felt some tingling in her right foot. At that time, she was advised to go to the emergency department for evaluation. The emergency physician ordered an MRI of the lumbosacral (L/S) spine along with a contrast CT of her chest, abdomen, and pelvis. Imaging with bone scan revealed an L3 compression fracture and multiple osteoblastic lesions throughout the axial skeleton, but no evidence of cord compression. CTs revealed a dense spiculated mass 3x3 cm in the right breast, multiple enlarged right axillary LNs, and at least three hypodensities were seen in the liver (largest 2.5 cm).

How Is a Diagnosis Established?

- The presence of osteoblastic bone lesions should be considered cancer until proven otherwise. The differential diagnosis includes metastatic lesions from multiple solid tumors which are likely to form osteoblastic lesions (BC, lung cancer, colon cancer). With this extent of involvement, other benign lesions or cancers (multiple myeloma) which make lytic lesions are less likely.

- When establishing the diagnosis of metastatic cancer, a biopsy is usually required. If possible, *soft tissue* biopsy is preferred to bone biopsy, as the decalcification process can degrade the sample, precluding molecular profiling. It is also preferable to choose a distant, safe site to biopsy.

Patient's Diagnosis

- *The patient underwent interventional radiology (IR) biopsy of the largest liver lesion. The pathology report revealed metastatic adenocarcinoma that was positive for GATA3+, CK7+CK20-, TTF1-, ER+, and Mammoglobin+. The final diagnosis reported was metastatic carcinoma consistent with breast primary.*

What Further Molecular or Genomic Testing Is Required?

- Newly diagnosed BCs must undergo testing for predictive biomarkers. The testing for ER, PR, and overexpression of HER2 receptors are discussed in Case 5.1. Biopsies from metastatic cancer aren't routinely tested for Ki-67.

Patient's Molecular and Genomic Testing

- ER+ 6/8, PR+ 3/8, HER2-negative (IHC 1+, *not sent for reflex FISH testing*)

How Is This Tumor Staged?

- The AJCC TNM staging system is used to stage BC.
- Clinical stage is done prior to any treatment. Staging is based on either TNM staging or with prognostic staging, which included predictive biomarker information. Clinical staging requires a physical exam and imaging. For early-stage disease, breast imaging including mammogram, US, and sometimes MRI is performed. For high-risk early-stage or patients with de novo metastatic cancer CT scans, a nuclear bone scan should be ordered. In some circumstances, brain imaging or PET/CT can be considered (renal insufficiency or iodine allergies).

Patient's Clinical Stage

- *Patient's clinical stage is T2cN1M1 stage IV.*

What Are Appropriate Treatment Options?

- Metastatic BC is treatable but not curable. The goal of treatment is to prevent or slow the spread of cancer, relieve any pain, and extend survival with a good quality of life.
- There are two types of treatment: local therapy and systemic therapy.
  - Local therapy includes surgery, ablation, and radiation therapy. These modalities are generally used for early-stage BC but can be part of palliative treatment plans.
  - Systemic therapy treats the entire body. It includes ET, chemotherapy, and targeted therapy.
- Given this patient is not in visceral crisis and disease is metastatic, there is currently no indication for surgery to the primary breast mass and she should be started on systemic treatment with consideration of local treatment for palliation of her painful bone lesion.
- In metastatic HR+, HER2- BC, in absence of visceral crisis, AI in combination with CDK 4/6 inhibition has category 1 approval in the frontline setting. In premenopausal women,

this treatment also requires ovarian ablation or ovarian suppression with a luteinizing hormone releasing hormone (LHRH) agonist.

- ○ AIs are ET; they function by inhibiting an enzyme, aromatase, which transforms androgen into estrogen. They do not suppress estrogen made by the ovaries. Nonsteroidal AIs include anastrozole (Arimidex) and letrozole (Femara). Exemestane (Aromasin) is a steroidal AI.
- ○ CDK 4/6 inhibitors is a targeted therapy. This drug class inhibits kinase activity of CDK, which phosphorylates the retinoblastoma pathway, which is downstream from the ER. Inhibiting CDK 4/6 proteins block the transition from the G1 to the S phase of the cell cycle. CDK 4/6 inhibitors include palbociclib (Ibrance), ribociclib (Kisqali), and abemaciclib (Verzenio). With all CDK 4/6 regimens, premenopausal women must also receive ovarian ablation or suppression.
- There are three FDA-approved CDK 4/6 inhibitors which are approved in combination with ET. The keystone trials are summarized in the text that follows:
  - ○ PALOMA-2 was a Phase III trial of postmenopausal females with advanced HR+ BC treated with palbociclib plus letrozole after progression on prior ET ($n = 666$). The trial showed the combination with palbocicilb led to an improvement in PFS (24.8 vs. 14.5 months; HR 0.58, 95% CI 0.46 to 0.72) and an objective response rate (ORR; 42 vs. 35 %) compared with letrozole alone.[19]
  - ○ MONALEESA-2 was a Phase III trial of postmenopausal females with advanced HR+ BC treated with ribociclib and letrozole in the first-line setting ($n = 668$). At 26.4 months of median follow-up, the combination was associated with an improvement in PFS (25.3 vs. 16.0 months; HR for progression or death was 0.56, 95% CI 0.45 to 0.70) and improved ORR of 43% versus 29% compared with letrozole alone. OS was improved with combination therapy (63.9 months vs. 51.4 months; HR 0.76, CI 0.63 to 0.93, $P = 0.004$).[20]
  - ○ MONALEESA-7 was a Phase III placebo-controlled clinical trial of pre- or perimenopausal females with advanced HR+ BC treated with ribociclib or placebo with goserelin plus either a nonsteroidal AI or tamoxifen ($n = 672$) in the first line. An improvement in PFS was seen with the addition of ribociclib (median PFS, 24 vs. 13 months; HR 0.55, 95% CI 0.4 to 0.69). At 3.5 years, an improvement in OS was reported with ribociclib (70% vs. 46%; HR 0.71, 95% CI 0.54 to 0.95).[21]
  - ○ Monarch-3 was a Phase III trial of postmenopausal females with advanced HR+ BC treated with a combination of abemaciclib with a nonsteroidal AI (letrozole or anastrozole) versus AI alone as first-line treatment. The study found that the combination of abemaciclib and AI improved PFS, compared with AI alone (median not reached vs. 14.7 months, respectively; HR 0.54, 95% CI 0.41 to 0.72). The ORR was higher in the treatment arm compared with AI monotherapy (59% vs. 44%).[22]
  - ○ Of note, to date only ribociclib and abemaciclib have shown OS benefit in Phase III randomized studies.

Recommended Treatment Plan for This Patient

- *Ribociclib 600 mg daily on days 1 to 21 of a 28-day cycle in combination with letrozole 2.5 mg daily. She was referred to radiation oncology for local treatment of her painful bone lesion.*

What Are the Toxicities Associated With Cyclin-Dependent Kinase 4/6 Inhibitors?

- All three FDA-approved CDK 4/6 inhibitors have a similar side effect profile. The most commonly reported toxicities include neutropenia, leucopenia, thrombocytopenia,

anemia, diarrhea, vomiting, febrile neutropenia, nausea, increased alanine aminotransferase (ALT), increased aspartate aminotransferase (AST), decreased appetite, and alopecia.
- For most grade 3 or 4 toxicities, treatment interruptions are indicated with dose reduction on resumption of treatment. Some grade 4 toxicities require permanent discontinuation.
- There are some special considerations to note. Abemaciclib causes less neutropenia but more GI upset. Ribociclib can increase QTc; it requires monitoring and causes arrhythmias.

What Are Other Treatment Considerations?

- In the metastatic setting, genetic testing should be assessed in all patients. Germline mutations in *BRCA1/2* and other high-risk genes have approved therapeutic targeted agents.
- Next-generation sequencing (NGS) should be considered at progression.
- Patients with metastatic bone disease should also be treated with bisphosphonates and calcium/vitamin D after dental clearance. The available treatments are denosumab, zoledronic acid, or pamidronate.
- For patients without metastatic bone disease, a baseline DEXA scan should be performed for patients receiving an AI, especially those who are at an increased risk for osteoperosis (age greater than 65, family history, steroids).
- Routine surgical resection of the primary breast tumor is generally not indicated in the treatment of de novo stage IV disease but can be considered for local control on an individual case-by-case basis.

Patient's Treatment Course
- *The patient was referred to a dentist for bisphosphonate clearance and started on zoledronic acid; she was also instructed to take calcium and vitamin D supplementation.*

Treatment Duration

Treatment should be continued indefinitely until progression of disease or unacceptable toxicity is reached.

Case 5.5: Recurrent Stage IV Breast Cancer

A 58-year-old female with known de novo metastatic ER+, PR+, and HER2- BC presents for follow-up. She presented 12 months ago with a right breast mass and was diagnosed with metastatic BC. She had metastasis to the axillary LNs and a malignant pleural effusion. The patient was started on first-line therapy with a CDK 4/6 inhibitor and AI. The patient had a good clinical response with resolution of the pleural effusion and has been stable on this regimen. She experienced intermittent joint pains and had grade 1 neutropenia. She is in clinic for her follow-up scans. CT scans show progression of disease with new osseous metastatic disease in the ribs and thoracic spine. Laboratory exams are within normal limits and glucose is below 100. Physical exam shows palpable right breast mass 3 cm × 4 cm, multiple enlarged axillary nodes, and no tenderness to palpation in the ribs or thoracic spine.

What Further Molecular or Genomic Testing Is Required?

- All newly diagnosed metastatic HR+ BCs must undergo NGS to look for the presence of *PIK3CA* mutations, which are present in 20% to 40% of HR+ BC.[23]

- NGS of tissue or liquid biopsy should be sent to access for *PIK3CA* mutations. Bone biopsy should be avoided, as processing can led to false-negative test results.

Patient's Molecular and Genomic Testing
- *NGS was performed on peripheral blood (circulating tumor DNA/liquid biopsy); it was positive for PIK3CA activating mutation.*

What Is Phosphoinositide 3 Kinase?

- Phosphoinositide kinases (PIK) phosphorylate the inositol ring of phosphoinositide and funetion as signal transducers.[24]
- PIK are further subdivided into three families: phosphoinositide 3 kinase (PI3K), phosphoinositide 4 kinase, and phosphoinositide 5 kinase.
- PIK3 kinases are a receptor tyrosine kinase with PIP3 as the end product. PIP3 is a very important secondary messenger in the cell; it interacts with a group of serine-threonine protein kinases called the AKT family. When activated, the AKT pathway leads to cell growth signaling by directly affecting regulation of cell proliferation, survival, and motility.

What Are Phosphoinositide 3 Kinase Mutations?

- *PI3K* mutations are a common resistance mechanism for HR+ BC to ET. *PI3K* is downstream of the ER, activating mutations that lead to constitutive signaling despite upstream blocking of the hormone receptor (HR) with ET.
- The three most common driver mutations (H1047R, E542K, and E545 K) are found in 80% of PI3K mutant tumors.

What Are Appropriate Treatment Options?

- Alpelisib is an oral therapy that selectively inhibits class I *PI3K*.
- The SOLAR-1 trial led to the FDA approval of alpelisib in combination with fulvestrant for *PIC3CA*-mutated HR+ advanced BC.[25]
- In this trial at 20 months, PFS was improved with the combination of alpelisib with fulvestrant versus placebo-fulvestrant (PFS 11.1 months 95% CI 7.5 to 14.5 vs. 5.7 months 95% CI 3.7 to 7.4). There was no benefit of alpelisib in *wtPIK3CA* BC.

Recommended Treatment Plan for This Patient
- *Alpelisib 300 mg daily and fulvestrant 500 mg IM monthly*

What Are the Toxicities Associated With Alpelisib?

- Most frequent side effects were hyperglycemia, gastrointestinal issues, and rash.
- Hyperglycemia was the most frequent AE and is an expected off-target effect. Grade 3 and 4 hyperglycemia was common, 60% and 34%, respectively, and was the most common reason for discontinuation (6.3%).
- SOLAR-1 only included normoglycemic patients with glucose less than 140 and A1c less than 6.4%.
- Rash was reported in 30% of subjects, and frequently required treatment with H2 blocker.

How Are These Toxicities Managed?

- Hyperglycemia
  - Hyperglycemia is an off-target effect; it occurs shortly after starting therapy (less than 14 days).
  - Grade 2 hyperglycemia can be managed with lifestyle modification and low threshold to start metformin. Once metformin is started, it can be titrated to a maximum tolerated dose with close follow-up (every 2 weeks for first 6 weeks). If there is no improvement at 21 days, dose reduction is recommended. If the fasting blood glucose is persistently greater than 160, pioglitazone can be considered.
  - In grade 3 hyperglycemia, the drug should be interrupted, and the hyperglycemia treated as previously noted. Insulin is not recommended for treatment of long-term hyperglycemia associated with alpelisib.
  - If grade 3 or 4 hyperglycemia does not improve to grade 2 shortly after interruption, permanently discontinue alpelisib.
- Rash
  - Skin rash grading is dependent on the percentage of body surface area involved. Grade 1 and 2 rash do not require drug interruption or discontinuation, but should be treated with topical corticosteroids.
  - Grade 3 rash requires interruption of the alpelisib with treatment with topical and systemic steroids until improvement to grade 1 or resolution. Grade 4 rash requires permanent discontinuation of the drug.

REVIEW QUESTIONS

1. A 72-year-old female with a history of stage III hormone receptor-positive (HR+) breast cancer (BC) presents with 8 weeks of back pain, fatigue, and 5 lb weight loss. She has been on adjuvant anastrozole for 3 years but stopped about 8 months ago due to joint pains. Restaging nuclear medicine (NM) bone scan and CT of the chest, abdomen, and pelvis are completed and reveal diffuse bone metastasis and three lesions in the liver concerning for metastatic disease. CT-guided biopsy of the liver confirms estrogen receptor-positive (ER+), progesterone receptor-positive (PR+), HER2- metastatic BC. Her performance status is 1. Which of the choices in optimal as first-line therapy for metastatic BC?
   A. Tamoxifen
   B. Abemaciclib + fulvestrant
   C. Abemaciclib + letrozole
   D. Chemotherapy

2. A 58-year-old female is diagnosed with left-sided hormone receptor-positive (HR+) breast cancer (BC) after presenting with a palpable mass. Mammogram and breast ultrasound (US) showed a 3.5-cm irregular, spiculated mass and several suspicious lymph nodes (LNs; two non-movable LNs, ~1.5 cm each). A biopsy of the mass shows invasive ductal cancer (IDC), grade 2, estrogen receptor-positive (ER+), progesterone receptor-positive (PR+), HER2- BC and an LN biopsy is positive for metastatic BC. What staging studies are indicated at this time?
   A. PET/CT
   B. Breast MRI
   C. CT scan of the chest, abdomen, and pelvis and nuclear medicine (NM) bone scan
   D. Brain MRI
   E. No further imaging

3. A 38-year-old female with *BRCA2* mutation is found to have left hormone receptor-positive (HR+) stage IIb breast cancer (BC). She is treated with neoadjuvant chemotherapy (NAC) and then undergoes bilateral mastectomy and right sentinel lymph node biopsy (SLNB). Pathology shows multifocal residual disease with the largest area of 9 mm, invasive ductal cancer (IDC), grade 3, estrogen receptor-positive (ER+), progesterone receptor-positive (PR+), HER2-, and Ki-67 18%, 1 LN shows micrometastatic disease. She has finished radiation of the right axilla. She is coming in to discuss starting adjuvant endocrine therapy (ET). What do you recommend?
   A. Tamoxifen for 10 years
   B. Olaparib for 1 year + ET + overall survival (OS) for 5 to 10 years
   C. Letrozole + OS for 10 years
   D. No further treatment is needed

4. A 42-year-old premenopausal female is found to have stage III left-sided breast cancer (BC). She is treated with neoadjuvant chemotherapy (NAC) and then undergoes a left-sided mastectomy with axillary lymph node (LN) dissection. Pathology of her tumor reveals residual disease of 22 mm, invasive ductal cancer (IDC), grade III, estrogen receptor-positive (ER+), weakly progesterone receptor-positive (PR+), HER2-, and Ki-67 30%. Four of the eight LNs are positive. She is about to start radiation. She comes in to discuss adjuvant endocrine therapy (ET). What do you offer?
   A. Abemaciclib 2 years + letrozole/overall survival (OS) 5 years
   B. Tamoxifen 5 years
   C. Fulvestrant + OS 5 years
   D. Letrozole for 10 years
   E. A or D

5. A 47-year-old premenopausal female is diagnosed with stage III right-sided breast cancer (BC). The BC is 5 cm and she has at least 1 positive, fixed lymph node (LN). The pathology shows invasive ductal cancer (IDC), estrogen receptor-positive (ER+; 5/8), progesterone receptor-positive (PR+; 3/8), HER2- (IHC 1+), and Ki-67 is 43%. She is offered neoadjuvant chemotherapy. All of the following are true regarding the advantages of neoadjuvant chemotherapy (NAC) except:

   A. Neoadjuvant therapy can downsize the tumor, making breast-conserving therapy more likely
   B. The pathological response can provide prognostic information
   C. It may provide early systemic treatment for micrometastatic disease
   D. It improves overall survival (OS)

6. A 75-year-old healthy female is diagnosed with stage I right-sided breast cancer (BC) found on screening mammogram. She undergoes upfront surgery with a lumpectomy + sentinel lymph node biopsy (SLNB). Pathology shows invasive lobular cancer (ILC), grade 1, estrogen receptor-positive (ER+), progesterone receptor-positive (PR+), HER2-, Ki-67 3%, and 0/3 lymph node (LN) positive for metastasis. She comes in to discuss adjuvant therapy. Her performance status (PS) is 0 and she walks 30 minutes 5 days per week. What do you recommend?

   A. Start letrozole and refer her to radiation therapy
   B. Order oncotype diagnosis to help with your decision about adjuvant chemotherapy
   C. Offer radiation therapy or 5 years of aromatase inhibitor (AI)
   D. Due to her age, defer radiation therapy

7. A 67-year-old female with metastatic hormone receptor-positive (HR+), HER2- breast cancer (BC) is being seen for progression of disease. She was found to have de novo metastatic disease 18 months ago and has been on ribociclib and anastrozole. Routine restaging showed progression of bone and lymph node (LN) metastasis. You decide to order next-generation sequencing (NGS) sequencing to identify if there is a targetable *PIK3CA* mutation. What type of specimen do you order NGS sequencing on?

   A. Place intervention biopsy consult for bone biopsy
   B. Place pulmonary consult for endobronchial ultrasound (EBUS) to mediastinal LN biopsy
   C. You can just assume the patient has developed a mutation since she is progressing
   D. Order liquid biopsy on peripheral blood

8. You send next-generation sequencing (NGS) and the patient is found to have a *PIK3CA* mutation. You decide to start the patient on second-line alpelisib and fulvestrant. What is the main side effect you have to monitor for?

   A. Diarrhea
   B. Hyperglycemia
   C. Rash
   D. Neutropenia
   E. B and C
   F. A and B

ANSWERS AND RATIONALES

1. **C. Abemaciclib + letrozole.** Cyclin-dependent kinase (CDK) 4/6 inhibitor combined with endocrine therapy (ET) is the standard of care for metastatic HR+ BC and the first-line setting. In the past, clinicians had reservations about delaying chemotherapy to later lines when the patient had liver and other visceral metastasis. Monarch-3 (abemaciclib) and MONALEESA-2 (ribociclib) showed that postmenopausal patients delayed chemotherapy and was effective in patients with visceral metastasis.

2. **C. CT scan of the chest, abdomen, and pelvis and NM bone scan.** The patient has T2N2 BC (stage III). Patients with nodal disease, nonmovable should have staging imaging. This can be done with NM bone scan and CT of the chest, abdomen, and pelvis or PET/CT. MRI of the brain is only needed if the patient is having neurological complaints. Breast MRI could be considered for surgical planning or if the patient had lobular histology, which can be underrepresented with mammogram and US.

3. **B. Olaparib for 1 year + ET + overall survival (OS) for 5 to 10 years.** Patients with high-risk, hormone receptor-positive (HR+) HER2- or HR- HER2- early-stage BC with *BRCA1/2* mutations are at higher risk than matched *BRCA1/2*-negative patients for reoccurrence. In the OlympiA trial, patients with germline *BRCA1/2* and high-risk HER2- early-stage BC were treated with olaparib for 1 year versus placebo. Olaparib was well tolerated and the patient treated had significantly longer survival free of invasive or distant disease than placebo. This treatment choice should be offered to all patients who fall into this group.

4. **A. Abemaciclib 2 years + letrozole/overall survival (OS) 5 years.** This patient has a high risk for relapse (~20% will progress to metastatic disease), and this patient should be offered escalated therapy with cyclin dependent kinase (CDK) 4/6 inhibitor + ET. This does require additional monitoring and has side effects; at a minimum, this patient should be offered 10 years of adjuvant ET. In the Monarch-E trial, patients with high-risk disease as defined as 4+ positive LN, 1 to 3+ LNs + grade 3 disease, tumor size greater than 5 cm, or 1 to 3+ LN + Ki-67 20% or greater were treated with abemaciclib + ET for 2 years and then went on to finish 5 to 10 years of ET. The addition of 2 years of abemaciclib led to 40% reduction in distant relapse-free survival (DRFS) and 37% reduction in invasive disease-free survival (IDFS). Other CDK 4/6 inhibitors have not shown this clinical benefit, likely due to trials including lower risk disease.

5. **D. It improves overall survival (OS).** NAC does not provide OS benefit. There has been a shift in treatment over the last decade toward neoadjuvant treatment of stage II or III BCs. While this is the standard of care in triple-negative breast cancer (TNBC) and hormone receptor-negative (HR-) HER2+ BC, it is increasingly offered in HR+ BC. The clinical response and serial biomarker information allows for prognostication and potentially de-escalation of adjuvant treatment for personalized recurrence risk.

6. **C. Offer radiation therapy or 5 years of aromatase inhibitor (AI).** The goal of treatment in older patients is different than in younger patients. Life expectancy and other comorbidities are key factors in treatment decisions. In patients older than 70 years of age with T1/T2 ER+ LN- disease, it is possible to omit either radiation or endocrine therapy (ET).

7. **D. Order liquid biopsy on peripheral blood.** NGS testing can be performed on soft tissue or liquid biopsy. In this setting, the patient has known metastatic disease and doesn't require an additional tissue biopsy for testing. If any patient requires NGS or genomic testing, bone biopsy should be avoided as the decalcification solution used for processing of the specimen can affect the genomic test results.

8. **E. B and C.** While diarrhea is commonly a mild (grade 1/2) side effect of alpelisib, hyperglycemia and rash are more commonly moderate to severe. In SOLAR-1, about 40% of patients developed grade 3 to 4 hyperglycemia and 20%, grade 3 to 4 rash. Hyperglycemia is an expected off-target effect of *PI3K* inhibition. This adverse effect (AE) usually occurs early within the first 15 days of treatment and requires additional monitoring and often treatment. Patients should return for a visit in 2 weeks for glucose monitoring. If the patient is prediabetic, metformin can be started along with alpelisib. Per treatment guidelines for the hyperglycemia with this agent, insulin is less effective than pioglitazone.

REFERENCES

1. Ellis MJ, Tao Y, Luo J, et al. Outcome prediction for estrogen receptor-positive breast cancer based on postneoadjuvant endocrine therapy tumor characteristics. *J Natl Cancer Inst.* 2008;100(19):1380–1388. doi:10.1093/jnci/djn309

2. Rusz O, Vörös A, Varga Z, et al. One-year neoadjuvant endocrine therapy in breast cancer. *Pathol Oncol Res.* 2015;21(4):977–984. doi:10.1007/s12253-015-9911-1

3. Amin MB, Edge S, Greene F, et al., eds. *Cancer Staging Manual.* 8th ed. Springer; 2018.

4. Wolmark N, Wang J, Mamounas E, Bryant J, Fisher B. Preoperative chemotherapy in patients with operable breast cancer: nine-year results from national surgical adjuvant breast and bowel project B-18. *J Natl Cancer Inst Monogr.* 2001;30:96–102. doi:10.1093/oxfordjournals.jncimonographs.a003469

5. Lerebours F, Rivera S, Mouret-Reynier M-A, et al. Randomized phase 2 neoadjuvant trial evaluating anastrozole and fulvestrant efficacy for postmenopausal, estrogen receptor-positive, human epidermal growth factor receptor 2-negative breast cancer patients: results of the UNICANCER CARMINA 02 French trial (UCBG 0609). *Cancer.* 2016;122(19):3032–3040. doi:10.1002/cncr.30143

6. Cataliotti L, Buzdar AU, Noguchi S, et al. Comparison of anastrozole versus tamoxifen as preoperative therapy in postmenopausal women with hormone receptor-positive breast cancer: the pre-operative "arimidex" compared to tamoxifen (PROACT) trial. *Cancer.* 2006;106(10):2095–2103. doi:10.1002/cncr.21872

7. Madigan LI, Dinh P, Graham JD. Neoadjuvant endocrine therapy in locally advanced estrogen or progesterone receptor-positive breast cancer: determining the optimal endocrine agent and treatment duration in postmenopausal women—a literature review and proposed guidelines. *Breast Cancer Res.* 2020;22:7. doi:10.1186/s13058-020-01314-6

8. Sparano JA, Gray RJ, Makower, DF, et al. Adjuvant chemotherapy guided by a 21-gene expression assay in breast cancer. *N Engl J Med.* 2018;379(2):111–121. doi:10.1056/NEJMoa1804710

9. Breastcancer.org. Invasive ductal carcinoma: diagnosis, treatment, and more. Accessed January 12, 2022. https://www.breastcancer.org/symptoms/types/idc

10. Margolese RG, Hortobagyi GN, Buchholz TA. The role of radiation for invasive breast cancer. In: Kufe DW, Pollock RE, Weichselbaum RR, et al., eds. *Holland-Frei Cancer Medicine.* 6th ed. BC Decker; 2003. https://www.ncbi.nlm.nih.gov/books/NBK13034

11. Henry NL, Azzouz F, Desta Z, et al. Predictors of aromatase inhibitor discontinuation as a result of treatment-emergent symptoms in early-stage breast cancer. *J Clin Oncol.* 2012;30(9):936–942. doi:10.1200/JCO.2011.38.0261

12. Fontaine C, Meulemans A, Huizing M, et al. Tolerance of adjuvant letrozole outside of clinical trials. *Breast.* 2008;17(4):376–381. doi:10.1016/j.breast.2008.02.006

13. Garreau JR, Delamelena T, Walts D, Karamlou K, Johnson N. Side effects of aromatase inhibitors versus tamoxifen: the patients' perspective. *Am J Surg.* 2006;192(4):496–498. doi:10.1016/j.amjsurg.2006.06.018

14. Early Breast Cancer Trialists' Collaborative Group (EBCTCG). Aromatase inhibitors versus tamoxifen in early breast cancer: patient-level meta-analysis of the randomised trials. *Lancet.* 2015;386(10001):1341–1352. doi:10.1016/S0140-6736(15)61074-1

15. Robertson JFR, Paridaens RJ, Lichfield J, Bradbury I, Campbell C. Meta-analyses of phase 3 randomised controlled trials of third generation aromatase inhibitors versus tamoxifen as first-line endocrine therapy in postmenopausal women with hormone receptor-positive advanced breast cancer. *Eur J Cancer.* 2021;145:19–28. doi:10.1016/j.ejca.2020.11.038

16. Harbeck N, Rastogi P, Martin M, et al. Adjuvant abemaciclib combined with endocrine therapy for high-risk early breast cancer: updated efficacy and Ki-67 analysis from the monarchE study. *Ann Oncol.* 2021, 32(12):1571–1581. doi:10.1016/j.annonc.2021.09.015

17. Robson ME, Tung N, Conte P, et al. OlympiAD final overall survival and tolerability results: olaparib versus chemotherapy treatment of physician's choice in patients with a germline *BRCA* mutation and *HER2*-negative metastatic breast cancer. *Ann Oncol.* 2019;30(4):558–566. doi:10.1093/annonc/mdz012

18. Tutt AN, Garber JE, Kaufman B, et al. Adjuvant olaparib for patients with *BRCA1-* or *BRCA2*-mutated breast cancer. *N Engl J Med.* 2021;384:2394–2405. doi:10.1056/NEJMoa2105215
19. Finn RS, Martin M, Rugo HS, et al. Palbociclib and letrozole in advanced breast cancer. *N Engl J Med.* 2016;375:1925–1936. https://www.ncbi.nlm.nih.gov/pubmed/27959613
20. Hortobagyi GN, Stemmer SM, Burris HA, et al. Updated results from MONALEESA-2, a phase III trial of first-line ribociclib plus letrozole versus placebo plus letrozole in hormone receptor-positive, *HER2*-negative advanced breast cancer. *Ann Oncol.* 2018;29:1541–1547. doi:10.1093/annonc/mdy155
21. Tripathy D, Im S-A, Colleoni M, et al. Ribociclib plus endocrine therapy for premenopausal women with hormone-receptor-positive, advanced breast cancer (MONALEESA-7): a randomized phase 3 trial. *Lancet Oncol.* 2018;19:904–915. doi:10.1016/S1470-2045(18)30292-4
22. Goetz MP, Toi M, Campone M, et al. MONARCH 3: abemaciclib as initial therapy for advanced breast cancer. *J Clin Oncol.* 2017;35:3638–3646. doi:10.1200/JCO.2017.75.6155
23. André F, Ciruelos E, Rubovszky G, et al. Alpelisib for *PIK3CA*-mutated, hormone receptor–positive advanced breast cancer. *N Engl J Med.* 2019;380:1929–1940. doi:10.1056/NEJMoa1813904
24. Samuels Y, Waldman T. Oncogenic mutations of *PIK3CA* in human cancers. *Curr Top Microbiol Immunol.* 2010;347:21–41. doi:10.1007/82_2010_68
25. Bosch A, Li Z, Bergamaschi A, et al. *PI3K* inhibition results in enhanced estrogen receptor function and dependence in hormone receptor-positive breast cancer. *Sci Transl Med.* 2015;7:283ra51. doi:10.1126/scitranslmed.aaa4442

CHAPTER 6

Triple-Negative Breast Cancer

Richard Benjamin Young and Helen K. Chew

INTRODUCTION

Triple-negative breast cancer (TNBC) is a subtype of breast cancer (BC) traditionally defined by its lack of hormone receptor (HR; estrogen and progesterone) expression and human epidermal growth factor receptor 2 (HER2) expression/amplification. Per the American Society of Clinical Oncology (ASCO)/College of American Pathologists (CAP) guidelines,[1] BCs that stain less than 1% for estrogen receptors (ERs) and progesterone receptors (PRs) are considered HR-. HER2 negativity includes tumors that are not *HER2* amplified, those that stain 0 or 1+ by immunohistochemistry (IHC), or are HER2 equivocal by IHC 2+ and not *HER2* amplified.[2] Because these receptors represent some of the most viable targets for treatment, patients with TNBC until the recent past have encountered a relative dearth of therapy options outside of traditional cytotoxic chemotherapy, compared to HR+ and HER2+ populations. Fortunately, with the advent of checkpoint inhibitors and targeted molecular therapy, exciting promise is on the horizon for this difficult-to-treat disease.

TNBC represents approximately 10% to 20% of new BC diagnoses annually. TNBC is generally more aggressive and portends a poorer prognosis relative to other BC subtypes. Patient demographics suggest that TNBC is more likely diagnosed in patients less than 50 years of age, those with *BRCA1* mutations, and in Black and Hispanic populations.[3] Due to the lack of HR and HER2 targets, (neo)adjuvant chemotherapy is offered in patients with early-stage disease who are chemotherapy-eligible. Chemotherapy regimens may include anthracyclines, taxanes, and fluorouracil. However, checkpoint inhibitors in combination with chemotherapy and molecularly targeted agents are emerging as newer therapeutic options in the (neo)adjuvant and metastatic setting.

CASE SUMMARIES

Case 6.1: Localized Triple-Negative Breast Cancer

A 60-year-old patient presents to the medical oncology clinic after a new diagnosis of TNBC. One month ago during routine screening mammography, a new left breast lesion was appreciated. She subsequently underwent diagnostic bilateral mammography that showed a single lesion in the left breast measuring 0.8 cm. Follow-up ultrasound (US) confirmed an 8-mm lesion that was biopsied, confirming a grade 2 invasive ductal carcinoma. The tumor stained less than 1% for both ER and PR. HER2 was not amplified by fluorescent in situ hybridization (FISH). The patient is asymptomatic. She has well-controlled hypertension and family history is significant for a paternal aunt diagnosed with BC in her 70s. Physical exam reveals an approximate 1 cm firm, mobile, nontender mass at the 3 o'clock position of the left breast. No axillary or supraclavicular lymphadenopathy is appreciated. The remainder of the physical exam is unremarkable.

How Is a Diagnosis Established?

- In a patient with a suspicious breast mass on screening mammography, diagnostic mammogram and breast US are recommended to further classify the lesion as benign, probably benign (BI-RADS 2 or 3, respectively), or suspicious/highly suspicious (BI-RADS 4 or 5, respectively).[4] If a lesion is BI-RADS 4 or 5, core biopsy is recommended to establish a diagnosis. If there are suspicious ipsilateral axillary lymph nodes (LNs), fine needle aspiration (FNA) or core biopsy are recommended to accurately stage the patient. Pathology will provide the histological diagnosis; tumor grade; and ER, PR, and HER2 status.

How Is This Tumor Staged?

- Tumor staging is based on the American Joint Committee on Cancer (AJCC) eighth edition cancer staging system.[5] This includes anatomic staging based on tumor size (T), nodal involvement (N), and presence of distant metastases (M). The AJCC eighth edition now includes a clinical prognostic stage based on tumor grade, HR, and HER2 status.
- For early-stage disease in the absence of systemic symptoms, routine imaging for distant metastasis is not recommended.

Patient's Diagnosis and Clinical Stage

- *The patient's disease is confined to the left breast and she is without evidence of axillary or systemic involvement. Her BC is clinically staged IB, T1bN0M0.*

What Other Diagnostic Considerations Are There?

- TNBCs are enriched in *BRCA1* mutation carriers relative to the general population. Patients diagnosed with TNBC under the age of 60 should undergo genetic counseling and testing to determine germline *BRCA1/2* status.[6] The poly adenosine diphosphate ribose polymerase (PARP) inhibitor olaparib improved disease-free survival (DFS) compared to placebo in patients with germline *BRCA1/2* mutations and early-stage BC. Olaparib has not yet been FDA-approved in the adjuvant setting.[7]

Patient's BRCA Status

- *The patient undergoes genetic counseling and testing and no pathogenic mutations are found in a panel of genes associated with hereditary BC, including BRCA1/2.*

What Are Appropriate Treatment Options?

Local Therapy

Treatment goals for early-stage BC are focused on achieving successful surgical resection, accomplished via mastectomy or lumpectomy followed by whole breast radiation therapy (WBRT). The results of several randomized trials comparing outcomes of mastectomy versus lumpectomy with WBRT demonstrate equivalence in DFS and overall survival (OS) for women with early-stage BCs.[8] The decision to proceed with mastectomy versus lumpectomy with WBRT is made on an individual basis.

- Contraindications to lumpectomy with WBRT include pregnancy or planned pregnancy during radiation therapy, multicentric disease (involving more than one quadrant of the

breast), or prior radiation to the breast. Additionally, relative contraindications include mixed connective tissue disorders and tumor size greater than 5 cm.
- As the patient has clinically node-negative disease, a sentinel lymph node biopsy (SLNB) is adequate for nodal staging.

Systemic Therapy
- ASCO guidelines note that the role of neoadjuvant treatment is to downsize tumors to allow for surgical resection or improve the chances of a lumpectomy if the patient desires. Because chemotherapy is the only adjuvant therapy option for TNBC, it can be given before or after surgery. Prior studies not limited to TNBC have demonstrated equivalent DFS among patients receiving adjuvant or neoadjuvant chemotherapy with operable BC.[9] Neoadjuvant therapy can be offered to patients with nodal involvement or tumors of T1c size or greater. For patients with T1a or T1b *and* N0 disease, as in this case, there is limited data regarding the role of neoadjuvant versus adjuvant treatment.
- The choice of adjuvant chemotherapy regimens includes anthracyclines followed by taxanes (such as doxorubicin/cyclophosphamide followed by paclitaxel or AC-T) or a taxane-only regimen (such as docetaxel/cyclophosphamide or TC). Non-inferiority trials comparing AC-T like regimens to TC have yielded inconsistent results.[10,11]

Patient's Treatment and Pathological Staging
- *The patient undergoes lumpectomy and SLNB revealing a grade 2, 1.5 cm invasive ductal carcinoma with negative margins. One sentinel LN is benign. She has anatomic stage IA and clinical prognostic stage IB, T1cN0, TNBC. She receives adjuvant TC followed by WBRT.*

What Are the Toxicities Associated With Systemic Chemotherapy?

Cytotoxic chemotherapy is associated with cytopenias, including neutropenia, which may lead to rare fatal infections, anemia, and thrombocytopenia. Other side effects include alopecia, nausea and vomiting, constipation, diarrhea, mucositis, and cumulative fatigue, among others.

- Anthracyclines are associated with dose-related cardiotoxicity and rare secondary leukemias and myelodysplastic syndrome.
- Taxanes are associated with sensory neuropathy.

Other Considerations

- Well-established guidelines for surveillance in the first 5 years after BC treatment are available through the National Comprehensive Cancer Network (NCCN).[12] Following treatment, patients should be evaluated for a history and physical exam 1 to 4 times annually for the first 5 years, then once annually thereafter. Annual mammography is recommended except in the case of mastectomy. For all surgical cases, but especially those involving axillary lymph node dissection (ALND), postsurgical monitoring for lymphedema should be incorporated into regular follow-up exams. Just as during initial diagnosis and workup, in the absence of systemic signs or symptoms, routine imaging for metastasis and serological tumor marker evaluation are not recommended. Lastly, for patients who received anthracyclines, monitoring for late cardiac complications should be incorporated into routine practice.

Case 6.2: Locally Advanced Triple-Negative Breast Cancer

A 29-year-old woman is evaluated by her primary care physician (PCP) after palpating a right breast mass 1 month ago. She has no other past medical history but has a family history of BC in a paternal aunt at age 55. A right breast US was remarkable for a 4.9 cm × 4.5 cm × 3.4 cm hypoechoic, irregular mass. Diagnostic mammogram revealed dense breast tissue with vague asymmetry of the right breast. A US-guided core needle biopsy revealed poorly differentiated invasive mammary carcinoma, with no staining for ER or PR. HER2 was equivocal at 2+ staining by IHC but not amplified. She was referred to surgical and medical oncology for additional recommendations. Office exam is remarkable for a palpable, well-circumscribed, 6 cm × 6 cm fixed, firm mass at the 9 o'clock position of the right breast with right axillary adenopathy. No skin changes are appreciated, and the remainder of the physical exam is normal.

How Is a Diagnosis Established?

Patients with a suspicious, palpable mass should undergo bilateral diagnostic mammogram and breast US with image-guided core biopsy. Breast MRI should be considered in patients younger than 50 years to evaluate the extent of disease due to increased breast density. Confirmed invasive carcinoma of the breast should be further characterized by ER, PR, and HER2 tumor status. If there are suspicious axillary LNs, FNA or core biopsy should be performed to establish axillary metastasis.

- Breast MRI is not universally recommended for all newly diagnosed BCs. While providing high sensitivity for the extent of disease, particularly in dense breast, there are concerns that MRI may overestimate the extent of disease. Subsequently. increased frequency of mastectomy has been attributed to MRI use, and this imaging modality should be considered on a case-by-case basis.[13]

How Is This Tumor Staged?

- Tumor staging is based on the AJCC eighth edition cancer staging system.[5] This includes anatomic staging based on tumor size (T), nodal involvement (N), and presence of distant metastases (M). The AJCC eighth edition now includes a clinical prognostic stage based on tumor grade, HR, and HER2 status.
- With locally advanced disease, staging studies including CT scans of the chest, abdomen, and pelvis; and bone scan are recommended.

Patient's Diagnosis and Clinical Stage

- *The patient undergoes FNA of a suspicious right axillary lymph node, confirming metastatic carcinoma. Breast MRI confirms a 6-cm right breast mass with several suspicious right axillary LNs. CT scans of the chest, abdomen, and pelvis, and bone scan, reveal no distant metastasis. Her BC is clinically staged IIIA, T3N1M0.*

What Other Diagnostic Considerations Are There?

- TNBCs are enriched in *BRCA1* mutation carriers relative to the general population. Patients diagnosed with TNBC under the age of 60 should undergo genetic counseling and testing to determine germline *BRCA1/2* status.[6] This patient is 29 and has a paternal family history of BC. The PARP inhibitor olaparib improved DFS compared to placebo in patients with germline *BRCA1/2* mutations and early-stage BC. Olaparib has not yet been FDA-approved in the adjuvant setting.[7]

Patient's BRCA Status

- *The patient undergoes genetic counseling and testing, and a pathogenic mutation is found in BRCA1.*

What Are Appropriate Treatment Options?

Systemic Therapy

In patients with locally advanced disease, neoadjuvant therapy is indicated to improve surgical outcomes or to render inoperable tumors resectable. ASCO guidelines recommend that all patients with TNBC and clinically positive LNs and/or T1c disease be offered an anthracycline and taxane containing regimen preoperatively.[14]

- The addition of carboplatin to preoperative paclitaxel followed by anthracycline-based chemotherapy in two Phase II studies resulted in improved pathological complete response (pCR) rates.[15,16] However, these studies were underpowered to detect differences in DFS or OS with the addition of carboplatin.
- In KEYNOTE-522, patients with stage II to III TNBC were randomized to neoadjuvant pembrolizumab or placebo in combination with neoadjuvant paclitaxel and carboplatin followed by anthracycline-based chemotherapy. Among patients whose tumors were program death-ligand 1 (PD-L1)–positive, defined as a combined positive score (CPS) of 10 or greater, the addition of pembrolizumab improved pCR rates to 64.8% compared to 51.2% among those who received placebo plus chemotherapy.[17] Both groups subsequently received postsurgical adjuvant pembrolizumab or placebo. Therefore, preoperative pembrolizumab, carboplatin, and paclitaxel followed by pembrolizumab, cyclophosphamide, and doxorubicin, followed by adjuvant pembrolizumab, should be considered in this case.

Local Therapy

After completion of neoadjuvant chemotherapy, patients are assessed for surgical resection (lumpectomy or mastectomy) with or without radiation therapy. The results of several randomized trials comparing outcomes of mastectomy versus lumpectomy with WBRT demonstrate equivalence in DFS and OS for women with early-stage BCs.[8] The decision to proceed with mastectomy versus lumpectomy with WBRT is made on an individual basis and, in this case, is the response to preoperative therapy.

- Contraindications to lumpectomy with WBRT include pregnancy or planned pregnancy during radiation therapy, multicentric disease (involving more than one quadrant of the breast), or prior radiation to the breast. Additionally, relative contraindications include mixed connective tissue disorders and tumor size greater than 5 cm.
- ALND is considered standard of care for patients with clinically positive lymph node disease. However, ALND is associated with long-term risks of lymphedema after surgery.[18]
- Post-mastectomy radiation therapy should be offered in this young patient with node-positive disease.

Patient's Treatment

- *She receives preoperative paclitaxel, carboplatin, and pembrolizumab followed by doxorubicin/cyclophosphamide and pembrolizumab with a clinical response. She tolerates therapy well and proceeds to right mastectomy, ALND, and prophylactic left simple mastectomy. Pathology reveals a residual 1 cm high grade invasive carcinoma of the right breast and one of 12 axillary LNs contains metastatic disease. Pathology of the left breast is benign. Thus, she has a residual yT1bN1 BC. She plans to complete adjuvant pembrolizumab and receive right post-mastecomy radiation therapy.*

What Are Other Treatment Considerations?

Adjuvant Therapy

- The CREATE-X trial randomized patients with early-stage, HER2- BC who had residual disease after standard neoadjuvant chemotherapy to either 8 cycles of adjuvant

capecitabine or not. Results from the triple-negative subgroup demonstrated not only improvements in DFS (68.8% vs. 56.1%) but OS as well (78.8% vs. 70.3%). While the addition of capecitabine should be considered, CREATE-X was conducted prior to the availability of preoperative and adjuvant pembrolizumab.[19]
- The OlympiA trial randomized patients with early-stage HER2- BC and germline *BRCA1/2* mutations to a year of olaparib or placebo. The primary endpoint of DFS was significantly improved at 3 years in subjects who received olaparib, 85.9% versus 77.1%.[7] As noted with the CREATE-X trial, patients on the OlympiA trial did not receive neo-adjuvant pembrolizumab. In addition, olaparib has not yet been FDA-approved in the adjuvant setting.

Fertility Preservation

- In patients of childbearing potential, fertility counseling should be offered. Case-control and registry studies have shown that pregnancy after invasive BC therapy is not associated with increased risk of recurrence or death from BC.[20] Therefore, all patients should be educated about the impact of chemotherapy on childbearing potential and offered fertility counseling. In addition, the use of gonadotropin-releasing hormone (GnRH) during cyto-toxic chemotherapy is associated with improved ovarian function preservation compared to placebo.[21]

Post-Therapy Surveillance

- Well-established guidelines for surveillance in the first 5 years after BC treatment are available through the NCCN.[12] Following treatment, patients should be evaluated for a history and physical exam 1 to 4 times annually for the first 5 years, then once annually thereafter. Annual mammography is recommended except in the case of mastectomy. For all surgical cases, but especially those involving axillary LN dissection, postsurgical monitoring for lymphedema should be incorporated into regular follow-up exams. In the absence of systemic signs or symptoms, routine imaging for metastasis and serological tumor marker revaluation are not recommended. Lastly, for patients who received anthracyclines, monitoring for late cardiac complications should be incorporated into routine practice.

Case 6.3: Metastatic Triple-Negative Breast Cancer

A 56-year-old woman presents to the clinic to establish care and discuss recent abnormal imaging. She considers herself healthy and has had minimal medical care, including age-recommended cancer screening. She was seen by a PCP 6 weeks earlier for a 1-month history of dry cough and increasing shortness of breath. She was prescribed a course of antibiotics with only modest improvement in symptoms. Workup included plain radiograph of the chest which revealed bilateral lung nodules. Subsequent CT scan of the chest showed diffuse bilateral lung nodules, suspicious hypodensities in the liver, and a 2-cm right breast mass with right axillary and supraclavicular adenopathy. She was subsequently referred to the oncology clinic where she reports persistent cough and fatigue. She can now palpate a right breast mass. The patient is adopted and unaware of her family history. On physical exam, a 2.5 cm × 2 cm mobile mass is palpated at the 10 o'clock position of the right breast with axillary adenopathy and a 1 cm right supraclavicular LN. The patient's lungs are clear and the remainder of her exam is unremarkable.

How Is a Diagnosis Established?

- In this patient with a suspicious, palpable breast mass, diagnostic mammogram and breast US are recommended. Furthermore, her symptoms, physical exam, and imaging studies raise suspicion for distant metastases. Core needle biopsy is indicated for suspicious (BI-RADS category 4) or highly suggestive (BI-RADS category 5) lesions on breast imaging. Given her presentation, further CT scan of her abdomen and pelvis and bone scan are recommended to evaluate the extent of disease. In cases where there is high suspicion of metastatic disease, biopsy of a metastatic lesion is recommended. Pathology will provide the histological diagnosis; tumor grade; and ER, PR, and HER2 status of the primary breast and metastatic lesion. A complete blood count and comprehensive metabolic profile, including liver function tests, are indicated.

How Is the Tumor Staged?

- Tumor staging is based on the AJCC eighth edition cancer staging system.[5] This includes anatomic staging based on tumor size (T), nodal involvement (N), and presence of distant metastases (M).

Patient's Diagnosis and Clinical Stage

- *Diagnostic mammogram and US reveal a 2.0-cm, heterogenous mass, with irregular borders in the right breast with a suspicious right axillary lymph node, a BI-RADS 5 study. Core biopsy reveals a grade 3 invasive mammary carcinoma not otherwise specified (NOS), with no staining for ER, PR, or HER2. FISH demonstrated no HER2 amplification. CT of the abdomen/pelvis reveals multiple liver lesions in both lobes and osseous metastases in the lumbar spine. Bone scan reveals uptake in the pubic ramus, left 7th to 9th ribs, and lumbar spine. She undergoes a CT-guided biopsy of a liver lesion confirming metastatic carcinoma, with no staining for ER, PR, or HER2.*
- *She has stage IV, T2N1M1, TNBC.*

What Further Molecular or Genomic Testing Is Required?

- TNBCs are enriched in *BRCA1* mutation carriers relative to the general population. Patients diagnosed with TNBC under the age of 60 should undergo genetic counseling and testing to determine germline *BRCA1/2* status. For metastatic TNBC, IHC staining for PD-L1 expression is recommended to determine eligibility for pembrolizumab in combination with chemotherapy. A tumor PD-L1 CPS of 10 or greater is considered positive.
- NCCN category 2A recommendations for all cancer subtypes may include tumor *NTRK* fusion, microsatellite instability/mismatch repair (*MSI-H/MMR*), and tumor mutational burden.
- Tumor next-generation sequencing (NGS) may identify therapeutic targets on a clinical trial.

Patient's BRCA and Tumor Status

- *No pathogenic mutations are detected in a panel of genes associated with hereditary BC, including BRCA1/2. Her tumor PD-L1 CPS is greater than 10.*

What Are Appropriate Treatment Options?

Systemic Therapy

- KEYNOTE-355 randomized patients with untreated metastatic TNBC to pembrolizumab or placebo in combination with chemotherapy (paclitaxel, nab-paclitaxel, or carboplatin/gemcitabine).[22] The median co-primary endpoint of progression-free survival (PFS) was 7.5 months in patients receiving pembrolizumab versus 5.6 months in the placebo arm in the intent-to-treat population. However, in patients with tumors with PD-L1

CPS of 10 or greater, mPFS was 9.7 months versus 5.6 months, respectively. Therefore, pembrolizumab has been FDA-approved for the first-line treatment of metastatic TNBC with PD-L1 CPS of 10 or greater.

- Sacituzumab govitecan is an antibody-drug conjugate, with an antibody targeting the human trophoblast cell-surface antigen 2 (Trop-2) linked to the topoisomerase I inhibiter SN-38. In the Phase III ASCENT trial, patients who had received two or more lines of therapy for metastatic TNBC were randomized to sacituzumab govitecan or single-agent chemotherapy of physician's choice, including eribulin, vinorelbine, capecitabine, or gem-citabine.[23] The primary endpoint of PFS was a median of 5.6 months in patients treated with sacituzumab govitecan versus 1.7 months with single-agent chemotherapy; OS was 12.1 months in the sacituzumab govitecan group versus 6.7 months. Sacituzumab is FDA-approved in patients with metastatic TNBC who have received at least two prior therapies.
- In patients whose tumors are not PD-L1–positive, or have progressed on first-line ther-apy, sequential cytotoxic chemotherapy including anthracyclines, taxanes, platinums, capecitabine, eribuin, and ixabepilone, among others, are used.
- In any case of metastatic TNBC, clinical trials should be considered.

Therapy for Patients With BRCA Germline Mutations

- Germline mutations in BRCA1/2 impair homologous recombination, which causes genetic instability. Researchers in the Phase III TNT trial[24] sought to exploit this unique characteristic by examining the use of platinum-containing agents in patients with met-astatic TNBC and among those who harbored a germline BRCA mutation. Because homologous recombination helps repair the DNA damage caused by platinum-contain-ing agents, it was theorized that a more robust response would be observed when using carboplatin compared to docetaxel. Among patients with a germline BRCA mutation, the primary endpoint of overall response rate (ORR) was significantly improved in the carboplatin arm versus the docetaxel arm (68% vs. 33%). Although this patient did not harbor a BRCA mutation, platinum therapy should be considered in patients with germ-line BRCA mutations.
- In addition, the PARP inhibitors olaparib and talazoparib have demonstrated improved PFS compared to single-agent chemotherapy of physician's choice in patients with germ-line BRCA mutations with previously treated, HER2- metastatic BC.[25,26]

What Are the Toxicities Associated With Systemic Therapies?

Cytotoxic chemotherapy is associated with cytopenias, including neutropenia, which may lead to rare fatal infections; anemia; and thrombocytopenia. Other side effects include alopecia, nausea and vomiting, constipation, diarrhea, mucositis, and cumulative fatigue, among others.

- Anthracyclines are associated with dose-related cardiotoxicity and rare secondary leuke-mias and myelodysplastic syndrome.
- Taxanes are associated with sensory neuropathy.
- Platinum-containing regimens may be nephrotoxic and increase neuropathy.

Toxicities of immunotherapy, such as pembrolizumab, include endocrinopathies, interstitial lung disease, dermatitis, hepatitis, and colitis, among others. Monitoring for endocrine com-plications include serum TSH/T4 at least every other cycle. Grading of adverse effects (AE) is specific to the organ system affected and outlined by NCCN guidelines.[27] For all immune-mediated AEs, grading is on a 1 to 4 scale, with grade 3 complications indicating consideration to discontinue treatment.

Sacituzumab govitecan is associated with neutropenia, sometimes severe. Prophylactic growth factors may be considered. Other side effects include diarrhea, nausea and vomiting, fatigue, and alopecia. There is an increased risk of toxicities in individuals with reduced uridine diphosphate-glucuronosyl transferase (UGT1A1) activity.

The PARP inhibitors olaparib and talazoparib can cause nausea and abdominal pain, anemia and leukopenia, fatigue, and mild liver function test abnormalities. Rarely, these agents are associated with venous thromboembolism, pneumonitis, and myelodysplastic syndrome or acute myeloid leukemia.

What Are Other Treatment Considerations?

Bone Metastases

- In patients with bone metastases, there is an established role for antiresorptive agents, such as bisphosphonates and denosumab, in addition to cancer-directed therapy to reduce skeletal related events, including bone pain, fractures, and need for radiation therapy. Treatment is typically every month. However, several trials have established the non-inferiority of an every 3 months schedule after the first year of monthly treatment versus continuing on a monthly schedule.[28,29,30] Currently, the NCCN panel recommends dosing monthly for 1 year, followed by every 12 weeks. Prior to initiating therapy, dental clearance is required. Lastly, for focal, symptomatic bone lesions, palliative radiation therapy can be considered.

Disease Monitoring

- Treatment of metastatic disease is not curative. Therefore, serial imaging to assess response to therapy every 2 to 3 cycles is recommended. Imaging may be more frequent if there are concerns for disease progression.

Patient's Treatment

- *The patient is started on first-line nab-paclitaxel and pembrolizumab. She has an excellent response before evidence of progressive disease 15 months later. Further therapeutic options include cytotoxic chemotherapy, the drug-antibody conjugate sacituzimab govitecan, and clinical trials. As she does not have a germline BRCA mutation, PARP inhibitors are not a treatment option.*

REVIEW QUESTIONS

1. Per American Society of Clinical Oncology/College of American Pathologists (ASCO/CAP) guidelines, which of the following immunohistochemistry (IHC) panels in an invasive carcinoma of the breast would be considered triple negative?
   A. Estrogen receptor (ER) 0, progesterone receptor (PR) 5%, human epidermal growth factor receptor 2 (HER2) 0
   B. ER 0, PR 0, HER2 1+
   C. ER 2%, PR 0, HER2 0
   D. ER less than 1%, PR less than 1%, HER2 2+

2. A 55-year-old woman has metastatic triple-negative breast cancer (TNBC). No pathogenic germline mutations were found on genetic testing. All of the following therapies can be potentially considered except:
   A. Sacituzumab govitecan
   B. Carboplatin
   C. Doxorubicin
   D. Talazoparib
   E. Paclitaxel

3. A 65-year-old healthy woman presents with a painless left breast mass. Imaging reveals a clinical T2 N0 lesion and breast biopsy confirms an intermediate-grade triple-negative breast cancer (TNBC). She is asymptomatic and her exam is unremarkable except for a mobile 3-cm breast mass. You are considering preoperative anthracycline and taxane-based chemotherapy. What else should you order at this time?
   A. CT scans of the chest, abdomen/pelvis, and bone scan
   B. Brain MRI
   C. Echocardiogram
   D. Baseline Cancer Antigen (CA) 15–3
   E. A and B

4. The patient in question #3 asks about the addition of carboplatin to neoadjuvant paclitaxel. Which of the following is true regarding the addition of carboplatin?
   A. Carboplatin improved the rates of pathological complete response (pCR)
   B. Carboplatin improved disease-free survival (DFS)
   C. Carboplatin improved overall survival (OS)
   D. A and B
   E. A, B, and C

5. A 60-year-old woman was diagnosed with metastatic, programmed death-ligand 1 (PD-L1)–positive triple-negative breast cancer (TNBC) a year ago. No pathogenic germline mutations were found on genetic testing. She has disease progression after 11 months of paclitaxel and pembrolizumab. What would you recommend next?
   A. Sacituzumab govitecan
   B. Eribulin
   C. Olaparib
   D. Nab-paclitaxel

6. A 63-year-old woman started preoperative pembrolizumab and nab-paclitaxel 2 months ago. She presents for treatment but is noted to be short of breath and her oxygen saturation

is 90% on room air. Her lungs are clear. Chest x-ray reveals increased bilateral interstitial markings. What should you do next?

A. Proceed with paclitaxel and pembrolizumab and add steroids
B. Proceed with paclitaxel and pembrolizumab and start antibiotics
C. Hold paclitaxel and pembrolizumab
D. Hold paclitaxel and pembrolizumab and add steroids

7. A 53-year-old woman with a germline *BRCA2* mutation and metastatic triple-negative breast cancer (TNBC) presents to discuss treatment options for disease progression. She had previously received carboplatin and paclitaxel and most recently doxorubicin. Which of the following treatments would you recommend?

A. Olaparib
B. Vinorelbine
C. Eribulin
D. Capecitabine

8. A 61-year-old healthy woman was diagnosed with a left clinical stage III triple-negative breast cancer (TNBC). At that time, no pathogenic germline mutations were found on genetic testing. She receives preoperative weekly paclitaxel followed by doxorubicin and cyclophosphamide. She undergoes left mastectomy and axillary lymph node dissection (ALND), revealing a residual 1-cm tumor and two of eight axillary lymph nodes (LNs) with metastatic deposits. What do you recommend next?

A. Carboplatin × 4 cycles
B. Pembrolizumab × 1 year
C. Olaparib × 1 year
D. Capecitabine × 8 cycles

ANSWERS AND RATIONALES

1. **B. ER 0, PR 0, HER2 1+.** Per ASCO/CAP guidelines, triple-negative breast cancers (TNBCs) stain less than 1% each for ERs and PRs. HER2- tumors stain 0 or 1+ by IHC, or are HER2 equivocal by IHC 2+ and not *HER2* amplified.

2. **D. Talazoparib.** Poly adenosine diphosphate-ribose polymerase (PARP) inhibitors are only approved for metastatic, human epidermal growth factor receptor 2 (HER2)- breast cancer (BC) in individuals with germline *BRCA1/2* mutations. The other therapies are all potential future therapeutic options.

3. **C. Echocardiogram.** In the absence of symptoms or physical signs, patients with early-stage breast cancer (BC) do not need staging to rule out metastatic disease. Tumor markers in early-stage disease are not indicated. As the patient is 65 years old and will be receiving anthracyclines, a baseline echocardiogram is warranted.

4. **A. Carboplatin improved the rates of pathologic complete response (pCR).** In two Phase II trials, the addition of carboplatin to paclitaxel improved pCR, but the trials were not powered to detect differences in DFS or OS with the addition of carboplatin to preoperative therapy.

5. **B. Eribulin.** Sacituzumab govitecan is U.S. Food and Drug Administration (FDA)-approved in patients with metastatic TNBC after two or more lines of therapy. Olaparib is not indicated as she does not have a *BRCA* mutation. Nab-paclitaxel is not expected to have activity in a patient who has disease progression with paclitaxel.

6. **D. Hold paclitaxel and pembrolizumab and add steroids.** The patient has symptomatic pneumonitis, likely from pembrolizumab. Therefore, treatment should be held and the patient should receive steroids.

7. **A. Olaparib.** The OlympiAD trial demonstrated improved progression-free survival (PFS) with olaparib versus physician's treatment of choice of single-agent vinorelbine, eribulin, or capecitabine in patients previously treated for metastatic, human epidermal growth factor receptor 2 (HER2)- breast cancer (BC) who carried a germline *BRCA1/2* mutation.

8. **D. Capecitabine × 8 cycles.** The CREATE-X trial randomized patients with residual human epidermal growth factor receptor 2 (HER2)- breast cancer (BC) after standard neoadjuvant therapy to 8 cycles of capecitabine or usual care. Patients receiving capecitabine had improved progression-free survival (PFS). There is no current benefit to adjuvant carboplatin or to adjuvant pembrolizumab alone. As the patient does not have a germline *BRCA1/2* mutation, adjuvant olaparib is not indicated.

REFERENCES

1. Allison KH, Hammond MEH, Dowsett M, et al. Estrogen and progesterone receptor testing in breast cancer: ASCO/CAP guideline update. *J Clin Oncol.* 2020;38(12):1346–1366. doi:10.1200/JCO.19.02309
2. Wolff AC, Hammond MEH, Allison KH, et al. Human epidermal growth factor receptor 2 testing in breast cancer: American Society of Clinical Oncology/College of American Pathologists clinical practice guideline focused update. *J Clin Oncol.* 2018;36(20):2105–2122. doi:10.1200/JCO.2018.77.8738
3. Surveillance, Epidemiology, and End Results Program. Cancer stat facts: female breast cancer. National Cancer Institute. https://seer.cancer.gov/statfacts/html/breast.html
4. D'Orsi CJSE, Mendelson EB, Morris EA, et al. *ACR BI-RADS® Atlas: Breast Imaging Reporting and Data System.* 5th ed. American College of Radiology; 2013.

5. Giuliano AE, Edge SB, Hortobagyi GN. Eighth edition of the AJCC cancer staging manual: breast cancer. *Ann Surg Oncol.* 2018;25(7):1783–1785. doi:10.1245/s10434-018-6486-6

6. Daly MB, Pilarski R, Axilbund JE, et al. Genetic/familial high-risk assessment: breast and ovarian, version 1.2014. *J Natl Compr Canc Netw.* 2014;12(9):1326–1338. doi:10.6004/jnccn.2014.0127

7. Tutt AN, Garber JE, Kaufman B, et al. Adjuvant olaparib for patients with *BRCA1*- or *BRCA2*-mutated breast cancer. *N Engl J Med.* 2021;384(25):2394–2405. doi:10.1056/NEJMoa2105215

8. Fisher B, Wolmark N, Redmond C, Deutsch M, Fisher ER. Findings from NSABP Protocol No. B-04: comparison of radical mastectomy with alternative treatments. II. The clinical and biologic significance of medial-central breast cancers. *Cancer.* 1981;48(8):1863–1872. doi:10.1002/1097-0142(19811015)48:8<1863::aid-cncr2820480825>3.0.co;2-u

9. Rastogi P, Anderson SJ, Bear HD, et al. Preoperative chemotherapy: updates of national surgical adjuvant breast and bowel project protocols B-18 and B-27. *J Clin Oncol.* 2008;26(5):778–785. doi:10.1200/JCO.2007.15.0235

10. Blum JL, Flynn PJ, Yothers G, et al. Anthracyclines in early breast cancer: the ABC trials—USOR 06-090, NSABP B-46-I/USOR 07132, and NSABP B-49 (NRG Oncology). *J Clin Oncol.* 2017;35(23):2647–2655. doi:10.1200/JCO.2016.71.4147

11. Nitz U, Gluz O, Clemens M, et al. West German study planB trial: adjuvant four cycles of epirubicin and cyclophosphamide plus docetaxel versus six cycles of docetaxel and cyclophosphamide in HER2-negative early breast cancer. *J Clin Oncol.* 2019;37(10):799–808. doi:10.1200/JCO.18.00028

12. Tevaarwerk A, Denlinger CS, Sanft T, et al. Survivorship, version 1.2021. *J Natl Compr Canc Netw.* 2021;19(6):676–685. doi:10.6004/jnccn.2021.0028

13. Katipamula R, Degnim AC, Hoskin T, et al. Trends in mastectomy rates at the Mayo Clinic Rochester: effect of surgical year and preoperative magnetic resonance imaging. *J Clin Oncol.* 2009;27(25):4082–4088. doi:10.1200/JCO.2008.19.4225

14. Gralow JR, Burstein HJ, Wood W, et al. Preoperative therapy in invasive breast cancer: pathologic assessment and systemic therapy issues in operable disease. *J Clin Oncol.* 2008;26(5):814–819. doi:10.1200/JCO.2007.15.3510

15. Sikov WM, Berry DA, Perou CM, et al. Impact of the addition of carboplatin and/or bevacizumab to neo-adjuvant once-per-week paclitaxel followed by dose-dense doxorubicin and cyclophosphamide on pathologic complete response rates in stage II to III triple-negative breast cancer: CALGB 40603 (Alliance). *J Clin Oncol.* 2015;33(1):13–21. doi:10.1200/JCO.2014.57.0572

16. von Minckwitz G, Schneeweiss A, Loibl S, et al. Neoadjuvant carboplatin in patients with triple-negative and HER2-positive early breast cancer (GeparSixto; GBG 66): a randomised phase 2 trial. *Lancet Oncol.* 2014;15(7):747–756. doi:10.1016/S1470-2045(14)70160-3

17. Schmid P, Cortés J, Dent R, et al. KEYNOTE-522: phase III study of pembrolizumab (pembro) + chemotherapy (chemo) vs placebo + chemo as neoadjuvant therapy followed by pembro vs placebo as adjuvant therapy for triple-negative breast cancer (TNBC). *J Clin Oncol.* 2018;36(15_suppl):TPS602. doi:10.1200/JCO.2018.36.15_suppl.TPS602

18. Deutsch M, Land S, Begovic M, Sharif S. The incidence of arm edema in women with breast cancer randomized on the national surgical adjuvant breast and bowel project study B-04 to radical mastectomy versus total mastectomy and radiotherapy versus total mastectomy alone. *Int J Radiat Oncol Biol Phys.* 2008;70(4):1020–1024. doi:10.1016/j.ijrobp.2007.07.2376

19. Masuda N, Lee S-J, Ohtani S, et al. Adjuvant capecitabine for breast cancer after preoperative chemotherapy. *N Engl J Med.* 2017;376(22):2147–2159. doi:10.1056/NEJMoa1612645

20. Kranick JA, Schaefer C, Rowell C, et al. Is pregnancy after breast cancer safe? *Breast J.* 2010;16(4):404–411. doi:10.1111/j.1524-4741.2010.00939.x

21. Moore HC, Unger JM, Phillips K-A, et al. Goserelin for ovarian protection during breast-cancer adjuvant chemotherapy. *N Engl J Med.* 2015;372(10):923–932. doi:10.1056/NEJMoa1413204

22. Cortes J, Cescon DW, Rugo HS, et al. Pembrolizumab plus chemotherapy versus placebo plus chemotherapy for previously untreated locally recurrent inoperable or metastatic triple-negative breast cancer (KEYNOTE-355): a randomised, placebo-controlled, double-blind, phase 3 clinical trial. *Lancet.* 2020;396(10265):1817–1828. doi:10.1016/S0140-6736(20)32531-9

23. Bardia A, Hurvitz SA, Tolaney SM, et al. Sacituzumab govitecan in metastatic triple-negative breast cancer. *N Engl J Med.* 2021;384(16):1529–1541. doi:10.1056/NEJMoa2028485

24. Tutt A, Tovey H, Cheang MCU, et al. Carboplatin in *BRCA1/2*-mutated and triple-negative breast cancer BRCAness subgroups: The TNT trial. *Nat Med.* 2018;24(5):628–637. doi:10.1038/s41591-018-0009-7

25. Robson ME, Tung N, Conte P, et al. OlympiAD final overall survival and tolerability results: olaparib versus chemotherapy treatment of physician's choice in patients with a germline *BRCA* mutation and HER2-negative metastatic breast cancer. *Ann Oncol.* 2019;30(4):558–566. doi:10.1093/annonc/mdz012

26. Litton JK, Rugo HS, Ettl J, et al. Talazoparib in patients with advanced breast cancer and a germline *BRCA* mutation. *N Engl J Med.* 2018;379(8):753–763. doi:10.1056/NEJMoa1802905

27. Thompson JA, Schneider BJ, Brahmer J, et al. NCCN guidelines insights: management of immunotherapy-related toxicities, version 1.2020. *J Natl Compr Canc Netw.* 2020;18(3):230–241. doi:10.6004/jnccn.2020.0012

28. Amadori D, Aglietta M, Alessi B, et al. Efficacy and safety of 12-weekly versus 4-weekly zoledronic acid for prolonged treatment of patients with bone metastases from breast cancer (ZOOM): a phase 3, open-label, randomised, non-inferiority trial. *Lancet Oncol.* 2013;14(7):663–670. doi:10.1016/S1470-2045(13)70174-8

29. Himelstein AL, Qin R, Novotny PJ, et al. CALGB 70604 (Alliance): a randomized phase III study of standard dosing vs. longer interval dosing of zoledronic acid in metastatic cancer. *J Clin Oncol.* 2015;33(15_suppl):9501. doi:10.1200/jco.2015.33.15_suppl.9501

30. Hortobagyi GN, Van Poznak C, Harker WG, et al. Continued treatment effect of zoledronic acid dosing every 12 vs 4 weeks in women with breast cancer metastatic to bone: the OPTIMIZE-2 randomized clinical trial. *JAMA Oncol.* 2017;3(7):906–912. doi:10.1001/jamaoncol.2016.6316

CHAPTER 7

Esophageal Cancer

Kamya Sankar, Charles B. Nguyen, and Bryan J. Schneider

INTRODUCTION

Esophageal cancer is the eighth most common cancer diagnosed worldwide and the sixth most common cause of cancer-related death. In the United States, there are 19,260 new cases annually, and 15,530 deaths from esophageal cancer, representing 2.6% of cancer-related deaths.[1] Despite advances in staging modalities and treatment, esophageal cancer continues to be associated with a high mortality rate.

The esophagus is divided into thirds: upper, middle, and lower (Figure 7.1). The American Joint Committee on Cancer (AJCC) further classifies the esophagus into regions based on distance from the upper incisors. The cervical esophagus is 15 to 20 cm from the incisors (level of the sternal notch). The upper thoracic esophagus is 20 to 25 cm from the incisors. The middle thoracic esophagus is defined as being 25 to 30 cm from the incisors. The lower thoracic esophagus is 30 cm from the incisors to the gastroesophageal junction.

There are two main histological subtypes of esophageal cancer: squamous cell carcinoma (SCC) and adenocarcinoma. Esophageal adenocarcinoma is the most common subtype in the United States and the Western world, and incidence has increased dramatically due to risk factors such as higher body mass index (BMI) and incidence of gastroesophageal reflux disease (GERD).[2] SCC remains the most common histological subtype worldwide but has decreased in incidence due to a reduction in alcohol and tobacco consumption.

Risk Factors

The risk factors for adenocarcinoma of the esophagus include GERD and Barrett's esophagus, with an annual 1% risk of progression from Barrett's esophagus to adenocarcinoma. Obesity is an independent risk factor for development of esophageal adenocarcinoma (relative risk of 1.7 for patients with BMI 25 to 30 kg/m², and increasing to 2.34 for those with BMI of 30 kg/m² or more).[3] Smoking increases the risk for esophageal adenocarcinoma, particularly in patients with Barrett's esophagus (relative risk 2.08 compared to nonsmokers), a risk that was found not to decrease over time after smoking cessation.[4] The strongest risk factors for SCC are alcohol and tobacco consumption. Other relatively rare predisposing conditions are longstanding achalasia, esophageal webs, tylosis, and human papillomavirus.

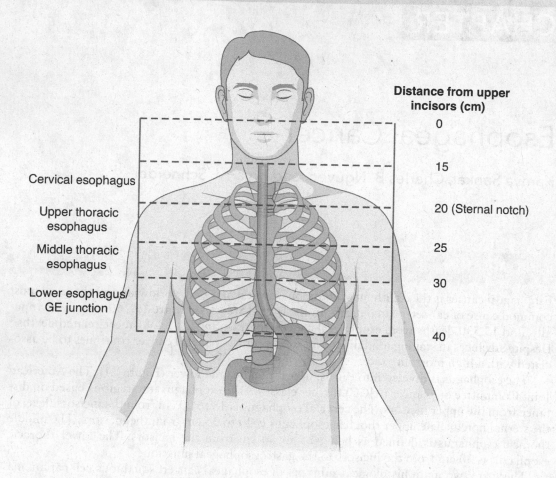

Figure 7.1 Anatomic classification of the esophagus.

Source: Adapted from Amin MB, Edge SB, Greene FL, et al, eds. *AJCC Cancer Staging Manual.* 8th ed. Springer Nature; 2017.

Clinical Presentation

Dysphagia and weight loss are the most common presenting symptoms of esophageal cancer. Swallowing difficulties are typically worse with meat and breads, and often progress to dysphagia with soft foods and liquids, which is typically when patients seek medical attention. Pain may also occur with swallowing. Anemia secondary to chronic gastrointestinal (GI) blood loss or frank GI bleeding can also be the first sign of esophageal cancer. Rarely, patients may present with cough or signs of aspiration, which may indicate a tracheoesophageal fistula.

Staging

The AJCC staging in the most recent (2017, eighth edition) revision includes tumors involving the esophagogastric junction (EGJ) with the tumor epicenter no more than 2 cm into the proximal stomach. Those with more than 2 cm into the proximal stomach are staged as gastric cancer. Regardless of histology and location in the esophagus, those with an epicenter within 2 cm of the EGJ share the same criteria for tumor size (T), nodal involvement (N), and metastases (M) designation (Table 7.1).[5] The prognostic stage then differs according to histology and time of staging (clinical vs. pathological vs. pathological post neoadjuvant therapy; Table 7.2).[5]

Table 7.1   Cancer Staging Categories for Cancer of the Esophagus and Esophagogastric Junction (AJCC Eighth Edition)

TNM	Description
Primary Tumor (T)	
T1	Tumor invades lamina propria (T1a), muscularis mucosae (T1a), or submucosa (T1b)
T2	Tumor invades muscularis propria
T3	Tumor invades adventitia
T4	Tumor invades adjacent structures
T4a	Resectable tumor invades pleura, pericardium, or diaphragm
T4b	Unresectable tumor invades adjacent structures such as aorta, vertebral body, trachea, etc.
Regional Lymph Nodes (N)	
N1	Metastasis in 1–2 regional LNs
N2	Metastasis in 3–6 regional LNs
N3	Metastasis in 7 or more regional LNs
Distant Metastasis (M)	
M0	No distant metastasis
M1	Distant metastasis

AJCC, American Joint Committee on Cancer; LNs, lymph nodes

Source: Data from Amin MB, Edge SB, Greene FL, et al, eds. *AJCC Cancer Staging Manual.* 8th ed. Springer Nature; 2017.

CASE SUMMARIES

Case 7.1: Locally Advanced, Resectable Esophageal Adenocarcinoma

A 62-year-old man with a history of 25 pack-years of tobacco use, GERD, and Barrett's esophagus presented for evaluation of dysphagia. He previously underwent endoscopic surveillance for Barrett's esophagus 2 years ago which showed low-grade dysplasia. He now reported progressive dysphagia to mostly solid foods, 10-pound unintentional weight loss, but no nausea, vomiting, hematemesis, or melena. The physical exam was notable for mild cachexia, no lymphadenopathy, and a normal abdominal exam. A barium swallow was obtained which identified a distal esophageal mass without complete obstruction.

How Is Esophageal Adenocarcinoma Diagnosed?

- Esophagogastroduodenoscopy (EGD) is the primary diagnostic modality which allows for direct biopsy and pathological analysis of the tumor.

Case Update
- An EGD was subsequently performed with biopsy of the mass revealing adenocarcinoma in the lower third of the esophagus, 38 cm from the incisors.

What Additional Workup Is Needed?

- A CT of the chest, abdomen, and pelvis with oral and intravenous (IV) contrast is the preferred initial imaging modality to exclude distant metastases (M1).

Table 7.2 Clinical (cTNM) Stage Groups per AJCC/UICC Eighth Edition Staging Manual for Esophagus and Esophagogastric Junction Cancers

Stage	T	N	M
Squamous Cell Carcinoma			
0	Tis	N0	M0
I	T1	N0-1	M0
II	T2	N0-1	M0
	T3	N0	M0
III	T3	N1	M0
	T1-3	N2	M0
IVA	T4	N0-2	M0
	T1-4	N3	M0
IVB	T1-4	N0-3	M1
Adenocarcinoma			
0	Tis	N0	M0
I	T1	N0	M0
IIA	T1	N1	M0
IIB	T2	N0	M0
III	T2	N1	M0
	T3-4a	N0-1	M0
IVA	T1-4a	N2	M0
	T4b	N0-2	M0
	T1-4	N3	M0
IVB	T1-4	N0-3	M1

AJCC, American Joint Committee on Cancer; M, metastases; N, nodal involvement; T, tumor size; UICC, Union for International Cancer Control.

Source: Data from Amin MB, Edge SB, Greene FL, et al, eds. *AJCC Cancer Staging Manual.* 8th ed. Springer Nature; 2017.

- Fluorodeoxyglucose (FDG)-PET/CT is strongly preferred if initial imaging is negative for M1 disease due to increased sensitivity in detecting distant lesions.
- In patients without distant metastases, endoscopic ultrasound (EUS) is also recommended to assess for tumor depth and locoregional LN involvement.

Case Update

- CT of the chest, abdomen, and pelvis showed mural thickening of the distal esophagus proximal to the gastroesophageal junction. No pulmonary nodules or enlarged LNs were visualized. FDG-PET/CT revealed an FDG-avid distal esophageal mass but no evidence of local LN involvement or distant metastases. EUS staging: T3N0M0.

What Is the Patient's Clinical Stage Per the AJCC Eighth Edition Criteria?

- Stage II

What Is the General Treatment Modality for Locally Advanced Esophageal Adenocarcinoma Defined as Clinical Stage T3-4a or any Regional Node-Positive Disease?

- A multimodal approach with neoadjuvant chemotherapy and radiation (chemoradiotherapy; CRT) followed by esophagectomy is preferred in a patient who has good performance status and is a candidate for surgery.
- The preferred neoadjuvant chemotherapy regimen is carboplatin combined with paclitaxel. In the CROSS trial, patients with esophageal or gastroesophageal junction cancer (adenocarcinoma was the predominant histology among patients being studied) were randomized to neoadjuvant carboplatin and paclitaxel with concurrent radiation therapy followed by esophagectomy (trimodal therapy) versus surgery alone. The median survival for patients receiving neoadjuvant CRT plus surgery was 49.4 months compared to 24 months in patients treated with surgery alone.[6] Additionally, patients who received trimodal therapy had lower rates of recurrence.[7] After completion of CRT, restaging FDG-PET/CT may be obtained to assess treatment response. If imaging reveals stable disease or treatment response, the patient can proceed directly to esophagectomy.
- If a complete surgical resection is achieved, adjuvant therapy with nivolumab for 12 months is recommended for patients who do not have a complete pathological response based on the results of the Phase III CheckMate-577 trial. Patients with resected (R0) locally advanced esophageal adenocarcinoma who had received neoadjuvant CRT and had residual pathological disease identified in the resected esophagus and/or regional LNs were randomized to 12 months of adjuvant nivolumab or placebo. A significant improvement in median disease-free survival was identified in patients who received adjuvant nivolumab (22.4 vs. 11 months, hazard ratio [HR] 0.69, 95% confidence interval [CI] 0.56 to 0.86, p less than 0.001).[8] No adjuvant therapy is recommended presently if the patient achieves a complete pathological response post-resection.
- Perioperative chemotherapy with fluorouracil, leucovorin, oxaliplatin, and docetaxel (FLOT) may be an alternative strategy to neoadjuvant CRT. In the FLOT4 trial, patients were randomized to receive 3 cycles of epirubicin, cisplatin, and fluorouracil (ECF) before and after surgery or FLOT for 4 cycles pre- and post-resection. This Phase III trial demonstrated a superior median overall survival (OS) in patients receiving FLOT (50 months) compared to ECF (35 months).[9] However, FLOT was associated with a higher rate of grade 3 and 4 infections, diarrhea, and neuropathy compared to ECF. Thus, FLOT is not administered with concurrent radiation therapy but may be considered perioperatively in patients who cannot receive radiotherapy.
- If a patient underwent an R0 esophagectomy without neoadjuvant therapy for locally advanced adenocarcinoma, postoperative therapy with fluorouracil, leucovorin, and concurrent radiation therapy is recommended.[10] In the INT-0116 trial, patients with T3+ or node-positive disease who received fluorouracil, leucovorin, and radiation following R0 resection were noted to have improved OS and relapse-free survival compared to observation alone (median OS 36 vs. 27 months, HR 1.35, 95% CI 1.05 to 1.66, $p = 0.005$).[11]
- A nonsurgical approach with combined chemotherapy and radiation therapy can be considered in patients who are poor surgical candidates or do not have access to an experienced thoracic surgeon. A higher dose of radiation (50.4 Gy) is typically given in combination with platinum/5-fluorouracil (FU)–based chemotherapy. However, there is limited data comparing definitive chemoradiation with trimodal therapy.

Case Update
- After discussing the treatment options with his oncologist, the patient preferred to undergo neoadjuvant CRT with carboplatin, paclitaxel, and radiation therapy.

Post-CRT FDG-PET/CT revealed an interval reduction in the size of the esophageal mass. He subsequently underwent an esophagectomy with negative surgical margins (R0) and on pathological review, residual disease in the resected esophagus (ypT2) was identified. The patient recovers well from his surgery and was started on nivolumab for adjuvant therapy.

What Surveillance Should the Patient Now Be On?

- Close clinical follow-up and monitoring for symptoms of progression should be done after completion of therapy. CT imaging and endoscopy can be performed as clinically indicated.
- The role of serum tumor markers in surveillance of esophageal cancer has not been defined and is not recommended.

Case 7.2: Locally Advanced Esophageal Squamous Cell Carcinoma

A 72-year-old female with medical history notable for hypertension and prior chronic alcohol use, with a good performance status presented with 7 months of early satiety and excessive belching. She denied dysphagia, odynophagia, or weight loss. A CT of the abdomen/pelvis revealed circumferential thickening of the distal esophagus. An FDG-PET/CT showed hypermetabolic uptake in the distal esophageal mass and mediastinal adenopathy but no distant metastases. EUS identified a tumor extending into the adventitia and three abnormal para-esophageal LNs (clinical stage III, T3N2M0), the biopsy of which revealed SCC.

What Is the General Treatment Approach for Locally Advanced Squamous Cell Carcinoma of the Lower Esophagus?

- Locally advanced, resectable SCC of the lower esophagus is managed similarly to locally advanced esophageal adenocarcinoma. As mentioned earlier, neoadjuvant carboplatin, paclitaxel, and concurrent radiation followed by esophagectomy (trimodal therapy) is the preferred approach for locally advanced esophageal adenocarcinoma based on the CROSS trial. The results of this trial are also applicable to locally advanced esophageal SCC as approximately 23% of cases included in the study were SCC. Patients with SCC who received trimodal therapy had an increased rate of achieving pathological complete response at the time of surgery (49%) compared to patients with adenocarcinoma (23%).[6] Thus, patients with SCC of the lower esophagus should undergo neoadjuvant CRT with carboplatin/paclitaxel. An interval re-staging FDG-PET/CT may be obtained after completing CRT and prior to proceeding with esophagectomy.
- Adjuvant therapy recommendations for SCC of the lower esophagus are similar to adenocarcinoma. Following CRT and esophagectomy, patients should receive 12 months of adjuvant nivolumab if a complete pathological response is not attained based on the CheckMate-577 trial.[8]
- Unlike locally advanced esophageal adenocarcinoma, there are no data to support perioperative chemotherapy for locally advanced esophageal SCC.

Case 7.3: Locally Advanced Cervical Esophageal Squamous Cell Carcinoma

A 71-year-old man with prior tobacco use and coronary artery disease presented with several months of dysphagia and difficulty swallowing his medications. He described a sensation of pills being stuck in his upper throat associated with nausea. The patient reported no vomiting, regurgitation, or weight loss. He underwent an EGD which identified diffuse mucosal changes in the upper esophagus above the suprasternal notch with mild luminal narrowing. Biopsy revealed poorly differentiated SCC. Staging CT and FDG-PET/CT scans showed no evidence of distant metastasis. EUS staging demonstrated two abnormal paratracheal LNs (EUS clinical stage III: T3N1M0). The patient had a good performance status and presented to the oncology clinic to discuss treatment options.

How Is Squamous Cell Carcinoma of the Cervical Esophagus Managed?

- Cervical esophageal SCC is managed differently than SCC of the middle and lower esophagus. As discussed earlier, treatment for locally advanced esophageal SCC includes neoadjuvant CRT, followed by esophagectomy and adjuvant nivolumab (if pathological residual disease is identified at the time of surgery). In contrast, cervical esophageal SCC is managed similarly to SCC of the head and neck with definitive CRT only. Surgery is not recommended as R0 resection is difficult to achieve due to anatomic limitations and decreased quality of life outcomes. Along with concurrent radiation therapy, chemotherapy options for cervical esophageal SCC include carboplatin with paclitaxel or fluorouracil with either oxaliplatin or cisplatin.

Case 7.4: Metastatic Esophageal Adenocarcinoma

An 81-year-old veteran with past medical history notable for hypertension, atrial fibrillation, and GERD presented to his primary care physician (PCP) with 6 months of dysphagia, unintentional 30-lb weight loss, and fatigue. On examination, he had conjunctival pallor, anicteric sclera, and mild tenderness to palpation in the epigastric region. Bloodwork revealed a hemoglobin of 10.1 mg/dL and a mild transaminitis. CT scan of the chest, abdomen, and pelvis was ordered in addition to a gastroenterology referral for endoscopy.

At the time of endoscopy, the patient was found to have circumferential narrowing at the distal esophagus with a friable and ulcerated mass. Biopsies were taken and showed a well-differentiated adenocarcinoma. The CT scan demonstrated a 5 × 6 cm mass at the distal esophagus, and three low-attenuating hypodense lesions in the liver, measuring up to 1.2 cm. An ultrasound (US)-guided liver biopsy confirmed metastatic esophageal adenocarcinoma. He had an Eastern Cooperative Oncology Group (ECOG) performance status of 1.

What Molecular or Genomic Testing Is Required?

- For all patients with inoperable locally advanced, recurrent, or metastatic adenocarcinoma of the esophagus or EGJ, the following biomarkers should be tested:
  - Assessment for human epidermal growth factor receptor 2 (*HER2*) overexpression using immunohistochemistry (IHC). Fluorescent in situ hybridization (FISH) or other in situ hybridization methods are used if IHC yields equivocal results.
  - Testing for microsatellite instability (MSI) by polymerase chain reaction (PCR) or mismatch repair (MMR) testing by IHC for those who are candidates for treatment with PD-1 inhibitors.
  - PD-L1 testing should be performed in locally advanced (when not a candidate for local therapies such as surgery or definitive concurrent CRT), recurrent, or metastatic esophageal or EGJ cancers for patients who are candidates for treatment with PD-1 inhibitors with or without chemotherapy. The PD-L1 combined positive score (CPS) has been shown to be predictive of response to PD-1 inhibitors in esophageal, EGJ, and gastric cancers.

Case Update
- The patient's diagnostic biopsy was sent for molecular testing and revealed: PD-L1 CPS 5%, HER2-, microsatellite stable.

What Are the Appropriate Frontline Treatment Options for Metastatic Esophageal Adenocarcinoma?

- Determination of treatment for a patient with metastatic esophageal cancer begins with a discussion between the physician and patient regarding goals of care. The patient must understand that the disease is incurable, and therefore any offered treatment is with the intention of improving symptoms (that is, malignant dysphagia), improve quality of life, and prolong survival.
- Many studies have demonstrated the significant survival benefit with use of palliative systemic chemotherapy as compared to supportive care alone in the treatment of metastatic esophageal cancer.
- *Chemotherapy.* The first-line therapy for metastatic esophageal adenocarcinoma[12,13] includes two drug combinations with platinum (cisplatin or oxaliplatin) along with fluoropyrimidine (infusional 5-FU or capecitabine). Other chemotherapy agents which have been studied and known to have activity in esophageal cancer include taxanes (paclitaxel and docetaxel) and irinotecan.
  - Several randomized Phase III trials have directly compared oxaliplatin-containing regimens with cisplatin-containing regimens, and all have shown comparable efficacy when oxaliplatin is substituted for cisplatin in two or three drug combination regimens in patients with unresectable locally advanced or metastatic esophagogastric cancer. Further, a meta-analysis including three of these trials showed that oxaliplatin-based regimens when compared to cisplatin-containing regimens were associated with improved progression-free survival (PFS) and OS, while having less myelosuppression and alopecia but with more neurotoxicity and diarrhea.
  - Therefore, oxaliplatin has become the most commonly used platinum agent in combination chemotherapy regimens for advanced esophagogastric cancers.
  - Three drug combination chemotherapy regimens that are typically not recommended as trials have shown two drug regimens achieve similar efficacy with less toxicity. For example, in the CALGB 80403 study, a randomized Phase II trial comparing ECF with FOLFOX, both arms in combination with cetuximab concluded similar response rates, PFS, and OS, in both regimens.[14]
  - Based on these data, FOLFOX (infusional 5-FU with leucovorin and oxaliplatin) or CapeOX (capecitabine and oxaliplatin) are the most commonly used combination chemotherapy regimens in the frontline setting for patients with metastatic esophageal cancer who are candidates for cytotoxic chemotherapy.
- *Immunotherapy*: Several clinical trials have evaluated the use of immune checkpoint inhibitors alone or in combination with chemotherapy in the frontline setting in different populations of patients with esophageal cancer.
  - Based on results from KEYNOTE-590, pembrolizumab in combination with platinum and fluoropyrimidine-based chemotherapy was approved for patients with metastatic or locally advanced esophageal or EGJ cancer who are not candidates for surgical resection or definitive chemoradiation in March 2021.
    - In KEYNOTE-590, a Phase III placebo-controlled randomized trial, patients with previously untreated locally advanced, unresectable, or metastatic esophageal cancer were randomly assigned to pembrolizumab or placebo in combination with 5-FU/cisplatin chemotherapy. All primary endpoints were met including a significant improvement in PFS (median PFS 6.3 vs. 5.8 months, HR 0.65, 95% CI 0.55 to 0.76, p less than 0.0001) and OS (median OS 12.4 vs. 9.8 months, HR 0.73, 95% CI 0.62 to 0.86, p less than 0.0001) in all randomized patients in the pembrolizumab group.[15]

- ○ Based on the results of CheckMate-649, nivolumab in combination with 5-FU/platinum-based chemotherapy was approved for the frontline treatment of metastatic or unresectable locally advanced esophagogastric adenocarcinoma irrespective of PD-L1 expression in April 2021.
  - In CheckMate-649, patients with treatment-naive HER2- advanced/unresectable or metastatic gastric, EGJ, or esophageal adenocarcinoma were randomly assigned to nivolumab plus chemotherapy or chemotherapy alone (oxaliplatin plus either leucovorin plus infusional 5-FU or capecitabine). This study met its primary endpoint of significantly improving median PFS and OS in the subset of patients with PD-L1 CPS of 5 or greater (median PFS 7.7 vs. 6.0 months, HR 0.68, 98% CI 0.56 to 0.81, p less than 0.0001; median OS 14.4 vs. 11.1 months, HR 0.71, 98% CI 0.59 to 0.86, p less than 0.0001).[16] The OS benefit was also seen when all CPS groups were combined, but there was no OS benefit seen in those patients with CPS less than 1.
  - Therefore, though nivolumab has been approved in combination with a fluoropyrimidine and platinum-containing regimen for metastatic gastric or gastroesophageal junction cancer and esophageal adenocarcinoma irrespective of PD-L1 CPS, the study results suggest that the benefits of immunotherapy in combination with chemotherapy have not been established in the PD-L1 CPS less than 1 group.

Case Update: Recommended Treatment Plan
- Patient initiated treatment with nivolumab 360 mg IV on day 1, oxaliplatin 130 mg/m² on day 1, and capecitabine 1000 mg/m² PO BID on days 1 to 14, given every 21 days.

What Are Toxicities to Consider With Systemic Chemoimmunotherapy in Metastatic Esophageal Adenocarcinoma?

- Nivolumab can be associated with fatigue, infusion-related reactions, and immune-related toxicities including rash, diarrhea/colitis, thyroiditis, hepatitis, hypophysitis, and pneumonitis. Rare immune-mediated toxicities include acute kidney injury, myocarditis, autoimmune hemolytic anemia, red cell aplasia, encephalitis, and myasthenia gravis.
- Fluoropyrimidine chemotherapeutic agents are associated with fatigue, myelosuppression, nausea, mucositis, diarrhea, and hand–foot syndrome.
- Oxaliplatin is associated with nausea, neuropathy, myelosuppression, and nephrotoxicity.

What Are Second-Line Treatment Options for Patients With Metastatic Esophageal Adenocarcinoma Who Progress on Frontline Chemotherapy or Chemoimmunotherapy?

- If patients have not previously received immunotherapy:
  - ○ <u>Second-line</u>: Pembrolizumab may be offered to patients whose tumors demonstrate MSI-H, dMMR, or tumor mutational burden (TMB) high (10 mutations/megabase).
- If patient has previously received and progressed on immunotherapy:
  - ○ <u>Second-line</u>: Ramucirumab (adenocarcinoma only) with or without paclitaxel, docetaxel, paclitaxel, irinotecan with or without ramucirumab (adenocarcinoma only), or fluorouracil with irinotecan.
  - ○ <u>Third-line</u>: Trifluridine and tipiracil may be used as third-line or subsequent therapy for EGJ adenocarcinoma.

- If next-generation sequencing (NGS) has been performed, patients with *NTRK* gene fusion are candidates for treatment with entrectinib or larotrectinib.

Case 7.5: Human Epidermal Growth Factor Receptor 2-Positive Metastatic Esophageal Cancer

A 57-year-old female with a history of iron deficiency anemia, hypertension, hyperlipidemia, and GERD presented to her PCP with abdominal pain and bloating. An EGD/EUS demonstrated a fungating ulcerated mass of the gastroesophageal junction (38 to 43 cm from incisors), with invasion of the adventitia, and no lymphadenopathy. She underwent neoadjuvant chemoradiation with weekly carboplatin and paclitaxel followed by a total esophagectomy (ypT3N2M0). Six months later, CT C/A/P demonstrated new bilateral lung nodules, right pleural thickening, hypodense liver lesions, and abdominal lymphadenopathy. Liver biopsy revealed adenocarcinoma compatible with metastasis from esophageal primary. Further molecular testing showed HER2 IHC 3+ and PD-L1 CPS 5%. MRI of the brain was negative for intracranial metastases.

How Is Human Epidermal Growth Factor Receptor 2 Tested for in Esophageal Cancer?

- IHC staining for *HER2* should be performed first. A positive result is IHC 3+ and a negative result is 0 to 1+.
- When IHC results are equivocal (2+), FISH should be performed.
  - FISH positivity is defined by HER2/chromosome enumeration probe 17 (CEP17) ratio of 2 or greater.

What Are the Frontline Treatment Options for Human Epidermal Growth Factor Receptor 2 Overexpressing Metastatic Esophageal Cancer?

- *Anti-HER2 therapy:* Trastuzumab is a monoclonal antibody which binds to the extracellular domain of HER2 protein. The benefit of trastuzumab in advanced HER2+ adenocarcinoma of the EGJ or stomach was shown by the ToGA trial which compared standard fluoropyrimidine/platinum-based chemotherapy with or without trastuzumab in the frontline setting.
  - The median OS (primary endpoint) was significantly better in the arm with trastuzumab in combination with chemotherapy (13.8 vs. 11.1 months, HR 0.74, 95% CI 0.6 to 0.91).[17]
- *Immunotherapy:* Immunotherapy agents have also been studied in the frontline setting in HER2-overexpressing esophageal cancers. In the multicenter Phase III KEYNOTE-811 trial, treatment-naive patients with HER2+ metastatic EGJ or gastric adenocarcinoma were randomized to receive trastuzumab plus fluoropyrimidine/platinum-based chemotherapy plus pembrolizumab or placebo.
  - Interim analysis demonstrated that the objective response rate (ORR; primary endpoint) was significantly higher with pembrolizumab (74% vs. 42%) with a higher percentage of complete responders (11% vs. 3%). Based on these data, pembrolizumab is now approved in combination with trastuzumab and fluoropyrimidine plus platinum-containing chemotherapy for patients with locally advanced unresectable or metastatic esophageal or EGJ cancers.

Case Update: Recommended Treatment Plan

- Trastuzumab in combination with chemoimmunotherapy was recommended. The patient received pembrolizumab and trastuzumab in combination with platinum plus fluoropyrimidine, per the KEYNOTE-811 regimen.

What Are the Second-Line Treatment Options for Patients With Human Epidermal Growth Factor Receptor 2-Positive Metastatic Esophageal Cancer?

- Trastuzumab deruxtecan is an antibody–drug conjugate (anti-HER2 antibody linked to a cytotoxic topoisomerase I inhibitor) and is recommended for patients who progress on frontline trastuzumab-based therapy. The Phase II DESTINY-Gastric01 study randomized patients with confirmed HER2+ gastric or EGJ adenocarcinoma to either trastuzumab deruxtecan or physician's choice chemotherapy after progressing on at least two previous therapies including trastuzumab. The objective response and OS were significantly higher in the trastuzumab deruxtecan group (objective response 51% vs. 14%, p less than 0.001; median OS 12.5 vs. 8.4 months, HR 0.59, 95% CI 0.39 to 0.88, $p = 0.01$).
- Other chemotherapy and/or immunotherapy second-line regimens listed in the previous section may be considered as well if second line anti-HER2—based therapy is unsuccessful.
- Continuing trastuzumab beyond progression is not recommended.[18]

REVIEW QUESTIONS

1. A 60-year-old man presents with dysphagia. His primary care provider (PCP) ordered an upper endoscopy that revealed a mass at the distal esophagus and biopsy showed adeno-carcinoma. A CT scan showed multiple liver lesions, and these are avid on follow-up fluo-rodeoxyglucose (FDG)-PET scan. A biopsy of a liver lesion confirms metastatic disease. Which of the additional tests should be added to the pathology assessment?
   A. *ERCC1* expression level
   B. Human epidermal growth factor receptor 2 (*HER2*) immunohistochemistry (IHC)
   C. Epidermal growth factor expression (*EGFR*)
   D. *MET* immunohistochemistry (IHC)

2. A 44-year-old man was diagnosed with squamous cell carcinoma (SCC) of the upper esophagus. Gastric biopsies during the esophagogastroduodenoscopy (EGD) revealed presence of *Helicobacter pylori* infection. His history is also positive for alcohol use and tobacco use, as well as long-standing gastroesophageal reflux disease (GERD). Physical exam reveals an obese man (body mass index [BMI] = 35). He inquires about his risk factors which led to this cancer. Which of the following modifiable risk factors put him at risk for his malignancy?
   A. Obesity
   B. *H. pylori* infection
   C. Smoking and alcohol use
   D. GERD

3. A 60-year-old woman with a history of gastroesophageal reflux disease (GERD) complicated by Barrett's esophagus is now diagnosed with gastroesophageal junction adenocarcinoma metastatic to the lung, programmed death-ligand 1 (PD-L1) combined positive score (CPS) 10%, human epidermal growth factor receptor 2 (*HER2*) immunohistochemistry (IHC) 1+. Her glomerular filtration rate is 40. Her Eastern Cooperative Oncology Group (ECOG) performance status is 0. After discussing the various options, which of the following regimens should she receive?
   A. Epirubicin, oxaliplatin, and capecitabine
   B. Cisplatin and 5-fluorouracil (5-FU)
   C. Capecitabine and oxaliplatin
   D. Capecitabine, oxaliplatin, and nivolumab

4. A 51-year-old man was recently diagnosed with a mass in the middle third of his esophagus. Biopsy was positive for adenocarcinoma. CT and fluorodeoxyglucose (FDG)-PET were negative for distant metastatic disease. Staging by endoscopic ultrasound (EUS) was T3N1M0 with a single regional lymph node (LN) identified. Which treatment regimen do you recommend?
   A. Preoperative chemotherapy followed by surgery followed by postoperative radiation
   B. Radiation alone
   C. Preoperative chemoradiation followed by surgery and subsequent adjuvant immuno-therapy if pathological residual disease is identified in the resected esophagus/LNs
   D. Preoperative chemoradiotherapy (CRT) followed by surgery

5. A 45-year-old man with long-standing history of tobacco and alcohol use presents to his physician with dysphagia and odynophagia. An esophagogastroduodenoscopy (EGD) reveals a mass in the upper esophagus above the sternal notch. Biopsy shows squamous cell carcinoma (SCC). An endoscopic ultrasound (EUS) identifies T2N1 disease.

fluorodeoxyglucose (FDG)-PET/CT is negative for distant metastases. What is the next best step in management of this patient?

A. Concurrent chemoradiotherapy (CRT) alone
B. Neoadjuvant chemoradiation followed by surgery followed by immunotherapy
C. Concurrent CRT plus immunotherapy
D. Chemotherapy followed by radiation therapy

6. A 68-year-old woman is diagnosed with metastatic esophageal adenocarcinoma, by liver biopsy. Human epidermal growth factor receptor 2 (*HER2*) immunohistochemistry (IHC) is 3+, microsatellite stable, tumor mutational burden (TMB) 5 mutations/megabase, programmed death-ligand 1 (PD-L1) combined positive score (CPS) 10. She received treatment with trastuzumab, pembrolizumab, capecitabine, and oxaliplatin. Six months later, a fluorodeoxyglucose (FDG)-PET/CT shows new liver lesions, lytic lesions in the ribs, scapula, and L3 vertebral body. Which of the following options is the next best treatment option for this patient?

A. Nivolumab
B. Ramucirumab
C. Trastuzumab deruxtecan
D. Docetaxel

7. A 49-year-old man with a history of untreated gastroesophageal reflux disease (GERD) presents to his primary care physician (PCP) reporting melena. An esophagogastroduodenoscopy (EGD)/endoscopic ultrasound (EUS) is performed and reveals a mass in the gastroesophageal junction abutting the diaphragm, without any suspicious lymphadenopathy. Biopsy shows adenocarcinoma. An fluorodeoxyglucose (FDG)-PET/CT shows no distant metastases. What is the next best step in management?

A. Offer palliative chemotherapy alone for unresectable disease
B. Offer sequential chemotherapy followed by radiation for unresectable disease
C. Offer neoadjuvant radiation for resectable disease
D. Offer neoadjuvant chemoradiation for resectable disease

8. Which of the following is not a risk factor for developing squamous cell carcinoma (SCC) of the esophagus?

A. Barrett's esophagus
B. Alcohol and tobacco use
C. Esophageal achalasia
D. Plummer–Vinson syndrome

9. A 55-year-old woman is diagnosed with metastatic esophageal adenocarcinoma with involvement of lymph node (LN), lung, and liver. Human epidermal growth factor receptor 2 (*HER2*) immunohistochemistry (IHC) is 3+ and programmed death-ligand 1 (PD-L1) combined positive score (CPS) is 10%. Her performance status is robust, and she has no significant comorbidities. What do you recommend for treatment?

A. Capecitabine and oxaliplatin
B. Pembrolizumab
C. Capecitabine, oxaliplatin, pembrolizumab, and trastuzumab
D. Trastuzumab and pembrolizumab

10. A 61-year-old man with programmed death-ligand 1 (PD-L1) combined positive score (CPS) 5%, human epidermal growth factor receptor 2 (HER2)-negative metastatic esophageal adenocarcinoma completes 6 cycles of capecitabine, oxaliplatin, and nivolumab. Re-staging scans demonstrate progression of disease in the lymph nodes (LNs) along with

two new hepatic lesions. His Eastern Cooperative Oncology Group (ECOG) performance status remains 1, and he is interested in therapy. What do you offer next?

A. Pembrolizumab
B. 5-fluorouracil (5-FU) plus bevacizumab
C. Ramucirumab plus paclitaxel
D. Cetuximab

ANSWERS AND RATIONALES

1. **B. Human epidermal growth factor receptor 2 (*HER2*) immunohistochemistry (IHC).** *HER2* IHC must be performed for all locally advanced unresectable or metastatic esophageal or esophagogastric junction (EGJ) cancer. If the *HER2* IHC results are equivocal, fluorescent in situ hybridization (FISH) must be performed. *HER2* testing drives therapy in locally advanced unresectable and metastatic esophageal cancer. Anti-HER2 therapy is a part of the frontline and subsequent line therapy regimens for HER2+ tumors.

2. **C. Smoking and alcohol use.** Tobacco and alcohol consumption have been found to be the strongest risk factors for development of esophageal SCC worldwide. The incidence of esophageal SCC is thought to have decreased over the last several years due to a worldwide decline of tobacco and alcohol consumption over time.

3. **D. Capecitabine, oxaliplatin, and nivolumab.** Frontline immunotherapy in combination with platinum plus fluoropyrimidine doublet was approved for esophageal adenocarcinoma, based on a randomized Phase III trial showing benefit in progression-free survival (PFS) and overall survival (OS) as compared to chemotherapy alone. The most significant survival benefit was noted in patients with PD-L1 CPS greater than 5%. This patient with PD-L1 CPS 10% without significant other comorbidities and good performance status would qualify for frontline immunotherapy in combination with chemotherapy.

4. **C. Preoperative chemoradiation followed by surgery and subsequent adjuvant immunotherapy if pathological residual disease is identified in the resected esophagus/LNs.** Neoadjuvant therapy with carboplatin and paclitaxel with concurrent radiation therapy followed by esophagectomy (trimodal therapy) was demonstrated to have an improved overall survival (OS) compared to surgery alone in the CROSS trial. If an R0 resection is obtained at the time of surgery, and pathological residual disease is identified, adjuvant therapy with 12 months of nivolumab is recommended based on the CheckMate-577 trial which showed improvement in median disease-free survival (DFS). Note that adjuvant therapy is not recommended if a pathological complete response is obtained after esophagectomy.

5. **A. Concurrent chemoradiotherapy (CRT) alone.** The management of SCC of the cervical esophagus is the same as SCC of the head and neck with definitive CRT alone. Surgery is generally avoided due to complex anatomy of the cervical esophagus and increased morbidity associated with surgery.

6. **C. Trastuzumab deruxtecan.** Trastuzumab deruxtecan, an antibody drug conjugate, is approved as second-line therapy for patients with metastatic HER2+ esophageal cancer who progress after frontline trastuzumab-containing therapy. This is based on a randomized Phase II study where trastuzumab deruxtecan was noted to have superior objective response rate (ORR) and progression-free survival (PFS) as compared to standard chemotherapy.

7. **D. Offer neoadjuvant chemoradiation for resectable disease.** Trimodality therapy (neoadjuvant chemotherapy with concurrernt radiation followed by surgery) was shown to improve overall survival (OS) as compared to surgery alone in the CROSS trial, in locally advanced esophageal adenocarcinoma, defined as clinical T3-4a or any regional node-positive disease. This patient with T4a N0 disease is a candidate for surgery after neoadjuvant concurrent chemoradiation.

8. **A. Barrett's esophagus.** Barrett's esophagus is a known risk factor for development of esophageal adenocarcinoma. Patients with Barrett's esophagus have an annual 1% risk of progression to adenocarcinoma. All other risk factors listed are risk factors associated with esophageal SCC (that is, tobacco, alcohol, achalasia, and Plummer–Vinson syndrome).

9. **C. Capecitabine, oxaliplatin, pembrolizumab, and trastuzumab.** Anti-HER2 therapy in combination with chemotherapy and immunotherapy is approved for newly diagnosed metastatic HER2+ esophageal adenocarcinoma based on outcomes in the KEYNOTE-811 trial. Immunotherapy alone would not be appropriate in the first-line setting despite a high PD-L1 CPS.

10. **C. Ramucirumab plus paclitaxel.** Following progression on first-line therapy, in patients who have previously received immunotherapy, ramucirumab with or without paclitaxel is approved. Other options in the second-line setting in patients who have previously received immunotherapy include docetaxel, paclitaxel, irinotecan, fluorouracil plus irinotecan, and irinotecan with or without ramucirumab.

REFERENCES

1. Siegel RL, Miller KD, Fuchs HE, Jemal A. Cancer statistics [Correction in *CA Cancer J Clin.* 2021;71(4):359. doi:10.3322/caac.21669]. *CA Cancer J Clin.* 2021;71(1):7–33. doi:10.3322/caac.21654
2. Pohl H, Sirovich B, Welch HG. Esophageal adenocarcinoma incidence: are we reaching the peak? *Cancer Epidemiol Biomarkers Prev.* 2010;19(6):1468–1470. doi:10.1158/1055-9965.EPI-10-0012
3. Turati F, Tramacere I, La Vecchia C, Negri E. A meta-analysis of body mass index and esophageal and gastric cardia adenocarcinoma. *Ann Oncol.* 2013;24(3):609–617. doi:10.1093/annonc/mds244
4. Cook MB, Kamangar F, Whiteman DC, et al. Cigarette smoking and adenocarcinomas of the esophagus and esophagogastric junction: a pooled analysis from the international BEACON consortium. *J Natl Cancer Inst.* 2010;102(17):1344–1353. doi:10.1093/jnci/djq289
5. Rice TW, Patil DT, Blackstone EH. 8th edition AJCC/UICC staging of cancers of the esophagus and esophagogastric junction: application to clinical practice. *Ann Cardiothorac Surg.* 2017;6(2):119–130. doi:10.21037/acs.2017.03.14
6. van Hagen P, Hulshof MC, van Lanschot JJ, et al. Preoperative chemoradiotherapy for esophageal or junctional cancer. *N Engl J Med.* 2012;366(22):2074–2084. doi:10.1056/NEJMoa1112088
7. Oppedijk V, van der Gaast A, van Lanschot JJ, et al. Patterns of recurrence after surgery alone versus preoperative chemoradiotherapy and surgery in the CROSS trials. *J Clin Oncol.* 2014;32(5):385–391. doi:10.1200/JCO.2013.51.2186
8. Kelly RJ, Ajani JA, Kuzdzal J, et al. Adjuvant nivolumab in resected esophageal or gastroesophageal junction cancer. *N Engl J Med.* 2021;384(13):1191–1203. doi:10.1056/NEJMoa2032125
9. Al-Batran S-E, Homann N, Pauligk C, et al. Perioperative chemotherapy with fluorouracil plus leucovorin, oxaliplatin, and docetaxel versus fluorouracil or capecitabine plus cisplatin and epirubicin for locally advanced, resectable gastric or gastro-oesophageal junction adenocarcinoma (FLOT4): a randomised, phase 2/3 trial. *Lancet.* 2019;393(10184):1948–1957. doi:10.1016/S0140-6736(18)32557-1
10. Macdonald JS, Smalley SR, Benedetti J, et al. Chemoradiotherapy after surgery compared with surgery alone for adenocarcinoma of the stomach or gastroesophageal junction. *N Engl J Med.* 2001;345(10):725–730. doi:10.1056/NEJMoa010187
11. Smalley SR, Benedetti JK, Haller DG, et al. Updated analysis of SWOG-directed intergroup study 0116: a phase III trial of adjuvant radiochemotherapy versus observation after curative gastric cancer resection. *J Clin Oncol.* 2012;30(19):2327–2333. doi:10.1200/JCO.2011.36.7136
12. Cunningham D, Okines AF, Ashley S. Capecitabine and oxaliplatin for advanced esophagogastric cancer. *N Engl J Med.* 2010;362(9):858–859. doi:10.1056/NEJMc0911925
13. Yamada Y, Higuchi K, Nishikawa K, et al. Phase III study comparing oxaliplatin plus S-1 with cisplatin plus S-1 in chemotherapy-naive patients with advanced gastric cancer. *Ann Oncol.* 2015;26(1):141–148. doi:10.1093/annonc/mdu472
14. Enzinger PC, Burtness BA, Niedzwiecki D, et al. CALGB 80403 (Alliance)/E1206: a randomized phase II study of three chemotherapy regimens plus cetuximab in metastatic esophageal and gastroesophageal junction cancers. *J Clin Oncol.* 2016;34(23):2736–2742. doi:10.1200/JCO.2015.65.5092

15. Sun JM, Shen L, Shah MA, et al. Pembrolizumab plus chemotherapy versus chemotherapy alone for first-line treatment of advanced oesophageal cancer (KEYNOTE-590): a randomised, placebo-controlled, phase 3 study. *Lancet.* 2021;398(10302):759–771. doi:10.1016/S0140-6736(21)01234-4

16. Janjigian YY, Shitara K, Moehler M, et al. First-line nivolumab plus chemotherapy versus chemotherapy alone for advanced gastric, gastro-oesophageal junction, and oesophageal adenocarcinoma (CheckMate 649): a randomised, open-label, phase 3 trial. *Lancet.* 2021;398(10294):27–40. doi:10.1016/S0140-6736(21)00797-2

17. Bang Y-J, Van Cutsem E, Feyereislova A, et al. Trastuzumab in combination with chemotherapy versus chemotherapy alone for treatment of HER2-positive advanced gastric or gastro-oesophageal junction cancer (ToGA): a phase 3, open-label, randomised controlled trial. *Lancet.* 2010;376(9742):687–697. doi:10.1016/S0140-6736(10)61121-X

18. Thuss-Patience PC, Shah MA, Ohtsu A, et al. Trastuzumab emtansine versus taxane use for previously treated HER2-positive locally advanced or metastatic gastric or gastro-oesophageal junction adenocarcinoma (GATSBY): an international randomised, open-label, adaptive, phase 2/3 study. *Lancet Oncol.* 2017;18(5):640–653. doi:10.1016/S1470-2045(17)30111-0

CHAPTER 8

Gastric Cancer

Karen Riggins and Huili Zhu

INTRODUCTION

Gastric cancer is the fifth most common cancer in the world and the third-leading cause of cancer-related deaths.[1] In 2020, there were more than 1 million cases and 768,000 gastric cancer-related deaths worldwide.[2] While there is global variation with the highest of incidences occurring among Eastern Asian and Eastern European populations, both disease incidence and mortality have continued to steadily decline over the past 70 years.[1] This decline is felt to be due in part to better hygiene, improved food conservation,[3] heathier dietary habits,[4] and *Helicobacter pylori* eradication.[5] Despite declines in mortality owing to preventive measures, gastric cancer continues to have a poor prognosis.

Even with new advancements, gastric cancer represents a heterogeneous and complex challenge in cancer care. Management involves a multidisciplinary approach including a combination of surgery, chemotherapy, radiation therapy, and supportive care to optimize survival outcome. An evidence-based multimodality treatment approach is recommended. This chapter will use a case-based approach to address standard treatment strategies in the comprehensive management of gastric cancer patients. Gastric cancer will be explored in three scenarios: (a) resectable locoregional gastric cancer, (b) unresectable locally advanced gastric cancer, and (c) metastatic gastric cancer.

CASE SUMMARIES

Case 8.1: Resectable Gastric Cancer

A 55-year-old male presents to the ED after having two episodes of coffee ground emesis. He was told that he had iron deficiency anemia 1 year ago but, at the time, he felt well and did not follow up with his primary care doctor. For the past 6 months, he has complained of worsening fatigue, early satiety, and ongoing reflux requiring management with over-the-counter antacids. He does not drink alcohol or smoke cigarettes but he is significantly obese with a body mass index (BMI) of 37. He has no family history of medical problems. On arrival to the ED, he was slightly tachycardic and appeared pale. He had mild tenderness to palpation in the epigastrum. The rest of the exam was unremarkable. A complete blood count (CBC) revealed an Hgb of 5.6 with a mean corpuscular volume (MCV) of 78. After transfusion with 2 units of red blood cells (RBCs), a CT of the chest, abdomen, and pelvis was ordered for further workup.

How Is a Diagnosis Established?

- The diagnosis of gastric cancer requires the direct visualization under anesthesia by esophagogastroduodenoscopy (EGD) with biopsy.
- Endoscopic ultrasound (EUS) is important in the staging of localized disease to determine the depth and extent of local invasion and lymph node (LN) involvement in patients with nonmetastatic disease.
- CT of the chest, abdomen, and pelvis (CAP) with oral and intravenous (IV) contrast is needed to evaluate the extent of disease.
- PET/CT evaluation may be beneficial in the assessment of metastatic disease and nodal involvement in patients without clear evidence of distant metastases.
- Diagnostic laparoscopy (DL) with cytology is more controversial but indicated for medically fit patients who are considered for resection. A DL can detect radiographically occult disease. Additionally, cytological examination of peritoneal lavage fluid can predict peritoneal dissemination or recurrence in gastric cancer patients.[6] If positive peritoneal cytology is found, it confers a poor prognosis and the patient is considered at higher risk for peritoneal failure.

Patient's Diagnosis

- *EGD under anesthesia finds an oozing friable ulcerated mass in the gastric cardia. EUS shows suspected malignant neoplasm of proximal gastric cardia and fundus with extension through the submucosa and into the muscularis propria without definitive evidence of malignant lymphadenopathy or ascites. Multiple biopsies were taken.*
- *Differential includes adenocarcinoma (makes up 90% of all gastric cancers), sarcoma, gastrointestinal stromal tumor (GIST), neuroendocrine tumor, and lymphoma. Gastric adenocarcinomas are classified based on location (cardia vs. noncardia) and histology (intestinal, diffuse, or atypical by Lauren criteria[7] or tubular, papillary, mucinous, and poorly cohesive [including signet ring cell carcinoma], and uncommon histological variants by the World Health Organization [WHO]).[8]*
- *Cardia gastric cancer is positively associated with gastroesophageal reflux disease (GERD) symptoms[9] and central obesity.[10] Furthermore, intestinal histology type is most common among patients with risk factors of GERD and obesity.*
- *The patient's biopsy reveals intestinal type adenocarcinoma and is likely the end-result of an inflammatory process that progresses from chronic gastritis to atrophic gastritis and finally to intestinal metaplasia and dysplasia.[5]*
- *The EUS shows a hypoechoic ulcerative mass with thickening at the mucosal layer with extension through the submucosa and into the muscularis propria without ascites or gastrohepatic or celiac lymphadenopathy.*
- *Whole body PET/CT shows hypermetabolic ulcerative mass along the greater curvature of the gastric cardia measuring approximately 3.3 x 1.3 x 2.1 cm.*
- *A DL is not concerning for metastatic spread.*

What Further Molecular or Genomic Testing Is Required?

- Evaluating the mismatch repair (MMR) system through universal testing for microsatellite instability (MSI) by polymerase chain reaction (PCR)/next-generation sequencing (NGS) or MMR by immunohistochemistry (IHC) is recommended in all newly diagnosed patients.
- Additional human epidermal growth factor receptor 2 (HER2) and programmed death-ligand 1 (PD-L1) testing is indicated for metastatic adenocarcinoma.

Patient's Molecular and Genomic Testing

- *Biopsy IHC revealed proficient mismatch repair (pMMR) and PCR analysis was consistent with MSI-stable disease.*

How Is This Tumor Staged?

- The American Joint Committee on Cancer (AJCC) tumor, lymph node, metastasis (TNM) system staging classification (8th ed., 2017) is used to stage gastric cancer.
- For cancers involving the cardia, the EGD helps define the Siewert-Stein classification as type II or type III, which depends on the level of involvement of the gastroesophageal junction.[11]
- Tumors are further staged using EUS, PET/CT imaging, and DL findings.
- Gastric cancers that invade the muscularis propria are considered a T2, as seen in this patient. The EUS provides valuable information by showing the depth of tumor invasion (T), presence of abnormal or enlarged LNs concerning for cancer involvement (N), and can suggest metastatic spread based on visualization of nearby lesions or the presence of ascites (M).
- The DL was without visualized metastatic disease and the peritoneal washings were negative for malignant cells.

Patient's Clinical Stage
- The patient's stage is cT2N0M0.

What Are Appropriate Treatment Options?

- This patient has a tumor that is locoregional resectable gastric cancer and his performance status suggests that he is a good surgical candidate.
- Management of early-stage gastric cancer involves a multimodality treatment approach. Utilization of perioperative chemotherapy and chemoradiation has been shown to improve the outcome of surgically resected gastric cancers in most patients.
- Endoscopic resection is essential and only indicated for very early-stage cancers with limited cT1a or cT1b tumors.
- Perioperative chemotherapy is recommended and preferred above surgery alone for resectable gastric cancer with lesions cT2 or higher.[12,13]
- Multiple studies have shown that perioperative treatment improves in overall survival (OS) when compared to surgery alone.
  - The MAGIC study (published in 2006) was the first landmark trial which showed OS improvement with perioperative chemotherapy in resectable gastric (74%), gastroesophageal junction (GEJ; 11% to 12%), and lower esophageal adenocarcinoma (14% to 15%) compared to surgery alone. Patients received 3 cycles of epirubicin, cisplatin, and 5-fluorouracil (5-FU)/capecitabine (ECF/ECX) before and after resection. Perioperative chemotherapy showed a significant improvement in 5-year OS (36%) with hazard ratio (HR) for death of 0.75 (95% confidence interval [CI] 0.60 to 0.93, $p = 0.0009$) as compared to surgery alone (23%).[13]
  - The SWOG/INT 0116 trial (published in 2001) was a Phase III study that demonstrated significantly improved OS and 3-year recurrence-free survival (RFS) in patients receiving bolus 5-FU plus leucovorin with radiation therapy after surgical resection compared to those receiving surgery alone. OS and RFS data demonstrate continued strong benefit from postoperative chemoradiation. The HR for OS is 1.32 (95% CI, 1.10 to 1.60; $p = .0046$). The HR for RFS is 1.51 (95% CI, 1.25 to 1.83; p less than .001).[14]
  - ARTIST 1 trial (published in 2001) sought to determine whether adjuvant chemoradiation benefits patients who already have curative-intent gastrectomy with D2 lymphadenectomy. Patients who underwent curative-intent gastrectomy with D2 lymphadenectomy were randomized either to surgery followed by chemotherapy or surgery followed by chemoradiation. On initial reporting, 3-year disease-free survival (DFS) was similar between the two groups; however, at 10-year follow-up, the study

finally demonstrated significantly improved OS and 3-year RFS in patients receiving adjuvant chemoradiation compared to those receiving surgery alone. It is to be noted that this study faces criticism as only a small number ($n = 54$) of patients underwent D2 lymphadenectomies so it is difficult to draw any definitive conclusions on the benefit of chemoradiation in patients' D2 lymphadenectomy.[15,16]

- The CLASSIC trial (published in 2012) was designed to compare 6 months of adjuvant capecitabine plus oxaliplatin versus observation after D2 gastrectomy for patients with stage II or III gastric cancer. The estimated 5-year DFS was 68% (95% CI 63 to 73) in the adjuvant capecitabine and oxaliplatin group versus 53% (47 to 58) in the observation alone group. Estimated 5-year OS was 78% (95% CI 74 to 82) in the adjuvant capecitabine and oxaliplatin group versus 69% (64 to 73) in the observation group. The 5-year OS rate was 78% in the adjuvant capecitabine and oxaliplatin group and only 69% in the observation group.[17]

- CRITICS trial (published in 2018) was designed to compare OS between patients with stage IB to IVA resectable gastric or gastroesophageal adenocarcinoma treated with preoperative chemotherapy followed by surgery and postoperative chemotherapy versus postoperative chemoradiation.[18] Postoperative chemoradiation did not improve OS as compared to postoperative chemotherapy after adequate preoperative chemotherapy and surgery.[19]

- In the II/III FLOT4/AIO trial (published in 2020), the group found that perioperative therapy with the docetaxel-based triplet FLOT (fluorouracil [5-FU]/leucovorin, oxaliplatin, and docetaxel) was associated with improved OS compared to ECF/ECX (epirubicin and cisplatin plus either 5-FU or capecitabine) in patients with resectable locally advanced gastric or GEJ adenocarcinoma. Median OS was improved with FLOT versus ECF (50 vs. 35 months; HR, 0.77; $p = 0.012$), with a projected improvement in 5-year OS (45% vs. 36%). PFS was also improved with FLOT (30 vs. 18 months; HR, 0.75; $p = 0.0036$%).[20] The FLOT4 study has established FLOT as the new standard of care for perioperative chemotherapy in patients with resectable gastric cancer who can tolerate a triplet chemotherapy regimen.

- ARTIST 2 trial (published in 2021) compared adjuvant regimens: oral S-1 for 1 year, S-1 plus oxaliplatin (SOX) for 6 months, and SOX plus chemoradiotherapy in patients with curatively D2-resected, stage II/III, node-positive gastric cancer. Studies showed that adjuvant SOX or SOXRT was effective in prolonging DFS, when compared with S-1 monotherapy. Additionally, the addition of radiotherapy to SOX did not significantly reduce the rate of recurrence after D2 gastrectomy.[21]

What Are the Goals of Surgical Resection?

- Surgery is an integral part of any curative intent management for resectable gastric tumors. For distally located tumors, resection can be achieved through distal subtotal or total gastrectomy. Proximally located tumors or tumors near the GEJ can be considered for proximal subtotal gastrectomy. Tumors having poorly differentiated histology or associated with Barrett's esophagus require total gastrectomy.

- Margin-negative (R0) gastrectomy and adequate lymphadenectomy removal of at least 16 LNs at a high-volume center are the cornerstones of multimodal treatment for operable gastric cancer.[22,23] R1 and R2 resections indicate microscopic and macroscopic residual disease and require postoperative chemoradiation with fluoropyrimidine.

- There has been much controversy regarding the extent of LN dissection in gastric cancer resection. Limited D1 nodal dissection includes perigastric LNs, classical extended D2 nodal dissection includes nodes along the celiac axis in addition to perigastric nodes as well as splenectomy and distal pancreatectomy, and D3 dissections involve perigastric, celiac axis, and para-aortic LN stations. The surgical approach to LN dissection has differed between the East and the West. Japan and Eastern countries prefer D2 and Western countries prefer the modified D2 approach which excludes splenectomy and distal pancreatectomy.

- The seminal Dutch D1D2 trial (published in 2004) sought to compare D1 and D2 dissections. The initial results of the trial showed higher postoperative morbidity (43% vs. 4%, p less than 0.001) and mortality (10% vs. 4%, p less than 0.004) in the D2 lymphadenectomy group compared with the D1 group without any difference in 5-year OS.[24] The 15-year follow-up showed that disease-specific survival was significantly higher in patients receiving D2 versus D1 lymphadenectomy, but there was no improvement in OS.[25]

Recommended Treatment Plan for This Patient

- FLOT every 14 days for 4 cycles followed by D2 subtotal gastrectomy with modified D2 resection from a high volume center followed by 4 more cycles of FLOT.

What Is Required for This Patient's Follow-Up and Survivorship?

- Post treatment contrast-enhanced CT imaging following adjuvant therapy will establish a new baseline for surveillance monitoring.
- Gastric cancer survivors should be monitored for adequate nutrition following treatment.
- Gastric cancer survivors who undergo surgical resection must be counseled on the short- and long-term digestive complications following gastric resections including indigestion, early satiety, and dumping symptoms.
- Patients who underwent distal or total gastrostomies should be additionally monitored for vitamin B12 and iron deficiencies.
- For patients who are under endoscopic resection, endoscopy is recommended every 6 months for 1 year, then annually for up to 5 years. However, patients who undergo surgical resection are not required to routinely undergo repeat EGD; endoscopy is to be completed as clinically indicated in these gastric cancer survivors.

Case 8.2: Unresectable Locally Advanced Gastric Cancer

A 60-year-old male with a history of coronary artery disease complicated by cerebrovascular accident last year with only minimal residual right-sided deficits presents to his primary care doctor with a 4-month history of nausea, vomiting, and a 30-pound weight loss. He had remained active and still is able to perform his activities of daily living without assistance until his symptoms worsened 3 weeks ago. Now, he has been unable to keep down most of his meals and, as a result, he has become weak and has required help at home for his daily activities. On exam, he appears cachectic with temporal wasting. Abdominal exam is remarkable for palpable abdominal mass near the epigastrum. His PCP prescribed ondansetron and ordered CT CAP, which showed marked gastric distention concerning for partial gastric outlet obstruction (GOO) with thickening at the pylorus with infiltration of the proximal duodenum, pancreatic head, and superior mesenteric vein with multiple bulky LNs. He was sent to the ED where Gastroenterology was consulted. An EGD/EUS was performed and showed a normal GEJ; however, upon entering the stomach a large amount of solid food was seen. An ulcerated mass in the pylorus approximately 4.6 cm in size was visualized that completely surrounded the pylorus and was the suspected source of obstruction; a biopsy was taken which later confirmed gastric adenocarcinoma, diffuse type histology. Further PET/CT imaging and DL confirmed clinical stage cT4bN2M0 gastric cancer.

How Is a Diagnosis Established?

- In addition to the CT CAP, EGD/EUS, and biopsy, a fluorodeoxyglucose (FDG)-PET/CT evaluation is suggested if there is no evidence of metastatic disease.
- Given the extent of disease, a DL with cytology is reasonable.

Patient's Diagnosis

- *EGD/EUS: Gastric tumor was circumferential and involving all layers of the gastric wall. The tumor penetrated through the serosa with extension to the duodenal wall and head of the pancreas with abutment of the superior mesenteric vein. Four perigastric LNs were enlarged.*

How Is This Tumor Staged?

- Gastric cancers that invade through serosa into adjacent organs are considered cT4b. The presence of 4 enlarged LNs is consistent with N2 involvement.
- The absence of metastatic disease as determined by PET/CT and DL exclude metastatic disease.

Patient's Clinical Stage

- *The patient's stage is cT4bN2M0.*

What Further Molecular or Genomic Testing Is Required?

- Unlike in early-stage resectable disease, patients with unresectable disease should be tested for HER2 and PD-L1 as targeted therapy is indicated in this setting.
- NGS should also be considered.

Patient's Molecular and Genomic Testing

- *Biopsy was MSI-stable, HER2+ (3+ immunohistochemistry), and PD-L1 expression CPS greater than 10.*

How Do You Manage the Acute Complication of Gastric Outlet Obstruction in Locally Advanced Gastric Cancer?

- GOO is a common and serious symptom in patients with advanced disease which can cause nausea, vomiting, and further malnutrition if untreated. It must be promptly addressed to avoid further complications and impact on performance status.
- Malignant GOO can be palliatively managed with surgical gastrojejunostomy or through the endoscopic placement of an enteral metallic stent.[26,27] In a meta-analysis of trials comparing stent placement and gastrojejunostomy, there was no significant difference in efficacy or complications. However, stenting was associated with a trend toward shorter hospital stay, faster relief of obstructive symptoms, and more re-intervention compared to surgically treated patients.[27]
- Radiation therapy or chemotherapy can also be useful to relieve GOO, but the benefit is not immediate. Finally, palliative management with a venting gastrostomy can be considered for patients with limited life expectancy.

Patient Management

- *Given the acute and symptomatic presentation and marginal performance status, this patient underwent urgent GOO management with endoscopic placement of an enteral metallic stent.*

What Are Appropriate First-Line Treatment Options in This Patient With Unresectable Locally Advanced Gastric Cancer?

- In locally advanced gastric cancer, determining resectability with curative intent is a key decision that requires multidisciplinary discussion (see Figure 8.1). Gastric cancer is considered unresectable when there is evidence of metastatic disease including positive peritoneal cytology, local disease infiltration of the root of the mesentery or para-aortic LN, or invasion or encasement of major vascular structures (excluding the splenic vessels). Comorbidities and performance status must also be taken into consideration.
- Palliative management with chemoradiation or systemic chemotherapy is indicated for unresectable locally advanced disease for patients with a good performance status (Karnofsky Performance Status Scale [KPS] score of 60% or greater or Eastern Cooperative Oncology Group [ECOG] PS score of 2 or lower).
- If chemotherapy is chosen, doublet therapy with a platinum and fluoropyrimidine is preferred over triplet therapy given the lower toxicity profile.
- For adenocarcinomas with HER2 overexpression, trastuzumab should be added to first-line chemotherapy based on results of the ToGa trial.[28]
- Nivolumab in combination with fluoropyrimidine and platinum-containing regimens is now indicated as first-line therapy for patients with unresectable locally advanced or metastatic gastric cancer overexpression of PD-L1 and a combined positive score (CPS) of 5 or more. The CheckMate-649 trial showed that nivolumab in combination with leucovorin, 5-fluorouracil, and oxaliplatin (FOLFOX) or capecitabine and oxaliplatin (CapeOX) resulted in a significant improvement in survival in treatment-naïve patients who had PD-L1–positive advanced gastric cancer, GEJ cancer, and esophageal adenocarcinoma versus chemotherapy alone. Patients who had a PD-L1 CPS of 5 or greater had a OS of 14.4 months in the combination group (95% CI, 13.1 to 16.2) compared with 11.1 months with chemotherapy alone (95% CI, 10 to 12.1; HR, 0.71; 98.4% CI, 0.59 to 0.86; p less than .0001).[29]
- Pembrolizumab in combination with chemotherapy is also indicated in the first-line setting for unresectable locally advanced or metastatic patients in combination with chemotherapy and trastuzumab for HER2+ disease based on KEYNOTE-811 results that showed the overall response rate (ORR) was 74% (95% CI = 66 to 82) in the pembrolizumab, traztuzumab, chemotherapy (5-FU plus cisplatin or capecitabine) arm and 52% (95% CI = 43 to 61) in the traztuzumab, chemotherapy arm (one-sided p value less than .0001, statistically significant).[30]

Recommended Treatment Plan for This Patient
- Given his HER2 overexpression (3+ IHC), traztuzumab in combination with FOLFOX was recommended.

Case 8.3: Metastatic Gastric Adenocarcinoma

A 43-year-old female presents with 5 months of progressively worsening nausea, vomiting, abdominal pain, and unintentional weight loss of 25 pounds. She was recently diagnosed and treated for H. pylori with triple therapy but when her symptoms did not improve, she was seen by her primary care physician (PCP) for follow-up. A CT scan of the chest, abdomen, and pelvis was ordered and showed prominent wall thickening of the gastric body as well as omental nodularity and a 4.2 x 3.8 cm liver nodule in segment IV concerning for metastatic disease. She was referred to medical oncology for assistance with further workup and evaluation. She is a mother of three and has good functional status. Outside of her gastrointestinal (GI) symptoms, she was otherwise healthy without any history of surgeries, or any tobacco and alcohol use. She has no family history of cancer.

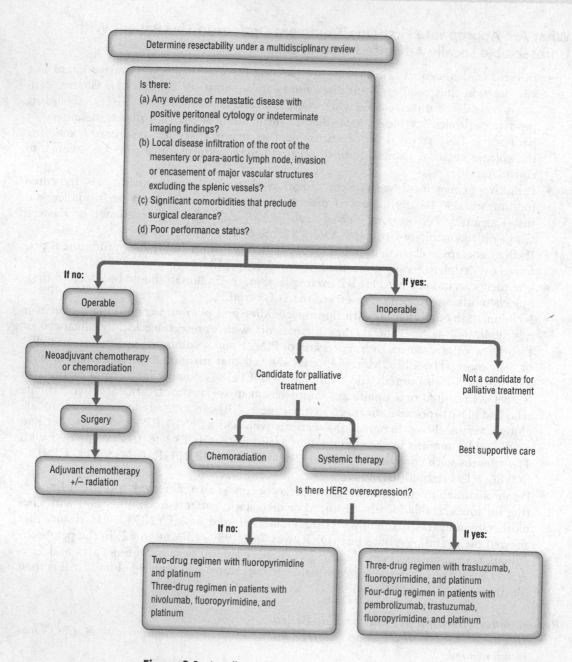

Figure 8.1 Locally advanced gastric cancer management

How Is a Diagnosis Established?

- Direct visualization under anesthesia by EGD with biopsy is indicated.
- A biopsy of a suspected metastatic lesion can be performed as indicated to confirm both stage and diagnosis in this case.
- Given CT CAP findings and concern for metastatic disease, a PET/CT is not necessary at this time.
- If metastasis is proven, a DL is not indicated in this case.

Patient's Diagnosis

- *EGD/EUS: Gastric tumor was an ulcerated mass 4 × 5.4 cm in diameter involving the gastric body along the greater curvature. Mass involved all layers of the gastric wall. The tumor penetrated the muscularis propria but did not involve any surrounding solid organs or vasculature. Three perigastric LNs were enlarged.*
- *The gastric and liver biopsy both revealed poorly differentiated adenocarcinoma with mucinous and signet ring cell features.*

What Further Molecular or Genomic Testing Is Required?

- HER2: Tumor specimen from all patients with advanced gastric cancer should be assessed for HER2 status.[31]
- MSI/MMR: Testing for MSI or MMR status should be performed by IHC in all newly diagnosed gastric cancers.[32]
- PD-L1: Testing for PD-L1 may be considered in locally advanced, recurrent, or metastatic gastric cancers.

Patient's Molecular and Genomic Testing

- *MSI-stable, HER2-, PD-L1–negative with CPS less than 1*

How Is This Tumor Staged?

- The AJCC eighth edition staging system (2017) is used to stage gastric cancers based on TNM staging: T is determined by the depth of tumor invasion and the N by number of positive regional LN groups as determined by EGD/EUS. M is determined by metastasis as visualized by radiographic imaging and confirmed by interventional radiology (IR)-guided liver biopsy.
- The primary tumor penetrated the muscularis propria representing T3 disease and was associated with three locoregionally enlarged LNs representing N2; this, along with confirmed liver metastasis, made her clinical stage T3N2M1.

Patient's Clinical Stage

- *The patient's stage is T3N2M1, stage IV.*

What Are Appropriate Treatment Options?

- Advanced-stage gastric cancer confers a poor prognosis with survival ranging from approximately 4 months with best supportive care to 12 months with chemotherapy.[33]
- Palliative treatment can be offered for patients with incurable metastatic disease with an appropriate performance status (KPS of 60% or greater or ECOG performance score of 2 or less).
- Two-drug cytotoxic regimens are preferred for patients with advanced disease because of lower toxicity in patients who are candidates for palliative therapy.
- First-line systemic treatment is chemotherapy with platinum plus a fluoropyrimidine backbone, and oxaliplatin is generally preferred over cisplatin due to lower toxicity.[34,35]
- For patients with HER2 overexpression, HER2-directed therapy is recommended based on the ToGA trial where trastuzumab in combination with cisplatin-based chemotherapy in HER2+ advanced gastric cancer had increased median OS (13.8 months) when compared with chemotherapy alone (11.1 months).[36]
- There have been multiple trials evaluating immunotherapy in advanced gastric cancer.

- For patients with PD-L1 expression, immunotherapy in combination with chemotherapy is indicated based on the KEYNOTE-062 trial where pembrolizumab plus chemotherapy did not prolong OS/PFS in PD-L1+ patients, but pembrolizumab monotherapy did improve OS in patients with high PD-L1 expression (CPS of 10 or greater).[37]
- In the CheckMate-649 trial, nivolumab in combination with chemotherapy had superior OS/PFS than chemotherapy alone in advanced gastric cancer with CPS of 5 or greater. Patients with CPS or 1 or more also showed OS/PFS benefit compared to chemotherapy alone.[29]
- Second-line treatment options for metastatic gastric cancer are based on a number of trials (Table 8.1).

Patient's Treatment

- *She was started on systemic chemotherapy with FOLFOX x 12 cycles and then transitioned to 5-FU maintenance with stable disease to date.*

What Are the Toxicities Associated With Therapy?

- Peripheral neuropathy is considered one of the most clinically significant side effects of platinum-based therapies.[47]
- Duloxetine is the only agent recommended by the American Society of Clinical Oncology (ASCO) in the management of chemotherapy-induced peripheral neuropathy (CIPN).[48]
- As compared with cisplatin, oxaliplatin is associated with lower incidences of grade 3 or 4 neutropenia, alopecia, renal toxicity, and thromboembolism but with a slightly higher grade 3 or 4 diarrhea and neuropathy.[49]
- Given prolonged use of cytotoxic therapy and increased risk of chemotherapy-related toxicity, maintenance therapy should be considered after induction fluoropyrimidine and platinum-based therapy. Maintenance therapy is associated with an improved toxicity profile and appears to have comparable efficacy to continuous treatment in metastatic gastric cancer.[50]

What Are Other Treatment Considerations?

- In older and/or frail patients, dose reduction in chemotherapy may provide better tolerance without compromising outcomes.[51]
- Research and clinical trials are underway to evaluate the efficacy of PD-1 inhibitor, CLDN18 inhibitor, novel anti-HER2 agents, poly adenosine diphosphate-ribose polymerase (PARP) inhibitor, and more in combination with first-line chemotherapy in treatment of advanced gastric cancer.

Table 8.1 Second-Line Treatment Options for Metastatic Gastric Cancer

Second-Line Trial	Number of Patients/ Trial Phase	Second Line-Chemotherapy Agent	Treatment Indication	Survival Results
Assersohn et al.[38]	38/II	5-FU (400 mg/m^2)/ leucovorin (125 mg/m^2) + irinotecan (180 mg/m^2) followed by 5-FU (1200 mg/m^2) q2w	Advanced gastric or gastroesophageal junction adenocarcinoma with one prior chemotherapy involving platinum	OS: 6.4 months PFS: 3.7 months
COUGAR-02[39]	168/III	Docetaxel (75 mg/m^2) q3w vs. Active symptom control	Advanced gastric cancer that had progressed on or within 6 months of treatment with a platinum-fluoropyrimidine combination	OS: 5.2 vs. 3.6 months HR 0.67, $p = 0.01$
Kang et al.[40]	202/III	Docetaxel 60 mg/m^2 q3w or irinotecan 150 mg/m^2 q2w vs. Best supportive care	Advanced gastric cancer with one or two prior chemotherapy regimens involving both fluoropyrimidines and platinum	OS: 5.3 vs. 3.8 months HR 0.657, $p = 0.007$
REGARD[41]	355/III	Ramucirumab (8 mg/kg) q2w vs. Placebo	Advanced gastric or gastroesophageal junction adenocarcinoma with one prior chemotherapy involving both fluoropyrimidine and platinum	OS: 5.2 vs. 3.8 months HR 0.776, $p = 0.047$ PFS: 2.1 vs. 1.3 months HR 0.483, $p < 0.0001$
RAINBOW[42]	665/III	Paclitaxel (80 mg/m^2) q1w + ramucirumab (8 mg/kg) q2w vs. Paclitaxel (80 mg/m^2) q1w + placebo	Advanced gastric or gastroesophageal junction adenocarcinoma with one prior chemotherapy involving both fluoropyrimidine and platinum	OS: 9.6 vs. 7.4 months HR 0.807, $p = 0.017$ PFS: 4.4 vs. 2.9 months HR 0.635, $p < 0.0001$
TAGS[43]	507/III	Trifluridine/tipiracil (35 mg/m^2 twice daily on days 1–5 and days 8–12 every 28 days) plus best supportive care vs. Placebo plus best supportive care	Advanced gastric cancer with at least two prior chemotherapy lines	OS: 5.7 vs. 3.6 months HR 0.69, $p = 0.00029$, (two-sided $p = 0.00058$)

(continued)

Table 8.1   Second-Line Treatment Options for Metastatic Gastric Cancer (*continued*)

Second-Line Trial	Number of Patients/ Trial Phase	Second Line-Chemotherapy Agent	Treatment Indication	Survival Results
KEYNOTE-061[44]	395/III	Pembrolizumab, 200 mg, intravenously every 3 weeks vs. Paclitaxel 80 mg/m² on day 1, 8, and 15 of a 28-day cycle	Advanced gastric or gastroesophageal adenocarcinoma with PD-L1 CPS ≥1 and at least two previous regimens which included a fluoropyrimidine and a platinum agent	OS: 9.1 months vs. 8.3 months; HR 0.82, $p = 0.04$
DESTINY-Gastric01[45]	187/II	Trastuzumab deruxtecan (6.4 mg per kilogram of body weight every 3 weeks) vs. Chemotherapy, physician's choice	Advanced gastric or gastroesophageal junction adenocarcinoma with at least two previous regimens, which included a fluoropyrimidine, a platinum agent, and trastuzumab (or approved biosimilar agent)	OS: 12.5 vs. 8.4 months; HR 0.59, $p = 0.01$
STARTRK-2[46]	54/I-II	Entrectinib orally at a dose of at least 600 mg once per day in a capsule	Patients with metastatic or locally advanced *NTRK* fusion-positive solid tumors	31 (57%; 95% CI 43·2–70·8) patients had an objective response: (7%) were complete responses and (50%) were partial responses. Median duration of response was 10 months (95% CI 7·1 to not estimable)

CI, confidence interval; CPS, combined positive score; HR, hazard ratio; OS, overall survival; PD-L1, programmed death-ligand 1; PFS, progression-free survival; q, every; w, week.

REVIEW QUESTIONS

1. A 62-year-old male with a 40 pack per year smoking history and coronary artery disease was diagnosed with proficient mismatch repair (MMR) locally advanced gastric cancer (cT3N0) of the gastric body amendable to resection. Which of the following is not an appropriate treatment option?
   A. Neoadjuvant chemotherapy followed by partial gastrectomy D2 and adjuvant chemotherapy
   B. Neoadjuvant chemoradiation followed by partial gastrectomy D2 and adjuvant chemotherapy
   C. Neoadjuvant chemotherapy followed by total gastrectomy D1 and adjuvant chemoradiation
   D. Endoscopic resection followed by observation
   E. Upfront partial gastrectomy followed by chemoradiation

2. A 50-year-old male comes to see you to discuss adjuvant therapy for recently diagnosed gastric cancer. He underwent neoadjuvant chemotherapy (with 5-fluorouracil and oxaliplatin [FOLFOX]) followed by partial gastrectomy for a tumor located at the antrum. The final pathology revealed a stage III (T3N1) gastric cancer and he had an R1 partial gastrectomy with D2 resection. What do you recommend for this patient?
   A. Observation
   B. Adjuvant oxaliplatin
   C. Adjuvant chemoradiation with 5-fluorouracil
   D. Adjuvant chemoradiation with oxaliplatin
   E. Nivolumab and 5-fluorouracil followed by chemoradiation

3. For gastric cancer resection, what is the acceptable number of lymph nodes (LNs) that should be examined/removed for an adequate lymphadenectomy with gastric resection?
   A. 6
   B. 10
   C. 11
   D. 12
   E. 16

4. A 65-year-old female presented with nausea and vomiting. She was referred by her primary care physician (PCP) to a local gastroenterologist who performed an esophagogastroduodenoscopy (EGD) that revealed a nonobstructive mass at the pylorus. A biopsy revealed adenocarcinoma, intestinal type. What additional workup is not indicated?
   A. Endoscopic ultrasound (EUS)
   B. PET/CT
   C. Diagnostic laparoscopy (DL)
   D. CT of the chest, abdomen, and pelvis
   E. Nuclear medicine (NM) bone scan

5. What biomarkers are indicated in the metastatic setting?
   A. Human epidermal growth factor receptor 2 (HER2) amplification
   B. Mismatch repair (MMR) status
   C. TP53 mutation
   D. *NTRK* gene fusion
   E. Programmed death-ligand 1 (PD-L1) expression

6. A 42-year-old male with unresectable proficient mismatch repair (pMMR) human epidermal growth factor receptor 2-negative (HER2-) locally advanced gastric cancer comes to discuss his options for first-line therapy. He has an Eastern Cooperative Oncology Group (ECOG) 1 and his programmed death-ligand 1 (PD-L1) combined positive score (CPS) is greater than 5. What would be an acceptable first-line therapy for this patient?
   A. Fam-trastuzumab deruxtecan-nxki
   B. Nivolumab, capecitabine, and oxaliplatin
   C. Pembrolizumab
   D. 5-flourouracil, alone
   E. Ramacirumab and nivolumab

7. A 33-year-old male with a history of gastroesophageal reflux disease (GERD) and now newly diagnosed stage IIb (cT3N0) proficient mismatch repair (pMMR) gastric adenocarcinoma of the cardia presents to his medical oncologist to discuss treatment options. He was recently discussed at the multidisciplinary tumor board where recommendations were made to initiate neoadjuvant chemotherapy prior to surgical resection. He has a good performance status and no prior history of peripheral neuropathy. What would be considered the optimal treatment in this case?
   A. 5-fluorauicil and leucovorin
   B. Cisplatin, capecitabine, and oxaliplatin
   C. Epirubicin, cisplatin, 5-flurauracil, and leucovorin
   D. 5-flurauracil, leucovorin, oxilaplatin, and doxetaxel
   E. Oxaliplatin and bevacizumab

8. A 62-year-old female with no prior medical history was found to have gastric cancer involving antrum of the stomach, and multiple fluorodeoxyglucose (FDG)-avid gastric lymph nodes (LNs) and liver nodules. Her human epidermal growth factor receptor 2 (HER2)/neu is 3+ on immunohistochemistry (IHC). She has good liver and renal function, and her baseline echocardiogram shows a left ventricular ejection fraction of 65%. She has an Eastern Cooperative Oncology Group (ECOG) performance status of 0. Which of the following treatment regimens would be most appropriate?
   A. Epirubicin, cisplatin, 5-fluorouracil
   B. Epirubicin, cisplatin, 5-fluorouracil, and trastuzumab
   C. Cisplatin, 5-fluorouracil, and lapatinib
   D. Cisplatin, 5-fluorouracil, and trastuzumab
   E. 5-fluorouracil

9. A 58-year-old male with a 6-month history of progressively worsening symptoms of epigastric abdominal pain, weight loss, and early satiety was diagnosed with metastatic, human epidermal growth factor receptor 2-negative (HER2-) gastric cancer. He was treated with 3 months of 5-fluorouracil and oxaliplatin; however, repeat imaging showed progression of disease. Of note, he is negative for NTRK gene fusions and has a programmed death-ligand 1 (PD-L1) combined positive score (CPS) of 0. Which of the following would be most appropriate as second-line treatment?
   A. Trastuzumab deruxtecan
   B. Ramucirumab and paclitaxel
   C. Capecitabine and cisplatin
   D. Entrectinib
   E. Pembrolizumab

10. Which of the following is not a correct statement regarding survivorship follow-up?
    A. Gastric cancer survivors must be monitored for vitamin B12 deficiency following total gastrectomy
    B. Gastric cancer survivors who have partial gastrectomy must undergo an annual esophagogastroduodenoscopy (EGD) for up to 5 years following treatment with chemoradiation.
    C. Gastric cancer survivors should be monitored for malnutrition
    D. Gastric cancer survivors should be screened for iron deficiency following total gastrectomy
    E. Gastric cancer survivors who have endoscopic resection need to undergo endoscopy every 6 months for 1 year then annually for up to 5 years

ANSWERS AND RATIONALES

1. **D. Endoscopic resection followed by observation.** This is not appropriate therapy for this tumor. Endoscopic resection is only indicated for T1a and T1b early-stage tumors. For all other resectable tumors cT2 and higher, perioperative chemotherapy is recommended and preferred above surgery alone for resectable gastric cancer.

2. **C. Adjuvant chemoradiation with 5-fluorouracil.** R1 margins indicate microscopic residual disease; this is associated with a poor prognosis. Adjuvant chemoradiation with a fluoropyrimidine is recommended to optimize local control.

3. **E. 16.** Margin-negative (R0) gastrectomy and adequate lymphadenectomy removal of at least 16 LNs at a high-volume center are the cornerstones of multimodal treatment for operable gastric cancer.

4. **E. Nuclear medicine (NM) bone scan.** An NM bone scan to evaluate bone disease is not indicated as a part of the initial workup for locoregional gastric cancer.

5. **C. TP53 mutation.** Assessment of MMR status, HER2 amplification, *NTRK* gene fusion, and PD-L1 expression are all biomarkers that help to guide treatment in the metastatic setting. While the TP53 mutation is the most frequent mutation in gastric cancer, it is not currently a predictive biomarker that impacts the decision for the treatment plan.

6. **B. Nivolumab, capecitabine, and oxaliplatin.** Based on the CheckMate-649 study, first-line nivolumab, capecitabine, and oxaliplatin has improved overall survival (OS) in patients who had a PD-L1 CPS of 5 or greater compared to chemotherapy alone (14.4 months versus 11.1 months; hazard ratio [HR], 0.71; 98.4% confidence interval [CI], 0.59 to 0.86; P less than .0001).

7. **D. 5-flurauracil, leucovorin, oxilaplatin, and doxetaxel.** The FLOT4/AIO trial showed that FLOT (fluorouracil [5-FU]/leucovorin, oxaliplatin, and docetaxel) was associated with improved overall survival (OS) compared to ECF/ECX (epirubicin and cisplatin plus either 5-FU or capecitabine) in patients with resectable locally advanced gastric or gastro-esophageal junction adenocarcinoma with a median OS, which was improved with FLOT versus ECF (50 vs. 35 months; hazard ratio [HR], 0.77; p = 0.012) and improved progression-free survival (PFS; 30 vs. 18 months; HR, 0.75; p = 0.0036%) in the FLOT cohort.

8. **D. Cisplatin, 5-fluorouracil, and trastuzumab.** This patient has metastatic gastric cancer with a good performance status and good baseline cardiac, renal, and hepatic functions. Based on the Phase III ToGA trial, HER2+ patients should receive trastuzumab in addition to fluoropyrimidine and platinum-containing regimen. It is not recommended to take trastuzumab in combination with anthracycline due to cardiotoxicity.

9. **B. Ramucirumab and paclitaxel.** This patient with metastatic gastric cancer progressed on first-line treatment of 5-fluorouracil and oxaliplatin. Capecitabine and cisplatin combination is another reasonable first-line regimen; however, this patient has progressed. Because he is negative for HER2 expression, *NTRK* gene fusions, and PD-L1 expression, he is not a candidate for trastuzumab deruxtecan, entrectinib, nor pembrolizumab, respectively.

10. **B. Gastric cancer survivors who have partial gastrectomy must undergo an annual esophagogastroduodenoscopy (EGD) for up to 5 years following treatment with chemoradiation.** Endoscopy is to be completed as clinically indicated. Patients who undergo surgical resection are not required to routinely undergo repeat EGD. However, patients who undergo endoscopic resection, endoscopy is recommended every 6 months for 1 year then annually for up to 5 years.

REFERENCES

1. Sung H, Ferlay J, Siegel RL, et al. Global cancer statistics 2020: GLOBOCAN estimates of incidence and mortality worldwide for 36 cancers in 185 countries. *CA Cancer J Clin.* 2021;71(3):209–249. doi:10.3322/caac.21660
2. Etemadi A, Safiri S, Sepanlou SG, et al. The global, regional, and national burden of stomach cancer in 195 countries, 1990–2017: a systematic analysis for the global burden of disease study 2017. *Lancet Gastroenterol Hepatol.* 2020;5(1):42–54. doi:10.1016/S2468-1253(19)30328-0
3. Yan S, Gan Y, Song X, et al. Association between refrigerator use and the risk of gastric cancer: a systematic review and meta-analysis of observational studies. *PLoS One.* 2018;13(8):e0203120. doi:10.1371/journal.pone.0203120
4. Buckland G, Travier N, Huerta JM, et al. Healthy lifestyle index and risk of gastric adenocarcinoma in the EPIC cohort study. *Int J Cancer.* 2015;137(3):598–606. doi:10.1002/ijc.29411
5. Parsonnet J, Friedman GD, Vandersteen DP, et al. *Helicobacter pylori* infection and the risk of gastric carcinoma. *N Engl J Med.* 1991;325(16):1127–1131. doi:10.1056/NEJM199110173251603
6. Oh CA, Bae JM, Oh SJ, et al. Long-term results and prognostic factors of gastric cancer patients with only positive peritoneal lavage cytology. *J Surg Oncol.* 2012;105:393–399. doi:10.1002/jso.22091
7. Lauren P. The two histological main types of gastric carcinoma: diffuse and so called intestinal-type carcinoma: an attempt at a histo-clinical classification. *Acta Pathol Microbiol Scand.* 1965;34:31–49. doi:10.1111/apm.1965.64.1.31
8. Bosman FT, Carneiro F, Hruban RH, Theise ND, eds. WHO *Classification of Tumours of the Digestive System.* IARC; 2010.
9. Chow WH, Finkle WD, McLaughlin JK, et al. The relation of gastroesophageal reflux disease and its treatment to adenocarcinomas of the esophagus and gastric cardia. *JAMA.* 1995;274(6):474–477.
10. Hoyo C, Cook MB, Kamangar F, et al. Body mass index in relation to oesophageal and oesophagogastric junction adenocarcinomas: a pooled analysis from the International BEACON Consortium. *Int J Epidemiol.* 2012;41(6):1706–1718. doi:10.1093/ije/dys176
11. Siewert JR, Stein HJ. Carcinoma of the gastroesophageal junction—classification, pathology and extent of resection. *Dis Esophagus.* 1996;9(3):173–182. doi:10.1093/dote/9.3.173
12. Ychou M, Boige V, Pignon J-P, et al. Perioperative chemotherapy compared with surgery alone for resectable gastroesophageal adenocarcinoma: an FNCLCC and FFCD multicenter phase III trial. *J Clin Oncol.* 2011;29:1715–1721. doi:10.1200/JCO.2010.33.0597
13. Cunningham D, Allum WH, Stenning SP, et al. Perioperative chemotherapy versus surgery alone for resectable gastroesophageal cancer. *N Engl J Med.* 2006;355(1):11–20. doi:10.1056/NEJMoa055531
14. Macdonald JS, Smalley SR, Benedetti J, et al. Chemoradiotherapy after surgery compared with surgery alone for adenocarcinoma of the stomach or gastroesophageal junction. *N Engl J Med.* 2001;345:725–730. doi:10.1056/NEJMoa010187
15. Lee J, Lim DH, Kim S, et al. Phase III trial comparing capecitabine plus cisplatin versus capecitabine plus cisplatin with concurrent capecitabine radiotherapy in completely resected gastric cancer with D2 lymph node dissection: the ARTIST trial. *J Clin Oncol.* 2012;30(3):268–273. doi:10.1200/JCO.2011.39.1953
16. Park SH, Sohn TS, Lee J, et al. Phase III trial to compare adjuvant chemotherapy with capecitabine and cisplatin versus concurrent chemoradiotherapy in gastric cancer: final report of the adjuvant chemoradiotherapy in stomach tumors trial, including survival and subset analyses. *J Clin Oncol.* 2015;33(28):3130–3136. doi:10.1200/JCO.2014.58.3930
17. Bang Y-J, Kim Y-W, Yang H-K, et al. Adjuvant capecitabine and oxaliplatin for gastric cancer after D2 gastrectomy (CLASSIC): a phase 3 open-label, randomised controlled trial. *Lancet.* 2012;379:315–321. doi:10.1016/S0140-6736(11)61873-4
18. Dikken JL, van Sandick JW, Maurits Swellengrebel HA, et al. Neo-adjuvant chemotherapy followed by surgery and chemotherapy or by surgery and chemoradiotherapy for patients with resectable gastric cancer (CRITICS). *BMC Cancer.* 2011;11:329. doi:10.1186/1471-2407-11-329
19. Cats A, Jansen E, van Grieken N, et al. Chemotherapy versus chemoradiotherapy after surgery and preoperative chemotherapy for resectable gastric cancer (CRITICS): an international, open-label, randomised phase 3 trial. *Lancet Oncol.* 2018;19(5):616–628. doi:10.1016/S1470-2045(18)30132-3
20. Al-Batran S-E, Homann N, Pauligk C, et al. Perioperative chemotherapy with fluorouracil plus leucovorin, oxaliplatin, and docetaxel versus fluorouracil or capecitabine plus cisplatin and epirubicin for locally advanced, resectable gastric or gastro-oesophageal junction adenocarcinoma (FLOT4): a randomised, phase 2/3 trial. *Lancet.* 2019;393(10184):1948–1957. doi:10.1016/S0140-6736(18)32557-1
21. Park SH, Lim DH, Sohn TS, et al. A randomized phase III trial comparing adjuvant single-agent S1, S-1 with oxaliplatin, and postoperative chemoradiation with S-1 and oxaliplatin in patients with node-positive gastric cancer after D2 resection: the ARTIST 2 trial. *Ann Oncol.* 2021;32(3):368–374. doi:10.1016/j.annonc.2020.11.017

22. Karpeh MS, Leon L, Klimstra D, Brennan MF. Lymph node staging in gastric cancer: is location more important than number? An analysis of 1038 patients. *Ann. Surg.* 2000;232(3):362–371. doi:10.1097/00000658-200009000-00008

23. Edge SB, Compton CC. The American Joint Committee on Cancer: the 7th edition of the AJCC cancer staging manual and the future of TNM. *Ann Surg Oncol.* 2010;17(6):1471–1474. doi:10.1245/s10434-010-0985-4

24. Hartgrink HH, Van de Velde CJ, Putter H, et al. Extended lymph node dissection for gastric cancer: who may benefit? Final results of the randomized dutch gastric cancer group trial. *J Clin Oncol.* 2004;22:2069–2077.

25. Songun I, Putter H., Kranenbarg EM-K, et al. Surgical treatment of gastric cancer: 15-year follow-up results of the randomised nationwide Dutch D1D2 trial. *Lancet Oncol.* 2010;11(5):439–449. doi:10.1016/S1470-2045(10)70070-X

26. Miyazaki Y, Takiguchi S, Takahashi T, et al. Treatment of gastric outlet obstruction that results from unresectable gastric cancer: current evidence. *World J Gastrointest Endosc.* 2016;8(3):165–172. doi:10.4253/wjge.v8.i3.165

27. Jeurnink SM, van Eijck CHJ, Steyerberg EW, et al. Stent versus gastrojejunostomy for the palliation of gastric outlet obstruction: a systematic review. *BMC Gastroenterol.* 2007;7(1):Article No. 18. doi:10.1186/1471-230X-7-18

28. Bang Y-J, Van Cutsem E, Feyereislova A, et al. Trastuzumab in combination with chemotherapy versus chemotherapy alone for treatment of HER2-positive advanced gastric or gastro-oesophageal junction cancer (ToGA): a phase 3, open-label, randomised controlled trial. *Lancet.* 2010;376(9742):687–697. doi:10.1016/S0140-6736(10)61121-X

29. Janjigian YY, Shitara K, Moehler M, et al. First-line nivolumab plus chemotherapy versus chemotherapy alone for advanced gastric, gastro-oesophageal junction, and oesophageal adenocarcinoma (CheckMate 649): a randomised, open-label, phase 3 trial. *Lancet.* 2021;398(10294):27–40. doi:10.1016/S0140-6736(21)00797-2

30. Chung HC, Bang Y-J, Fuchs CS, et al. First-line pembrolizumab/placebo plus trastuzumab and chemotherapy in HER2-positive advanced gastric cancer: KEYNOTE-811. *Future Oncol.* 2021;17(5): 491–501. doi:10.2217/fon-2020-0737

31. Bartley AN, Washington MK, Colasacco C, et al. HER2 testing and clinical decision making in gastroesophageal adenocarcinoma: guideline from the College of American Pathologists, American Society for Clinical Pathology, and the American Society of Clinical Oncology. *J Clin Oncol.* 2017;35(4):446–464. doi:10.1200/JCO.2016.69.4836

32. Kato S, Okamura R, Baumgartner JM, et al. Analysis of circulating tumor DNA and clinical correlates in patients with esophageal, gastroesophageal junction, and gastric adenocarcinoma. *Clin Cancer Res.* 2018;24(24):6248–6256. doi:10.1158/1078-0432.CCR-18-1128

33. van Cutsem E, Sagaert X, Topal B, et al. Gastric cancer. *Lancet.* 2016;388:2654–2664. doi:10.1016/S0140-6736(16)30354-3

34. Enzinger PC, Burtness BA, Niedzwiecki D, et al. CALGB 80403 (Alliance)/E1206: a randomized phase II study of three chemotherapy regimens plus cetuximab in metastatic esophageal and gastroesophageal junction cancers. *J Clin Oncol.* 2016;34(23):2736–2742. doi:10.1200/JCO.2015.65.5092

35. Al-Batran S-E, Hartmann JT, Probst S, et al. Phase III trial in metastatic gastroesophageal adenocarcinoma with fluorouracil, leucovorin plus either oxaliplatin or cisplatin: a study of the Arbeitsgemeinschaft Internistische Onkologie. *J Clin Oncol.* 2008;26(9):1435–1442. doi:10.1200/JCO.2007.13.9378

36. Bang Y-J, Van Cutsem E, Feyereislova A, et al. Trastuzumab in combination with chemotherapy versus chemotherapy alone for treatment of HER2-positive advanced gastric or gastro-oesophageal junction cancer (ToGA): a phase 3, open-label, randomised controlled trial. *Lancet.* 2010;376(9742):687–697. doi:10.1016/S0140-6736(10)61121-X

37. Shitara K, Van Cutsem E, Bang Y-J, et al. Efficacy and safety of pembrolizumab or pembrolizumab plus chemotherapy vs chemotherapy alone for patients with first-line, advanced gastric cancer: the KEYNOTE-062 phase 3 randomized clinical trial. *JAMA Oncol.* 2020;6:1571–1580. doi:10.1001/jamaoncol.2020.3370

38. Assersohn L, Brown G, Cunningham D, et al. Phase II study of irinotecan and 5-fluorouracil/leucovorin in patients with primary refractory or relapsed advanced oesophageal and gastric carcinoma. *Ann Oncol.* 2004;15(1):64–69. doi:10.1093/annonc/mdh007

39. Ford HE, Marshall A, Bridgewater JA, et al. Docetaxel versus active symptom control for refractory oesophagogastric adenocarcinoma (COUGAR-02): an open-label, phase 3 randomised controlled trial. *Lancet Oncol.* 2014;15(1):78–86. doi:10.1016/S1470-2045(13)70549-7

40. Kang JH, Lee SI, Lim DH, et al. Salvage chemotherapy for pretreated gastric cancer: a randomized phase III trial comparing chemotherapy plus best supportive care with best supportive care alone. *J Clin Oncol.* 2012;30(13):1513–1518. doi:10.1200/JCO.2011.39.4585

41. Fuchs CS, Tomasek J, Yong CJ, et al. Ramucirumab monotherapy for previously treated advanced gastric or gastro-oesophageal junction adenocarcinoma (REGARD): an international, randomised, multicentre, placebo-controlled, phase 3 trial. *Lancet.* 2014;383(9911):31–39. doi:10.1016/S0140-6736(13)61719-5

42. Wilke H, Muro K, Van Cutsem E, et al. Ramucirumab plus paclitaxel versus placebo plus paclitaxel in patients with previously treated advanced gastric or gastro-oesophageal junction adenocarcinoma (RAINBOW): a double-blind, randomised phase 3 trial. *Lancet Oncol.* 2014;15(11):1224–1235. doi:10.1016/S1470-2045(14)70420-6

43. Shitara K, Doi T, Dvorkin M, et al. Trifluridine/tipiracil versus placebo in patients with heavily pretreated metastatic gastric cancer (TAGS): a randomised, double-blind, placebo-controlled, phase 3 trial. *Lancet Oncol.* 2018;19(11):1437–1448. doi:10.1016/S1470-2045(18)30739-3

44. Fuchs CS, Doi T, Jang RW, et al. Safety and efficacy of pembrolizumab monotherapy in patients with previously treated advanced gastric and gastroesophageal junction cancer: phase 2 clinical KEYNOTE-059 trial. *JAMA Oncol.* 2018;4(5):e180013. doi:10.1001/jamaoncol.2018.0013

45. Shitara K, Bang Y-J, Iwasa S, et al. Trastuzumab deruxtecan in previously treated HER2-positive gastric cancer. *N Engl J Med.* 2020;382(25):2419–2430. doi:10.1056/NEJMoa2004413

46. Doebele RC, Drilon A, Paz-Ares L, et al. Entrectinib in patients with advanced or metastatic *NTRK* fusion-positive solid tumours: integrated analysis of three phase 1–2 trials. *Lancet Oncolo.* 2020;21(2):271–282. doi:10.1016/S1470-2045(19)30691-6

47. Kanat O, Ertas H, Caner B. Platinum-induced neurotoxicity: a review of possible mechanisms. *World J Clin Oncol.* 2017;8(4):329–335. doi:10.5306/wjco.v8.i4.329

48. Hershman DL, Lacchetti C, Dworkin RH, et al. Prevention and management of chemotherapy-induced peripheral neuropathy in survivors of adult cancers: American Society of Clinical Oncology clinical practice guideline. *J Clin Oncol.* 2014;32(18):1941–1967. doi:10.1200/JCO.2013.54.0914

49. Cunningham D, Starling N, Rao S, et al. Capecitabine and oxaliplatin for advanced esophagogastric cancer. *N Engl J Med.* 2008;358(1):36–46. doi:10.1056/NEJMoa073149

50. Walden D, Sonbol MB, Buckner Petty S, et al. Maintenance therapy in first-line gastric and gastroesophageal junction adenocarcinoma: a retrospective analysis. *Front Oncol.* 2021;11:641044. doi:10.3389/fonc.2021.641044

51. Hall PS, Swinson D, Cairns DA, et al. Efficacy of reduced-intensity chemotherapy with oxaliplatin and capecitabine on quality of life and cancer control among older and frail patients with advanced gastroesophageal cancer: the GO2 phase 3 randomized clinical trial. *JAMA Oncol.* 2021;7(6):869–877. doi:10.1001/jamaoncol.2021.0848

CHAPTER 9

Pancreatic Cancer

Huili Zhu, Zachary Phillip Yeung, Benjamin Musher, and Shalini Makawita

INTRODUCTION

Pancreatic cancer (PC) is the third-leading cause of cancer mortality in the United States and seventh-leading cause worldwide. Most recent analysis of Surveillance, Epidemiology, and End Results (SEER) data suggests a rising incidence of PC with approximately 60,000 new diagnoses and 48,000 deaths annually.[1] Major risk factors include cigarette smoking, obesity, physical inactivity, hereditary and chronic pancreatitis, and genetic predisposition such as inherited PC syndromes. Five-year survival rate is 10%, and this has been unchanged in the past 30 years. The high mortality rate is largely due to late presentation. Even when PC presents in early stages, it is often not curable. Only about 15% to 20% of the patients present with resectable disease, 30% with locally advanced disease, and 50% with metastatic disease.[2] Five-year survival after margin-negative surgical resection is approximately 30% for node-negative and only 10% for node-positive disease.[3] Additional challenges that contribute to PC's high mortality include lack of molecular targets and immunologic activity, and its being more resistant to chemotherapy/radiation than other cancers. The following four cases will delve into these factors as well as provide a comprehensive review of the management and treatment of PC.

CASE SUMMARIES

Case 9.1: Resectable Pancreatic Cancer

A 61-year-old man with a 50 pack-year history of smoking, obesity (body mass index [BMI] 31), and hypertension presented with 3 months of belching, fatigue, loss of appetite, and weight loss (10 pounds). Ten days before presentation, he noticed darkening of his urine, floating khaki-colored stool, yellowing of his eyes then skin, generalized pruritus, and mild abdominal discomfort. He denied fevers, chills, vomiting, dyspnea, or leg swelling. He drank alcohol socially but stopped in his 40s. He worked full time as an accountant and had no known family history of cancer. In his spare time, he did carpentry and biked in his neighborhood. Physical examination was remarkable for icteric sclerae, jaundice, and periumbilical tenderness without hepatomegaly or abdominal distention. Initial laboratory evaluation revealed a total bilirubin of 5, alkaline phosphatase of 140, aspartate aminotransferase (AST) of 87, alanine aminotransferase (ALT) of 115, carcinoembryonic antigen (CEA) of 1.5, and carbohydrate antigen (CA) 19-9 of 217. The patient was referred to interventional gastroenterology.

How Is a Diagnosis Established?

- For suspected PC, CT with pancreas protocol (arterial and portal venous phases with thin slices) or MRI with gadolinium is recommended to visualize the pancreatic mass, assess involvement of adjacent vasculature (superior mesenteric vein [SMV], portal veins [PVs], celiac axis, hepatic artery, and superior mesenteric artery [SMA]), and evaluate for intra-abdominal metastases. Once a diagnosis has been established, imaging of the chest and pelvis should be performed.
- MRI and cholangiopancreatography can further characterize indeterminate lesions within the liver but are not routinely required.
- Endoscopic ultrasound (EUS) is used to confirm malignancy in localized disease, provide material for molecular testing, define the tumor/vasculature relationships, and evaluate regional nodal involvement. EUS-guided fine-needle core biopsy (FNB) is preferred over aspiration for better yield.
- Endoscopic retrograde cholangiopancreatography (ERCP) with stent placement should be performed in patients with biliary obstruction. If a plastic stent is placed initially, it should be replaced with a metal stent if the tumor is unresectable or the patient will be receiving neoadjuvant therapy (NAT).
- For biomarker evaluation of PC, serum CA 19-9 is the most validated for early detection and surveillance, but it is also elevated in benign pancreatic and hepatobiliary diseases (for example, pancreatitis, biliary obstruction). Therefore, CA 19-9 is not a recommended diagnostic tool but can be valuable to prognosticate and monitor established PC. CEA, when expressed, may also be useful and is not affected by biliary obstruction or pancreatitis.

Patient's Diagnosis

- CT of the abdomen and pelvis with iodine contrast (pancreas protocol) revealed a 2.6-cm heterogeneous mass in the head of the pancreas causing marked dilation of the common and intrahepatic bile ducts. The SMA, common hepatic artery (CHA), celiac axis, SMV, and PV were free from tumor involvement. No liver masses, lymphadenopathy, ascites, or omental/peritoneal nodules were appreciated.
- EUS revealed a mass in the head of the pancreas without vascular involvement or lymphadenopathy, and biopsy confirmed adenocarcinoma.

What Further Molecular or Genomic Testing Is Required?

- Familial risk for PC accounts for as many as 15% of cases, and 5% to 10% of patients are proven to harbor a pathogenic germline variant that increases susceptibility to PC, most commonly BRCA2, BRCA1, ATM, and PALB2.
- National Comprehensive Cancer Network (NCCN) guidelines recommend germline testing for all patients with newly diagnosed PC to guide chemotherapy selections and facilitate genetic counseling of family members.[4]
- The U.S. Preventative Services Task Force recommends against routine screening for PC in the absence of a genetic syndrome or a strong family history.
- Comprehensive tumor tissue molecular profiling has identified hallmark driver genes in PC including KRAS, CDKN2A, TP53, and SMAD4. Underlying genomic instability associated with DNA repair mechanisms, including homologous recombination resulting in synthetic lethality, increases susceptibility of tumors with pathogenic variants to platinum-based therapy and poly (ADP-ribose) polymerase inhibitors.

Patient's Molecular and Genomic Testing

- Next-generation sequencing (NGS) of biopsy specimen: pathogenic mutations in TP53 (p.Y220C, loss of function) and KRAS (p.G12R, gain of function); microsatellite stable.

How Is This Tumor Staged?

Per the American Joint Committee on Cancer (AJCC) tumor, lymph node, metastasis (TNM) system eighth edition staging system for pancreatic ductal adenocarcinoma:

- Stage I disease includes a tumor measuring less than 4 cm without arterial or lymph node (LN) involvement.
- Stage II disease includes a primary tumor greater than 4 cm and/or involvement of one to three regional LNs.
- Stage III includes any size tumor that has spread to four or more regional LNs and/or involves the celiac axis or SMA.
- Stage IV includes distant (nonregional) spread.

While TNM staging of PC allows for prognostication, clinical decision-making relies on anatomic resectability and a patient's suitability for undergoing surgery. To be considered anatomically resectable, a PC must not involve the celiac axis, CHA, or SMA, but it may abut the SMV and/or PV by 180 degrees or less and without venous distortion or thrombosis. Borderline resectable disease includes tumors with more extensive venous involvement and/or limited arterial involvement (less than 180 degree involvement of the celiac axis, CHA, and/or SMA). Locally advanced unresectable disease includes tumors with greater than 180-degrees arterial involvement and/or long-segment venous thrombosis that would preclude reconstruction.

Patient's Clinical Stage
- *The patient's stage is T2N0M0 (IB).*

What Are Appropriate Treatment Options?

- The goals of surgery include R0 (negative microscopic margin) resection of the primary tumor and regional LNs, as well as minimization of postoperative morbidity.
- Given the complexities of radiographic interpretation and surgical planning, multidisciplinary discussion and evaluation in high volume centers of excellence is strongly recommended.
- Surgery should be performed by experienced pancreatobiliary surgeons at high-volume centers since higher surgical volume is associated with fewer postoperative complications, higher rates of R0 resection, and longer overall survival (OS).[5]
- Patient factors, such as functional status and comorbidities, must be assessed to optimize surgical outcomes, especially in the geriatric population.

Patient's Surgery
- *The case was presented at a multidisciplinary tumor board, with a consensus recommendation to proceed with upfront pancreatoduodenectomy (Whipple procedure). The patient underwent a minimally invasive Whipple procedure at a high-volume center and recovered without major complications. Pathological evaluation revealed a 3.0-cm adenocarcinoma with negative resection margins (R0 resection) and 0/42 involved LNs. Final pathological stage was T2N0M0 (stage IB).*

What Are Other Treatment Considerations?

- Even with successful R0 resection, recurrence rates are very high (greater than 90%) due to the presence of micrometastases at diagnosis, so additional therapy is recommended in all patients who undergo resection. NCCN guidelines recommend that adjuvant therapy (AT) be initiated when the patient has recovered from surgery.[1]
- Table 9.1 lists the major clinical trials of AT for resected PC.

- CONKO-001[6] showed a 6.7-month improvement in median disease-free survival (DFS), 2.6-month improvement in OS, and 10.3% improvement in 5-year survival (hazard ratio [HR], 0.76; 95% confidence interval [CI]; 0.61 to 0.95; $P = 0.01$) of single-agent gemcitabine compared to observation.
- RTOG 97-04[7] showed that, in all-comers with resected PC, adjuvant gemcitabine plus 5-FU-based chemoradiation did not improve survival over 5-FU plus 5-FU-based chemoradiation. In the subset of pancreatic head tumors, 3-year OS was higher in the gemcitabine arm (31% vs. 21%, HR = 0.79, CI = 0.63 to 0.99, $P = 0.047$).
- ESPAC-3(v2)[8] showed no significant difference in OS between adjuvant 5-FU/leucovorin (23 months) and gemcitabine (23.6 months; HR, 0.94 [95%CI, 0.81 to 1.08]; $P = 0.39$).
- ESPAC-4[9] showed a 2.5-month improvement in OS for patients who received adjuvant gemcitabine plus capecitabine compared to gemcitabine alone (HR, 0.82 [95% CI, 0.68 to 0.98]; $P = 0.032$).
- PRODIGE-24[10] showed a 19.4-month improvement in median OS (mOS; HR, 0.66 [95% CI, 0.49 to 0.89]) and 12.7-month improvement in metastasis-free survival of modified regimen of folinic acid, fluorouracil, irinotecan, and oxaliplatin (FOLFIRINOX) over gemcitabine (HR, 0.59 [95% CI, 0.46 to 0.76]).
- APACT[11] showed no difference in DFS but did show a 4.7-month improvement in interim OS of gemcitabine/nab-paclitaxel compared to gemcitabine alone (HR, 0.82 [95% CI, 0.680 to 0.996]; $P = 0.045$).
- Of note, the mOS of single-agent gemcitabine was 22 to 23 months in CONKO-001/ ESPAC-3, 26 months in ESPAC-4, and 35 to 36 months in PRODIGE and APACT. The progressive improvement in mOS with single-agent gemcitabine in these trials may have arisen from more careful patient selection (including a higher proportion of patients with potentially resectable disease undergoing NAT), more effective therapies for relapsed disease, and improved supportive care.

Table 9.1   Adjuvant Therapy Clinical Trials Summary

Trial	Year	Number of Patients	Control Arm	Experimental Arm	Median Survival (Months) Control vs. Experiment	P-Value
GITSG[29]	1985	43	Observation	5-FU/RT + 5-FU	10.9 vs. 21.0	0.03
EORTC[29]	1999	114	Observation	5-FU/RT	17.1 vs. 12.6	0.09
ESPAC-1[29]	2004	289	Observation	5-FU/LV	15.6 vs. 20.1	0.003
RTOG 9704[8]	2008	388	5-FU/RT	Gemcitabine/RT	16.9 vs. 20.5	0.05
ESPAC-3[9]	2009	1149	5-FU/LV	Gemcitabine	23.0 vs. 23.6	0.39
ESPAC-4[10]	2017	732	Gemcitabine	Gemcitabine/ Capecitabine	25.5 vs. 28.0	0.032
CONKO-001[7]	2012	368	Observation	Gemcitabine	20.2 vs. 22.1	0.01
JASPAC 01[29]	2013	378	Gemcitabine	S-1	25.5 vs. 46.5	<0.0001
PRODIGE 24[11]	2018	493	Gemcitabine	mFOLFIRINOX	34.8 vs. 54.4	N/A
APACT[12]	2019	866	Gemcitabine	Gemcitabine/ nab-paclitaxel	36.2 vs. 40.5	0.045

5-FU, fluorouracil; LV, leucovorin; mFOLFIRINOX, modified regimen of folinic acid, fluorouracil, irinotecan, and oxaliplatin; RT, radiotherapy.

- CONKO-005[12] showed no improvement in DFS nor OS when erlotinib was added to adjuvant gemcitabine.
- NAT for resectable disease is still under clinical investigation[13] but has been adopted as standard in many high-volume academic centers. NCCN guidelines[1] recommend consideration of NAT in high-risk patients, including those with extreme elevations in CA 19-9, large primary tumors, large regional LNs, excessive weight loss, and severe pain.

Patient's Adjuvant Therapy

- *The patient had returned to biking and woodworking within 8 weeks after surgery, so he started a 6-month course of adjuvant mFOLFIRINOX.*

What Is Required for This Patient's Follow-Up and Survivorship?

- History and physical examination for symptom assessment every 3 to 6 months for 2 years then every 6 to 12 months as clinically indicated is needed.
- Consider monitoring CA 19-9 levels, particularly in cases where initial levels were elevated.
- Consider CT of the chest, abdomen, and pelvis with contrast as indicated by symptoms or rising CA 19-9 levels.

Case 9.2: Borderline Resectable Pancreatic Cancer

A 67-year-old woman with a 14 pack-year history of smoking, hypertension, treated H. pylori infection, and major depressive disorder presented to her primary physician for progressive abdominal pain. She denied changes in the color of her skin or stools, nausea, or weight loss. Surgical history was only notable for hysterectomy. Family history was negative for cancer. She lived alone and was independent of her activities of daily living. She reported no underlying neuropathy.

How Is a Diagnosis Established?

- Similar imaging and biopsy modalities are used as described with Case 9.1.

Patient's Diagnosis

- *CT scan of the abdomen and pelvis showed a 3.8-cm ill-defined mass in the pancreatic head that involved the SMV and PV near the splenoportal confluence causing distortion of the PV. Three peripancreatic nodes were noted. No other suspicious masses or lesions were seen.*
- *EUS-guided biopsy showed invasive, moderately differentiated adenocarcinoma.*

- Criteria defining borderline resectable pancreatic cancer (BRPC):
  - Arterial:
    - Pancreatic head or uncinate process: contact with the CHA without extension to the celiac artery or hepatic artery bifurcation. Contact with the SMA should be 180 degrees or less.
    - Body or tail of the pancreas: contact with the celiac artery 180 degrees or less, or contact greater than 180 degrees without involvement of the aorta and with intact and uninvolved gastroduodenal artery.
  - Venous:
    - Contact with the SMV or PV greater than 180 degrees, or contact 180 degrees or less with contour irregularity, thrombosis of the vein, or involvement with the inferior vena cava (IVC) but with enough proximal and distal suitable for resection and reconstruction.

What Further Molecular or Genomic Testing Is Required?

- This is as noted with Case 9.1.

Patient's Molecular and Genomic Testing

- Germline testing: no pathogenic germline variants identified
- NGS of biopsy specimen: pathogenic mutations in CKDN2A (p.H83Y, loss of function), TP53 (p.K132R, loss of function), and KRAS p.G12D (gain of function); microsatellite stable

How Is This Tumor Staged?

- This tumor is staged as noted with Case 9.1 with the following additional considerations:
- Staging laparoscopy can be considered in select high-risk patients with no radiographic evidence of metastatic disease to detect occult metastases in the abdominal cavity. High risk is defined by high CA 19-9, bulky primary tumor and/or regional nodes, as well as heavy symptom burden.
- Surgery should incorporate intraoperative staging at the time of resection to rule out peritoneal, liver, and distant LN metastases.

Patient's Clinical Stage

- The patient's stage is T4N1M0 (III).
- A CT of the chest showed no pulmonary metastasis; diagnostic laparoscopy showed no peritoneal or liver lesions; and cytology of peritoneal washings showed no malignant cells.

What Are Appropriate Treatment Options?

- In addition to increasing the rate of R0 resection in BRPC, administering chemotherapy before aggressive surgery increases the proportion of patients with potentially resectable disease who will receive systemic therapy at all (since many patients who undergo upfront resection never receive AT). NAT also allows the clinician to assess in vivo sensitivity of the tumor to standard chemotherapy as well as experimental agents. Finally, attacking micrometastatic disease upfront helps the multidisciplinary team select those patients who do not have occult chemoresistant disease and who therefore stand to benefit most from primary tumor resection.
- Multicenter prospective Phase II and III data have shown that completing NAT in patients with BRPC is feasible and increases the probability of R0 resection from 33% to about 80%.[14,15]
- NAT regimens for BRPC include mFOLFIRINOX, gemcitabine/nab-paclitaxel, or gemcitabine/capecitabine with or without subsequent chemoradiation.
- The PREOPANC study,[16] which randomized 246 patients with BRPC to upfront surgery followed by adjuvant gemcitabine or neoadjuvant gemcitabine and chemoradiation followed by surgery, showed that the NAT led to improved DFS, R0 resection, and OS.
- ESPAC-5F,[17] which randomized 90 patients with BRPC to upfront surgery or one of three NAT regimens (gemcitabine/capecitabine, FOLFIRINOX, or concurrent capecitabine/radiation), showed improved 1-year survival with NAT but was not powered to compare the neoadjuvant arms.
- In patients with known BRCA1/2 or PALB2 mutations, a platinum-containing regimen (FOLFIRINOX or gemcitabine/cisplatin) with or without subsequent chemoradiation is preferred.[18]
- CT re-staging should be performed after therapy to reassess tumor-vessel relationships and resectability, but radiographic response may not correlate with pathological response. Ideally, surgery is performed 4 to 8 weeks after completion of NAT.

Patient's Treatment and Course
- A multidisciplinary tumor board recommended NAT for her BRPC. She started FOLFIRINOX given her good performance status.
- Re-staging CT after 4 biweekly cycles showed smaller peripancreatic nodes and a smaller pancreas tumor with less venous distortion. She received another 4 cycles, with CT showing ongoing response in her primary tumor and an absence of metastatic disease. Her case was re-presented at the multidisciplinary tumor board. In light of her radiographic tumor response and the onset of persistent neuropathy in her fingers and toes, her team recommended that she proceed to surgery. She underwent a Whipple procedure, with pathology showing a 1.5-cm tumor, 0/12 involved nodes, negative margins, and histological evidence of tumor response (ypT1N0, R0 resection). She recovered without significant postoperative complications and received 4 additional cycles of FOLFIRINOX with dose-reduced oxaliplatin.

Case 9.3: Locally Advanced Pancreatic Cancer

A 72-year-old male with hypertension, type 2 diabetes, hyperlipidemia, and a 30 pack-year smoking history presented to his primary doctor with early satiety, weight loss, and painless jaundice. He worked as a construction worker in his youth and reported no family history of cancer. Initial blood work showed a total bilirubin of 7, alkaline phosphatase of 85, and CA 19-9 of 152 U/mL. He underwent ERCP with placement of metal stent. He had an excellent performance status (ECOG 0).

How Is a Diagnosis Established?

- Similar imaging and biopsy modalities are used as described with Case 9.1.

Patient's Diagnosis
- CT of the abdomen showed a 4.3-cm pancreatic head mass encasing the celiac axis and abutting the aorta, as well as two enlarged pancreaticoduodenal LNs. Further imaging showed no evidence of metastases in the lungs, liver, or abdominal cavity.
- EUS demonstrated the presence of a mass in the pancreatic head and regional lymphadenopathy. FNB confirmed pancreatic adenocarcinoma.

What Further Molecular or Genomic Testing Is Required?

- The testing is as noted with Case 9.1.

Patient's Molecular and Genomic Testing
- *Germline testing:* no pathogenic germline variants identified
- *NGS of biopsy specimen:* pathogenic mutations in TP53 (p.L330fs, loss of function), SMAD4 (p.R445*, loss of function), CDKN2A copy number loss, and KRAS (p.G12V, gain of function); microsatellite stable

How Is This Tumor Staged?

- The tumor is staged as noted with Cases 9.1 and 9.2.
- Locally advanced pancreatic cancer (LAPC) is defined by increasing 180-degree abutment of the SMA or celiac artery; any contact of both the celiac artery and aorta; and/or involvement of the SMV or PV extensive enough to preclude reconstruction.

Patient's Clinical Stage

- *The stage is T4N1M0 (stage III).*
- *Diagnostic laparotomy showed no peritoneal or liver lesions, and cytology from peritoneal cavity washings showed no malignant cells.*

What Are Appropriate Treatment Options?

- Consider referral to an academic institution for enrollment into clinical trials.
- Therapy for LAPC mimics that of BRPC, with the goal of treating microscopic as well as gross disease.
- Rendering LAPC resectable with currently approved therapy remains highly unlikely but should be reconsidered upon subsequent re-staging.
- Although consolidative radiation with or without chemotherapy is often recommended after induction chemotherapy, its benefit in LAPC has still not been proven. In the LAP07 trial,[19] 223 patients with LAPC whose disease was well-controlled after 4 months of induction chemotherapy were randomized to chemoradiation or continuation of chemotherapy. Chemoradiation lowered the risk of local progression but did not improve mOS over continuing chemotherapy.

Patient's Treatment

- *He was referred to an academic cancer center for consideration of a clinical trial.*

Case 9.4: Metastatic Pancreatic Cancer

A 60-year-old female with diabetes and hypertension presented with 2 months of abdominal pain, poor appetite, and unintentional weight loss of 20 pounds. Her prior surgeries included appendectomy and tubal ligation. She was independent in all her daily activities and lived with her husband and son. She was a lifetime nonsmoker and did not drink alcohol. Her maternal grandmother was diagnosed with breast cancer at age 65. Laboratory workup showed a total bilirubin of 2.2, alkaline phosphatase of 74, CEA of 12, and CA 19-9 of 1100 U/mL.

How Is a Diagnosis Established?

- Similar imaging modalities are used as described with Case 9.1.

Patient's Diagnosis

- *A CT pancreas protocol of the abdomen and pelvis showed a 3.5-cm pancreatic uncinate mass encasing the SMA and SMV and numerous hypodense hepatic lesions.*
- *Biopsy of a 2-cm liver lesion confirmed metastatic adenocarcinoma of the pancreas.*

What Further Molecular or Genomic Testing Is Required?

- The testing required is as noted with Case 9.1.
- The POLO study[20] showed that the PARP inhibitor olaparib improved progression-free survival (PFS) and OS over placebo when used as maintenance therapy after induction of platinum-based chemotherapy in patients with metastatic PC and germline *BRCA* mutations.

Patient's Molecular and Genomic Testing

- *Germline testing: mutation in BRCA2*
- *NGS of biopsy specimen: pathogenic mutations in ARID1A (p.G2107fs, loss of function), TP53 (p.G244C, loss of function), SETD2 (p.S821fs, loss of function), KDM6A (p.E44*, loss of function), and KRAS (p.G12D, gain of function); microsatellite stable*

How Is This Tumor Staged?

- This tumor is staged as noted with Case 9.1 with the following additional considerations.
- In the setting of metastatic disease, biopsy of a metastatic lesion may be completed to establish tissue diagnosis of metastasis and for molecular profiling.

Patient's Stage
- T2N0M1 (stage IV)

What Are Appropriate Treatment Options?

- Consider referral to an academic institution for enrollment into clinical trials.
- Chemotherapy has been proven to improve survival, symptom control, and quality of life in patients with metastatic PC. In appropriately fit treatment-naive patients, combination chemotherapy is preferred over single-agent therapy.
- In the Phase III randomized-controlled PRODIGE trial,[21] FOLFIRINOX yielded superior PFS (6.4 vs. 3.3 months, HR 0.47; P less than 0.001) and OS (11.1 months vs. 6.8 months, HR 0.57; P less than 0.001) when compared to single-agent gemcitabine in patients with untreated metastatic PC who had an ECOG PS of 0-1.
- In the Phase III randomized-controlled MPACT III,[22] nab-paclitaxel plus gemcitabine yielded superior PFS (5.5 vs. 3.7 months, HR 0.69; P less than 0.001) and OS (8.5 vs. 6.7 months, HR 0.72; P less than 0.001) over single-agent gemcitabine in patients with untreated metastatic PC who had ECOG performance status of 0 to 2.
- Therefore, both FOLFIRINOX and nab-paclitaxel/gemcitabine are acceptable options for first-line treatment of metastatic PC, as they have not been compared head-to-head. Treatment recommendation should be based on performance status and patient/physician preference.
- In NAPOLI-1,[23] a Phase III study in metastatic PC patients previously treated with gemcitabine-based chemotherapy, nanoliposomal irinotecan plus fluorouracil, and folinic acid yielded superior mOS (6.1 vs. 4.2 months, HR 0.67; P = 0.012) over fluorouracil and folinic acid.
- NAPOLI-3[24] is an ongoing randomized, Phase III study comparing fluorouracil, liposomal irinotecan, and oxaliplatin to nab-paclitaxel/gemcitabine in patients with treatment-naïve metastatic PC.
- Clinical trials are investigating combinations of standard chemotherapy and novel agents.

Patient's Treatment
- The patient received 6 months of FOLFIRINOX and interval imaging revealed a substantial decrease in the size of her pancreatic tumor and liver metastases. Based on her germline BRCA2 mutation and the data reported from the POLO trial, she was switched to maintenance olaparib.

What Are Toxicities Associated With Chemotherapy?

- The most common toxicities associated with FOLFIRINOX are fatigue, neutropenia, nausea, diarrhea, and sensory neuropathy.
- The most common toxicities associated with gemcitabine/nab-paclitaxel include myelosuppression, fatigue, alopecia, nausea, and peripheral neuropathy.

What Encompasses Best Supportive Care?

- All patients with newly diagnosed PC, regardless of stage, are at high risk for developing cancer-related symptoms (for example, pain, weight loss, nausea, fatigue, constipation, diarrhea, and depression) as well as side effects from treatment. They need to be supported aggressively to improve survival, alleviate suffering, and optimize quality of life.

- Many studies have shown the benefits of palliative care alongside disease-modifying treatments for advanced cancers.[25] All patients with advanced PC should be considered for referral to a palliative care physician, nutritionist, and counselor/psychologist.
- Palliative care should be directed to one or more of the following sequelae of PC: biliary obstruction, gastric outlet/duodenal obstruction, tumor-associated abdominal pain, pancreatic insufficiency, venous thromboembolism (VTE), malnutrition, depression, and anxiety.
- Palliative radiotherapy and celiac plexus neurolysis can alleviate tumor-related pain refractory to opioids. Metal biliary stents are preferred over plastic stents due to their durability. Duodenal stenting or surgical gastrojejunostomy can restore oral intake in patients with gastric outlet obstruction.
- VTE is common among patients with PC. CONKO-004[26] demonstrated that primary prophylaxis with enoxaparin decreased the incidence of symptomatic VTE by 9% in patients with advanced PC undergoing chemotherapy, but it had no effect on PFS or OS. Thus, starting all such patients on prophylactic anticoagulation is not currently standard practice. Rather, clinicians should maintain a high level of suspicion for VTE in any PC patient complaining of asymmetric lower extremity swelling and/or respiratory symptoms.

Future Directions

- Current efforts are underway to explore targeted therapy options outside PARP inhibition. Systemic therapies targeting *NTRK* fusions[27,28] and microsatellite instability (MSI) have gained tumor-agnostic approval, but these alterations are extremely rare in PC. Agents directed against *KRAS* have recently shown some activity against *KRASG12C*-mutated tumors and are under further investigation. Thus far, agents targeting stroma (hyaluronidase and hedgehog inhibitors) have not shown benefit, but newer agents are in development.
- Randomized trials testing SM88, an oral tyrosine derivative thought to dysregulate metabolism, and CPI 613, which hyperstimulates an endogenous redox mechanism for KDGH enzyme and leads to reactive oxygen species-signaling associated apoptosis, have recently finished accrual.
- Pathogenic variants with actionable somatic alterations have been identified in young-onset PC patients.[29] Recent guidelines have shifted toward universal germline testing and somatic profiling in all patients, irrespective of family history.
- Although immunotherapy has not yet proven efficacious in the vast majority of PCs, studies are underway to identify subsets of patients who may respond to known immunotherapeutic agents and to develop novel agents that may convert PC from an immunoresistant to an immunoresponsive tumor. The Phase II POLAR trial is evaluating the safety of pembrolizumab plus olaparib in metastatic PC patients and stratifying subjects by mutational status.
- Circulating tumor DNA analysis, tumor subtyping, and immune profiling are being used to identify patients who may be candidates for chemoimmunotherapy.

REVIEW QUESTIONS

1. A 55-year-old male with recently diagnosed type 2 diabetes mellitus presents with painless jaundice. Alkaline phosphatase is 820, and total bilirubin is 13.5 g/dL. He undergoes pancreas protocol CT that demonstrates a 2.6-cm hypodense mass in the pancreatic head resulting in biliary obstruction. The mass does not contact the superior mesenteric, celiac, or hepatic arteries. There is less than 180 degrees abutment of the superior mesenteric vein. No sites of distant disease are found. He undergoes an endoscopic retrograde cholangiopancreatography (ERCP) with successful biliary stenting and improvement in his serum bilirubin. endoscopic ultrasound (EUS)-guided fine-needle core biopsy (FNB) reveals pancreatic adenocarcinoma. His serum carbohydrate antigen (CA) 19.9 level is 120 U/mL, and he has an Eastern Cooperative Oncology Group (ECOG) performance status (PS) of 1. What is the next step in management of this patient?
   A. Surgery +/- neoadjuvant chemotherapy
   B. Chemoradiation with 5-fluorouracil or capecitabine
   C. Consideration for clinical trial
   D. Stereotactic body radiation therapy (SBRT)
   E. Both option A and C

2. The patient in question 1 undergoes a successful pancreaticoduodenectomy (Whipple) with R0 resection. Pathology shows a 1.8-cm pancreatic ductal adenocarcinoma 0/40 examined lymph nodes (LNs) negative for malignancy. He has fully recovered 6 weeks after surgery and presents to the medical oncology clinic for a recommendation about adjuvant therapy. His postoperative carbohydrate antigen (CA) 19.9 is less than 35, and his Eastern Cooperative Oncology Group (ECOG) performance status (PS) is 0. He has no baseline neuropathy. Which of the following statements is false?
   A. The addition of capecitabine to gemcitabine did not show superiority when compared to gemcitabine alone in patients with resected pancreatic cancer (PC)
   B. The patient should be offered modified FOLFIRINOX for 6 months given his excellent ECOG PS
   C. Adjuvant chemotherapy is recommended, and radiation therapy may also be considered for close or positive margins
   D. Erlotinib showed no disease-free survival (DFS) or overall survival (OS) benefit when added to gemcitabine in the CONKO-005 study

3. Which of the following is false in the management of pancreatic adenocarcinoma?
   A. Universal germline genetic testing is recommended for all patients with a new PC diagnosis
   B. A patient with solid tumor contact of greater than 180 degrees with the superior mesenteric artery (SMA) is considered borderline resectable
   C. A patient with solid tumor contact of greater than 180 degrees with the celiac axis is considered locally advanced
   D. Diagnostic staging laparoscopy can be considered for ruling out occult metastatic disease not detected on imaging

4. A 48-year-old male with borderline resectable pancreatic adenocarcinoma is undergoing neoadjuvant chemotherapy. He has completed 5 cycles of FOLFIRINOX chemotherapy. At diagnosis, he required biliary duct stenting via endoscopic retrograde cholangio-pancreatography (ERCP) which was replaced with a covered metal stent prior to starting chemotherapy. His carbohydrate antigen (CA) 19.9 at diagnosis is 515 U/mL and has decreased with therapy to 125 U/mL. He has been tolerating his chemotherapy well with minimal toxicity. He presents for clearance prior to cycle 6 with right upper quadrant pain and scleral icterus. His total bilirubin is 4.5 and his alkaline phosphatase is elevated. What is the next best course of action?
   A. Proceed with cycle 6 of chemotherapy
   B. Change therapy to gemcitabine/nab-paclitaxel
   C. Notify the patient he has disease progression and is no longer borderline resectable
   D. Obtain urgent ultrasound of the liver and ERCP and hold chemotherapy
   E. Refer to surgery to expedite his Whipple procedure

5. A 58-year-old female with diabetes mellitus (DM) presented to an urgent care facility for epigastric pain. CT of the abdomen shows a 4.6-cm mass in the pancreatic body encasing the superior mesenteric artery (SMA) and carbohydrate antigen (CA) by greater than 180 degrees. Tumor thrombus is noted in the portal vein (PV). CT of the chest and pelvis reveals no additional sites of disease, and endoscopic ultrasound (EUS)-guided biopsy confirms adenocarcinoma of the pancreas. She has decreased appetite and moderate abdominal pain that is well-controlled with hydrocodone. She has stopped going to work but is able to do housework and run errands on her own. Her complete blood count (CBC) and comprehensive metabolic panel (CMP) are within normal limits, and CA 19.9 is elevated at 422 U/mL. What is the most appropriate management?
   A. She is resectable and should go for an upfront Whipple procedure
   B. She is borderline resectable and should start neoadjuvant chemotherapy
   C. She is borderline resectable and should start neoadjuvant chemoradiation therapy
   D. She is unresectable. Evaluate for chemotherapy (+/- RT) and clinical trial options
   E. She is unresectable and therefore does not require germline genetic testing

6. A 54-year-old female with a personal history of breast cancer (BC) treated 10 years ago is diagnosed with metastatic pancreatic adenocarcinoma. Germline genetic testing shows a pathogenic mutation in *BRCA2*. Her Eastern Cooperative Oncology Group (ECOG) performance status is 1. What is the most appropriate management?
   A. Gemcitabine and nab-paclitaxel until disease progression
   B. First-line platinum-based therapy for 4 to 6 months and, if no disease progression, maintenance olaparib
   C. Given the *BRCA2* mutation, she should receive the poly adenosine diphosphate-ribose polymerase (PARP) inhibitor olaparib as first-line therapy
   D. First-line platinum-based therapy for 4 to 6 months and, if no disease progression, maintenance pembrolizumab

ANSWERS AND RATIONALES

1. **E. Both option A and C.** This patient has a resectable pancreatic cancer (PC) with a good performance status and has undergone successful decompression of their biliary tree. They should be considered for surgical resection at a high-volume center. Patients should be evaluated for clinical trial options at each stage of their treatment and discussed in multidisciplinary tumor boards. Neoadjuvant chemotherapy is still under investigation in resectable disease; however, it is being used more commonly as the standard at high-volume academic centers. Of note—if the patient had a plastic biliary stent placed, this should be replaced with a metal stent prior to start of chemotherapy.

2. **A. The addition of capecitabine to gemcitabine did not show superiority when compared to gemcitabine alone in patients with resected pancreatic cancer (PC).** Statement A is false as the ESPAC-4 study compared 6 months of gemcitabine alone versus gemcitabine + capecitabine in patients with resected PC. At a median follow-up of 43.2 months, an improvement in mOS was seen in the combination arm (hazard ratio [HR], 0.82; 95% confidence interval [CI] 0.68-0.98, P =0.032). A 60-month follow-up analysis continued to show a small OS benefit. doi:10.1200/JCO.2020.38.15_suppl.4516>

3. **B. A patient with solid tumor contact of greater than 180 degrees with the superior mesenteric artery (SMA) is considered borderline resectable.** Statement B is false. A patient with solid tumor contact of the SMA greater than 180 degrees is considered locally advanced and not borderline resectable. Universal germline genetic testing is now recommended in the National Comprehensive Cancer Network (NCCN) guidelines for all pancreatic cancer patients and diagnostic staging laparoscopy can be considered for ruling out occult metastasis not detected on imaging. The ESPAC-4 study compared 6 months of gemcitabine alone versus gemcitabine + capecitabine in patients with resected pancreatic cancer (PC). At a median follow-up of 43.2 months, an improvement in median overall survival (mOS) was seen in the combination arm (hazard ratio [HR], 0.82; 95% confidence interval [CI] 0.68 to 0.98, P = 0.032). A 60-month follow-up analysis continued to show a small overall survival (OS) benefit. (doi:10.1200/JCO.2020.38.15_suppl.4516 *J Clin Oncol.* 2020;38(15_suppl):4516–4516.)

4. **D. Obtain urgent ultrasound of the liver and ERCP and hold chemotherapy.** Pancreatic cancer (PC) patients should be closely monitored for cholangitis and biliary stent re-occlusion during therapy. Symptoms of right upper quadrant pain, jaundice, dark urine, and elevation of serum alkaline phosphatase and/or bilirubin should prompt rapid evaluation for biliary obstruction. Antibiotics should be considered, particularly when suspicion for cholangitis is high. Given this patient's improvement in CA 19.9, it is less likely that he is progressing.

5. **D. She is unresectable. Evaluate for chemotherapy (+/– RT) and clinical trial options.** Given greater than 180-degree involvement of the SMA, her tumor is unresectable. CA greater than 180 without aortic or gastroduodenal artery involvement and thrombus in the PV may not, in and of themselves, preclude resection as long as the venous anatomy is amenable to reconstruction. Decisions regarding resectability should be based on consensus at multidisciplinary meetings. Germline genetic testing is universally recommended for all patients with newly diagnosed pancreatic cancer (PC).

6. **B. First-line platinum-based therapy for 4 to 6 months and, if no disease progression, maintenance olaparib.** In the Phase III POLO trial, patients with metastatic pancreatic cancer (PC) in the context of a germline *BRCA* mutation whose disease was stable or responding after at least 16 weeks of platinum-based chemotherapy were randomized to

the PARP inhibitor olaparib or placebo. The study showed median progression-free survival (PFS) of 7.4 months in the olaparib maintenance arm compared to 3.8 months with placebo (hazard ratio [HR] 0.53; 95% confidence interval [CI] 0.35 to 0.82; P = 0.004). At the interim analysis, no overall survival (OS) benefit was noted.

REFERENCES

1. Surveillance, Epidemiology, and End Results Program. Cancer stat facts: pancreatic cancer. National Cancer Institute. https://seer.cancer.gov/statfacts/html/pancreas.html
2. Siegel RL, Miller KD, Fuchs HE, Jemal A. Cancer statistics. *CA Cancer J Clin.* 2021;71(1):7–33. doi:10.3322/caac.21654
3. Allen PJ, Kuk D, Fernandez-del Castillo C, et al. Multi-institutional validation study of the American Joint Commission on cancer changes for T and N staging in patients with pancreatic adenocarcinoma. *Ann Surg.* 2017;265(1):185–191. doi:10.1097/SLA.0000000000001763
4. National Comprehensive Cancer Network. NCCN clinical practice guidelines in oncology. Pancreatic adenocarcinoma. Version 2.2021. November 16, 2021.
5. Bilimoria KY, Bentrem DJ, Ko CY, et al. Multimodality therapy for pancreatic cancer in the U.S.: utilization, outcomes, and the effect of hospital volume. *Cancer.* 2007;110(6):1227–1234. doi:10.1002/cncr.22916
6. Tempero MA., Reni M, Riess H. APACT: phase III, multicenter, international, open-label, randomized trial of adjuvant nab-paclitaxel plus gemcitabine vs gemcitabine for surgically resected pancreatic adenocarcinoma [abstract]. *J Clin Oncol.* 2019;37(15 suppl):4000. doi:10.1200/JCO.2019.37.15_suppl.4000
7. Neoptolemos JP, Palmer DH, Ghaneh P, et al. Comparison of adjuvant gemcitabine and capecitabine with gemcitabine monotherapy in patients with resected pancreatic cancer (ESPAC-4): a multicentre, open-label, randomised, phase 3 trial. *Lancet.* 2017; 389(10073):1011–1024. doi:10.1016/S0140-6736(16)32409-6
8. Oettle H, Neuhaus P, Hochhaus A, et al. Adjuvant chemotherapy with gemcitabine and long-term outcomes among patients with resected pancreatic cancer: the CONKO-001 randomized trial. *JAMA.* 2013;310(14):1473–1481. doi:10.1001/jama.2013.279201
9. Regine WF, Winter KA, Abrams RA, et al. Fluorouracil vs gemcitabine chemotherapy before and after fluorouracil-based chemoradiation following resection of pancreatic adenocarcinoma: a randomized controlled trial. *JAMA.* 2008;299(9):1019–1026. doi:10.1001/jama.299.9.1019
10. Neoptolemos J, Büchler M, Stocken DD, et al. ESPAC-3(v2): a multicenter, international, open-label, randomized, controlled phase III trial of adjuvant 5-fluorouracil/folinic acid (5-FU/FA) versus gemcitabine (GEM) in patients with resected pancreatic ductal adenocarcinoma. *J Clin Oncol.* 2009;27(18 suppl). doi:10.1200/jco.2009.27.18_suppl.lba4505
11. Conroy T, Hammet P, Hebbar M, et al. Unicancer GI PRODIGE 24/CCTG PA.6 trial: a multicenter international randomized phase III trial of adjuvant mFOLFIRINOX versus gemcitabine in patients with resected pancreatic ductal adenocarcinomas [abstract]. *J Clin Oncol.* 2018;36(18 suppl):Abstract LBA4001. doi:10.1200/JCO.2018.36.18_suppl.LBA4001
12. Sinn M, Bahra M, Liersch T, et al. CONKO-005: adjuvant chemotherapy with gemcitabine plus erlotinib versus gemcitabine alone in patients after R0 resection of pancreatic cancer: a multicenter randomized phase III trial. *J Clin Oncol.* 2017;35(29):3330–3337. doi:10.1200/JCO.2017.72.6463
13. Sohal DPS, Duong M, Ahmad SA, et al. Efficacy of perioperative chemotherapy for resectable pancreatic adenocarcinoma: a phase 2 randomized clinical trial. *JAMA Oncol.* 2021;7(3):421–427. doi:10.1001/jamaoncol.2020.7328
14. Katz MH, Fleming JB, Bhosale P, et al. Response of borderline resectable pancreatic cancer to neoadjuvant therapy is not reflected by radiographic indicators. *Cancer.* 2012;118(23):5749–5756. doi:10.1002/cncr.27636
15. Chawla A, Molina G, Pak LM, et al. Neoadjuvant therapy is associated with improved survival in borderline-resectable pancreatic cancer. *Ann Surg Oncol.* 2020;27(4):1191–1200. doi:10.1245/s10434-019-08087-z
16. Van Eijck CH, Versteijne E, Suker M, et al. Preoperative chemoradiotherapy to improve overall survival in pancreatic cancer: long-term results of the multicenter randomized phase III PREOPANC trial. *J Clin Oncol.* 2021;39(15_suppl):4016. doi:10.1200/JCO.2021.39.15_suppl.4016
17. Ghaneh PDHP, Palmer DH, Cicconi S, et al. ESPAC-5F: four-arm, prospective, multicenter, international randomized phase II trial of immediate surgery compared with neoadjuvant gemcitabine plus capecitabine (GEMCAP) or FOLFIRINOX or chemoradiotherapy (CRT) in patients with borderline resectable pancreatic cancer. *J Clin Oncol.* 2020;38(15_suppl):4505. doi:10.1200/JCO.2020.38.15_suppl.4505
18. Waddell N, Pajic M, Patch A-M, et al. Whole genomes redefine the mutational landscape of pancreatic cancer. *Nature.* 2015;518(7540):495–501. doi:10.1038/nature14169

19. Hammel P, Huguet F, van Laethem J-L, et al. Effect of chemoradiotherapy vs chemotherapy on survival in patients with locally advanced pancreatic cancer controlled after 4 months of gemcitabine with or without erlotinib: the LAP07 randomized clinical trial. *JAMA*. 2016;315(17):1844–1853. doi:10.1001/jama.2016.4324

20. Golan T, Hammel P, Reni M, et al. Maintenance olaparib for germline *BRCA*-mutated metastatic pancreatic cancer. *N Engl J Med*. 2019;381(4):317–327. doi:10.1056/NEJMoa1903387

21. Conroy T, Desseigne F, Ychou M, et al. FOLFIRINOX versus gemcitabine for metastatic pancreatic cancer. *N Engl J Med*. 2011;364(19):1817–1825. doi:10.1056/NEJMoa1011923

22. Von Hoff DD, Ervin T, Arena FP, et al. Increased survival in pancreatic cancer with nab-paclitaxel plus gemcitabine. *N Engl J Med*. 2013;369(18):1691–1703. doi:10.1056/NEJMoa1304369

23. Wang-Gillam A, Li C-P, Bodoky G, et al. Nanoliposomal irinotecan with fluorouracil and folinic acid in metastatic pancreatic cancer after previous gemcitabine-based therapy (NAPOLI-1): a global, randomised, open-label, phase 3 trial. *Lancet*. 2016;387(10018):545–557. doi:10.1016/S0140-6736(15)00986-1

24. Wainberg ZA, Bekaii-Saab TS, Hubner R, et al. NAPOLI-3: an open-label, randomized, phase III study of first-line liposomal irinotecan+ 5-fluorouracil/leucovorin+ oxaliplatin versus nab-paclitaxel+ gemcitabine in patients with metastatic pancreatic ductal adenocarcinoma. *J Clin Concol*. 2020;38(15_suppl):TPS4661. doi:10.1200/JCO.2020.38.15_suppl.TPS4661

25. Temel JS, Greer JA, El-Jawahri A, et al. Effects of early integrated palliative care in patients with lung and GI cancer: a randomized clinical trial. *J Clin Oncol*. 2017;35(8):834–841. doi:10.1200/JCO.2016.70.5046

26. Pelzer U, Opitz B, Deutschinoff G, et al. Efficacy of prophylactic low-molecular weight heparin for ambulatory patients with advanced pancreatic cancer: outcomes from the CONKO-004 trial. *J Clin Oncol*. 2015;33(18):2028–2034. doi:10.1200/JCO.2014.55.1481

27. Drilon A, Laetsch TW, Kummar S, et al. Efficacy of larotrectinib in TRK fusion positive cancers in adults and children. *N Engl J Med*. 2018;378:731–739. doi:10.1056/NEJMoa1714448

28. Doebele RC, Drilon A, Paz-Ares L, et al. Entrectinib in patients with advanced or metastatic *NTRK* fusion-positive solid tumours: integrated analysis of three phase 1-2 trials. *Lancet Oncol*. 2020;21:271–282. doi:10.1016/S1170-2045(19)30691-6

29. Varghese AM, Singh I, Singh R, et al. Early-onset pancreas cancer: clinical descriptors, genomics, and outcomes. *J Natl Cancer Inst*. 2021;111(9):1194–1202. doi:10.1093/jnci/djab038

CHAPTER 10

Neuroendocrine Cancer

Tannaz Armaghany and Zachary Phillip Yeung

INTRODUCTION

Neuroendocrine neoplasms (NENs) are a diverse set of malignancies that can arise from endocrine cells throughout the body. They most commonly present as tumors of the gastrointestinal (GI) tract, lungs, bronchi, thymus, and pancreas. Age-adjusted incidence of this family of tumors within the most recent Surveillance, Epidemiology, and End Results (SEER) data is about 6.98 cases per 100,000 people and is thought to be increasing over time due to improved classification and proliferation of endoscopic cancer screening.[1] Most NENs are thought to be sporadic, and risk factors for a majority of NENs outside genetic syndromes are poorly understood. These tumors share common characteristics; however, unique features related to the primary site of the tumor and the produced hormones from these neoplasms distinguish the different subtypes. NENs can be found incidentally due to nonspecific symptoms related to mass effect or constitutional symptoms such as weight loss but may also have symptoms attributable to functional hypersecretion of hormones, which necessitate biochemical testing. GI NENs may present with symptoms of intermittent flushing and diarrhea, whereas pulmonary NENs have been associated with bronchospasm and wheezing. Hypertension (HTN) distinguishes pheochromocytoma and paraganglioma. Other tumors secreting insulin, glucagon, gastrin, and other peptides present with symptoms related to the hormone produced. For accurate diagnosis on pathology, both specimen differentiation and grade reporting are necessary on pathology. The exception is poorly differentiated neuroendocrine tumors (NETs) that are by default considered high grade (G3). Differentiation is the degree of pathological resemblance of the tumor tissue to the tissue of origin. Grade is assessed by the mitotic rate and proliferative index (Ki-67). Both indices measure aggressiveness and speed of growth. Mitotic rate measures the number of mitoses/2 mm^2 (equaling 10 high-power fields at 40× magnification and an ocular field diameter of 0.5 mm). The Ki-67 proliferation index value is determined by counting at least 500 cells in the regions of highest labeling (hot-spots). The 2019 World Health Organization (WHO) classification of the digestive system for NETs is shown in Table 10.1. This classification recognizes high-grade (G3) well-differentiated gastroentropancreatic (GEP)-NETs as a new category and all poorly differentiated neuroendocrine carcinomas (NECs) as high grade by default. All G1, G2, and G3 well-differentiated NENs are staged by the 2017 American Joint Committee on Cancer (AJCC) eighth edition of cancer staging. Poorly differentiated NETs are staged similar to small cell lung cancer (SCLC) using the 2017 AJCC eighth edition for SCLC (Table 10.1).

Table 10.1　2019 WHO Classification of NENs

Tumor Nomenclature	Mitotic Count/10 HPF (Mitosis/2 mm²)	Proliferation Index % (Ki-67)
Well-Differentiated NET		
Low grade (G1)	<2	<3
Intermediate grade (G2)	2–20	3–20
High grade (G3)	>20	>20
Poorly Differentiated (NEC)		
Large cell type (LCNEC)	>20	>20
Small cell type (SCNEC)	>20	>20
MiNEN (variable grade) Well or poorly differentiated	Variable	Variable

LCNEC, large cell neuroendocrine carcinoma; MiNEN, mixed neuroendocrine-nonneuroendocrine neoplasm; NEC, neuroendocrine carcinoma; NENs, neuroendocrine neoplasms; NET, neuroendocrine tumor; SCNEC, small cell neuroendocrine carcinoma; WHO; World Health Organization.

Source: National Comprehensive Cancer Network. *National Comprehensive Cancer Network. Clinical Practice Guidlines in Oncolopy. Neuroendocrine and Adrenal Tumors.* Version 4.2021. December 14, 2021. https://www.nccn.org/guidelines/guidelines-detail?category=1&id=1448; Halfdanarson TR, Strosberg JR, Tang, L, et al. The North American Neuroendocrine Tumor Society (NANETS) consensus guidelines for surveillance and medical management of pancreatic neuroendocrine tumors. *Pancreas.* 2020;49(7):863–881. doi:10.1097/MPA.0000000000001597

CASE SUMMARIES

Case 10.1: Gastric Neuroendocrine Neoplasm

A 69-year-old male with past medical history (PMH) of HTN, diabetes mellitus (DM), autoimmune thyroiditis, gastroesophageal reflux disease (GERD), and smoking history presented to his primary care provider (PCP) with chronic abdominal pain and dyspepsia. A short 2-month course of proton pump inhibitors (PPI) did not relieve his symptoms. A CT of the abdomen with oral and IV contrast showed a single gastric polyp and otherwise normal. Physical exam was normal. Routine complete blood count (CBC) and comprehensive metabolic panel (CMP) was normal. His medication consisted of enalapril, metformin, protonix, valsartan, and aspirin.

An esophagogastroduodenoscopy (EGD) discovered a peduncular polyp and at least 20 mucosal nodules, 10 to 20 mm in size, in the gastric body along the greater curvature. Some were ulcerated. Multiple biopsies were taken from the lesions and gastric mucosa and pathology revealed atrophic oxyntic mucosa with neuroendocrine cell hyperplasia, microcarcinoids (well-differentiated NETs), chronic gastritis, and intestinal metaplasia consistent with autoimmune atrophic gastritis. Immunostains were positive for chromogranin, less than 1 mitotic figures/10 high power field (HPF) with Ki-67 proliferative index less than 2% consistent with grade I, gastric-NET. A repeat EGD was subsequently performed to remove the larger lesions. Two lesions, each more than 2 cm, were removed by endoscopic mucosal resection (EMR). Pathology revealed the same but a higher Ki-67 of 4% and a positive margin.

For fasting serum gastrin measurement, the patient was asked to hold PPI for 1 week. Gastrin level was 1300 pg/mL.

What Are the Subtypes of Gastric Neuroendocrine Tumors?

Gastric neuroendocrine tumors (g-NETs) are divided into three subtypes:

- **Type 1 gastric NET (T1 g-NET):** This subtype is associated with antrum sparing auto-immune atrophic gastritis and sometimes pernicious anemia. A unique feature in this subtype is gastric hypoacidity due to absent or decreased acid-producing parietal cells that in turn induce a high gastrin production. These tumors are considered nonfunctional because excess gastrin does not cause a clinical presentation. The lesions are usually small (5 to 20 mm) and present as multifocal submucosal nodules or multifocal polypoid lesions with a small central ulceration in the gastric mucosa.
- **Type 2 gastric NET (T2 g-NET):** Also known as gastrinoma and Zollinger–Ellison syndrome (ZES) because of the excess secretion of gastrin that is responsible for the clinical presentation, the ZES triad includes (a) gastric acid hypersecretion, (b) fasting serum hypergastrinemia, and (c) peptic ulcer disease and diarrhea. This type presents with multiple gastric ulcers or ulcers in uncommon locations of the GI luminal tract secondary low gastric PH.
- **Type 3 gastric NET (T3 g-NET):** This is an aggressive subtype.

How Is This Cancer Staged?[2]

- Endoscopic staging is utilized for tissue diagnosis and defining tumor (T) and nodal (N) status.
- Tumors are staged using CT, MRI, or somatostatin receptor (SSR) PET scan (68Ga or Cu) if clinically indicated.

How Is Diagnosis Established for Gastric Neuroendocrine Neoplasm?[4,5]

- EGD with careful review of the background gastric mucosa is essential. Endoscopic ultrasonography (EUS) is utilized to screen for submucosal lesions and biopsies from gastric mucosa, fundus, body, antrum, duodenum, and the tumor are needed.
- Gastric mucosa looks normal or atrophic in type 1, normal or hypertrophic in type 2, and normal in type 3.
- Conventional imaging (CT or MRI scan) has a limited role in detecting small type 1 and 2 lesions and are not recommended, unless enlarged lymph nodes (LNs) or liver lesions are suspected on EGD/EUS, or high-risk lesions (type 3) or advanced disease is suspected.
- The majority of T2 g-NETs originate from the duodenum or pancreas but sometimes are obscured and not found on EUS or by cross-sectional and functional imaging. In these cases, laparoscopic exploration is performed to locate the tumor.
- Gastric PH measurement might be required in certain circumstances for T2 g-NETs and may assist with the diagnosis when the primary mass is not found on scans or EGD. In this scenario, serum gastrin and gastric PH are measured simultaneously. A serum gastrin value greater than 10 times the upper limit of normal (1000 pg/mL) in the presence of a gastric pH below 2 is diagnostic for ZES. A secretin stimulation test can be used to confirm gastrinoma. Physiologic secretin decreases the secretion of gastrin but in gastrinoma it fails to do so.
- Serum fasting gastrin level is measured after PPI is held for at least 1 week and H2 blockers are held for at least 24 hours. Holding PPI in ZES is not advised unless H2 blockers are given to prevent fulminant ulcer flare and bleeding.
- Somatostatin receptor analogue (SSRA) functional imaging such as OctreoScan and PET imaging (Ga68 DOTATE, Ga68 DOTANOC, Cu64 DOTATAE) is not used in type 1 (lesions are usually small and under the detection of a PET scan) but are used in type 2 and 3 for staging purposes and to evaluate for SSRA-directed nuclear medicine therapy (Lu 17 PRRT or Y90 PRRT) indication. One of these functional scans is required to be positive in order to treat with peptide receptor radionuclide therapy.

Is Biochemical Testing Required for the Disease?

- Fasting serum gastrin is measured for the initial diagnosis and during follow-up while on treatment and surveillance for T2 g-NET and T3 g-NET. The high gastrin level for T1 g-NET is secondary to atrophic gastritis; it is not due to the NET and not considered a tumor marker in this subtype.

What Molecular or Genetic Markers Are Used In Current Clinical Practice?

- Currently there are no defined prognostic or predictive molecular markers used in clinical practice.
- Multiple endocrine neoplasia type 1 ([MEN1] or Werner syndrome) are associated with gastrinoma (T2-g-NET) in 20% to 60% of the cases. Genetic counseling and germline testing for MEN1 are recommended for T2 g-NETs. A careful personal and family history in first-, second-, and third-degree family is recommended to assess genetic risk for hereditary endocrine neoplasia syndromes (mainly for type 2). Somatic MEN gene alteration is also seen in NETs and should not be mistaken with germline mutations.

How Do Various Types of Gastric Neuroendocrine Neoplasm Present?

- T1 g-NET presents with high gastric PH and a high serum fasting gastrin level. These indolent cancers are asymptomatic if confined to the gastric mucosa. They are incidentally found when workup is done for dyspepsia. Low vitamin B12 level, macrocytic anemia, and pernicious anemia are specific for T1 g-NET. Weight loss, abdominal pain, vomiting, and loss of appetite are related to the underlying gastric atrophy and seen in this type. T1 g-NETs are indolent tumors, and the risk of metastasis is 10% in lesions less than 2 cm.[6-8]
- T2 g-NET presents with low gastric PH, high fasting gastrin, and multiple indolent tumors, which are slightly larger in size than T1 g-NET. They are considered functional tumors and also rarely (5%) found in other sites, including the stomach, liver, ovary, and lung.[9] T2 g-NETs are associated with germline MEN1 (25%) but can occur as sporadic tumors. This disease presents with diarrhea secondary to high acid in the GI tract. Patients also have GERD, as well as multiple and recurrent gastric ulcers (ZES).
- T3 g-NET presents with normal gastric PH and normal fasting serum gastrin, and is considered functional due to the secretion of hormones such as serotonin or histamine and the most aggressive type among g-NETs. Well-differentiated T3 g-NET presents with *atypical carcinoid syndrome* (CS) with flushing and intense pruritis and bronchospasm.
- T3 g-NECs are the more aggressive subtypes of gastric type 3 tumors, and they present with abdominal pain, bleeding from a large single fungating gastric mass, and distant metastasis.

Patient's Diagnosis

- *The EGD showed chronic atrophic gastritis with multiple 10- to 20-mm submucosal nodules consistent with NET. His fasting serum gastrin level was high while being off PPI. Some of the g-NET nodules were ulcerated and he had no peptic ulcers. His fasting serum gastrin was physiologically elevated due to chronic atrophic gastritis mainly and to the addition of PPI. His clinical picture was most consistent with nonfunctional, type I, intermediate grade (G2) well-differentiated g-NET.*

How Is the Type 1 Gastric Neuroendocrine Tumor Managed and What Are Treatment Options?

- Lesions less than 5 mm are observed with repeated surveillance endoscopy.
- Lesions of 5 mm or greater are endoscopically removed by EMR or endoscopic submucosal dissection (ESD). SSRAs such as Sandostatin LAR or lanreotide can be used in

patients with multiple small lesions that cannot all be removed endoscopically or have repeated recurrences after EMR or ESD. SSRA controls the tumor growth by decreasing the secretion of gastrin.

- Antrectomy to suppress the excess gastrin is debated due to complete antrectomy being an uncertain procedure; therefore, partial or total gastrectomy is more commonly performed.
- Gastrectomy is indicated also with submucosal tumors, T2 lesions, tumors that are repeatedly recurrent after EMR or ESD, LN involvement, or positive margin after local resection of a polyp or lesion.[4,10]
- Metastatectomy and removal of the primary tumor in all subtypes of g-NET is advised (excluding NEC) if total resection can be achieved with surgery.
- Local therapy for liver metastasis including TACE (transcatheter arterial chemoembolization) or TARE (trans-arterial radioembolization) or thermo-ablation is considered for palliative control of tumor function or tumor growth.
- If the liver is the only or the main metastatic region, liver-directed therapy is a treatment option for decreasing the liver tumor burden prior to debulking surgery if greater than 80% of the whole tumor bulk can be surgically removed.
- SSRA (lanreotide and Sandostatin) are considered first-line therapy for all types of g-NETs.
- Upon progression on SSRA, PRRT using liver-directed ^{90}Yttrium or ^{177}Lutetium (^{177}Lu-Dotatate) labeled may be considered for all types of gastric g-NETs. G-NECs are treated differently.

What Are the Toxicities Associated With Systemic Therapy Options?

- See under pancreatic neuroendocrine tumors (pNETs).

How Are Patients Followed Up for Surveillance?

- See under pNETs.

Case 10.1 Follow-Up

- *Case 10.1 was discussed in GI multidisciplinary tumor board. Due to the presence of numerous 2 cm or greater remaining lesions in the gastric mucosa and the positive margin after EMR, partial gastrectomy was recommended. A negative CT of the chest ruled out distant metastatic lesions prior to surgery. A partial gastrectomy and lymphadenectomy were performed. During surgery multiple subcentimeter suspicious liver lesions were visualized that prompted segment 4 and 7 hepatic lobe biopsy for metastatic pathological workup. Final surgical pathology revealed multiple 1- to 2-cm lesions, all consistent with well-differentiated intermediate grade (highest Ki-67 4%) NETs in the gastric body arising in a background of diffuse atrophic gastritis, 2/16 positive LNs, and synaptophysin. Chromogranin was positive on immunohistochemistry (IHC). The liver tissue showed grade 2 (Ki-67 4%). The final stage was mpT2N1M1a (m = multiple). Monthly SSRA (lanreotide or Sandostatin LAR) injections versus close observation was discussed, and he decided to receive monthly SSRA injections.*

Case 10.2: Pancreatic Neuroendocrine Neoplasm

A 52-year-old female presented to medical oncology with progressive stage IV well-differentiated pNET. Her PMH is significant for hyperlipidemia and papillary thyroid cancer. At age 43 she had undergone subtotal thyroidectomy and has been in remission since then. She was found to have a solid mass in the tail of the pancreas incidentally at age 41. EUS-guided biopsy of the pancreatic mass was consistent with well-differentiated pNET. Routine labs and tumor markers were normal. Contrast-enhanced CT of the chest/abdomen and an OctreoScan showed a single 2.5-cm pancreatic lesion without local lymphadenopathy or distant metastasis. Distal pancreatomy and splenectomy was performed, and pathology reported a single 2.2-cm mass confined to the pancreas, well differentiated, low grade (G1), with mitotic rate 1 mitosis per HPF, Ki-67 was 4%, 1/19 nodes were positive for nodal metastasis, with negative margins with positive lymphovascular invasion. She remained without evidence of cancer until 2 years later when a repeat OctreoScan showed a suspicious metastatic lesion in the liver. Liver biopsy revealed pNET recurrence with well-differentiated metastatic PNET to the liver. Ki-67 was 14% and she was started on monthly Sandostatin. Repeat scans show progression in the liver after 13 months of Sandostatin.

How Are Pancreatic Neuroendocrine Neoplasms Classified?

- PNET classification follows the 2019 WHO classification of the digestive system seen in Table 10.1.
- PNETs are also divided into functional and nonfunctional tumors. Functional tumors are regarded as tumors in which a hormone-related syndrome is present due to excess secretion of a specific hormone. A positive IHC on staining (for example, gastrin, glucagon, and so forth) without the clinical presentation of the associated syndrome is not considered a functional tumor.

What Is the Specific Pathology for Each Disease?

- The pathology report should include three essential items: differentiation (well vs. poor), IHC staining, and grade. IHC staining includes synaptophysin and chromogranin staining. All pNETs strongly and diffusely stain for synaptophysin and most, but not all, express chromogranin. Lower percentages of pancreatic neuroendocrine carcinomas (pNECs) stain positive for these markers (as low as 50% to 60%).
- Ki-67 proliferation index and/or mitotic index report both measure the grade and can show discrepancy between each other and between the matched primary and metastatic lesion specimens. If there is discrepancy between the two, the final grade is assigned based on the highest measurement and the prognosis follows the highest grade. Ki-67 proliferation index correlates with the size of the tumor; therefore, it is recommended to measure the Ki-67 from the largest metastasis.[3]
- Ki-67 and/or mitotic rate cannot distinguish between high-grade pNET and pNECs without report on differentiation.

How Is the Disease Diagnosed?

- It is essential to distinguish between PNET and pNEC.
- EGD/EUS is a very effective procedure to obtain tissue diagnosis for pNENs.
- Interventional radiology-guided biopsy of the liver, lung, bone, and LN can provide tissue diagnosis of metastatic sites.
- Multiphase cross-sectional imaging with IV contrast CT scan and/or MRI that includes the primary site provides appropriate staging.
- Functional SSR imaging is utilized for evaluation of distant disease. This is essential to predict the likelihood of effectiveness of SSR-directed therapies (PRRT).
- SSR-based imaging includes octreotide SPECT, Ga68-DOTATAE (NETSPOT), Ga68-DOTATOC, or Cu64-DOTATAE. SSR-PET/MRI is another option. Octreotide SPECT is significantly less sensitive than the SSR-PET scan. A lesion is considered SSR-positive if the update of the tracer is above the uptake of the liver.[2]

- Fluorodeoxyglucose (FDG) PET scan is used only in cases diagnosed or suspected of PNEC or high-grade NET when the tumor is growing rapidly and showing aggressive behavior.

Is Biochemical Testing Required for the Disease?

- Serum biochemical hormone testing is decided by the presence of the hormonal clinical presentation and not advised in asymptomatic patients. Testing for a nonspecific tumor marker such as chromogranin A (CgA) is not routinely recommended in PNETs and has no role in management. CgA can be falsely elevated in the setting of atrophic gastritis, renal insufficiency, and the use of PPI.
- In functional tumors, the relevant hormonal circulating biomarker is measured in the context of the clinical presentation and followed over time; for example, VIP in VIPOMA, or gastrin in gastrinoma.

What Molecular Markers Are Used In Current Clinical Practice for Pancreatic Neuroendocrine Tumors?

- Death-domain associated protein (DAXX) and alpha-thalassemia/intellectual disability syndrome X-linked (ATRX) and MEN1 molecular markers distinguish pNETs from pNECs. DAXX and ATRX are totally absent in pNECs. On the other hand, a fraction of pNETs irrespective of their grade (G1, G2, G3) harbor mutations in *TP53*, *Rb1*, and *SMAD4*. This molecular data can be utilized to assist in distinguishing high-grade PNET from pNEC in puzzling cases in clinical practice. IHC for DAXX, ATRX (loss of expression of either indicative of NET), *p53* (mutant-pattern staining indicative of NEC), and *Rb* (loss of expression indicative of NEC) can be used to facilitate the distinction of these two distinct entities.
- Currently, due to the lack of predictive and prognostic value of the tested genes and the absence of actionable targets for the majority of PNETs, routine next-generation sequencing (NGS) is not recommended. The only exception is the uncommon G3 pNEN subtype that might harbor actionable mutations such as microsatellite instability (MSI) or *NTRK* mutations.[3]

Does the Disease Have Specific Germline Mutations to Warrant Genetic Counseling?

- In patients who are known to have MEN1 mutation or have clinical presentation suspicious for germline mutation (hypercalcemia, pituitary, or adrenal adenoma, and so forth), genetic counseling and relevant germline mutation testing is recommended.

How Does the Disease Present?

- Nonfunctional pNETs are diagnosed either incidentally or they present later in the course of disease with symptoms related to local tumor effect or distant metastasis. Uncommonly nonfunctional PNETs can present with metachronous hormonal syndromes later in their course by evolving into hormone secretors and produce insulinoma, VIPoma, gastrinoma, and glucagonoma.[11]
- Functional tumors present with various hormonal symptoms. The diagnosis is delayed primarily due to their hormonal syndrome mimicking other more common disease presentations.

- Hormonal syndromes can be related to abnormal secretion of insulin (insulinoma causing hypoglycemia), gastrin (gastrinoma, with peptic ulcers), vasoactive intestinal polypeptide VIP (VIPoma, with severe diarrhea and hypokalemia), glucagon (glucagonoma with hyperglycemia and necrolytic migratory erythema rash), somatostatin (somatostatinoma, with hyperglycemia), ACTH hormone (ACTHoma with ectopic Cushing's syndrome), and some more rare types such as serotoninoma and calcitoninoma.
- PNETs associated with MEN1 mutation present with symptoms related to any of the involved organs. Hypercalcemia due to hyperparathyroidism is the first presenting symptom in most of the cases and it presents mostly by 30 years old.

How Is a Pancreatic Neuroendocrine Tumor Managed and What Are the Treatment Options?

- Sporadic pNETs are surgically removed by enucleation or surgical resection of the tumor and LN dissection.
- In nonfunctional pNETs in the setting of MEN1, either resection with enucleation or surgical resection in addition to lymphadenectomy in considered. In this scenario, the Whipple procedure is rarely indicated. If the nonfunctional pNET is less than 2 to 2.5 cm in size, observation and close radiographic monitoring is an acceptable alternative.[3]
- Resectable pNETs in older adults and patients with comorbidities can be observed.
- Advanced unresectable or metastatic asymptomatic nonfunctional patients with low volume disease can be closely watched without treatment with re-staging imaging every 3 to 4 months.
- Local liver therapies include hepatic artery bland embolization, chemoembolization (TACE), or radioembolization (^{90}Y), and are utilized when tumor shrinkage or hormonal control is required.
- If the disease is progressive after the initial observational period, if there is a high disease burden, or the pNET is functional and hormonal control is required, a systemic option is used. These options include SSRAs such as lanreotide or Sandostatin, sunitinib, everolimus, and, in cases with liver-predominant metastasis, local liver treatments options.
- First-line systemic treatment options for pNETs include sunitinib, everolimus, and SSRA. All three are cytostatic and have low response rates (RRs).
- Sunitinib showed statistically significant improvement in median progression-free survival (mPFS) benefit compared to placebo in PNETS. (11 vs. 5.5, hazard ratio [HR] 0.42 [0.26 to 0.66], P less than 0.001).[12]
- RADIANT 2 study compared everolimus to placebo. In the study, 429 functional GEP-NET patients were randomized in 1:1 fashion. Both arms were on Sandostatin, and they all had CS. The mPFS benefit compared to placebo was 16.4 versus 11.3, HR 0.77 (0.59 to 1.00), P = 0.26.
- RADIANT 3 study compared everolimus to placebo in pNETs. In the study, 410 patients were randomized in 1:1 fashion. The mPFS was 11 versus 4.6, HR 0.35 (0.27 to 0.45), P less than 0.001. The overall RR was 5%.[13]
- The use of lanreotide as the first-line standard of care option is established based on CLARINET study.[14] This study revealed an antiproliferative effect and progression-free survival (PFS) benefit of lanreotide in GEP-NETs. This was a randomized, double-blinded, multinational study that enrolled well to moderately differentiated, nonfunctional, SSR-positive NETs (Ki-67 less than 10%). The primary tumors were from GEP-NET and unknown primary origin and they all had positive SSR uptake on functional imaging. Patients were randomized to 120 mg of lanreotide versus placebo injections every 4 weeks. Two hundred patients were equally assigned to either arm. The arms had close to

an equal number of pNETs (45%), midgut plus hindgut (43%), and unknown primary (13%). This study met the primary objective of PFS with HR of 0.47 and $P = 0.0002$. mPFS was 18 months versus median had not reached in the lanreotide arm at the time of publication.

- The effectiveness of SSR-directed therapies in the setting of negative functional imaging is controversial.
- Treatment with Lutathera radioisotope (Lutetium Lu 177 Dotatate), also known as PRRT, is indicated in second-line treatment after progression of midgut tumors. A Phase III randomized open label clinical trial (NETTER-1) enrolled 229 patients with well differentiated, G1 and G2 metastatic midgut NETs. Patients were randomly assigned to Lu-Dotatate (116 patients) plus 30 mg Sandostatin versus high-dose Sandostatin at 60 mg as the control arm every 4 weeks. PFS at 20 months was 65% in the PRRT arm versus 10.8 months in the control arm.[15] It is important to remember that pNETs were not part of this trial; however, adequate evidence for the benefit of Lutathera has rendered PRRT as a valuable treatment modality for advanced and progressive pNETs.
- Several retrospective trials have shown the benefit of Lutathera in pNETs.
- Brabander et al. retrospectively evaluated a large group of bronchial and GEP-NETs and their outcome with Lutathera. Among 443 evaluable patients, 113 had pNETs. mPFS, median overall survival (mOS), and objective response rate (ORR) were 30 months, 71 months, and 55%, respectively.[16]
- Ezziddin et al. retrospectively evaluated 68 inoperable progressive metastatic G1/G2 pNETs after 4 cycles of Lutathera. Lutathera was the first-line treatment in 51% of the patients. mPFS, mOS, and ORR were 34 months, 53 months, and 72%, respectively.[17]
- SSR uptake on functional imaging (Ga68 PET, Cu 67 PET, indium 111-SPECT) is required for consideration of PRRT.
- If OctreoScan is totally negative, a more sensitive test (G68 PET or Cu 67 PET) is required to rule out a true negative G1/G2 pNET.
- A true negative functional imaging for G1/G2 pNET is rare; this should prompt another biopsy to rule out G3 pNET.
- PRRT is also associated with significant quality of life improvement, symptomatic improvement, and decrease in plasma hormone levels (80%) in functional pNETs.[18,19]
- Capecitabine and temozolomide (CAPTEM) have both been studied retrospectively and prospectively in the setting of well-differentiated pNETs and well-differentiated G1, G2, and G3 neuoendocrine tumors. This combination is recommended in symptomatic and large bulky tumors in cases where tumor shrinkage is required for disease control.
- A retrospective analysis of 143 patients treated with CAPTEM showed a mPFS of 17 months with an impressive 54% RR and 73.2 months mOS.
- ECOG 2211 was a prospective trial of temozolomide versus temozolomide + capecitabine that showed statistically significant improvement in mPFS (14.4 vs. 22.7, HR, 0.58; $P = 0.02$) and mOS (38 vs. not reached, HR, 0.41; $P = 0.01$) with the combination.[20]

How Are Advanced Unresectable or Metastatic Well-Differentiated G3 Pancreatic Neuroendocrine Tumors Managed?

- Well-differentiated low-grade (G1/2) NET can evolve into grade 3 NET and show a more aggressive behavior. This is known from the similar molecular markers that they share (ATRX, DAXX, and MEN1).
- Locoregional disease is treated by radical surgery.
- Metastatic or locally advanced or unresectable disease is treated with temozolomide-based chemotherapy (temozolomide + capecitabine) at first line.

- Everolimus can be considered when decrease of tumor bulk is not a critical matter.
- If SSR imaging is positive, conventional (octreotide LAR or lanreotide) or radiolabeled (Lutathera) SSRAs can be considered.
- Prophylactic brain radiation in nonmetastatic stage IV is not recommended due to low frequency of central nervous system (CNS) metastasis.
- Immune checkpoint inhibitor immunotherapy that targets both programmed cell death-1 (PD-1) and cytotoxic T lymphocyte associated antigen 4 checkpoints are indicated in second-line treatment or platinum-refractory patients. Cases with deficient mismatch repair (dMMR), high levels of microsatellite instability (MSI-H), or high levels of tumor mutational burden (TMB; 10 to 15 mutations/mega base) are much more responsive to immunotherapy.
- These cases do not respond well to platinum-based chemotherapy and are only known to be reasonably effective if ki-67 index is greater than 55.
- Carlsen et al performed a retrospective analysis of grade 3 NETs, treated with Lutathera in first, second, and third line. PRRT showed promise in these patients. A total of 149 patients were included; of these, 89 (60%) were pancreatic, 34 (23%) were GI, and 26 (17) were unknown primary. PRRT was given in 30 (20%) patients in the first line, 62 (42%) patients in the second line, and 57(38%) patients in the late lines.[21]
- Cytoreductive tumor debulking surgery is considered for palliation for non-aggressive tumors even if there is evidence of extrahepatic disease. Nonrandomized trials have shown benefit with cytoreductive liver surgery in NETs from various primaries if 70% to 90% of the cancer can be removed; this included PNETs.[22]

Case 10.2 Follow-Up

- *The patient in Case 10.2 has nonfunctional pNET. She was started on daily 37.5 mg sunitinib, which was discontinued after 4 months due to intolerance. She received 4 cycles of Lutathera followed by standard Sandostatin the day after each treatment. Her disease was stable for 9 months and later she lost follow up. She presented to the ED a year later with severe mid back pain. A thoracolumbar-spine MRI revealed T4 to L2 metastatic lesions, a bulky tumor in T5 with surrounding cord edema. She was started on IV dexamethasone and Neurosurgery was immediately consulted. T5 corpectomy and spine stabilization was performed. Re-staging CT of the chest and abdomen with contrast showed enlarged mediastinal lymphadenopathy and mild progression of liver metastasis. Tissue from the spine pathology showed well-differentiated grade 3 (Ki-67 35%) NET believed to be from original pancreatic origin. She had a palliative spine and was started on CAPTEM.*

What Are the Toxicities Associated With Systemic Therapy Options?

- Lanreotide: abdominal pain, Vitamin B12 deficiency, thyroid dysfunction
- Everolimus: aphthous oral ulcers, diarrhea, hyperglycemia, cytopenia, and pneumonitis
- Sunitinib: HTN, palmar-plantar erythrodysesthesia (hand–foot syndrome), diarrhea, fatigue, and cytopenia
- Capecitabine/temozolomide: neutropenia (13% G3/4) and thrombocytopenia (8% G3/4)
- PRRT: cytopenia (typically resolve before the next treatment within 8 weeks) and myeloid neoplasm are considered long-term side effects (9 to 125 months) and include myelodysplastic syndrome (MDS) and/or acute leukemia in 2% to 3% myelodysplastic.[16]

What Are the Prognostic Markers and How Do They Impact Treatment and/or Survival?

- Prognostic markers include stage, differentiation, and grade. Poorly differentiated tumors have a poor prognosis. Grade has a significant impact on survival in well-differentiated

NETs. G1 well-differentiated pNET is an indolent disease, whereas well-differentiated G3 is considered an aggressive tumor. The prognosis of well-differentiated G2 falls between well-differentiated G1 and G2.[1]

How Are Patients Followed Up for Surveillance?

- The frequency of interventions regarding surveillance of resected pNETS depends on the initial presentation, resected tumor bulk, functionality, and grade. National Comprehensive Cancer Network (NCCN) guidelines are followed.[2]

Case 10.3: Midgut Neuroendocrine Tumor and Carcinoid Syndrome

A 53-year-old prior schoolteacher female with PMH of migraine headache, obesity, and HTN presented with intermittent facial flushing, randomly most noticeable with stress and watery diarrhea 7 to 8 times a day for the last 5 years. Dermatology diagnosed her with rosacea. She had to quit her job due to unrelenting diarrhea in the last year. She has visited with a gastroenterologist for diarrhea workup, and upper and lower gastroenterology endoscopies did not reveal any abnormalities. She was diagnosed with irritable bowel syndrome and used intermittent Imodium without response. A notable finding was dark red flushing of the face. A CT of the abdomen with IV contrast showed a 5-cm mid-abdominal mass with calcifications and a liver segment 2 mass. An OctreoScan showed enhancement in the mesentery as well as the liver mass. She is referred to surgical and medical oncology. Her working diagnosis is stage IV functional midgut NET.

What Is the Specific Pathology?

- There are no specific pathological features associated with midgut carcinoid tumors and they are similar to GEP-NETs on pathological review.

How Is the Disease Diagnosed?

- The diagnosis is established with a tissue biopsy from the affected organ (primary or metastatic) in addition to consideration of the constellation of hormonal symptoms related to carcinoid tumor if functional.

What Biomarkers Are Used in Current Clinical Practice?

- Urine 24-hour 5-HIAA and serotonin are measured in patients with known typical CS.

What Molecular Markers Are Used Currently in Clinical Practice?

- There are no standard molecular markers used for clinical management of mid- or hindgut NETs.

Does the Disease Have Specific Germline Mutations to Warrant Genetic Counseling?

- There are currently no germline mutations associated with these tumors and genetic counseling is not required.

How Does the Disease Present?

- The CS presentation depends on the type of the excess biochemical production.
- Although not an absolute demarcation, there is a correlation between the symptoms and the primary location of the tumor.
- The classic presentations of CS secondary to well-differentiated low grade small bowel (SB) NETs are flushing, diarrhea, and liable blood pressure episodes (hypotension or HTN).
- CS in SB is secondary to excess production of serotonin from the SB tumor enterochromaffin-like (ECL) cells.
- The typical flushing is in the face and upper torso without sweating (dry flush) that worsens with stress, exercise, alcohol, and some food products such as cheese and nuts; it commonly happens without any trigger. The color of the flushed skin is anywhere from pink to dark red, and in patients with long lasting exposure to high levels of serum serotonin, the skin can stay permanently red even after appropriate treatment.
- Excess serum serotonin is also responsible for watery diarrhea, and it can be anywhere from a few to 20–30 times a day. The diarrhea is watery with high frequency, not responsive to home remedies. These patients are known to decrease social interaction and even quit their jobs due to unrelenting diarrhea.
- Most of the excess circulating serotonin produced by NETs is eliminated from the blood by the first pass metabolism of the liver unless there is the presence of liver metastasis. Carcinoid syndrome due to excess serotonin happens with the presence of liver metastasis.
- SB obstruction is a common presentation of SB NETs. This is not only related to the presence of luminal tumor but also to the mesenteric fibrotic desmoid reaction that these tumors produce in the mesentery. This phenomenon is also responsible for bowel angina due to compromised bowel blood circulation caused by the surrounding inflammatory fibrosis.
- The diagnosis of CS is frequently and significantly delayed due to misdiagnosis.
- CS mimics several more common medical conditions. Facial flushing is mistaken for rosacea, menopause, and stress-related skin changes, and diarrhea is mistaken for irritable bowel syndrome, inflammatory bowel disease (early Crohn's or ulcerative colitis), food intolerance, GI infections, and malabsorption. Wheezing, shortness of breath (SOB), and itching are mistaken for seasonal or environmental allergies, respiratory infections, and congestive heart failure (CHF).

How Is a Midgut Neuroendocrine Tumor Managed and What Are Treatment Options?

- Locoregional jejunal/ileal/colon primary tumors are resected with bowel resection and regional lymphadenectomy.
- Nonmetastatic duodenal NETs are treated with endoscopic resection and local excision, plus lymphadenectomy or Whipple procedure.
- Appendiceal NETs are managed with simple appendectomy if the tumor is 2 cm or less.
- If the appendiceal tumor is greater than 2 cm or regional nodes are known to be or suspected to be positive, or the margin of resection with simple appendectomy is positive, hemicolectomy + lymphadenectomy + appendectomy is performed.
- Rectal NETs are managed with local resection if low grade and less than 1 cm; otherwise, they undergo trans-anal resection if T1 and LAR or abdominoperineal resections (APR) in larger and node-positive tumors.
- Debulking surgery can be considered in patients in which their primary and metastatic disease can be completely resected.

- Asymptomatic and low tumor burden tumors can be monitored with imaging and relevant tumor markers if totally asymptomatic.
- In the absence of measurable disease on imaging after debulking surgery and the lack of symptoms related to the original tumor or the excess hormone in the setting of normal serum biochemical markers, adjuvant treatment has not been shown to provide any benefit.
- Screening echocardiogram and/or measurement of N-terminal pro-brain natriuretic peptide (BNP) for carcinoid heart disease is considered in this population, especially when the serotonin levels stay high for an extended amount of time.
- There is no consensus for the indication or frequency of screening for carcinoid heart (CH) disease in these patients. Echocardiogram and/or measurement of N-terminal pro-BNP are used for this purpose.
- The North American Neuroendocrine Society (NANETS) recommends at minimum all patients with significant elevation of serum serotonin or 5-hydroxyindoleacetic acid (5-HIAA) undergo annual echocardiography and patients with known CH disease should be monitored more closely.[3]

Case 10.3 Follow-Up

- *The patient in Case 10.3 was staged at pT3N2M1a. She was followed up with scans, physical exam, and tumor markers (5-HIAA and serotonin) every 3 months and remained with no evidence of disease for 2 years. Later, her disease recurred with watery diarrhea, flushing, and increase of tumor makers. A multiphase abdominal CT scan with contrast confirmed recurrence with bilateral (BL) liver metastasis, and biochemical testing showed serum serotonin of 1200 with elevated 24-hour urine 5-HIAA. A liver fine needle aspiration (FNA) biopsy was taken for the purpose of grading the current tumor, and it showed intermediate grade with a Ki-67 index of 15% (unchanged from 2 years ago). She was started on 120 mg of lanreotide injections every 4 weeks that controlled her symptoms for another 15 months. A screening ECHO cardiogram was performed that showed thickening of both the tricuspid and pulmonary valve and moderate-to-severe tricuspid regurgitation, and a mildly thickened right ventricle most consistent with CH. Clinically she did not have evidence of CHF. Repeat scans show progression of the disease.*

What Are the Appropriate Treatment Options at This Stage?

- Debulking surgery is an acceptable approach as the primary and most/all of the metastatic tissue can be removed in bulky and functional tumors.
- Nonbulking and asymptomatic tumors can be closely monitored with exam and serial scans.
- Local liver therapy with TACE or Y-90 are viable options in symptomatic cases if the bulk of the tumor is believed to be in the liver.
- SSR analogues (lanreotide short-acting octreotide and long-acting octreotide) are the first line of treatment for CS and are used in nonfunctional tumors for tumor control.
- Somatostatin analogues (SSAs) are known to have antiproliferative effects on GEP-NETs: The Phase III PROMID study randomized metastatic midgut patients to receive long-acting octreotide (Sandostatin) versus placebo. This trial showed PFS benefit but no OS benefit. The trial allowed for cross-over, which might have cofounded the OS results. The extent of the liver tumor burden was a predictor of survival.[23]
- The Phase III CLARINET study randomized GEP-NETS to lanreotide versus placebo. Close to one-third of the patients were from midgut origin. This study required a positive functional scan and nonfunctional tumors to be enrolled. All patients had a Ki-67 index of less than 10%. Lanreotide showed improved PFS in this population.[14]

- Telotristat is a tryptophan hydroxylase inhibitor indicated for the treatment of CS diarrhea in combination with SSA therapy in adults inadequately controlled by SSA therapy. The primary endpoint was the frequency of bowel movements on average in 12 weeks. It was studied in a double-blinded placebo-controlled trial of 90 patients with metastatic NET and CS. Placebo or telotristat 250 mg was given to patients three times daily for 12 weeks while staying on Sandostatin or lanreotide. Concomitant antidiarrheal medications such as Imodium and diphenoxylate/atropine, pancreatic enzymes, and opioid analgesics used for diarrhea or pain were allowed. A reduction in overall average bowel movements from baseline of at least two bowel movements per day was seen in 33% of patients randomized to telotristat and 4% of patients randomized to placebo.
- Everolimus showed efficacy in GI-NETs with CS in the RADIANT-2 trial. In this trial, 429 patients were randomized to 30 mg octreotide LAR (Sandostatin) every 4 weeks with or without 10 mg/day everolimus. This trial showed an mPFS improvement of 16.4 versus 11.3, HR 0.77 (0.59 to 1.00), $P = 0.26$. The OS was not different, which might have been confounded by the cross-over.
- Pazopanib was studied under the Alliance A021202 study. This Phase II trial randomized 171 patients with progressive nonpancreatic NETs to pazopanib versus placebo. Midgut tumors were 66% of the whole population. mPFS in patients receiving pazopanib ($n = 97$) was 11.6 months compared with 8.5 months in those receiving placebo ($n = 74$, HR 0.53, $P = 0.0005$). OS was not improved, which might have been confounded due to cross-over.[24]
- Bevacizumab has been studied as a single agent (RR 18%), and in combination with octreotide (RR 12%). Octreotide + bevacizumab showed no mPFS improvement in comparison to octreotide + interferon in a SWOG randomized trial (16.6 vs. 15.4 months). Radiographic RR was improved in the bevacizumab arm (12 vs. 4%).[25]
- PRRT is a viable option after first line for advanced mid- and hindgut tumors. The pivotal trial, NETTER-1, was an open label Phase III international trial comparing high-dose monthly Sandostatin (60 mg) as the control group to 4 cycles of 200 mCi ^{177}Lu-Dotatate (Lutathera) every 8 weeks. In the study, 231 patients were included in the final analysis. ^{177}Lu-Dotatate significantly reduced the risk of progression of disease or death and improved health-related quality of life compared with high-dose long-acting octreotide in patients with advanced, progressive, well-differentiated midgut NETs. At 6 years follow-up, the final OS did not reach a statistical significance difference, but the median OS was 48.0 months in the ^{177}Lu-Dotatate group and 36.3 months in the control group. A 11.7-month difference in mOS with ^{177}Lu-Dotatate is considered clinically relevant.
- Lutathera is administered along with a solution containing lysine and arginine amino acids to prevent kidney toxicity. Repeat treatment with Lutathera can be considered if the disease progression happened at minimum after 12 months. In this scenario, only 2 cycles of PRRT are administered.
- Interferon was administered before SSRA drugs were available. Due to serious toxicities, this treatment is not recommended unless there are no other viable options remaining.[2]
- The combination of PRRT + everolimus is under investigation currently.
- The role of CAPTEM in this low-grade advance midgut and hindgut NET is controversial.
- The patients with CH are referred to Cardiothoracic Surgery and Cardiology.
- Pulmonary +/- tricuspid valve replacement is performed in ventricle function preserved patients.
- CH is secondary to right- and left-side heart valve injury secondary to very high levels of serum serotonin in patients with CS. Recurrent CH is rarely seen in the bioprosthetic valves in patients with uncontrolled CS who have persistent very high serum serotonin levels.

What Are the Toxicities Associated With Systemic Therapy Options?

- See under pNET.

What Are the Prognostic Markers and How Do They Impact Treatment and/or Survival?

- The prognosis is driven by tumor grade and bulk of disease in these well-differentiated tumors.

Case 10.3 Further Follow-Up

- *The patient in Case 10.3 had serum serotonin and a 24-hour urine 5HIAA measurement that resulted as 1500 ng/mL and 25 mg (normal greater than 15), respectively. A Ga68 PET scan showed significant uptake in the known lesions and ruled out other metastatic deposits. The case was discussed in a multidisciplinary GI tumor board, and surgical resection of the primary tumor and liver metastasis was recommended. She was started on monthly lanreotide injections and PRN Lomotil, and 4 weeks later she safely had debulking surgery. At the time of her surgery, her diarrhea and flushing had improved and her serotonin and 24-hour urine 5-HIAA had decreased, but was still higher than normal. A screening ECHO was done for cardiac workup, and it was reported as poor quality, but her left ventricular ejection fraction (LVEF) was 60% and she was cleared for surgery. The surgery included removal of all the gross and visible cancer, which included SB and associated regional lymphadenectomy, as well as segment 2 liver with hepatectomy. Prophylactic octreotide infusion was provided to prevent carcinoid crises.[26]*

The Patient's Pathology Report

- *Final pathology revealed well-differentiated, ileal primary NET that invades through muscularis propria into subserosa without penetrating the overlying serosa. The primary tumor is 2 cm in size with 18 out of 30 LNs positive as part of a 6-cm mesenteric mass, mitotic index 1/10 HPF (Ki-67 index 8%), and margins of both the liver and bowel were negative for tumor. IHC was positive for chromogranin and negative for synaptophysin. The patient's flushing resolved, and diarrhea improved. Her serum serotonin and 24-hour 5-HIAA normalized. Her persistent diarrhea post-surgery was believed to be secondary to SB syndrome rather than CS. She was followed up with scans and biomarkers every 3 months for 9 months when she lost follow-up. She returned with recurrent CS and liver and bone metastasis seen on repeat Ga68 PET scan. The next step systemic options are SSRA, PRRT, or everolimus. There is extrahepatic disease seen in the bone; therefore, local liver-directed therapies were not considered. She was started on Lutathera and lanreotide. CS was greatly controlled with the first and second cycles. She was also referred to Cardiology and Cardiothoracic Surgery, where she had pulmonary and tricuspid valve replacement with bio-prosthesis. The surgery took place after the carcinoid tumor was maximally controlled and perioperative octreotide infusion was provided to prevent carcinoid crises.*

What Are the Side Effects of Various Treatments?

- See treatment-related side effects under Case 10.2.

How Are Patients Followed Up for Surveillance?

- See surveillance strategy under Case 10.2.

Case 10.4: Poorly Differentiated Neuroendocrine Carcinoma

A 43-year-old man with 15 pack-years of cigarette smoking history presented to the hospital with abdominal and back pain. He was in his usual state of health until about 5 weeks prior to presentation when he developed abdominal pain, early satiety, belching, hiccups, progressive nausea and vomiting, and 48 pounds weight loss in the last 3 months. No relevant family history.

CT of the chest, abdomen, and pelvis demonstrated multiple masses measuring up to 9 cm involving the body and pylorus of the stomach with encasement of the second portion of the duodenum with significant lymphadenopathy of the gastrohepatic nodes and innumerable liver lesions measuring up to 8 cm in size. Small subcentimeter pulmonary nodules are seen bilaterally in multiple lobes. An additional 1-cm lesion is also seen at L2 in the spine. MRI of the C/T/L (cervical/thoracic/lumbar) spine showed no signal change in the cord but showed small lesions in L1 to L3. Physical examination shows temporal wasting, as well as right upper quadrant (RUQ) abdominal tenderness to palpation. Spine and neurological exam were normal. Labs were remarkable for albumin of 2.9, and total bilirubin of 2.1, 1.9 of which was direct. Hemoglobin (Hgb) was 10.9. International normalized ratio (INR) was 1.3.

EGD showed gastric outlet obstruction from extrinsic compression and further extrinsic narrowing at D2 that was confirmed with EUS. Biopsy of the largest segment VII liver lesion by interventional radiology demonstrated poorly differentiated NEC with greater than 20 mitosis per 10 HPF, Ki-67 80%. IHC was positive for synaptophysin, chromogranin, CK7, CAM 5.2, and CK5/6.

What Is the Specific Pathology for Each Disease and How Is it Staged?

- The most important step is to separate GEP-NEC from GEP-NETs.
- In contrast to NETs, NECs have less resemblance to the non-neoplastic neuroendocrine cells.
- NECs are all poorly differentiated on pathology and, almost always, strongly and diffusely stain positive for synaptophysin.
- IHC for these are needed to assure the case is not confused with other poorly differentiated carcinomas.
- GEP-NECs are divided into two histological distinct entities: small cell (40%) and large cell NECs (60%).[27,28] They are all considered high grade by default and grading measurement and report with mitotic index or Ki-67 proliferative index is not necessary in unequivocal cases.
- There is no Ki-67 index cutoff within the G3 range that absolutely separates NECs versus NETs. A high Ki-67 (greater than 55%) is more likely to be NEC, but rates in the 20% to 55% range can be seen with both NET and NEC.
- Mitotic rate greater than 20 per 10 HPF usually indicates an NEC.
- Given the propensity for early spread beyond the initial site, baseline staging necessitates either CT scan of the chest with contrasted CT or MRI of the abdomen and pelvis.
- The incidence of brain metastasis in GEP-NEC is lower than SCLC. Screening brain imaging (CT scan or MRI) is not routinely recommended and is driven by symptoms.
- SSR imaging is negative in more than 50% of cases and not considered routine.[29]
- FDG-PET is positive in more than 90% of the cases.[30]

How Is Pacreatic Neuroendocrine Carcinoma Diagnosed?

- The diagnosis is established with EGD/EUS biopsy of the pancreatic mass or the metastatic lesion.

Is Biochemical Testing Required for the Disease?

- Tumor markers are not measured in pNECs as these are negative most of the time.

What Molecular Markers Are Used in Current Clinical Practice?

- Given the rarity of these tumors, NCCN guidelines suggest testing for biomarkers such as MSI, MMR, and TMB to evaluate for targeted therapy options.[2]
- There is a distinction between some molecular markers between GEP-NECs and GEP-NETs and GEP-NECs and lung-NECs; these can potentially be used to finalize a diagnosis in puzzling cases.
- *Rb* loss and *KRAS* mutation have been found to be predictors of the response to platinum-based chemotherapy in pNECs.
- The association of these molecular markers on non-pancreatic GI NECs partially holds in some subtype, but this is not all inclusive.
- Hijioka et al.[31] studied the association between these tumor markers and response to platinum-based chemotherapy in pNECs and pNETs and stratified the clinicopathological and molecular features in 70 patients, G3 pNENs, from 31 institutions. Of these, 21 (30%) were pNETs and 49 (70%) were pNECs. pNETs showed a lower median Ki-67 index (28.5%) than pNECs (80%), no *Rb* loss, no *p53* loss, and no *KRAS* mutation. pNEN-G3 were stratified based on *Rb* and *KRAS*. PNENs with Rb loss and mutated *KRAS* showed statistically significant higher RR to platinum-based chemotherapy than those without. *Rb* and *KRAS* were proposed as predictive markers of response to platinum-based chemotherapy.
- GEP-NEC has a lower rate of mutations in the *TP53* gene and alterations in expression of the *RB1* gene than SCLC.
- *KRAS* mutations are found in 50% of pNECs but are rare in SCLC. Conversely, SCLC has a greater than 90% incidence of loss of *RB1* gene function, compared with 60% in pancreatic small cell NEC.

Does the Disease Have Specific Germline Mutations to Warrant Genetic Counseling?

- pNECs are not associated with germline mutations and genetic counseling is not recommended.

How Does the Disease Present?

- These cancers present with an aggressive behavior and bulky tumor burden, which is typical for poorly differentiated NEC.
- GEP-NECs usually present with advanced widespread disease.
- Brain metastasis is seen less commonly than the lung NEC's counterpart.[32]
- NECs are rarely functional and are not associated with genetic syndromes.
- NECs have a significantly lower OS rate (almost half) in comparison to grade 3 NETs (11 to 27 months) versus 41 to 99 months).[33-37]

How Is Pancreatic Neuroendocrine Carcinoma Managed and What Are the Treatment Options?

- The treatment paradigm of GEP-NECs follows the same treatment as SCLC.
- The treatment is the same among the various GI primaries (midgut, hindgut, pancreatic).
- Patients with early and locoregional esophageal, anal, and rectum NECs are treated with platinum-based chemotherapy plus radiation. APR after chemoradiation is highly individualized.
- Nonmetastatic pNECs are treated similarly to GEP-NECs with radial surgery followed by adjuvant platinum-based chemotherapy. Platinum-based neoadjuvant chemotherapy followed by radial surgery is frequently considered.

- GEP-NECs have a lower ORR to platinum-based chemotherapy in comparison to lung -NECs.[38]
- RR to platinum-based first-line chemotherapy is associated with the level of Ki-67 proliferative index, which was shown in the NORDIC-NEC study.[39] This study evaluated predictive and prognostic factors in the treatment of advanced GI-NECs. Data from 252 patients with advanced NECs from 12 Nordic hospitals were retrospectively reviewed. Patients with Ki-67 less than 55% had a lower RR (15% vs. 42%, P less than 0.001), but better survival than patients with Ki-67 of 55% or greater (14 vs. 10 months, P less than 0.001).
- At this time PRRT is not considered for NECs. NECs usually have a low or no uptake on SSR imaging; hence, they do not respond to this treatment modality.
- In an uncommon NEC scenario, PRRT can be considered if there is low FDG-PET and high Krenning scale uptake on SSR PET imaging uptake. The Krenning scale ranges from grade 0 (no uptake by tumor) to grade 4 (very intense uptake by tumor), with higher grades indicating a higher level of expression of SSRs on nuclear imaging.
- Lutathera has shown tumor response in NECs in the second or third-line setting. PFS was 11 months for low NEC (Ki-67 of 55% or less) and 4 months for high NEC (Ki-67 greater than 55%).[29]

Follow-Up on Case 10.4

- *The patient in Case 10.4 was initiated on C1 of carboplatin/etoposide in the hospital. On day 2 of his first cycle, he was noted to have potassium of 5.6, creatinine of 1.4, and uric acid of 11. He was aggressively managed with fluids and rasburicase with resolution of his lab abnormalities. No further tumor lysis was observed with subsequent cycles. NGS was performed, which showed TP53 mutation, MSI-S, and TMB of 5%. PET reevaluation after 6 cycles showed NED. However, at 3 months surveillance, PET showed FDG-avid disease of the liver, lung, and abdominal lymphadenopathy. The decision was made to initiate nivolumab/ipilimumab. The patient unfortunately declined in functional status with increasing fatigue and weight loss and PET demonstrated progressive disease 12 weeks into immunotherapy, and he elected to transition to hospice.*

What Are the Prognostic Markers and How Do They Impact Treatment and/or Survival?

- Large cell GEP-NEC and small cell GEP-NEC have a similar prognosis.
- Similar to the lung NEC's counterpart, their prognosis is poor, and the majority relapse despite undergoing curative intent surgery even if found in early stages.[40]

How Are Patients Followed Up for Surveillance?

- These cancers are followed up similar to lung cancer on surveillance.

REVIEW QUESTIONS

1. A 57-year-old male with peptic ulcer disease on omeprazole presented to the ED with nausea, vomiting, epigastric pain, and diarrhea 30 times a day. Esophagogastroduodenoscopy (EGD) showed multiple gastric and duodenal ulcers in addition to multiple 0.5- to 1-cm size mucosal nodules. Pathology of the duodenal ulcer showed slough and inflammatory debris and no malignancy. The mucosal nodule showed neuroendocrine hyperplasia and grade I well-differentiated gastric neuroendocrine tumors (NETs; Ki-67 less than 1%). Gastrinoma was diagnosed based on the combination of serum fasting gastrin level of greater than 1000 (5500) and PH of less than 2 (1.2). A pancreatic protocol contrast-enhanced CT, EGD/endoscopic ultrasound (EUS), and a Ga68 PET scan did not identify any lesions. What is the next best step?
   A. Endoscopic removal of the gastric mucosal nodules that are greater than 2 cm in size and repeat endoscopy in 3 months
   B. Start Sandostatin LAR and repeat scans in 3 months
   C. Refer to surgery for exploratory laparotomy
   D. Refer to surgery for antral gastrectomy

2. The patient in question 1 had an exploratory laparotomy and was found to have three submucosal duodenal lesions, one very close to the ampulla and shotty peri-duodenal lymph node (LN). Whipple surgery and local lymphadenectomy were performed and multifocal well-differentiated, duodenal, and ampullary neuroendocrine tumors (NETs) were found, with the largest 1.5 cm in size; 2/15 LNs were positive, grade 2 (Ki-67 4%), less than 1 in 10 high power field (HPF) mitotic figures, and positive for CAM 5.2, synaptophysin, and chromogranin. All margins were negative. His gastrin level has decreased to 15. What is the next best step?
   A. Adjuvant lanreotide
   B. Adjuvant capecitabine + temozolomide
   C. Adjuvant cisplatin and etoposide
   D. Genetic counseling and testing for multiple endocrine neoplasia type 1 (MEN1) germline mutation

3. A 26-year-old female medical student with no past medical history (PMH) was brought to the ED by ambulance with a blood sugar of 27. She has had tingling in the extremities with activity, memory change, confusion, and mood swings for the last 4 weeks. Her husband called 911 after he could not wake her up from sleep. Her blood sugar was 27 per paramedics' testing; she was started on IV dextrose and brought to the ED. CT of the abdomen revealed a 2-cm hypervascular lesion in her pancreatic body. After stabilization, she had tumor enucleation and pathology, which revealed a well-differentiated grade I neuroendocrine tumor (NET), Ki-67 less than 2%. Suspicious liver lesions were biopsied in the OR, and these were consistent with liver metastasis from the pancreatice neuroendocrine tumor (pNET). She continued to have hypoglycemia after she was discharged from the hospital. A Ga68 PET scan was done that showed faint uptake in two small liver lesions (standardized uptake value [SUV] 5). In addition to starting her on diazoxide and endocrinology referral, what is the best next step?
   A. Capecitabine and temozolomide (CAPTEM) combination
   B. Lanreotide
   C. Everolimus
   D. Peptide receptor radionuclide therapy (PRRT)

4. A 55-year-old male with no past medical history (PMH) presented to the ED with weight loss, nausea, vomiting, and abdominal pain. He worked as an office clerk, did not smoke or drink alcohol, and went to the gym 2 times a week. An abdominal CT scan with contrast revealed a 4-cm hypervascular pancreatic body mass and a large burden of liver lesions without bile duct dilatation. Endoscopic ultrasound (EUS) biopsy from both the pancreatic mass and a liver lesion showed well-differentiated neuroendocrine tumors (NET), immunohistochemistry (IHC) staining positive for chromogranin, and synaptophysin on both the pancreatic and liver specimen. The pancreatic lesion and liver Ki-67 index was 15% (G2) and 45% (G3), respectively. CT scan of the chest showed no other lesion. Ga68 PET scan showed mild uptake in the pancreatic lesions but no uptake in the liver lesions. A fluorodeoxyglucose (FDG) PET showed uptake in the known liver lesions. What is the best systemic option in this case?
   A. Carboplatin and etoposide
   B. Lanreotide
   C. Everolimus
   D. Capecitabine and temozolomide

5. Select the correct statement from the list that follows:
   A. Lung carcinoids are associated with germline von Hippel Lindau (VHL) in 6% of the cases
   B. Adjuvant somatostatin receptor analogues (SSRAs) showed survival benefit in R0 resected, greater than 5 cm in size, and intermediate grade lung carcinoid patients
   C. Well-differentiated advanced lung primary carcinoid tumors are commonly present with carcinoid syndrome (CS)
   D. Molecular markers have no role in clinical practice in carcinoid tumors

6. A 65-year-old female with a newly diagnosed grade 2 rectal neuroendocrine tumor (NET) with bilateral liver metastasis has carcinoid syndrome (CS). Her symptoms are diarrhea 5 to 6 times per day and flushing. Her medications include octreotide LAR (Sandostatin), PRN Lomotil, and PRN Imodium telotristat. What is correct about telotristat (Xermelo)?
   A. It is indicated for both CS diarrhea and flushing per U.S. Food and Drug Administration (FDA) label
   B. Telotristat decreases the level of chromogranin
   C. Cardiac arrhythmia is the most serious side effect of telotristat
   D. Telotristat starts improving bowel movement in an average of 2 weeks
   E. There is no benefit with the combination of Sandostatin and telotristat

7. A 31-year male was diagnosed with hypercalcemia and primary hyperparathyroidism at age 17 who had undergone multi-gland resection and right forearm autograft. He was recently diagnosed with two hypervascular pancreatic masses, sizes 1.5 and 3 cm, on pancreatic protocol CT scan. Endoscopic ultrasound (EUS)-guided biopsy revealed low-grade, well-differentiated neuroendocrine tumor (NET). He had pancreatectomy and lymphadenectomy that showed the same. His serum hormones (insulin, proinsulin, c-peptide, gastrin, and vasoactive intestinal peptide [VIP]) were all normal. His sister and father had a similar clinical presentation. His sister was recently found to have a pituitary adenoma on screening MRI, and genetic testing confirmed a germline mutation, but the patient does not remember the details. What is the most likely germline mutation associated with this patient's syndrome?
   A. pVHL 3q25
   B. MEN1
   C. RET 10q
   D. CDKN18

8. A 26-year-old male with no past medical history (PMH) presents to his primary care physician (PCP) with 20 lbs. weight loss in the last 4 weeks and right upper quadrant (RUQ) abdominal pain referring to his back. After initial workup, a multiphasic abdominal MRI shows a 16.7-cm right suprarenal mass containing some necrosis and calcifications with arterial enhancement, venous washout, and a pseudocapsule and mass effect on the inferior vena cava (IVC) and adjacent liver. Endocrine showed normal serum cortisol and dexamethasone stimulation test, adrenocorticotropic hormone (ACTH), dehydroepiandrosterone (DHEA), androstenedione, testosterone, 17-OHP, estradiol, metanephrine, and catecholamines. He underwent a right adrenalectomy and pathology revealed a 17-cm, moderately differentiated, high-grade adenocarcinoma, necrotic and hemorrhagic; margins were all negative and no lymph nodes (LNs) were submitted. Ki-67 index was 40% and he was staged at pT2pNx. Distant metastases were ruled out prior to surgery. What is the next step?

A. Adjuvant lanreotide
B. Adjuvant mitotane
C. Observation
D. Adjuvant pembrolizumab

ANSWERS AND RATIONALES

1. **C. Refer to surgery for exploratory laparotomy.** Gastrin level greater than 1000 plus gastric PH level less than 2 measured at the same time is diagnostic of gastrinoma, also known as Zollinger-Ellison syndrome (ZES). Localization and resection of the gastrinoma is the next step in management to eradicate the tumor and to control hypergastrinemia. Majority of the gastrinomas that are not readily seen on endoscopy or scans are found in the gastrinoma triangle. Rarely they can be found in the ovary or lung. The NET nodules found in the gastric mucosa are secondary to the high gastrin level. Answers A and D are appropriate for early-stage type 1 gastrinoma. Answer B is appropriate for advanced type 1 gastrinoma.

2. **D. Genetic counseling and testing for multiple endocrine neoplasia type 1 (MEN1) germline mutation.** Similar to most of the well-differentiated NETs with very few exceptions (for example, high risk adrenocortical pheochromocytomas), adjuvant treatment in any form is not recommended in gastrinoma patients who have no evidence of disease radiographically and biochemically. This patient's tumor has been fully removed and his serum gastrin level has rapidly decreased to normal after surgery. Between 2% and 4% of gastrinomas have a germline MEN1 mutation and genetic counseling and screening for MEN1 is indicated.

3. **C. Everolimus.** Everolimus has shown survival benefit in pNETs based on the RADIANT 3 trial. Hyperglycemia is also a side effect of everolimus; in this case, it is favored due to hypoglycemia as the hallmark of insulinoma. Lanreotide can paradoxically induce hypoglycemia in somatostatin receptor (SSRT)-negative insulinoma patients and should be avoided in an uncontrolled insulinoma. CAPTEM is not used on the first-line setting unless grade 3 NET. PRRT is indicated in the second line.[41]

4. **D. Capecitabine and temozolomide.** A negative Ga68 PET, highly positive FDG-PET scans, and a high Ki-67 index confirm an aggressive tumor and cytotoxic chemotherapy is the best answer; however, the best treatment option for this uncommon and aggressive tumor is not defined yet. The patient is symptomatic and tumor shrinkage is required. Response to platinum-based chemotherapy has been reported in retrospective data. Patients with a Ki-67 index less than 55% have a lower response to platinum-based chemotherapy than patients with 55% or higher, but with a similar disease control rate.[39] Temozolomide-based therapy is considered the first best treatment option in this setting due to better overall response rate (ORR) based on multiple retrospective analyses. Response rate of up to 41% was seen in a multicenter analysis of the combination of capecitabine and temozolomide in week-differentiated G3 neuroendocrine tumors (NETs).[42] It is important to distinguish between well-differentiated G3 pancreatice neuroendocrine tumors (pNETs) and poorly differentiated pancreatic neuroendocrine carcinomas (pNECs). The pNECs have a higher response rate to platinum-based chemotherapy, and this combination is used in the first line.

5. **D. Molecular markers have no role in clinical practice in carcinoid tumors.** Lung neuroendocrine tumors (LNETs) are associated with germline multiple endocrine neoplasia type 1 (MEN1), as seen on 4.8% of cases. It is not associated with germline VHL. Adjuvant treatment has not shown benefit in patients who have total curative resection of LNETs. Carcinoid tumor is a rare presentation of lung carcinoids.

6. **D. Telotristat starts improving bowel movement in an average of 2 weeks.** Telotristat is a tryptophan hydroxylase inhibitor indicated for the treatment of CS diarrhea in combination with somatostatin analog (SSA) therapy in adults inadequately controlled by SSA therapy. It was studied in a double-blinded placebo-controlled trial of 90 patients with metastatic NET and CS. Placebo or Xermelo 250 mg was given to patients 3 times daily for 12 weeks while staying on Sandostatin or lanreotide. Concomitant anti-diarrheal medications such as Imodium and diphenoxylate/atropine, pancreatic enzymes, and opioid analgesics used for diarrhea or pain were allowed. A reduction in overall average bowel movements from baseline of at least two bowel movements per day was seen in 33% of patients randomized to telotristat and 4% of patients randomized to placebo. Flushing had improved in some patients; however, flushing was not considered an endpoint in this study. This drug decreased the level of serotonin and urine 5-HIAA. It takes an average of 2 weeks (1 to 3 weeks) for telotristat to start showing benefit. The most common side effect is constipation.

7. **B. MEN1.** The patient has MEN1 syndrome. Germline MEN1 mutation can be diagnosed without genetic testing based on the patient having two or more features of the disease, or if the patient has one feature and a first-degree relative with MEN1. The other answers are related to other germline mutations (Von Hipple Lindau, MEN2, and MEN4).

8. **B. Adjuvant mitotane.** The European Society of Endocrinology (ESE) and ENSAT 2018 guidelines recommend adjuvant mitotane treatment after resection of adenoid cystic carcinoma (ACC) in patients with a high risk of recurrence (that is, stage III, R1 resection, or Ki-67 greater than 10%).[43] ENSAT 2018 has not reached a consensus for the addition of chemotherapy in the adjuvant setting; however, there was agreement to consider this in patients with very high risk of relapse.[43] Lanreotide in the adjuvant setting has not shown to be beneficial in any of the nonendocrine neoplasms (NENs). Single-agent pembrolizumab provides a 23% response rate and medical overall survival of 25 months in advanced ACC.[44] The patient is high risk for recurrence due to a high Ki-67 index and observation is not recommended.

REFERENCES

1. Dasari A, Shen C, Halperin D, et al. Trends in the incidence, prevalence, and survival outcomes in patients with neuroendocrine tumors in the United States. *JAMA Oncol.* 2017;3(10):1335–1342. doi:10.1001/jamaoncol.2017.0589
2. National Comprehensive Cancer Network. *National Comprehensive Cancer Network. Clinical Practice Guidlines in Oncolopy. Neuroendocrine and Adrenal Tumors.* Version 4.2021, December 14, 2021. https://www.nccn.org/guidelines/guidelines-detail?category=1&id=1448
3. Halfdanarson TR, Strosberg JR, Tang, L, et al. The North American Neuroendocrine Tumor Society (NANETS) consensus guidelines for surveillance and medical management of pancreatic neuroendocrine tumors. *Pancreas.* 2020;49(7):863–881. doi:10.1097/MPA.0000000000001597
4. Delle Fave G, O'Toole D, Sundin A, et al. ENETS consensus guidelines update for gastroduodenal neuroendocrine neoplasms. *Neuroendocrinol.* 2016;103(2):119–124. doi:10.1159/000443168
5. Roberto GA, Rodrigues CMB, Peixoto RD, Younes RN. Gastric neuroendocrine tumor: a practical literature review. *World J Gastrointest Oncol.* 2020;12(8):850–856. doi:10.4251/wjgo.v12.i8.850
6. Rindi G, Bordi C, Rappel S, et al. Gastric carcinoids and neuroendocrine carcinomas: pathogenesis, pathology, and behavior. *World J Surg.* 1996;20(2):168–172. doi:10.1007/s002689900026
7. Merola E, Sbrozzi-Vanni A, Panzuto F, et al. Type I gastric carcinoids: a prospective study on endoscopic management and recurrence rate. *Neuroendocrinol.* 2012;95(3):207–213. doi:10.1159/000329043
8. Uygun A, Kadayifci A, Polat Z, et al. Long-term results of endoscopic resection for type I gastric neuroendocrine tumors. *J Surg Oncol.* 2014;109(2):71–74. doi:10.1002/jso.23477

9. Rossi RE, Elvevi A, Citterio D, et al. Gastrinoma and Zollinger Ellison syndrome: a roadmap for the management between new and old therapies. *World J Gastroenterol.* 2021;27(35):5890–5907. doi:10.3748/wjg.v27.i35.5890

10. Gladdy RA, Strong VE, Coit D, et al. Defining surgical indications for type I gastric carcinoid tumor. *Ann Surg Oncol.* 2009;16(11):3154–3160. doi:10.1245/s10434-009-0687-y

11. de Mestier L, Hentic O, Cros J, et al. Metachronous hormonal syndromes in patients with pancreatic neuroendocrine tumors: a case-series study. *Ann Intern Med.* 2015;162(10):682–689. doi:10.7326/M14-2132

12. Raymond E, Dahan L, Raoul J-L, et al. Sunitinib malate for the treatment of pancreatic neuroendocrine tumors. *N Engl J Med.* 2011;364(6):501–513. doi:10.1056/NEJMoa1003825

13. Yao JC, Shah MH, Ito T, et al. Everolimus for advanced pancreatic neuroendocrine tumors. *N Engl J Med.* 2011;364(6):514–523. doi:10.1056/NEJMoa1009290

14. Caplin ME, Pavel M, Ruszniewski P. Lanreotide in metastatic enteropancreatic neuroendocrine tumors [Comment]. *N Engl J Med.* 2014;371(16):1556–1557. doi:10.1056/NEJMc1409757

15. Strosberg J, El-Haddad G, Wolin E, et al. Phase 3 trial of ^{177}Lu-Dotatate for midgut neuroendocrine tumors. *N Engl J Med.* 2017;376(2):125–135. doi:10.1056/NEJMoa1607427

16. Brabander T, van der Zwan WA, Teunissen JJM, et al. Long-term efficacy, survival, and safety of [^{177}Lu-DOTA^0,Tyr^3]octreotate in patients with gastroenteropancreatic and bronchial neuroendocrine tumors. *Clin Cancer Res.* 2017;23(16):4617–4624. doi:10.1158/1078-0432.CCR-16-2743

17. Ezziddin S, Khalaf F, Vanezi M, et al. Outcome of peptide receptor radionuclide therapy with ^{177}Lu-octreotate in advanced grade 1/2 pancreatic neuroendocrine tumours. *Eur J Nucl Med Mol Imaging.* 2014;41(5):925–933. doi:10.1007/s00259-013-2677-3

18. Strosberg J, Wolin E, Chasen B, et al. Health-related quality of life in patients with progressive midgut neuroendocrine tumors treated with ^{177}Lu-Dotatate in the phase III NETTER trial. *J Clin Oncol.* 2018;36(25):2578–2584. doi:10.1200/JCO.2018.78.5865

19. Zandee WT, Brabander T, Blažević A, et al. Symptomatic and radiological response to 177Lu-DOTATATE for the treatment of functioning pancreatic neuroendocrine tumors. *J Clin Endocrinol Metab.* 2019;104(4):1336–1344. doi:10.1210/jc.2018-01991

20. Kunz PL, Catalano PJ, Nimeiri H, et al. A randomized study of temozolomide or temozolomide and capecitabine in patients with advanced pancreatic neuroendocrine tumors: a trial of the ECOG-ACRIN Cancer Research Group (E2211). *Clin Oncol.* 2018;36(15_suppl15):abstr 4004. doi:10.1200/JCO.2018.36.15_suppl.4004

21. Carlsen EA, Fazio N, Granberg D, et al. Peptide receptor radionuclide therapy in gastroenteropancreatic NEN G3: a multicenter cohort study. *Endocr Relat Cancer.* 2019;26(2):227–239. doi:10.1530/ERC-18-0424

22. Morgan RE, Pommier SJ, Pommier RF. Expanded criteria for debulking of liver metastasis also apply to pancreatic neuroendocrine tumors. *Surgery.* 2018;163(1):218–225. doi:10.1016/j.surg.2017.05.030

23. Rinke A, Wittenberg M, Schade-Brittinger C, et al. Placebo-controlled, double-blind, prospective, randomized study on the effect of octreotide LAR in the control of tumor growth in patients with metastatic neuroendocrine midgut tumors (PROMID): results of long-term survival. *Neuroendocrinology.* 2017;104(1):26–32. doi:10.1159/000443612

24. Bergsland EK, Mahoney MR, Asmis TR, et al. Prospective randomized phase II trial of pazopanib versus placebo in patients with progressive carcinoid tumors (CARC) (Alliance A021202). *J Clin Oncol.* 2019;37(15_suppl):4005. doi:10.1200/JCO.2019.37.15_suppl.4005

25. Yao JC, Guthrie KA, Moran C, et al. Phase III prospective randomized comparison trial of depot octreotide plus interferon alfa-2b versus depot octreotide plus bevacizumab in patients with advanced carcinoid tumors: SWOG S0518. *J Clin Oncol.* 2017;35(15):1695–1703. doi:10.1200/JCO.2016.70.4072

26. Woltering EA, Wright AE, Stevens MA, et al. Development of effective prophylaxis against intraoperative carcinoid crisis. *J Clin Anesth.* 2016;32:189–193. doi:10.1016/j.jclinane.2016.03.008

27. Basturk O, Tang L, Hruban RH, et al. Poorly differentiated neuroendocrine carcinomas of the pancreas: a clinicopathologic analysis of 44 cases. *Am J Surg Pathol.* 2014;38(4):437–447. doi:10.1097/PAS.0000000000000169

28. Volante M, Birocco N, Gatti G, et al. Extrapulmonary neuroendocrine small and large cell carcinomas: a review of controversial diagnostic and therapeutic issues. *Hum Pathol.* 2014;45(4):665–673. doi:10.1016/j.humpath.2013.03.016

29. Sorbye H, Kong G, Grozinsky-Glasberg S. PRRT in high-grade gastroenteropancreatic neuroendocrine neoplasms (WHO G3). *Endocr Relat Cancer.* 2020;27(3):R67–R77. doi:10.1530/ERC-19-0400

30. Walter T, Tougeron D, Baudin E, et al. Poorly differentiated gastro-entero-pancreatic neuroendocrine carcinomas: are they really heterogeneous? Insights from the FFCD-GTE national cohort. *Eur J Cancer.* 2017;79:158–165. doi:10.1016/j.ejca.2017.04.009

31. Hijioka S, Hosoda W, Matsuo K, et al. Rb loss and *KRAS* mutation are predictors of the response to platinum-based chemotherapy in pancreatic neuroendocrine neoplasm with grade 3: a Japanese multicenter pancreatic NEN-G3 study. *Clin Cancer Res.* 2017;23(16):4625–4632. doi:10.1158/1078-0432.CCR-16-3135

32. Brennan SM, Gregory DL, Stillie A, et al. Should extrapulmonary small cell cancer be managed like small cell lung cancer? *Cancer.* 2010;116(4):888–895. doi:10.1002/cncr.24858

33. Heetfeld M, Chougnet CN, Olsen IH, et al. Characteristics and treatment of patients with G3 gastroenteropancreatic neuroendocrine neoplasms. *Endocr Relat Cancer.* 2015;22(4):657–664. doi:10.1530/ERC-15-0119

34. Scoazec J-Y, Couvelard A, Monges G, et al. Well-differentiated grade 3 digestive neuroendocrine tumors: myth or reality—the PRONET study group. *J Clin Oncol.* 2012;30(15_suppl):4129. doi:10.1200/jco.2012.30.15_suppl.4129

35. Vélayoudom-Céphise F-L, Duvillard P, Foucan L, et al. Are G3 ENETS neuroendocrine neoplasms heterogeneous? *Endocr Relat Cancer.* 2013;20(5):649–657. doi:10.1530/ERC-13-0027

36. Basturk O, Yang Z, Tang LH, et al. The high-grade (WHO G3) pancreatic neuroendocrine tumor category is morphologically and biologically heterogenous and includes both well differentiated and poorly differentiated neoplasms. *Am J Surg Pathol.* 2015;39(5):683–690. doi:10.1097/PAS.0000000000000408

37. Walter T, Tougeron D, Baudin E, et al. Characteristics, prognosis and treatments of 294 patients with poorly differentiated neuroendocrine carcinoma: the FFCD-GTE national cohor. *J Clin Oncol.* 2015;33(15_suppl):4095. doi:10.1200/jco.2015.33.15_suppl.4095

38. Terashima T, Morizane C, Hiraoka N, et al. Comparison of chemotherapeutic treatment outcomes of advanced extrapulmonary neuroendocrine carcinomas and advanced small-cell lung carcinoma. *Neuroendocrinology.* 2012;96(4):324–332. doi:10.1159/000338794

39. Sorbye H, Welin S, Langer SW, et al. Predictive and prognostic factors for treatment and survival in 305 patients with advanced gastrointestinal neuroendocrine carcinoma (WHO G3): the NORDIC NEC study. *Ann Oncol.* 2013;24(1):152–160. doi:10.1093/annonc/mds276

40. Dasari A, Mehta K, Byers LA, et al. Comparative study of lung and extrapulmonary poorly differentiated neuroendocrine carcinomas: a SEER database analysis of 162,983 cases. *Cancer.* 2018;124(4):807–815. doi:10.1002/cncr.31124

41. Magalhães D, Sampaio IL, Ferreira G, et al. Peptide receptor radionuclide therapy with (177)Lu-DOTA-TATE as a promising treatment of malignant insulinoma: a series of case reports and literature review. *J Endocrinol Invest.* 2019;42(3):249–260. doi:10.1007/s40618-018-0911-3

42. Chan DL, Bergsland EK, Chan JA, et al. Temozolomide in grade 3 gastroenteropancreatic neuroendocrine neoplasms: a multicenter retrospective review. *Oncologist.* 2021;26(11):950–955. doi:10.1002/onco.13923

43. Fassnacht M, Dekkers OM, Else T, et al. European Society of Endocrinology clinical practice guidelines on the management of adrenocortical carcinoma in adults, in collaboration with the European Network for the Study of Adrenal Tumors. *Eur J Endocrinol.* 2018;179(4):G1–G46. doi:10.1530/EJE-18-0608

44. Raj N, Zheng Y, Kelly V, et al. PD-1 blockade in advanced adrenocortical carcinoma. *J Clin Oncol.* 2020;38(1):71–80. doi:10.1200/JCO.19.01586

CHAPTER 11

Hepatobiliary Cancer

Brian Pham and Edward J. Kim

INTRODUCTION

There were an estimated 42,230 new cases of hepatocellular and intrahepatic ductal carcinoma in 2021 with 30,230 deaths representing 5% of all cancer deaths.[1] Globally, hepatocellular carcinomas (HCC) are sixth in new cases and third in causes of death from cancer.[2] The incidence is highest in Asia due to the high prevalence of hepatitis B infection.

There are multiple risk factors for HCC but cirrhosis is the most common, with cirrhotic patients having an annual incidence rate of 1% to 8% of developing HCC over their lifetime.[3] There are multiple potential causes of cirrhosis, with underlying hepatitis B and C infection being the most common. It is important to note that patients with chronic hepatitis B can also develop HCC without cirrhosis. Hepatitis B is an oncogenic virus leading to HCC via multiple pathways which include integration of hepatitis B DNA and epigenetic remodeling altering oncogenic and tumor suppressor genes for malignant transformation. Also, the inhibition of the immune microenvironment promotes tumor formation via evasion of immune surveillance.[4] Recent antiviral medications for hepatitis C and vaccinations against hepatitis B have helped reduce the risk of developing HCC. Other risk factors for HCC that also stem from cirrhosis include alcohol and non-alcoholic fatty liver disease. Less common risk factors for HCC include hemochromatosis, aflatoxins, and alpha1-antitrypsin deficiency.

Surveillance is recommended in patients with cirrhosis and chronic hepatitis B without cirrhosis. A standard surveillance plan includes ultrasound of the liver once every 6 months with addition of diagnostic MRI or CT for any suspicious lesions.

CASE SUMMARIES

Case 11.1: Metastatic Hepatocellular Carcinoma

A 58-year-old Vietnamese man with a history of diabetes, hypertension, cirrhosis (Child-Pugh Score [CPS] A), and hepatitis B presented for evaluation of liver lesions. The patient had an abdominal ultrasound which revealed multiple liver lesions concerning for HCC. MRI of the abdomen was obtained confirming HCC. CT of the chest showed pulmonary lesions consistent with metastatic disease. The patient was asymptomatic.

How Is a Diagnosis Established?

- Imaging can be sufficient for diagnosis of HCC based on the liver imaging reporting and data systems (LI-RADS) classification in patients with cirrhosis or chronic hepatitis B. LI-RADS scores range from 1 to 5 with LI-RADS 5 lesions deemed to be "definitely HCC" if at least 1 cm in size and demonstrate both non-rim arterial phase hyperenhancement and nonperipheral washout in the portal venous or delayed phase. Lesions that do not meet these criteria require biopsy for tissue confirmation.[5]

Patient's Diagnosis
- *Patient was diagnosed via MRI with findings that included an LI-RADS 5 lesion consistent with HCC.*

What Further Molecular or Genomic Testing Is Required?

- There is no required molecular or genomic testing required for HCC.

Patient's Molecular and Genomic Testing
- *None*

How Is This Tumor Staged?

- The American Joint Committee on Cancer (AJCC) eighth edition staging system is used to stage HCC. However, there are other factors that must be considered to optimally guide therapy because the tumor, lymph node, metastasis (TNM) staging system does not account for underlying liver dysfunction.
- Multiple staging systems have been developed to better account for liver dysfunction in the background of HCC including the Barcelona Clinic Liver Cancer (BCLC), Okuda, and Cancer of the Liver Italian Program (CLIP).
- The BCLC staging system is the most widely used system and incorporates the CPS, performance status, tumor size, vascular invasion, and number of lesions.

Patient's Clinical Stage
- *BLCL stage C, AJCC stage IVB (T3N0M1)*

What Are Appropriate Treatment Options?

- Based on results from the SHARP trial which demonstrated improved overall survival with sorafenib compared to placebo (10.7 months vs. 7.9 months), sorafenib became the standard of care first-line systemic therapy in advanced HCC with CPS A with the U.S. Food and Drug Administration (FDA) approval in 2007.[6]
- Recent data from the IMbrave 150 trial established the combination of atezolizumab and bevacizumab as the new standard of care front-line therapy with statistically and clinically significant improvement in 12-month overall survival with atezolizumab and bevacizumab compared to sorafenib (67.2% vs. 54.6%).[7]
- Lenvatinib was assessed in a noninferiority design trial against sorafenib and found to be noninferior (median overall survival rate [OS] 13.6 vs. 12.3 months, respectively).[8] Therefore, lenvatinib is also an option as first-line therapy for unresectable HCC.
- There has been no direct head-to-head comparison between lenvatinib and atezolizumab with bevacizumab. However, a meta-analysis of atezolizumab with bevacizumab compared to sorafenib and lenvatinib again provided evidence of atezolizumab and bevacizumab as the front-line standard of care.[9]

Recommended Patient Treatment Plan
- *Atezolizumab and bevacizumab*

What Are the Toxicities Associated With Chemotherapy?

- Patients receiving atezolizumab need to be monitored for immune-related adverse events such as pneumonitis, dermatitis, colitis, hypothyroidism, and adrenal insufficiency.
- Bevacizumab-associated toxicities include hypertension and proteinuria, which must be monitored while on therapy. Notably, due to increased risk of bleeding from esophageal varices with bevacizumab, endoscopic evaluation is required prior to starting therapy and should ideally be done within 6 months prior to starting.
- Lenvatinib is associated with increased risk of diarrhea, hypertension, proteinuria, and hypothyroidism, whereas sorafenib demonstrates higher risk of palmar plantar erythrodysesthesia.[8]

What Are Other Treatment Considerations?

- The immune checkpoint inhibitors pembrolizumab and nivolumab have also been evaluated in treatment of patients with advanced HCC. In the first-line setting, the CheckMate 459 Phase III trial demonstrated treatment with nivolumab yielded a higher overall response rate than sorafenib, but this did not translate into a longer progression-free survival (PFS) or OS.[10] KEYNOTE -224 was a Phase II trial of pembrolizumab in 51 patients who had been treated previously with sorafenib. The overall response rate (ORR) was 16% and the median duration of response was not reached.[11] However, the KEYNOTE-240 Phase III demonstrated no significant OS or PFS benefit when pembrolizumab was compared to placebo in patients who had been treated with sorafenib.[12]
- Another immunotherapy option is the dual checkpoint inhibitor combination of nivolumab and the cytotoxic T-lymphocyte-associated protein 4 (CTLA-4) inhibitor ipilimumab after progression on sorafenib. The CheckMate 040 Phase I/II trial tested various dosing regimens of nivolumab and ipilumumab in patients previously treated with sorafenib, with nivolumab 1 mg/kg and ipilimumab 3 mg/kg every 3 weeks for 4 cycles followed by nivolumab maintenance providing optimal benefit, with median OS of 22.2 months and 32% ORR.[13]
- Alternatives to immunotherapy include other vascular endothelial growth factor (VEGF) inhibitors such as regorafenib and ramucirumab. The RESORCE trial compared regorafenib to placebo for those who progressed on sorafenib with median OS 10.6 months versus 7.8 months, respectively.[14] The REACH-2 Phase III trial compared ramucirumab with placebo for patients with high alpha-fetoprotein (AFP; AFP greater than 400) advanced HCC after sorafenib treatment and showed OS benefit of 8.5 months versus 7.3 months favoring ramucirumab.[15]
- Based on the CELESTIAL Phase III trial, cabozantinib was approved for patients in the second- or third-line setting after being previously treated with sorafenib. Cabozantinib versus placebo was superior with better median OS (10.2 months vs. 8 months) and PFS (5.2 months vs. 1.9. months).[16]
- The landscape for treatment options has shifted dramatically in a short amount of time and has led to new questions including optimal sequencing of the multiple new systemic therapies for advanced HCC. At this point in time, choosing between the various agents depends on prior therapy choices and toxicity experienced by each individual patient.

What Is Required for This Patient's Follow-Up?

- Surveillance for response to systemic therapy typically includes serial imaging every 2 to 3 months. This includes either multiphasic abdominal MR or multiphase abdominal CT for the liver or CT of the chest and MR/CT pelvis.
- AFP can be followed as a tumor marker for trends suggestive of disease status.

Biliary Tract Cancer

Biliary tract cancers (BTC) include both gallbladder and cholangiocarcinoma. Cholangio-carcinoma can be further divided into intrahepatic and extrahepatic cholangiocarcinoma. Intrahepatic cholangiocarcinoma includes tumors originating from the intrahepatic ducts to the bifurcation of the hepatic ducts. Extrahepatic cholangiocarcinoma begins at the common hepatic duct and extends to the ampulla of Vater. Globally, there has been an increased inci-dence of gallbladder and cholangiocarcinoma. The incidence has increased by 76% from 1990 to 2017 with 210,878 new cases in 2017.[17]

Risk factors for development of gallbladder adenocarcinoma include gallstones, pol-yps, porcelain gallbladder, primary sclerosing cholangitis (PSC), and chronic infection from *Salmonella* or *Helicobacter*. These factors all share a common pathway of inducing chronic inflammation of the gallbladder. The risk factors for cholangiocarcinoma include primary hepatobiliary disease, infections, and genetic disorders. Primary hepatobiliary diseases include PSC, chronic intrahepatic stone disease, and cirrhosis. In the United States and Europe, the more common risk factor for cholangiocarcinoma is PSC, although the mechanism underlying this risk is currently unclear. Hepatitis B/C, HIV, liver flukes, and *Helicobacter pylori* have all been associated with cholangiocarcinoma. Specifically, parasitic liver flukes in the genera Clonorchis and Opisthorchis are endemic in parts of Asia and lead to higher incidence of intra-hepatic cholangiocarcinoma in those regions. Lastly, genetic disorders such as cystic fibrosis, Lynch syndrome, BAP1 tumor predisposition syndrome, and multiple biliary papillomatosis increase the risk of cholangiocarcinoma.

Case 11.2: Locally Advanced Cholangiocarcinoma

A 56-year-old woman with a history of hypertension and diabetes mellitus presents with fatigue, weight loss, and abdominal pain. She was noted to have 15 lbs weight loss over 2 weeks and started having right upper quadrant (RUQ) pain at the same time. She underwent a CT of the abdomen and pelvis which revealed a 6-cm hypodense liver mass of the left lobe and biliary ductal dilation. Her labs were notable for aspartate aminotransferase 63 U/L, alkaline phospha-tase 121 U/L, alanine aminotransferase 48 U/L, total bilirubin of 2.3 mg/dL, direct bilirubin of 1.5 mg/dL, and CA 19-9 of 65. Subsequently, the patient underwent an endoscopic retrograde cholangio-pancreatography (ERCP) for stent placement and cytology from brushing confirmed adenocarcinoma. Further staging with CT of the chest did not reveal distant metastasis. The patient was deemed a surgical candidate and underwent a partial hepatectomy, cholecystectomy, and hepaticojejunostomy. Pathology confirmed adenocarcinoma of the liver lesion in addition to one positive lymph node (LN). The patient has now recovered from surgery and follows-up for any further treatment.

How Is a Diagnosis Established?

- Diagnosis is based on a constellation of studies as biliary tract tumors can be difficult to diagnose via biopsy alone. Tissue sampling from the biliary tract may not always yield enough tumor for a diagnosis. Imaging studies need to include a multi-phase liver CT or MRI of the abdomen/pelvis and a CT of the chest to complete staging. A magnetic resonance cholangiopancreatography (MRCP) and/or CT is preferred for diagnostic purposes instead of direct cholangiography as there is higher sensitivity, specificity, and diagnostic accuracy for hilar cholangiocarcinoma.

Patient's Diagnosis

- *Intrahepatic cholangiocarcinoma*

What Further Molecular or Genomic Testing Is Required?

- *No molecular or genomic testing is required.*

Patient's Molecular and Genomic Testing

- *None*

How Is This Tumor Staged?

- The AJCC eighth edition staging system is used to stage cholangiocancer. Staging for cholangiocarcinoma is divided into intrahepatic, perihilar, and distal bile duct tumors.

Patient's Clinical Stage

- *AJCC stage III T1bN1M0*

What Are Appropriate Treatment Options?

- For patients with resected tumor, the evidence for adjuvant therapy suggests overall benefit, but the optimal specific regimen has not been well-defined. There is a paucity of randomized Phase III clinical trials that adequately show the benefit of a specific regimen over another. Given the rarity and heterogeneity of BTC, robust randomized trials have been difficult to execute and complete.
- BILCAP was a randomized Phase III clinical trial in resected BTC evaluating capecitabine for 6 months versus observation. The primary endpoint of improved overall survival with capecitabine was not met in the intention to treat population. Median overall survival was 51.1 months with capecitabine and 36.4 months in the observation group, but the hazard ratio of 0.81 was not statistically significant. However, the per protocol treatment and preplanned sensitivity analysis showed a positive result with capecitabine, suggesting capecitabine may be a reasonable option for adjuvant therapy in resected BTC.[18]
- Gemcitabine combined with oxaliplatin was studied in the PRODIGE 12–ACCORD-18 UNICANCER GI study, but this failed to show a significant difference when compared to observation alone.[19]
- Adjuvant therapy with radiation alone or chemoradiation remains unclear as most studies were based on retrospective data or small Phase II trials. For node-positive or resection with positive margins in extrahepatic and gallbladder carcinoma, the SWOG S0809 trial demonstrated that 4 cycles of gemcitabine and capecitabine followed by concurrent radiation and capecitabine was feasible and yielded a median OS of 36 months with 65% 2-year survival.[20]

Recommended Patient Treatment Plan

- *8 cycles of capecitabine*

What Are the Toxicities Associated With Chemotherapy?

- Capecitabine was dosed at 1250 mg/m^2 twice daily in the BILCAP study but this dose was associated with significant toxicities, with 44% of the patients in the study developing at least one grade 3 toxicity. The most frequent toxicities observed were hand–foot syndrome, diarrhea, and fatigue.

What Are Other Treatment Considerations?

- Given the paucity of data and guidance for adjuvant therapy, patients should be discussed among a multidisciplinary team while also considering clinical trials.

Case 11.3: Metastatic Cholangiocarcinoma

A 68-year-old man presented to the ED for severe RUQ pain, abdominal bloating, and jaundice. Physical exam showed tender RUQ, jaundice, and scleral icterus. His labs were notable for an elevated alkaline phosphatase of 501 U/L, total bilirubin of 6.7 mg/dL, and direct bilirubin of 4.9 mg/dL. CA 19-9 was 33 and AFP was normal. The patient was found to have multiple liver lesions, enlarged LNs, intrahepatic ductal dilation, and peritoneal fluid on CT abdomen and pelvis. Liver lesions under imaging were not consistent with HCC based on the LI-RADS score. CT of the chest showed multiple pulmonary nodules concerning for metastatic spread. He underwent an ERCP with stent placement and his symptoms improved along with normalization of his total bilirubin and alkaline phosphatase. Biopsy of a pulmonary nodule and brushings from the ERCP confirmed adenocarcinoma.

How Is a Diagnosis Established?

- Refer to establishing diagnosis as seen in the locally advanced case.

Patient's Diagnosis
- *Intrahepatic cholangiocarcinoma*

What Further Molecular or Genomic Testing Is Required?

- Next-generation sequencing (NGS) is used for additional therapeutic targets.

How Is This Tumor Staged?

- The AJCC eighth edition staging system is used to stage BTC. Staging for BTC is divided into intrahepatic, perihilar, and distal bile duct tumors.

Patient's Clinical Stage
- *AJCC stage IV T2N1M1*

What Are Appropriate Treatment Options?

- The ABC-02 Phase III trial included both gallbladder and cholangiocarcinoma and demonstrated a median overall survival benefit with gemcitabine and cisplatin compared to gemcitabine alone (11.7 months vs. 8.1 months, respectively).[21] Gemcitabine/cisplatin is currently the standard of care front-line treatment for metastatic BTC.

- Other acceptable gemcitabine regimens that have been used in the front-line setting include gemcitabine with oxaliplatin (GEMOX). A Phase II study demonstrated a median OS of 7.6 months and 22% response rate.[22] A triplet regimen of gemcitabine, cisplatin, and albumin-bound paclitaxel appears promising based on a Phase II study demonstrating a median OS of 19.2 months.[23] Recently, the randomized Phase III SWOG trial S1815 comparing the triplet to gemcitabine/cisplatin completed accrual.
- Consideration can also be given for 5-fluorouracil-based regimens combined with either oxaliplatin or cisplatin.[24]

Recommended Patient Treatment Plan
- *Gemcitabine and cisplatin*

What Are the Toxicities Associated With Chemotherapy?

- Toxicities associated with gemcitabine include myelosuppression and elevated liver enzymes. Other rare and reported severe toxicities that would require immediate discontinuation include pulmonary toxicities, hemolytic uremic syndrome, and posterior reversible encephalopathy syndrome.
- Cisplatin is commonly associated with ototoxicity, nephrotoxicity, emesis, and peripheral neuropathy. Due to cisplatin-induced nephrotoxicity, careful consideration should be given for patients with chronic kidney disease or renal impairment weighing the potential risk versus benefit of administration. Additionally, age and functional status may contribute to poor tolerance of cisplatin.

What Are Other Treatment Considerations?

- After progression on first-line therapy with gemcitabine-based chemotherapy, the combination of 5-fluorouracil and oxaliplatin (FOLFOX) is the preferred option based on the ABC-06 trial which showed FOLFOX provides a median OS of 6.2 months compared to 5.3 months with supportive care alone.[25]
- Beyond standard chemotherapy, targeted agents have also been evaluated and approved in the second-line setting for select targets including isocitrate dehydrogenase (IDH) inhibitors, fibroblast growth factor receptor (FGFR) inhibitors, and neurotrophic tyrosine kinase (NTRK).
- Ivosidenib, an IDH-1 inhibitor, was approved for treatment of advanced cholangiocarcinoma based on the Phase III Clar1DHy trial showing prolonged survival and durable response. In patients with previously treated advanced cholangiocarcinoma, ivosidenib showed a median OS of 10.3 months compared to 7.3 months with placebo.[26]
- Pemigatinib and infigratinib are oral FGFR inhibitors approved for cholangiocarcinoma. Pemigatinib was approved based on the Phase II FIGHT-202 trial. Patients with FGFR2 fusion or rearrangement had an 80% disease control rate (objective response or stable disease).[27] Infigratinib was given FDA accelerated approval based on a Phase II trial of 108 patients with achievement of an ORR of 23% and median duration of response of 5 months.[28]
- A Phase I/II trial of larotrectinib, a TRK inhibitor, in 55 patients who had TRK fusion-positive cancer revealed an ORR was 75%. Based on this, larotrectinib was approved for solid tumors with an *NTRK* gene fusion.[29]
- Lastly, immunotherapy should be considered for patients whose tumors are microsatellite instability (MSI)-high or deficient in mismatch repair. In the Phase II KEYNOTE-158 study, there were 22 MSI-high cholangiocarcinoma patients with nine patients experiencing objective response after receiving pembrolizumab. Pembrolizumab is now FDA-approved for any MSI-high solid tumor.[30]

1. A 44-year-old man with a history of cirrhosis due to hepatitis C presents to establish care. He last had an ultrasound 8 months ago which was negative. He has no history of esophageal varices or ascites. His liver enzymes are within normal limits. What is the next step in management?
   A. Ultrasound now
   B. Ultrasound in 4 months
   C. CT of the abdomen/pelvis
   D. MRI of the abdomen
   E. Liver transplant evaluation

2. A 43-year-old Vietnamese man with a history of hepatitis B presents with right upper qudrant (RUQ) abdominal pain. Abdominal ultrasound reveals a suspicious focal liver lesion and 4-phase liver CT scan confirms a 3.5-cm lesion in a background of cirrhosis. The lesion has non-rim enhancement and there is washout on the delayed phase. Liver enzymes are normal but alpha-fetoprotein (AFP) is elevated at 202 ng/mL. What is the next step in management?
   A. Biopsy of the liver lesion
   B. Hepatectomy
   C. CT of the chest
   D. Referral for hepatology
   E. Liver transplant evaluation

3. A 66-year-old man with decompensated cirrhosis (Child Pugh Score [CPS] C) due to hepatitis B presents for follow-up after an ultrasound reveals three liver lesions. A follow-up MRI confirms three lesions, each less than 3 cm in size, consistent with hepatocellular carcinoma (HCC). Staging scans do not reveal any distant disease. What is the next step in management?
   A. Atezolizumab and bevacizumab
   B. Lenvatinib
   C. Sorafenib
   D. Transarterial chemoembolization (TACE)
   E. Liver transplant evaluation

4. A 54-year-old man with hereditary hemochromatosis complicated by cirrhosis presents with right upper qudrant (RUQ) pain. A CT scan of the abdomen confirms multiple suspicious lesions for hepatocellular carcinoma (HCC). A complete staging showed multiple pulmonary lesions consistent with metastatic spread. He is deemed a candidate for systemic therapy with atezolizumab and bevacizumab. What is the next step prior to initiation of therapy?
   A. Esophagogastroduodenoscopy (EGD)
   B. Bone scan for metastatic lesions
   C. Referral to hepatology
   D. Liver transplant evaluation
   E. Liver biopsy for MSI-high disease

5. A 64-year-old woman with a history of well-controlled diabetes complicated by mild peripheral neuropathy presents to the ED for severe right upper quadrant (RUQ) pain, jaundice, and fever. CT reveals multiple hypodense lesions in the liver. Her liver enzymes, total bilirubin, and direct bilirubin are elevated. She undergoes an endoscopic retrograde

cholangio-pancreatography (ERCP) with stent placement and brushings of the bile duct. Cytology from the brushings is consistent with adenocarcinoma. Complete staging reveals pulmonary metastases. Her liver enzymes and bilirubin levels normalize after stent placement and she is discharged from the hospital. Overall, she is able to return to her normal daily activities and is very active with her local walking group. She is interested in therapy. What is the next step in management?

A. Gemcitabine alone

B. Gemcitabine and cisplatin

C. 5-fluorouracil and oxaliplatin (FOLFOX)

D. 5-flurouracil, irinotecan, and oxalplatin (FOFIRINOX)

E. Referral to hospice

6. A 55-year-old man with a history of metastatic hepatocellular carcinoma (HCC) in the setting of cirrhosis complicated by multiple episodes of bleeding esophageal varices presents for follow-up after recently starting lenvatinib. The patient has overall tolerated therapy the last 2 months but today is noted to have a blood pressure of 178/100. Despite attempts to control the new hypertension with optimal medical management, his blood pressure remains elevated at greater than 160/100 (Grade 3). What is your next step in management?

A. Permanently discontinue lenvatinib

B. Refer to cardiology

C. Hold lenvatinib and potentially restart at lower dose

D. Change treatment to sorafenib

E. Change treatment to atezolizumab and bevacizumab

7. A 63-year-old man with a history of metastatic hepatocellular carcinoma (HCC), cirrhosis (Child-Pugh Score [CPS] A), and diabetes presents for follow-up. He has completed 3 cycles of atezolizumab and bevacizumab. He reports shortness of breath that started a few weeks ago. Chest x-ray done at the start of his symptoms was normal but due to worsening shortness of breath over the past week, CT of the chest is performed and reveals diffuse ground glass opacities. What is the next step in his management?

A. Referral to pulmonary

B. Pulmonary function test

C. Continue atezolizumab and bevacizumab

D. Continue bevacizumab alone

E. Hold atezolizumab and bevacizumab

ANSWERS AND RATIONALES

1. **A. Ultrasound now.** Patients with a history of cirrhosis are at increased risk for developing hepatocellular carcinoma. Screening with ultrasound should be completed every 6 months. This patient's last ultrasound was 8 months ago and so he is now overdue for imaging.

2. **C. CT of the chest.** Patient has an isolated liver lesion and is a candidate for local therapy if he does not have any evidence of distant metastases. There is no further need for a biopsy given liver imaging meets diagnostic imaging criteria for hepatocellular carcinoma.

3. **E. Liver transplant evaluation.** This patient has liver-limited HCC but in the setting of decompensated cirrhosis (CPS C). Currently available systemic therapies have only been tested and approved for patients with well-preserved liver function (CPS A). Liver-directed therapies may be an option, but any cancer treatment must be evaluated in the context of the competing mortality from his decompensated cirrhosis.

4. **A. Esophagogastroduodenoscopy (EGD).** Prior to initiation of bevacizumab therapy, patients should undergo an EGD to treat any esophageal varices because of the high risk for bleeding associated with bevacizumab.

5. **B. Gemcitabine and cisplatin.** The results of the ABC-02 trial established gemcitabine and cisplatin as the standard of care first-line treatment for gallbladder adenocarcinoma and cholangiocarcinoma based on greater overall survival rate compared to gemcitabine alone.

6. **C. Hold lenvatinib and potentially restart at lower dose.** A common side effect of lenvatinib is hypertension. This patient had persistent grade 3 hypertension despite optimal medical management. Therefore, the recommendation is to hold lenvatinib and potentially resume treatment at a lower dose if the hypertension improves to at least grade 2. Patients that develop grade 4 hypertension must discontinue lenvatinib permanently.

7. **E. Hold atezolizumab and bevacizumab.** This patient's symptoms and imaging are concerning for an immunotherapy-induced pneumonitis due to atezolizumab. Systemic steroids are indicated for grade 2 or higher immunotherapy-induced pneumonitis. There is no indication for bevacizumab monotherapy in metastatic HCC.

REFERENCES

1. Surveillance, Epidemiology, and End Results Program. Cancer stat facts: liver and intrahepatic bile duct cancer. National Cancer Institute. Accessed December 1, 2021. https://seer.cancer.gov/statfacts/html/livibd.html
2. Sung H, Ferlay J, Siegel RL, et al. Global cancer statistics 2020: GLOBOCAN estimates of incidence and mortality worldwide for 36 cancers in 185 countries. *CA: A Cancer J Clin.* 2021;71(3):209–249. doi:10.3322/caac.21660
3. Ioannou GN, Splan MF, Weiss NS, McDonald GB, Beretta L, Lee SP. Incidence and predictors of hepatocellular carcinoma in patients with cirrhosis. *Clin Gastroenterol Hepatol.* 2007;5(8):938–945.e4. doi:10.1016/j.cgh.2007.02.039
4. Jiang Y, Han Q, Zhao H, Zhang J. The mechanisms of HBV-induced hepatocellular carcinoma. *J Hepatocellular Carcinoma.* 2021;8:435–450. doi:10.2147/jhc.s307962
5. Lim J, Singal AG. Surveillance and diagnosis of hepatocellular carcinoma. *Clin Liver Dis.* 2019;13(1):2–5. doi:10.1002/cld.761
6. Llovet JM, Ricci S, Mazzaferro V, et al. Sorafenib in advanced hepatocellular carcinoma. *N Engl J Med.* 2008;359(4):378–390. doi:10.1056/nejmoa0708857
7. Finn RS, Qin S, Ikeda M, et al. Atezolizumab plus bevacizumab in unresectable hepatocellular carcinoma. *N Engl J Med.* 2020;382(20):1894–1905. doi:10.1056/nejmoa1915745

8. Kudo M, Finn RS, Qin S, et al. Lenvatinib versus sorafenib in first-line treatment of patients with unresectable hepatocellular carcinoma: a randomised phase 3 non-inferiority trial. *Lancet.* 2018;391(10126):1163–1173. doi:10.1016/s0140-6736(18)30207-1

9. Sonbol MB, Riaz IB, Naqvi SAA, et al. Systemic therapy and sequencing options in advanced hepatocellular carcinoma. *JAMA Oncol.* 2020;6(12):e204930. doi:10.1001/jamaoncol.2020.4930

10. Yau T, Park JW, Finn RS, et al. Nivolumab versus sorafenib in advanced hepatocellular carcinoma (CheckMate 459): a randomised, multicentre, open-label, phase 3 trial. *Lancet Oncol.* 2022;23(1):77–90. doi:10.1016/S1470-2045(21)00604-5

11. Zhu AX, Finn RS, Edeline J, et al. Pembrolizumab in patients with advanced hepatocellular carcinoma previously treated with sorafenib (KEYNOTE-224): a non-randomised, open-label phase 2 trial. *Lancet Oncol.* 2018;19(7):940–952. doi:10.1016/S1470-2045(18)30351-6

12. Finn RS, Ryoo B-Y, Merle P, et al. Pembrolizumab as second-line therapy in patients with advanced hepatocellular carcinoma in KEYNOTE-240: a randomized, double-blind, phase III trial. *J Clin Oncol.* 2020;38(3):193–202. doi:10.1200/jco.19.01307

13. Yau T, Kang Y-K, Kim T-Y, et al. Efficacy and safety of nivolumab plus ipilimumab in patients with advanced hepatocellular carcinoma previously treated with sorafenib: the CheckMate 040 randomized clinical trial. *JAMA Oncol.* 2020;6(11):e204564. doi:10.1001/jamaoncol.2020.4564

14. Bruix J, Qin S, Merle P, et al. Regorafenib for patients with hepatocellular carcinoma who progressed on sorafenib treatment (RESORCE): a randomised, double-blind, placebo-controlled, phase 3 trial. *Lancet.* 2017;389(10064):56–66. doi:10.1016/S0140-6736(16)32453-9

15. Zhu AX, Kang Y-K, Yen C-J, et al. Ramucirumab after sorafenib in patients with advanced hepatocellular carcinoma and increased α-fetoprotein concentrations (REACH-2): a randomised, double-blind, placebo-controlled, phase 3 trial. *Lancet Oncol.* 2019;20(2):282–296. doi:10.1016/S1470-2045(18)30937-9

16. Abou-Alfa GK, Meyer T, Cheng A L, et al. Cabozantinib in patients with advanced and progressing hepatocellular carcinoma. *N Engl J Med.* 2018;379(1):54–63. doi:10.1056/nejmoa1717002

17. Ouyang G, Liu Q, Wu Y, et al. The global, regional, and national burden of gallbladder and biliary tract cancer and its attributable risk factors in 195 countries and territories, 1990 to 2017: a systematic analysis for the global burden of disease study 2017. *Cancer.* 2021;127(13):2238–2250. doi:https://doi.org/10.1002/cncr.33476

18. Primrose JN, Fox RP, Palmer DH, et al. Capecitabine compared with observation in resected biliary tract cancer (BILCAP): a randomised, controlled, multicentre, phase 3 study. *Lancet Oncol.* 2019;20(5):663–673. doi:10.1016/s1470-2045(18)30915-x

19. Edeline J, Benabdelghani M, Bertaut A, et al. Gemcitabine and oxaliplatin chemotherapy or surveillance in resected biliary tract cancer (PRODIGE 12-ACCORD 18-UNICANCER GI): a randomized phase III study. *J Clin Oncol.* 2019;37(8):658–667. doi:10.1200/jco.18.00050

20. Ben-Josef E, Guthrie KA, El-Khoueiry AB, et al. SWOG S0809: a phase II intergroup trial of adjuvant capecitabine and gemcitabine followed by radiotherapy and concurrent capecitabine in extrahepatic cholangiocarcinoma and gallbladder carcinoma. *J Clin Oncol.* 2015;33(24):2617–2622. doi:10.1200/jco.2014.60.2219

21. Valle J, Wasan H, Palmer DH, et al. Cisplatin plus gemcitabine versus gemcitabine for biliary tract cancer. *N Engl J Med.* 2010;362(14):1273–1281. doi:10.1056/nejmoa0908721

22. André T, Tournigand C, Rosmorduc O, et al. Gemcitabine combined with oxaliplatin (GEMOX) in advanced biliary tract adenocarcinoma: a GERCOR study. *Annal Oncol.* 2004;15(9):1339–1343. doi:10.1093/annonc/mdh351

23. Shroff RT, Javle MM, Xiao L, et al. Gemcitabine, cisplatin, and nab-paclitaxel for the treatment of advanced biliary tract cancers. *JAMA Oncol.* 2019;5(6):824. doi:10.1001/jamaoncol.2019.0270

24. Novarino AM, Satolli MA, Chiappino I, et al. FOLFOX-4 regimen or single-agent gemcitabine as first-line chemotherapy in advanced biliary tract cancer. *Am J Clin Oncol.* 2013;36(5):466–471. doi:10.1097/COC.0b013e31825691c3

25. Lamarca A, Palmer DH, Wasan HS, et al. Second-line FOLFOX chemotherapy versus active symptom control for advanced biliary tract cancer (ABC-06): a phase 3, open-label, randomised, controlled trial. *Lancet Oncol.* 2021;22(5):690–701. doi:10.1016/s1470-2045(21)00027-9

26. Zhu AX, Macarulla T, Javle MM, et al. Final overall survival efficacy results of ivosidenib for patients with advanced cholangiocarcinoma with IDH1 mutation. *JAMA Oncol.* 2021;7(11):1669. doi:10.1001/jamaoncol.2021.3836

27. Abou-Alfa GK, Sahai V, Hollebecque A, et al. Pemigatinib for previously treated, locally advanced or metastatic cholangiocarcinoma: a multicentre, open-label, phase 2 study. *Lancet Oncol.* 2020;21(5):671–684. doi:10.1016/s1470-2045(20)30109-1

28. Javle M, Lowery M, Shroff RT, et al. Phase II study of BGJ398 in patients with FGFR-altered advanced cholangiocarcinoma. *J Clin Oncol.* 2018;36(3):276–282. doi:10.1200/JCO.2017.75.5009

29. Drilon A, Laetsch TW, Kummar S, et al. Efficacy of larotrectinib in TRKFusion–positive cancers in adults and children. *N Engl J Med.* 2018;378(8):731–739. doi:10.1056/nejmoa1714448

30. Marabelle A, Le DT, Ascierto PA, et al. Efficacy of pembrolizumab in patients with noncolorectal high microsatellite instability/mismatch repair–deficient cancer: results from the phase II KEYNOTE-158 study. *J Clin Oncol.* 2020;38(1):1–10. doi:10.1200/jco.19.02105

CHAPTER 12

Colorectal Cancer

Brian Pham and Edward J. Kim

INTRODUCTION

Colorectal cancer (CRC) is the fourth most common cancer in the United States with an estimated 149,500 new cases in 2021; however, the estimated 52,980 deaths make it the second most common cause of cancer-related deaths.[1] The overall incidence and death rate has been declining, with an average of 2% decline yearly from 2009 to 2018, in part due to better surveillance methods and treatment options. However, this overall trend of decreasing incidence and mortality is reversed in patients under the age 50, with a 2% yearly increase from 1995 through 2016.[2] The exact cause of this trend remains unclear.

There are a multitude of risk factors for CRC including both genetic and environmental factors. Family history and genetic syndromes can increase CRC risk and alter screening recommendations. The most common genetic syndromes associated with CRC include Lynch syndrome and familial adenomatous polyposis (FAP), which both lead to an earlier onset of CRC compared to the normal population. Other factors that affect CRC and screening guidelines include those with a history of inflammatory bowel disease, cystic fibrosis, and prior abdomino-pelvic radiation. In terms of environmental or lifestyle factors, there have been observational studies which show factors that may increase CRC risk, but causality has been difficult to prove. Some of these include the use of tobacco, long-term consumption of processed meats, alcohol, and obesity. For risk reduction, increased physical activity, increased fiber intake, nonsteroidal anti-inflammatory drugs, and aspirin have all been reported as an association with decreased risk of CRC.

Fearon and Vogelstein first presented a multistep model of benign neoplasms or polyps transforming into invasive adenocarcinoma in 1990.[3] Normal epithelial glandular cells acquire genetic or epigenetic changes, causing this transformation into adenocarcinoma. These transformations into adenocarcinoma take many years to develop, and therefore screening guidelines recommend colonoscopy every 10 years for average risk patients. The majority of CRC develop from chromosomal instability (CIN) or microsatellite instability (MSI). CIN accounts for approximately 85% of CRC and is defined by loss or gain of whole or partial chromosome. There are various genes associated with CIN, but the most common in CRC is the adenomatous polyposis coli (*APC*) gene. *APC* is a tumor suppressor gene, and the loss of both alleles causes sporadic CRC. Single germline mutation of APC is seen in FAP and predisposes to increased development of polyps and CRC earlier in life. The other common cause of CRC is MSI caused by a defect in the DNA mismatch repair (MMR) process, which accounts for approximately 15% of CRC. The evaluation of MSI involves the loss of one or more of the four MMR proteins MLH1, MSH2, MSH6, and PMS2. Germline mutations in these MMR enzymes are seen in Lynch syndrome, which accelerates polyp formation into CRC.

CASE SUMMARIES

Case 12.1: Locally Advanced Colon Adenocarcinoma

A 45-year-old man with no significant past medical history (PMH) presented with 6 weeks of hematochezia. His primary care physician (PCP) referred him to Gastroenterology for further evaluation. A colonoscopy was performed, and a mass was found in the sigmoid colon. Biopsy confirmed colon adenocarcinoma with tumor invasion into the muscularis propria. CT of the chest, abdomen, and pelvis did not show evidence of any distant metastatic disease. The patient underwent surgical resection with four of 14 lymph nodes (LNs) found to be positive for involvement. The patient now presents to medical oncology for further management.

How Is a Diagnosis Established?

- Biopsy is confirmed from tissue via a colonoscopy.
- CT of the chest, abdomen, and pelvis with contrast are appropriate for complete staging.

Patient's Diagnosis
- *Tissue biopsy from colonoscopy confirmed colon adenocarcinoma with invasion into the muscularis propria.*

What Further Molecular or Genomic Testing Is Required?

- Tumor from all newly diagnosed colon cancer patients should undergo an evaluation for MSI or MMR protein expression.

Patient's Molecular and Genomic Testing
- *Immunohistochemistry (IHC) for MLH 1, MSH 2, MSH 6, and PMS 2 showed intact expression.*

How Is This Tumor Staged?

- The American Joint Committee on Cancer (AJCC) eighth edition staging system is used for staging colon cancer.
- Tumors are staged using clinical examination, colonoscopy, and CT of the chest, abdomen, and pelvis.
- A minimum of 12 LNs are needed to establish the nodal (N) stage.

Patient's Clinical Stage
- *Patient's stage is T2, N2a, M0 (stage IIIB).*

What Are Appropriate Treatment Options?

- Patients with node-positive disease (stage III) colon cancer are recommended to undergo adjuvant chemotherapy. Treatment with oxaliplatin and 5-fluorouracil (5-FU)-based chemotherapy is recommended. Adjuvant therapy should typically start within 8 weeks of surgery.
- The Intergroup 0035 trial initially established 5-FU as the standard for adjuvant therapy for resected stage III colon cancer after showing a reduced cancer mortality of 33% and

reduction of relapse by 41%.[4] Intergroup 0089 later led to adoption of 5-FU and leucovorin as the next standard first line of chemotherapy for stage III disease.[5]

- The results of the MOSAIC trial led to the addition of oxaliplatin to 5-FU based on improved overall survival (OS) for stage III resected colon cancer with 10-year OS of 71.7% versus 67.1% with fluoropyridine therapy alone.[6,7] This established adjuvant 5-FU and oxaliplatin (FOLFOX) chemotherapy as a standard of care regimen for stage III colon cancer.
- Capecitabine is a pro-drug of fluoruracil and may also be combined with oxaliplatin (XELOX). XELOX was compared to FOLFOX in a pooled analysis of four randomized controlled trials and showed similar disease-free survival (DFS) and OS, making it another acceptable option for patients.[8,9]

Recommended Treatment Plan for This Patient
- *Adjuvant FOLFOX chemotherapy for 6 months*

What Are the Toxicities Associated With Chemotherapy?

- Capecitabine and 5-FU have similar toxicities which include cytopenia, mucositis, diarrhea, and palmar plantar erythrodysesthesia.
- Common toxicities from oxaliplatin include cold hypersensitivity and peripheral neuropathy. If grade 3 or 4 peripheral neuropathy develops, oxaliplatin should be discontinued as a proportion of patients will have irreversible neuropathy affecting quality of life even after cessation of oxaliplatin.

What Are Other Treatment Considerations?

- Recently, the IDEA collaboration included six trials which all evaluated 6 versus 3 months of FOLFOX or XELOX as adjuvant treatment in over 12,000 stage III colon cancer patients. Although the overall final result failed to show a statistically significant non-inferiority of 3 versus 6 months, the outcomes were further evaluated to identify potential subgroups for whom 3 months could still be reasonable. For patients with lower risk T1 to T3, N1 disease, 3 months of adjuvant XELOX compared to 6 months showed a 5-year OS of 89.6% versus 88.9%, respectively. Therefore, it may be reasonable to offer 3 months of XELOX in favor of reducing toxicities from oxaliplatin-induced neuropathy. Although none of the six trials included in the IDEA collaboration were designed to directly compare FOLFOX and XELOX, it is notable that FOLFOX did not show equivalent similarity between 3 and 6 months in these low-risk patients. Patients with higher risk T4 or N2 disease had inferior DFS with only 3 months of FOLFOX compared to 6 months. Although adjuvant FOLFOX for 6 months is still the standard of care for all stage III colon cancer, reasonable consideration may be given for 3 months of XELOX in low-risk stage III colon cancer.[10,11]

What Is Required for This Patient's Follow-Up and Survivorship?
- *History and physical every 3 to 6 months for 2 years followed by every 6 months for a total of 5 years*
- *CT of the chest, abdomen, and pelvis every 12 months for a total of 5 years*
- *Carcinoembryonic antigen (CEA) every 3 to 6 months for 2 years, then every 6 months for a total of 5 years*
- *Colonoscopy screening 1 year after surgery unless obstructive lesions preoperatively, then would repeat colonoscopy in 3 to 6 months*

Case 12.2: Locally Advanced Rectal Cancer

A 35-year-old man with no significant PMH presents for rectal pain. The patient has had tenesmus and rectal pain for several months with associated hematochezia intermittently the last several weeks. On physical exam, a rectal mass was palpated. He was referred to gastroenterology and underwent a colonoscopy which showed a large rectal mass of 12 cm. Biopsy of the mass confirmed rectal adenocarcinoma with intact expression of MMR proteins by IHC. MRI of the rectum showed the tumor mass 3 cm from the anal verge, extending 2 mm beyond the rectal wall into the mesorectal fat, no involvement of the mesorectal fascia, no extramural invasion, and two suspicious subcentimeter presacral and mesorectal LNs without extramesorectal LN involvement. CT of the chest showed no suspicious distant metastatic lesions.

How Is a Diagnosis Established?

- Tissue diagnosis is required which is usually obtained via a colonoscopy.

Patient's Diagnosis
- *Rectal adenocarcinoma*

What Further Molecular or Genomic Testing Is Required?

- Tumors from all newly diagnosed patients with rectal cancer are evaluated for MSI or MMR protein expression.

Patient's Molecular and Genomic Testing
- *IHC for MLH 1, MSH 2, MSH 6, and PMS 2 showed intact expression.*

How Is This Tumor Staged?

- The AJCC eighth edition staging system is used for staging rectal cancer.
- Tumors are staged using clinical examination; colonoscopy; CT of the chest, pelvis, and abdomen; and MRI of the pelvis. PET/CT scans are not indicated.
- Consider endorectal ultrasound if MRI of the pelvis is contraindicated.

Patient's Clinical Stage
- *The patient's stage is cT3, N1b, M0 (stage IIIB).*

What Are Appropriate Treatment Options?

- The treatment for locally advanced rectal adenocarcinoma continues to evolve at a rapid pace with multiple options that can now be considered. The standard of care approach continues to involve a tri-modality approach with chemotherapy, radiation, and surgery. The optimal sequencing of chemoradiation (CRT) and systemic chemotherapy continues to be evaluated. The historically standard approach for those with high-risk node-positive disease has been neoadjuvant CRT followed by surgery and then adjuvant systemic chemotherapy.
- The CAO/ARO/AIO-094 trial demonstrated lower rates of locoregional recurrence and lower toxicities with neoadjuvant CRT. This led to the standard sequencing of neoadjuvant CRT, surgery, and adjuvant chemotherapy. Neoadjuvant CRT consists of 5-FU or capecitabine concurrently with radiation therapy.[12–15]
- Recently, total neoadjuvant therapy (TNT) has become an alternative approach for treatment of locally advanced rectal adenocarcinoma, especially for those with T4,

node-positive, and low-lying rectal tumors. TNT changes the timing of chemotherapy from the adjuvant to the neoadjuvant setting with the goal of earlier systemic treatment of potential micro-metastatic disease, opportunity to evaluate treatment response, and potentially reduce toxicity, thereby increasing adherence to completion of treatment. The duration and timing of systemic chemotherapy before or after CRT requires further prospective trials to determine best outcomes.

- Phase II trial from the German CAO/ARO/AIO-12 trial compared TNT approaches of induction chemotherapy followed by CRT versus consolidation chemotherapy after CRT. Induction chemotherapy and CRT resulted in better adherence to chemotherapy but failed to meet the primary endpoint of the hypothesized 25% pathological complete response (pCR).[16]
- The PRODIGE 23 trial tested intensive chemotherapy with 3 months of 5-FU, oxaliplatin, and irinotecan (FOLFIRINOX) followed by CRT, surgery, and then postoperative FOLFOX. This approach was compared to the standard approach of CRT, surgery, and 6 months of adjuvant chemotherapy. The experimental arm yielded a 3-year DFS of 76% compared to 69% with the standard approach.[17]
- The Phase III RAPIDO trial investigated a TNT approach with short course of radiotherapy (5 x 5 Gy over a maximum of 8 days) followed by chemotherapy prior to surgery in comparison to the approach of standard CRT (28 fractions of 1.8 Gy or 25 fractions of 2.0 Gy with concomitant capecitabine), surgery, and adjuvant chemotherapy. This study showed a TNT approach using short course radiotherapy had lower rates of disease-related treatment failure defined as locoregional recurrence, treatment-related death, distant metastasis, or new primary colorectal tumor.[18] Overall, the TNT approach has shown a benefit for locally advanced rectal tumors and requires further evaluation to optimize the duration and timing of systemic chemotherapy.

Recommended Treatment Plan for This Patient
- FOLFOX *then chemoRT with infusional 5-FU followed by surgery*

What Are the Toxicities Associated With Chemotherapy?

- See toxicities noted previously for 5-FU and oxaliplatin.

What Is Required for This Patient's Follow-Up and Survivorship?
- History, physical, and CEA every 3 to 6 months for 2 years, then every 6 months for a total of 5 years.
- CT of the chest, abdomen, and pelvis every 3 to 6 months for 2 years, then every 6 to 12 months for a total of 5 years.
- Colonoscopy 1 year after surgery except for those who had an obstructive lesion which would require a colonoscopy in 3 to 6 months after surgery.

Case 12.3: Unresectable Metastatic Colon Adenocarcinoma

A 68-year-old woman with history of stage IIIA sigmoid adenocarcinoma of the colon presents for surveillance follow-up 4 years following initial diagnosis. She was initially diagnosed through a screening colonoscopy and underwent a low anterior resection followed by capecitabine and oxaliplatin for 6 months. She tolerated therapy well with only mild peripheral neuropathy which resolved. On surveillance follow-up she was noted to have an elevated CEA of 14.5 which had previously been normal. CT of the chest, abdomen, and pelvis showed multiple pulmonary lung nodules and mediastinal lymphadenopathy. Lung biopsy confirmed metastatic adenocarcinoma of colorectal origin. She currently has no acute symptoms, and her physical exam was normal.

How Is a Diagnosis Established?

- Fine needle aspiration (FNA) biopsy of the pulmonary nodule confirmed metastatic colon adenocarcinoma.
- CT of the chest, abdomen, and pelvis with contrast are appropriate for surveillance and detection of metastatic lesions.

Patient's Diagnosis

- CT of the chest showed multiple cavitary pulmonary nodules too numerous to count and superior mediastinal node measuring 1.5 cm × 0.6 cm.
- CT-guided lung biopsy: Right upper lung nodule positive for metastatic colonic adenocarcinoma negative for thyroid transcription factor 1 (TTF-1), Napsin A, and positive for CK20 and CDX2.

What Further Molecular or Genomic Testing Is Required?

- All patients with metastatic colon cancer should have their tumor evaluated for mutations in genes KRAS, NRAS, and BRAF, as well MMR deficiency.

Patient's Molecular and Genomic Testing

- IHC for MLH 1, MSH 2, MSH 6, and PMS 2 showed intact expression next-generation sequencing (NGS) confirmed microsatellite stable, tumor mutational burden (TMB) of 8 mut/Mb, and wild type KRAS, NRAS, and BRAF.

How Is This Tumor Staged?

- The AJCC eighth edition staging system is used for staging colon cancer.
- Tumors are staged using clinical examination, colonoscopy, and CT of the chest, abdomen, and pelvis.

Patient's Original Clinical Stage

- The patient's stage is T1, N2a, M0 (stage IIIa), now with metastatic disease.

What Are Appropriate Treatment Options?

- Doublet chemotherapy has been considered the backbone of treatment of metastatic colon cancer in combination with targeted therapies against epidermal growth factor receptor (EGFR) or vascular endothelial growth factor (VEGF). Single-agent fluoropyridine-based chemotherapy was the standard of care before the addition of oxaliplatin and irinotecan was shown to have superior benefit and OS. Fluorouracil (5-FU) and oxaliplatin (FOLFOX) or 5-FU and irinotecan (FOLFIRI) are standard of care first-line therapy treatments. There is no significant OS benefit in patients treated with either FOLFOX or FOLFIRI. The choice between regimens depends on the toxicity profile.[19–24]
- Oral prodrug, capecitabine, converts into 5-FU after enzymatic conversion and has similar efficacy compared to infusional 5-FU when combined with oxaliplatin. CAPEOX (capecitabine and oxaliplatin) compared to FOLFOX had similar OS and progression-free survival (PFS) when used.[25,26]
- Compared to doublet chemotherapy, another option that can be considered is the triplet regimen 5-FU, oxaliplatin, irinotecan, and leucovorin (FOLFOXIRI). Compared to FOLFIRI, FOLFOXIRI had higher median OS (mOS; 22.6 vs. 16 months). However, the toxicity profile was higher with increased grade 2 to 3 peripheral neurotoxicity and grade 3 to 4 neutropenia seen in the FOLFOXIRI group. The higher toxicity profile has slowed adoption of FOLFOXIRI as the standard of care first-line regimen with most oncologists still preferring to use one of the doublet regimens.[23,27,28]

- Bevacizumab, which targets VEGF, can be used in the first-line setting with FOLFOX or FOLFIRI. Patients with right-sided colon cancer appear to benefit more with bevacizumab compared to left-sided colon cancer.[29,30]
- Cetuximab and panitumumab target EGFR and can be combined with first-line therapy in patients with wild type *KRAS* and *NRAS*. In addition, patients with left-sided colon cancer appear to have greater overall benefit from anti-EGFR agents compared to VEGF inhibitors. Anti-EGFR therapy does not appear to benefit patients with right-sided colon cancer.[31]

Recommended Treatment Plan for This Patient
- *FOLFOX + cetuximab*

What Are the Toxicities Associated With Chemotherapy?

- 5-FU-associated toxicities include mucositis, diarrhea, and palmer-planter erythrodysesthesia.
- Oxaliplatin toxicities include peripheral neuropathy, cold hypersensitivity, and laryngopharyngeal dysesthesias. Oxaliplatin is less emetogenic than cisplatin and does not share the same risk for nephrogenic toxicity. Rarely, oxaliplatin hypersensitivity can occur and typically presents with symptoms of anaphylaxis during infusion.
- Irinotecan toxicities include diarrhea, neutropenia, and alopecia.
- Bevacizumab and other VEGF inhibitors can cause hypertension, arterial thrombosis, and proteinuria. It can also interfere with wound healing and should be avoided for at least 4 weeks before and after elective surgery.
- Typical EGFR inhibitor toxicities are papulopustular rashes, hypomagnesemia, conjunctivitis, and diarrhea.

What Are Other Treatment Considerations?

- For patients with deficient mismatch repair (dMMR)/MSI-high (microsatellite instable) CRC, immune checkpoint inhibitors are a preferred option. The KEYNOTE-177 Phase III trial compared pembrolizumab with 5-FU–based chemotherapy with or without cetuximab or bevacizumab in the first-line setting. The PFS was significantly longer in the pembrolizumab arm at 16.2 months versus 8.2 months compared to the chemotherapy arm. The estimated mean survival at 24 months follow-up for pembrolizumab versus chemotherapy was 13.7 months versus 10.8 months.[32]
- Patients with a *BRAF*-mutated CRC demonstrate a more aggressive tumor type with worse prognosis due to generally more treatment-resistant disease, including to anti-EGFR agents.[33] The triplet FOLFOXIRI may be considered for first-line treatment in patients with very good performance status based in part on the TRIBE study which showed FOLFOXIRI/bevacizumab yielded a mOS of 19 months versus 10 months with FOLFIRI/bevacizumab. It is important to note, however, that the *BRAF*-mutated tumors represented only a very small subset of the study population (7% in both arms).[27] A portion of *BRAF*-mutated patients will also be MSI-high and immunotherapy can be considered as another first-line option as previously discussed for this subset of patients. Additionally, recent data in *BRAF* V600E patients from the Phase III BEACON trial compared a triplet combination of encorafenib, binimetinib, and cetuximab, a doublet of encorafenib and cetuximab, and physician's choice of either cetuximab and irinotecan or cetuximab and FOLFIRI. The final results showed mOS was 9.3 months in both the doublet and triplet arms compared to 5.9 months with control.[34] Thus, encorafenib and cetuximab with or without binimetinib should be standard for previously treated *BRAF* V600 patients.

REVIEW QUESTIONS

1. A 68-year-old man with a history of diabetes, congestive heart failure (CHF), and hypertension (HTN) undergoes a screening colonoscopy. Biopsy of a 4.5-cm sigmoid colon mass is positive for adenocarcinoma. He undergoes a hemi-colectomy to resect the mass and 7 of 13 lymph nodes (LNs) are positive for involvement with adenocarcinoma. What is the best therapy after hemi-colectomy?
   A. 5-fluorouracil (5-FU) and oxaliplatin (FOLFOX)
   B. 5-FU and irinotecan (FOLFIRI)
   C. 5-FU, oxaliplatin, and irinotecan (FOLFOXIRI)
   D. Gemcitabine
   E. Observation

2. A 69-year-old woman with a history of hypertension (HTN), hyperlipidemia, chronic kidney disease (CKD) stage III, and diabetes presents for severe emesis, abdominal distention, and abdominal pain. CT of the abdomen finds a large mass obstructing the ascending colon along with multiple hepatic lesions and ascites. She undergoes a diverting ostomy for relief of the obstruction. Biopsy of the liver lesions and the primary mass confirms synchronous metastatic colon adenocarcinoma. Subsequent staging does not show any other sites of metastasis. What is the next step in her management?
   A. Start 5-fluorouracil (5-FU), oxaliplatin, and irinotecan (FOLFOXIRI)
   B. Obtain next-generation sequencing (NGS)
   C. Start 5-FU and oxaliplatin (FOLFOX) + bevacizumab
   D. Refer to hospice
   E. Start FOLFOX

3. A 66-year-old African American woman with a history of rheumatoid arthritis, diabetes complicated by severe peripheral neuropathy, and gout presents with abdominal pain in the right upper quadrant. Liver ultrasound finds multiple hypodense lesions. Further CT scans of the chest, abdomen, and pelvis find small volume ascites and enlarged lymph nodes (LNs). Biopsy of a liver lesion shows adenocarcinoma. Colonoscopy reveals a 3-cm sigmoid mass with biopsy confirming adenocarcinoma. Next-generation sequencing (NGS) demonstrates the tumor is microsatellite stable, *KRAS/NRAS/BRAF* wild type, and has a tumor mutational burden (TMB) of 3 mut/Mb. What is the next step in her management?
   A. Start liver transplant evaluation and resection of the sigmoid mass
   B. Refer to surgery
   C. Start 5-fluorouracil (5-FU) and oxaliplatin (FOLFOX) and cetuximab
   D. Start FOLFOX and bevacizumab
   E. Start 5-FU and irinotecan (FOLFIRI) and cetuximab

4. A 51-year-old woman with no significant past medical history (PMH) presents for an annual wellness visit. She undergoes a screening colonoscopy that finds a pedunculated polyp in the transverse colon which is removed completely as a single specimen. Pathological evaluation of the polyp shows a grade 1 invasive carcinoma invading the submucosa but not into the muscularis propria with negative resection margins and no lymphovascular invasion. What is the appropriate management for her stage of disease?
   A. Adjuvant 5-fluorouracil (5-FU) and oxaliplatin (FOLFOX)
   B. Adjuvant 5-FU and irinotecan (FOLFIRI)
   C. Colectomy
   D. Observation alone
   E. Colonoscopy 1 year after resection

5. A 35-year-old man diagnosed with stage III colon cancer presents for follow-up after resection and adjuvant chemotherapy. He wants to advise his family on colon cancer screening. He has a 33-year-old brother and two sons. What is your recommendation?
   A. Advise the brother for screening now and for the sons to wait until they are 50 years old
   B. Advise the sons for screening at the age of 25 and for the brother at age 40
   C. Advise the screening for the brother now and the sons at age 25
   D. Advise all family members to screen at age 45
   E. Advise all family members to screen at age 50

6. A 55-year-old man presents to the ED for abdominal pain, emesis, and constipation for 6 days. CT of the abdomen/pelvis reveals a large obstructing mass in the descending colon with surrounding enlarged lymph nodes (LNs). He undergoes an emergent hemi-colectomy. What is the next step in management?
   A. PET/CT
   B. Surveillance with yearly colonoscopy
   C. Observation for 8 weeks and referral to medical oncology
   D. CT of the chest
   E. Referral to radiation oncology

7. A 59-year-old woman with colon cancer metastatic to both lobes of the liver presents for follow-up. Her cancer is *KRAS/NRAS/BRAF* wild-type and microsatellite stable. She completed 8 cycles of 5-fluorouracil (5-FU) and oxaliplatin (FOLFOX) with cetuximab and a recent CT scan shows clear progression of the disease. What is the next step in management?
   A. Regorafenib
   B. 5-FU and irinotecan (FOLFIRI)
   C. CAPEOX
   D. 5-FU, oxaliplatin, and irinotecan (FOLFOXIRI)
   E. Pembrolizumab

8. A 64-year-old man with a history of gout, hyperlipidemia, and hypertension (HTN) presents for evaluation of his newly diagnosed metastatic colon cancer. Testing reveals the tumor is microsatellite instability (MSI)-high with 40 mt/Mb, *KRAS* mutated, and *BRAF* wild type. What do you recommend for initial therapy?
   A. 5-fluorouracil (5-FU) and irinotecan (FOLFIRI)
   B. 5-FU and oxaliplatin (FOLFOX) + bevacizumab
   C. 5-FU, oxaliplatin, and irinotecan (FOLFOXIRI)
   D. CAPEOX
   E. Pembrolizumab

9. A 46-year-old man with a history of hypertension (HTN) presents to medical oncology after recent hemi-colectomy for a colon adenocarcinoma. CT scans show no distant metastases. Pathological evaluation of the tumor reveals invasion through the muscularis propria with 12 of 16 lymph nodes (LNs) involved by cancer. Additional testing shows the tumor is microsatellite stable. He is recovering well from his surgery and would like to get started on adjuvant therapy but would like the shortest duration of therapy possible. What is your recommendation?
   A. Capecitabine plus oxaliplatin (XELOX) for 3 months
   B. XELOX for 9 months
   C. 5-fluorouracil (5-FU) and oxaliplatin (FOLFOX) for 3 months
   D. FOLFOX for 6 months
   E. FOLFOX for 9 months

10. A 55-year-old woman with stage IV colon adenocarcinoma presents for follow-up. Her tumor is *KRAS/NRAS/BRAF* wild-type and she was started on 5-fluorouracil (5-FU) and irinotecan (FOLFIRI) and cetuximab. She presents after cycle 1 with new acneiform rash on her face, head, and neck. What is the cause of her rash?

    A. Infusional 5-FU
    B. Bolus 5-FU
    C. Irinotecan
    D. Cetuximab

ANSWERS AND RATIONALES

1. **A. 5-FU and oxaliplatin (FOLFOX).** This patient has stage III disease and requires adjuvant chemotherapy after hemi-colectomy. Higher disease-free survival (DFS) and overall survival (OS) were seen with doublet therapy with 5-FU and oxaliplatin. FOLFIRI is contraindicated in the adjuvant setting due to clinical trial evidence of increased risk of death.

2. **E. Start FOLFOX.** This patient has metastatic disease and needs systemic treatment. Although molecular profiling for *KRAS/NRAS/BRAF* and mismatch repair (MMR) status are recommended to guide optimal therapy, treatment should not be delayed. Although KRAS/NRAS status helps determine the potential benefit from anti-epidermal growth factor receptor (EGFR) therapies, this patient's right-sided tumor predicts less benefit with anti-EGFR therapy. Anti-vascular endothelial growth factor (VEGF) therapies are preferred for right-sided primary tumors, but the patient had recent surgery and anti-VEGF agents are contraindicated in the immediate peri-operative setting due to interference with wound healing. The patient may ultimately qualify for single-agent immunotherapy if her tumor is deficient in MMR protein expression and thus microsatellite instability (MSI)-high, but this only represents about 5% of patients who present with metastatic disease.

3. **E. 5-FU and irinotecan (FOLFIRI) and cetuximab.** For patients with *KRAS/NRAS/BRAF* wild-type disease, cetuximab has been approved for front-line therapy in addition to doublet chemotherapy with either FOLFOX or FOLFIRI. Additionally, this patient has a left-sided tumor which predicts greater overall benefit from anti-epidermal growth factor receptor (EGFR) therapy compared to anti-vascular endothelial growth factor (VEGF). Therefore, the preferred targeted agent to add to chemotherapy would be cetuximab over bevacizumab. For this patient, FOLFIRI is the preferred doublet over FOLFOX because of her severe neuropathy from diabetes which limits the use of neuro-toxic oxaliplatin.

4. **E. Colonoscopy 1 year after resection.** This patient has a T1 stage I colon cancer. For stage I disease, the standard of care is resection of the tumor without need for adjuvant systemic therapy. Additionally, if the polyp is pedunculated, resection via colonoscopy alone without subsequent surgery is adequate provided there are negative margins and the polyp is not removed in piece-meal fashion. Therefore, this patient who had complete removal of her pedunculated polyp can now simply undergo surveillance at 1 year with colonoscopy.

5. **C. Advise the screening for the brother now and the sons at age 25.** All first-degree relatives of patients with a diagnosis of colon cancer should be screened including those who are 40 years or older or 10 years younger than the patient's age at their time of diagnosis.

6. **D. CT of the chest.** Complete staging is required to determine the patient's prognosis and optimal management. There is no routine indication for PET/CT and it should not be used to replace staging with CT.

7. **B. 5-FU and irinotecan (FOLFIRI).** The patient has progressed on oxaliplatin-based combination, and standard of care second-line therapy is irinotecan-based regimen. There is no data for continuing oxaliplatin-based doublet regimens after progression; therefore, FOLFOXIRI and CAPEOX would not be recommended. Regorafenib could be considered for a later line of therapy. Pembrolizumab is not an option for this patient who has microsatellite stable disease.

8. **E. Pembrolizumab.** Based on the KEYNOTE-177 trial, patients with MSI-high disease who received pembrolizumab benefitted with longer progression-free survival (PFS) compared

to patients who received chemotherapy. Therefore, patients with MSI-high disease should be considered for front-line pembrolizumab monotherapy.

9. **D. 5-FU and oxaliplatin (FOLFOX) for 6 months.** This patient has N2 disease based on the finding of four or more involved LNs. The IDEA collaboration tested de-escalation of adjuvant therapy with reduction in duration of therapy to 3 months from the standard 6 months. The study failed to confirm non-inferiority of the shortened duration of adjuvant therapy in the subset of patients with higher risk disease. Therefore, this patient should receive a recommended 6 months of adjuvant therapy.

10. **D. Cetuximab.** This patient's new skin rash is most likely from anti-epidermal growth factor receptor (EGFR) therapy with cetuximab. This side effect can be treated with topical steroids and oral doxycycline.

REFERENCES

1. Surveillance Research Program NCI. SEER*Explorer: an interactive website for SEER cancer statistics [Internet]. Accessed December 1, 2021 https://seer.cancer.gov/explorer

2. Siegel RL, Miller KD, Fuchs HE, Jemal A. Cancer statistics, 2021. *CA: Cancer J Cli.* 2021;71(1):7–33. doi:10.3322/caac.21654

3. Fearon ER, Vogelstein B. A genetic model for colorectal tumorigenesis. *Cell.* 1990;61(5):759–767. doi:10.1016/0092-8674(90)90186-i

4. Moertel CG, Fleming TR, Macdonald JS, et al. Intergroup study of fluorouracil plus levamisole as adjuvant therapy for stage II/Dukes' B2 colon cancer. *J Clin Oncol.* 1995;13(12):2936–2943. doi:10.1200/JCO.1995.13.12.2936

5. Haller DG, Catalano PJ, Macdonald JS, et al. Phase III study of fluorouracil, leucovorin, and levamisole in high-risk stage II and III colon cancer: final report of intergroup 0089. *J Clin Oncol.* 2005;23(34):8671–8678. doi:10.1200/jco.2004.00.5686

6. André T, de Gramont A, Vernerey D, et al. Adjuvant fluorouracil, leucovorin, and·oxaliplatin in stage II to III colon cancer: updated 10-year survival and outcomes according to *BRAF* mutation and mismatch repair status of the MOSAIC study. *J Clin Oncol.* 2015;33(35):4176–4187. doi:10.1200/jco.2015.63.4238

7. André T, Boni C, Navarro M, et al. Improved overall survival with oxaliplatin, fluorouracil, and leucovorin as adjuvant treatment in stage II or III colon cancer in the MOSAIC trial. *J Clin Oncol.* 2009;27(19):3109–3116. doi:10.1200/jco.2008.20.6771

8. Haller DG, Tabernero J, Maroun J, et al. Capecitabine plus oxaliplatin compared with fluorouracil and folinic acid as adjuvant therapy for stage III colon cancer. *J Clin Oncol.* 2011;29(11):1465–1471. doi:10.1200/jco.2010.33.6297

9. Schmoll H-J, Twelves C, Sun W, et al. Effect of adjuvant capecitabine or fluorouracil, with or without oxaliplatin, on survival outcomes in stage III colon cancer and the effect of oxaliplatin on post-relapse survival: a pooled analysis of individual patient data from four randomised controlled trials. *Lancet Oncol.* 2014;15(13):1481–1492. doi:10.1016/s1470-2045(14)70486-3

10. André T, Meyerhardt J, Iveson T, et al. Effect of duration of adjuvant chemotherapy for patients with stage III colon cancer (IDEA collaboration): final results from a prospective, pooled analysis of six randomised, phase 3 trials. *Lancet Oncol.* 2020;21(12):1620–1629. doi:10.1016/S1470-2045(20)30527-1

11. Grothey A, Sobrero AF, Shields AF, et al. Duration of adjuvant chemotherapy for stage III colon cancer. *N Engl J Med.* 2018;378(13):1177–1188. doi:10.1056/nejmoa1713709

12. Sauer R, Fietkau R, Wittekind C, et al. Adjuvant vs. neoadjuvant radiochemotherapy for locally advanced rectal cancer: the German trial CAO/ARO/AIO-94. *Colorectal Dis.* 2003;5(5):406–415. doi:10.1046/j.1463-1318.2003.00509.x

13. Sauer R, Becker H, Hohenberger W, et al. Preoperative versus postoperative chemoradiotherapy for rectal cancer. *N Engl J Med.* 2004;351(17):1731–1740. doi:10.1056/NEJMoa040694

14. Roh MS, Colangelo LH, O'Connell MJ, et al. Preoperative multimodality therapy improves disease-free survival in patients with carcinoma of the rectum: NSABP R-03. *J Clin Oncol.* 2009;27(31):5124–5130. doi:10.1200/jco.2009.22.0467

15. Sauer R, Liersch T, Merkel S, et al. Preoperative versus postoperative chemoradiotherapy for locally advanced rectal cancer: results of the German CAO/ARO/AIO-94 randomized phase III trial after a median follow-up of 11 years. *J Clin Oncol.* 2012;30(16):1926–1933. doi:10.1200/jco.2011.40.1836

16. Fokas E, Allgäuer M, Polat B, et al. Randomized phase II trial of chemoradiotherapy plus induction or consolidation chemotherapy as total neoadjuvant therapy for locally advanced rectal cancer: CAO/ARO/AIO-12. *J Clin Oncol.* 2019;37(34):3212–3222. doi:10.1200/jco.19.00308

17. Conroy T, Bosset JF, Etienne PL, et al. Neoadjuvant chemotherapy with FOLFIRINOX and preoperative chemoradiotherapy for patients with locally advanced rectal cancer (UNICANCER-PRODIGE 23): a multicentre, randomised, open-label, phase 3 trial. *Lancet Oncol.* 2021;22(5):702–715. doi:10.1016/S1470-2045(21)00079-6

18. Bahadoer RR, Dijkstra EA, van Etten B, et al. Short-course radiotherapy followed by chemotherapy before total mesorectal excision (TME) versus preoperative chemoradiotherapy, TME, and optional adjuvant chemotherapy in locally advanced rectal cancer (RAPIDO): a randomised, open-label, phase 3 trial. *Lancet Oncol.* 2021;22(1):29–42. doi:10.1016/s1470-2045(20)30555-6

19. de Gramont A, Figer A, Seymour M, et al. Leucovorin and fluorouracil with or without oxaliplatin as first-line treatment in advanced colorectal cancer. *J Clin Oncol.* 2000;18(16):2938–2947. doi:10.1200/jco.2000.18.16.2938

20. Cheeseman SL, Joel SP, Chester JD, et al. A 'modified de Gramont' regimen of fluorouracil, alone and with oxaliplatin, for advanced colorectal cancer. *Br J Cancer.* 2002;87(4):393–399. doi:10.1038/sj.bjc.6600467

21. Maindrault-Goebel F, de Gramont A, Louvet C, et al. Evaluation of oxaliplatin dose intensity in bimonthly leucovorin and 48-hour 5-fluorouracil continuous infusion regimens (FOLFOX) in pretreated metastatic colorectal cancer. Oncology multidisciplinary research group (GERCOR). *Ann Oncol.* 2000;11(11):1477–1483. doi:10.1023/a:1026520812351

22. Tournigand C, André T, Achille E, et al. FOLFIRI followed by FOLFOX6 or the reverse sequence in advanced colorectal cancer: a randomized GERCOR study. *J Clin Oncol.* 2004;22(2):229–237. doi:10.1200/JCO.2004.05.113

23. Falcone A, Ricci S, Brunetti I, et al. Phase III trial of infusional fluorouracil, leucovorin, oxaliplatin, and irinotecan (FOLFOXIRI) compared with infusional fluorouracil, leucovorin, and irinotecan (FOLFIRI) as first-line treatment for metastatic colorectal cancer: the gruppo oncologico nord ovest. *J Clin Oncol.* 2007;25(13):1670–1676. doi:10.1200/JCO.2006.09.0928

24. André T, Louvet C, Maindrault-Goebel F, et al. CP1-11 (irinotecan) addition to bimonthly, high-dose leucovorin and bolus and continuous-infusion 5-fluorouracil (FOLFIRI) for pretreated metastatic colorectal cancer. GERCOR. *Eur J Cancer.* 1999;35(9):1343–1347. doi:10.1016/s0959-8049(99)00150-1

25. Hoff PM, Ansari R, Batist G, et al. Comparison of oral capecitabine versus intravenous fluorouracil plus leucovorin as first-line treatment in 605 patients with metastatic colorectal cancer: results of a randomized phase III study. *J Clin Oncol.* 2001;19(8):2282–2292. doi:10.1200/JCO.2001.19.8.2282

26. Cassidy J, Clarke S, Díaz-Rubio E, et al. XELOX *vs* FOLFOX-4 as first-line therapy for metastatic colorectal cancer: NO16966 updated results. *Br J Cancer.* 2011;105(1):58–64. doi:10.1038/bjc.2011.201

27. Cremolini C, Loupakis F, Antoniotti C, et al. FOLFOXIRI plus bevacizumab versus FOLFIRI plus bevacizumab as first-line treatment of patients with metastatic colorectal cancer: updated overall survival and molecular subgroup analyses of the open-label, phase 3 TRIBE study. *Lancet Oncol.* 2015;16(13):1306–1315. doi:10.1016/S1470-2045(15)00122-9

28. Cremolini C, Antoniotti C, Lonardi S, et al. Activity and safety of cetuximab plus modified FOLFOXIRI followed by maintenance with cetuximab or bevacizumab for *RAS* and *BRAF* wild-type metastatic colorectal cancer: a randomized phase 2 clinical trial. *JAMA Oncol.* 2018;4(4):529–536. doi:10.1001/jamaoncol.2017.5314

29. Saltz LB, Clarke S, Díaz-Rubio E, et al. Bevacizumab in combination with oxaliplatin-based chemotherapy as first-line therapy in metastatic colorectal cancer: a randomized phase III study. *J Clin Oncol.* 2008;26(12):2013–2019. doi:10.1200/JCO.2007.14.9930

30. Hurwitz H, Fehrenbacher L, Novotny W, et al. Bevacizumab plus irinotecan, fluorouracil, and leucovorin for metastatic colorectal cancer. *N Engl J Med.* 2004;350(23):2335–2342. doi:10.1056/NEJMoa032691

31. Venook AP, Niedzwiecki D, Lenz HJ, et al. Effect of first-line chemotherapy combined with cetuximab or bevacizumab on overall survival in patients with *KRAS* wild-type advanced or metastatic colorectal cancer: a randomized clinical trial. *JAMA.* 2017;317(23):2392–2401. doi:10.1001/jama.2017.7105

32. André T, Shiu K-K, Kim TW, et al. Pembrolizumab in microsatellite-instability–high advanced colorectal cancer. *N Engl J Med.* 2020;383(23):2207–2218. doi:10.1056/nejmoa2017699

33. Pietrantonio F, Petrelli F, Coinu A, et al. Predictive role of *BRAF* mutations in patients with advanced colorectal cancer receiving cetuximab and panitumumab: a meta-analysis. *Eur J Cancer.* 2015;51(5):587–594. doi:10.1016/j.ejca.2015.01.054

34. Tabernero J, Grothey A, Van Cutsem E, et al. Encorafenib plus cetuximab as a new standard of care for previously treated BRAF V600E–mutant metastatic colorectal cancer: updated survival results and subgroup analyses from the BEACON study. *J Clin Oncol.* 2021;39(4):273–284. doi:10.1200/jco.20.02088

CHAPTER 13

Anal Cancer

Arathi Mohan and John C. Krauss

INTRODUCTION

Anal cancers are an uncommon gastrointestinal (GI) malignancy accounting for 2.7% of digestive system cancers. The most common histology by far is squamous cell carcinoma of the anus (SCCA). Other malignancies may occur in the anal region including adenocarcinoma, melanoma, neuroendocrine tumors (NETs), and lymphoma but are quite uncommon. These cancers are managead according to histology specific guidelines. This chapter will focus on the management of SCCA.

The vast majority (86% to 97%) of SCCA are associated with human papilloma virus (HPV), most commonly with high-risk subtypes including HPV-16 and HPV-18.[1] HPV infection is associated with carcinogenesis along a pathway in which high-grade anal intraepithelial neoplasia (AIN) precedes SCCA.[2] Risk factors for HPV infection include history of receptive anal intercourse; high number of lifetime sexual partners; history of sexually transmitted diseases; immunosuppression (for example, immunosuppressive medication after solid organ transplantation or for autoimmune disorders and HIV infection); history of cervical, vulvar, or vaginal cancer; and smoking.

There are no national guidelines regarding anal cancer screening in high-risk individuals. Some recommend screening HIV-positive men having sex with men, HIV-positive women with history of cervical or vulvar dysplasia, and anyone with a history of anal or genital condyloma. Screening is performed by rectal examination and a cytological smear of the anus. Abnormal cytology is followed by high-resolution anoscopy with biopsy if needed.

The 9-valent HPV vaccine is indicated for men and women ages 9 to 45 for the prevention of anal cancer and head and neck cancer, and for women for the prevention of cervical cancer, as well as a variety of other HPV-related precancerous conditions. Compared to the 4-valent HPV vaccine, 9-valent HPV vaccine is predicted to prevent an additional 464 cases of anal cancer annually.[3] The Advisory Committee on Immunization Practices (ACIP) recommends routine use of the 9-valent vaccine in children aged 11 to 12 years and a catch-up vaccination for individuals through 26 years of age who have not been previously vaccinated.[4-7] In 2020, only 59% of adolescents in the United States were up to date with HPV vaccination, with coverage for Tdap being 90%. Vaccine hesitancy and refusal has several causes, and the sexual transmission of HPV has been another reason for parents and young adults to not receive the HPV vaccine.[8]

The anal canal is a 4-cm long transitional mucosa between glandular rectal epithelium and keratinizing stratified squamous epithelium of the skin. Anatomic landmarks include the dentate line, the halfway point of the anal canal, above which is transitional mucosa and below non-keratinizing squamous mucosa. Squamous mucosa of the anal canal merges at the anal verge, the distal end of the canal with true epidermal tissue of the perianal skin. Most anal cancers are SCCs, but historically, they have also been called epidermoid, cloacogenic, transitional, and basaloid carcinomas. Perianal skin cancers are treated as primary cutaneous SCCs if distinctly separated from the anal verge.

SCCA tumors tend to present with local or local-regional disease but do have the potential for distant metastasis. The major prognostic factors are tumor size and nodal status. The staging of SCCA, unlike most GI malignancies, is not dependent on the degree of tumor tissue penetration of the anal canal, but rather on the size of the primary tumor. Staging according to the American Joint Committee on Cancer (AJCC) is outlined in Table 13.1. The 5-year relative survival rates based on SEER stage are as follows: localized (83%), regional (67%), distant (36%), and unstaged (63%).[9]

Table 13.1 American Joint Committee on Cancer Staging System for Anal Carcinoma

Stage	Definition
I	Tumor confined to anal canal, ≤2 cm (T1)
IIA	Tumor confined to anal canal, >2 cm — <5 cm (T2)
IIB	Tumor confined to anal canal, >5 cm (T3)
IIIA	Tumor <5 cm (T1–T2) with metastasis to regional LNs (N1)
IIIB	Tumor invading into adjacent organs (T4) without metastasis to regional LNs
IIIC	Tumor >5 cm or invading into adjacent organs (T3–T4) with metastasis to regional LNs (N1)
IV	Tumor of any size with distant metastases (M1)

LNs, lymph nodes

Source: Data from Amin MB, Edge SB, Greene FL, et al, eds. *AJCC Cancer Staging Manual.* 8th ed. Springer Nature; 2017.

CASE SUMMARIES

Case 13.1: Locally Advanced Anal Cancer

A 61-year-old HIV-negative woman presented with 2 months of anal pain. Anoscopy revealed a 6-cm mass in the anal canal centered just distal to the dentate line. Biopsy showed a poorly differentiated, invasive SCC.

What Studies Are Needed to Complete Staging?

- Thorough examination is performed including digital rectal examination (DRE), anoscopy, and palpation of inguinal lymph nodes (LNs) with fine needle aspiration (FNA)/biopsy of LNs that are enlarged by clinical exam or imaging.
- CT of the chest and abdomen and CT or MRI of the pelvis, which can provide further information on whether the tumor is invading adjacent organs or whether there is LN involvement. Assessment of T stage, though, is primarily from clinical examination.
- PET/CT can be considered for assessment of metastatic lymph nodes but is not a substitute for diagnostic CT imaging.
- Gynecologic examination is performed, including cervical cancer screening, due to association of anal cancer and HPV.

The Patient's CT Chest/Abdomen/Pelvis

- *A CT of the chest, abdomen, and pelvis revealed enlarged perirectal and internal iliac LNs in addition to the anal tumor. CT of the chest did not have evidence of metastatic disease.*

What Is the Stage of Her Anal Cancer?

- Tumor size is greater than 5 cm (T3) and there is metastasis to regional LNs (N1), stage IIIC (T3N1).

What Are Recommended Treatment Modalities for Stage I to III Anal Cancer?

- Chemotherapy and radiation (CRT) are the standard of care. Two cycles of 5-fluorouracil (5-FU) and mitomycin C (MMC) are combined with a minimum radiation therapy (RT) dose of 45 Gy to the primary cancer, with larger tumors (T2 to T4) or node-positive patients receiving an additional dose of 9 to 14 Gy.
- Historically, anal cancer was treated with primary abdominoperineal resection (APR). However, high rates of local recurrence, morbidity of permanent colostomy, and poor survival led to development of CRT.[10] CRT preserves anal function and is associated with superior locoregional control and survival.
- A Phase III EORTC study questioned the need for chemotherapy comparing RT alone to CRT (5-FU & MMC). The CRT-treated patients had higher rates of complete response (80% vs. 54%), better colostomy-free survival, and improved locoregional control.[11]
- A Phase III UKCCR study (ACT I) trial also demonstrated CRT (5-FU & MMC) had superior local control compared to RT alone. A 13-year follow-up of that study showed continued benefit for CRT including an overall survival (OS) advantage (median overall survival [mOS] 5.4 years RT arm vs. 7.6 years in CRT arm).[12,13]
- The benefit of combination chemotherapy with RT (5-FU & MMC vs. 5-FU only) was shown in a Phase III intergroup study. Patients receiving CRT with combination 5-FU and MMC had a lower colostomy rate (9% vs. 22%; $P = 0.002$) and a higher disease-free survival (DFS; 73% vs. 51%; $P = 0.0003$) as compared with patients receiving CRT with 5-FU alone. There was no difference in OS and toxicity was higher in the MMC arm. The benefit of addition of MMC on colostomy rate was highest for large (T3/T4) tumors.[14]
- Cisplatin and 5-FU has been directly compared to 5-FU and MMC as the chemotherapy combined with radiation and was not superior.[15,16] Additionally, in this same study, two cycles of adjuvant cisplatin and 5-FU following completion of primary CRT did not improve outcomes.
- Stage I tumors can be considered for attenuated therapy, such as 5-FU with concurrent RT. This may be considered especially in older patients.
- There is an ongoing study, EA2182, *A Randomized Phase II Study of De-Intensified ChemoRadiation for Early-Stage Anal Squamous Cell Carcinoma (DECREASE; ClinicalTrials.gov Identifier: NCT04166318)* to assess whether de-intensification therapy can be used for early-stage anal cancer (T1-2N0).

The Patient's Treatment

- *The patient completes chemoradiotherapy; at 8 weeks on DRE, there is a persistent 2-cm nodule in the anal canal.*

When Is the Response to First-Line Chemoradiotherapy Assessed?

- Disease response is first assessed 8 to 12 weeks following completion of CRT. Patients are classified as having complete response, persistent disease, or progressive disease. If there is persistent disease, re-assessment occurs in 4-week intervals to monitor for continuing response, persistence, or progression. Regression can be seen for up to 6 months post completion of radiation therapy. A decision to proceed to salvage APR and colostomy may occur if there is biopsy-proven progressive disease.[17]

How Should Surveillance Be Conducted Following Primary Treatment?

- DRE at 8 to 12 weeks following CRT. With complete response, follow-up every 3 to 6 months with DRE, anoscopy, and LN exam for 5 years. Annual CT of the chest, abdomen, and pelvis is recommended for 3 years for patients with stage II to III disease.
- Monitor for late sequelae from CRT (for example, fecal incontinence, bowel dysfunction, sexual dysfunction, and urinary dysfunction).

The Patient's Follow-Up Physical Exam and Biopsy

- At 27 weeks following CRT, the patient was noted to have progressive disease on DRE, and she underwent a biopsy which confirmed progressive disease.

How Should Locoregional Failure After Primary Chemoradiotherapy Be Managed?

- Locoregional failure rates after CRT are up to 30%.[18,19]
- If no metastatic disease, salvage APR may be offered, with very select cases eligible for anal sphincter-sparing surgery.

Case 13.2: Very Early-Stage Anal Cancer Requiring Surgery Alone

An 82-year-old man presented to his primary care physician (PCP) with complaints of hemorrhoids for 3 months. He denies any pain with bowel movements but noted streaks of bright red blood when he wipes. On perianal examination, he was found to have a pedunculated, red, 2-cm perianal lesion abutting the anal verge. Biopsy was positive for a high-grade squamous intraepithelial lesion (HSIL; AIN3). Given the size and location, he underwent a local transanal excision with pathology showing superficially invasive SCC with negative margins.

What Are the Precursor Lesions for Anal Cancer?

- HPV-associated squamous proliferation is classified into two stages: low-grade squamous intraepithelial lesion (LSIL) and HSIL. Anal lesions can be classified according to the level of AIN where AIN I = LSIL and AIN II/III = HSIL.[20,21]
- HSIL are considered true precursor lesions to anal cancer and may progress to invasive SCCA. Rates of spontaneous regression for anal HSIL are not known but are less likely to occur as compared to anal LSIL.

How Should Precursor Lesions for Anal Cancer Be Managed?

- Low-grade dysplasia is treated with local therapies and surgery.
- AIN and superficially invasive SCC (SISCCA) local excision is indicated.[22]
- Recurrence rates are high, however, and routine surveillance is recommended with anoscopy.

What Additional Testing Should Be Discussed or Recommended?

- HIV testing if patient's HIV status is unknown. Risk of anal carcinoma has been reported to be higher in persons living with HIV/AIDS (PLWH).[23]

Case 13.3: Metastatic Anal Cancer

A 67-year-old woman was diagnosed with a T4N1 anal SCC in 2017. She completed CRT with MMC and 5-FU with a complete response noted 15 weeks after treatment. A year later, surveillance CT of the chest, abdomen, and pelvis noted bilateral pulmonary nodules and vulvar nodules with biopsy confirming recurrent anal SCC.

What Are the Most Common Sites for Distant Metastatic Disease?

- Liver, lungs, and extra-pelvic LNs

What Is the Risk of Metastatic Disease?

- A small minority of patients (~10%) will have metastatic cancer on initial presentation, and 10% to 20% of patients who have received curative therapy will have a metastatic relapse.[9,13,24] Larger tumor size and more advanced nodal stage are predictive factors for metastatic anal carcinoma.

What Is the Recommended First-Line Treatment for Metastatic Anal Cancer?

- InterAACT/EA2133 evaluated carboplatin and weekly paclitaxel versus cisplatin and 5-FU as first therapy for metastatic disease. Carboplatin/paclitaxel demonstrated a longer OS (20 vs. 12.3 months, $P = 0.014$), better tolerance with increased median number of cycles provided (6 vs. 4.5 cycles), and reduced G3/4 toxicities. Findings established carboplatin/paclitaxel as a standard, first-line treatment for metastatic anal cancer.[25]
- There is an ongoing study, EA2176, *A Randomized Phase III Study of Immune Checkpoint Inhibition With Chemotherapy in Treatment-Naïve Metastatic Anal Cancer (ClinicalTrials.gov Identifier: NCT04444921) Patients* to evaluate first-line combination therapy with chemotherapy and immunotherapy.

The Patient's Systemic Chemotherapy

Ms. CG receives carboplatin and paclitaxel for 6 months before progressive pulmonary disease was noted. She remains minimally symptomatic from disease and is interested in further therapy.

What Are Second-Line Treatment Options for Anal Cancer?

- The immune checkpoint inhibitors nivolumab and pembrolizumab are both approved second-line treatment options regardless of programmed death-ligand 1 (PD-L1) status of the tumor.[26,27]

REVIEW QUESTIONS

1. A 45-year-old HIV-positive man with no other past medical history (Eastern Cooperative Oncology Group [ECOG] performance status [PS] 0) presents with newly diagnosed stage II squamous cell carcinoma of the anus (SCCA). His last CD4 count a month ago was less than 200 and he has no history of opportunistic infections. What treatment would you recommend for him?
   A. Concurrent 5-fluorouracil (5-FU), mitomycin, and radiation therapy without dose reduction, but with weekly monitoring of blood counts and close monitoring for treatment-related toxicity
   B. Concurrent 5-FU and radiation, omitting mitomycin due to concern for cytopenias
   C. Concurrent 5-FU, mitomycin, and radiation therapy with 25% dose reduction of mitomycin
   D. Radiation alone as he is too high risk for chemotherapy toxicity with his CD4 count less than 200

2. A 65-year-old HIV-positive woman on highly active antiretroviral therapy (HAART) presents with stage II squamous cell carcinoma of the anus (SCCA) and is initiated on concurrent 5-fluorouracil (5-FU), mitomycin, and radiation therapy. Two weeks into treatment she develops thrombocytopenia (platelets less than 50,000), anemia (Hgb 7.0), and an acute kidney injury (AKI [Cr 2.5]). What do you consider a potential cause of the previously noted symptoms?
   A. Drug interaction between HAART and mitomycin C (MMC) causing MMC toxicity
   B. 5-FU toxicity secondary to dihydropyrimidine dehydrogenase deficiency
   C. MMC-induced microangiopathic hemolytic anemia
   D. Expected side effects with concurrent 5-FU and MMC and indicate a need for dose reductions

3. A 63-year-old man was diagnosed with stage IIIC squamous cell carcinoma of the anus (SCCA) and completed primary chemoradiotherapy 24 months ago. He has since recovered and states his life has returned to normal. At follow-up, a 3-cm inguinal lymph node (LN) is palpated and subsequently biopsied with pathology confirming recurrent squamous cell carcinoma (SCC). CT of his chest, abdomen, and pelvis are negative and anoscopy does not identify a local recurrence. How would you treat him?
   A. Refer to a surgeon for consideration of inguinal LN dissection
   B. Refer to a surgeon for consideration of inguinal LN dissection and abdominoperineal resections (APR)
   C. Start systemic chemotherapy with carboplatin/paclitaxel
   D. Observe as he is asymptomatic, and all therapy would be palliative in intent

4. A 58-year-old man presents for follow-up 14 weeks after completing chemoradiotherapy (CRT) with 5-fluorouracil (5-FU) and mitomycin for stage III primary squamous cell carcinoma of the anus (SCCA). His tumor is unchanged in size compared to evaluation immediately after CRT completion. He is very anxious and asks whether this means he will have to undergo surgery. You tell him the following:
   A. "The need for surgery cannot be determined at this time as tumor regression after CRT has been shown to continue for up to 26 weeks post-treatment completion"
   B. "The stable tumor size is concerning for persistent disease. I will refer you to a surgeon for an abdominoperineal resection (APR)"
   C. "I would like to biopsy the tumor to confirm that it is persistent disease"
   D. "I will refer you to a surgeon for local resection"

5. A 55-year-old man presented after palpating a mass within his anus which was confirmed to be squamous cell carcinoma (SCC) after biopsy. PET/CT revealed fluorodeoxyglucose (FDG)-avid left-sided perirectal and inguinal lymph adenopathy, the largest measuring 1.5 cm. There was no evidence of distant metastases. How would you complete his staging workup?
   A. Biopsy a left inguinal lymph node (LN) to confirm metastatic disease
   B. No further workup is necessary
   C. Complete surgical staging with abdominoperineal resections (APR) with total meso-rectal excision (TME)
   D. Biopsy perirectal lymph node (LN)

ANSWERS AND RATIONALES

1. **A. Concurrent 5-fluorouracil (5-FU), mitomycin, and radiation therapy without dose reduction, but with weekly monitoring of blood counts and close monitoring for treatment-related toxicity.** Modifications to anal cancer treatment should not be made solely based on a patient's HIV status. He is young, has good performance status, is otherwise healthy, and has had no complications from disease. A CD4 count less than 200 alone is not an indication for modification of standard of care treatment. A dose reduction in mitomycin C (MMC) could be considered if the patient has a history of opportunistic infections.

2. **C. MMC-induced microangiopathic hemolytic anemia.** Microangiopathic hemolytic anemia is a rare but potential side effect of MMC and can occur even after therapy with MMC has completed. Treatment involves stopping subsequent MMC and supportive care including consideration for steroids and plasmapheresis.

3. **A. Refer to a surgeon for consideration of inguinal LN dissection.** This patient has an inguinal recurrence without evidence of local recurrence. Patients who have already received groin irradiation should undergo an inguinal LN dissection. An APR in addition to an inguinal LN dissection would be considered if there is evidence of recurrent/persistent anal canal disease in addition to positive inguinal LNs.

4. **A. "The need for surgery cannot be determined at this time as tumor regression after CRT has been shown to continue for up to 26 weeks post-treatment completion."** The ACT II trial, in which 940 patients were randomized first to 5-FU with mitomycin or cisplatin and concurrent radiation, then randomized again to maintenance chemotherapy, assessed local disease responses at 11, 18, and 26 weeks. Analysis showed that 29% of those who were not in complete clinical response at 11 weeks were so at 26 weeks, supporting the view that anal squamous cell carcinoma (SCC) continues to regress up to 26 weeks post-completion of chemoradiotherapy.

5. **A. Biopsy a left inguinal lymph node (LN) to confirm metastatic disease.** Confirmation of metastatic disease within his LNs should always be considered when it could result in upstaging a patient as it could impact prognosis and treatment. Since an inguinal LN is easily accessible for a needle biopsy, that would be the best next step in workup of his disease to complete his staging. Surgical staging has no role in squamous cell carcinoma of the anus (SCCA).

REFERENCES

1. Ouhoummane N, Steben M, Coutlée F, et al. Squamous anal cancer: patient characteristics and HPV type distribution. *Cancer Epidemiol.* 2013;37(6):807–812. doi:10.1016/j.canep.2013.09.015
2. Smyczek P, Singh AE, Romanowski, B. Anal intraepithelial neoplasia: review and recommendations for screening and management. *Int J STD AIDS.* 2013;24(11):843–851. doi:10.1177/0956462413481527
3. Saraiya M, Unger ER, Thompson TD, et al. US assessment of HPV types in cancers: implications for current and 9-valent HPV vaccines. *J Natl Cancer Inst.* 2015;107(6):djv086. doi:10.1093/jnci/djv086
4. Markowitz LE, Dunne EF, Saraiya M, et al. Human papillomavirus vaccination: recommendations of the Advisory Committee on Immunization Practices (ACIP). *MMWR Recomm Rep.* 2014;63(RR-05):1–30. https://www.cdc.gov/mmwr/preview/mmwrhtml/rr6305a1.htm
5. Meites E, Kempe A, Markowitz LE. Use of a 2-dose schedule for human papillomavirus vaccination—updated recommendations of the Advisory Committee on Immunization Practices. *MMWR Morb Mortal Wkly Rep.* 2016;65(49):1405–1408. doi:10.15585/mmwr.mm6549a5
6. Meites E, Szilagyi PG, Chesson HW, et al. Human papillomavirus vaccination for adults: updated recommendations of the Advisory Committee on Immunization Practices. *MMWR Morb Mortal Wkly Rep.* 2019;68(32):698–702. doi:10.15585/mmwr.mm6832a3

7. Murthy N, Wodi AP, Bernstein H, et al. Advisory Committee on Immunization Practices recommended immunization schedule for adults aged 19 years or older—United States, 2022. *MMWR Morb Mortal Wkly Rep.* 2022;71:229–233. doi:10.15585/mmwr.mm7107a1

8. Pingali C, Yankey D, Elam-Evans LD, et al. National, regional, state, and selected local area vaccination coverage among adolescents aged 13–17 years—United States, 2020. *MMWR Morb Mortal Wkly Rep.* 2021;70(35):1183–1190. doi:10.15585/mmwr.mm7035a1

9. National Cancer Institute Surveillance, Epidemiology, and End Results Program. Anus, anul canal, anorectum SEER 5-year relative survival rates, 2012-2018. https://seer.cancer.gov/statistics-network/explorer/application.html?site=34&data_type=4&graph_type=5&compareBy=stage&chk_stage_104=104&chk_stage_105=105&chk_stage_106=106&chk_stage_107=107&series=9&sex=1&race=1&age_range=1&advopt_precision=1&advopt_show_ci=on

10. Ryan DP, Compton CC, Mayer RJ. Carcinoma of the anal canal. *N Engl J Med.* 2000;42(11):792–800. doi:10.1056/NEJM200003163421107

11. Bartelink H, Roelofsen F, Eschwege F, et al. Concomitant radiotherapy and chemotherapy is superior to radiotherapy alone in the treatment of locally advanced anal cancer: results of a phase III randomized trial of the European Organization for Research and Treatment of Cancer Radiotherapy and Gastrointestinal Cooperative Groups. *J Clin Oncol.* 1997;15(5):2040–2049. doi:10.1200/JCO.1997.15.5.2040

12. Northover J, Glynne-Jones R, Sebag-Montefiore D, et al. Chemoradiation for the treatment of epidermoid anal cancer: 13-year follow-up of the first randomised UKCCCR Anal Cancer Trial (ACT I). *Br J Cancer.* 2010;102(7):1123–1128. doi:10.1038/sj.bjc.6605605

13. UKCCCR Anal Cancer Trial Working Party. Epidermoid anal cancer: results from the UKCCCR randomised trial of radiotherapy alone versus radiotherapy, 5-fluorouracil, and mitomycin. UK Co-ordinating Committee on Cancer Research. *Lancet.* 1996;348(9034):1049–1054. doi:10.1016/S0140-6736(96)03409-5

14. Flam M, John M, Pajak TF, et al. Role of mitomycin in combination with fluorouracil and radiotherapy, and of salvage chemoradiation in the definitive nonsurgical treatment of epidermoid carcinoma of the anal canal: results of a phase III randomized intergroup study. *J Clin Oncol.* 1996;14(9):2527–2539. doi:10.1200/JCO.1996.14.9.2527

15. Gunderson LL, Winter KA, Ajani JA, et al. Long-term update of US GI intergroup RTOG 98-11 phase III trial for anal carcinoma: survival, relapse, and colostomy failure with concurrent chemoradiation involving fluorouracil/mitomycin versus fluorouracil/cisplatin. *J Clin Oncol.* 2012;30(35):4344–4351. doi:10.1200/JCO.2012.43.8085

16. James RD, Glynne-Jones R, Meadows HM, et al. Mitomycin or cisplatin chemoradiation with or without maintenance chemotherapy for treatment of squamous-cell carcinoma of the anus (ACT II): a randomised, phase 3, open-label, 2 × 2 factorial trial. *Lancet Oncol.* 2013;14(6):516–524. doi:10.1016/S1470-2045(13)70086-X

17. Glynne-Jones R, Sebag-Montefiore D, Meadows HM, et al. Best time to assess complete clinical response after chemoradiotherapy in squamous cell carcinoma of the anus (ACT II): a post-hoc analysis of randomised controlled phase 3 trial. *Lancet Oncol.* 2017;18(3):347–356. doi:10.1016/S1470-2045(17)30071-2

18. Schiller DE, Cummings BJ, Rai S, et al. Outcomes of salvage surgery for squamous cell carcinoma of the anal canal. *Ann Surg Oncol.* 2007;14(10):2780–2789. doi:10.1245/s10434-007-9491-8

19. Mullen JT, Rodriguez-Bigas MA, Chang GJ, et al. Results of surgical salvage after failed chemoradiation therapy for epidermoid carcinoma of the anal canal. *Ann Surg Oncol.* 2007;14(2):478–483. doi:10.1245/s10434-006-9221-7

20. Darragh TM, Colgan TJ, Cox JT, et al. The lower anogenital squamous terminology standardization project for HPV-associated lesions: background and consensus recommendations from the College of American Pathologists and the American Society for Colposcopy and Cervical Pathology. *Arch Pathol Lab Med.* 2012;136(10):1266–1297. doi:10.5858/arpa.LGT200570

21. Solomon D, Davey D, Kurman R, et al. The 2001 Bethesda System: terminology for reporting results of cervical cytology. *JAMA.* 2002;287(16):2114–2119. doi:10.1001/jama.287.16.2114

22. Richel O, de Vries HJ, van Noesel CJ, et al. Comparison of imiquimod, topical fluorouracil, and electrocautery for the treatment of anal intraepithelial neoplasia in HIV-positive men who have sex with men: an open-label, randomised controlled trial. *Lancet Oncol.* 2013;14(4):346–353. doi:10.1016/S1470-2045(13)70067-6

23. Frisch M, Biggar RJ, Goedert JJ. Human papillomavirus-associated cancers in patients with human immunodeficiency virus infection and acquired immunodeficiency syndrome. *J Natl Cancer Inst.* 2000;92(18):1500–1510. doi:10.1093/jnci/92.18.1500

24. Ryan D, Willet CG. Anal cancer. cancer of the lower gastrointestinal tract. *Atlas of Clinical Oncology.* American Cancer Society; 2001:196–213.

25. Rao S, Sclafani F, Eng C, et al. International rare cancers initiative multicenter randomized Phase II trial of cisplatin and fluorouracil versus carboplatin and paclitaxel in advanced anal cancer: interAAct. *J Clin Oncol.* 2020;38(22):2510–2518. doi:10.1200/JCO.19.03266

26. Morris VK, Salem ME, Nimeiri H, et al. Nivolumab for previously treated unresectable metastatic anal cancer (NCI9673): a multicentre, single-arm, phase 2 study. *Lancet Oncol.* 2017;18(4):446–453. doi:10.1016/S1470-2045(17)30104-3

27. Marabelle A, Cassier PA, Fakih M, et al. Pembrolizumab for previously treated advanced anal squamous cell carcinoma: pooled results from the KEYNOTE-028 and KEYNOTE-158 studies. *J Clin Oncol,* 2020;38(15_suppl):4020. doi:10.1200/JCO.2020.38.15_suppl.4020

CHAPTER 14

Prostate Cancer

Monica Tamil, Nagaishwarya Moka, Aihua Edward Yen, and Arpit Rao

INTRODUCTION

Prostate cancer is one of the most common cancers with approximately 1.4 million new cases and 375,000 deaths worldwide in 2020.[1] Despite occurrence of androgen receptor (AR)-driven disease biology in a majority of cases,[2-4] there is considerable heterogeneity in clinical presentation and trajectory. On the indolent end of the spectrum are men with localized, low Gleason score disease who can be safely managed with observation alone without any adverse impact on quality of life or survival.[5] On the aggressive end, patients can present with widespread de novo metastatic disease with a life expectancy of mere months.[6] Thus, it is critical for clinicians to accurately assess the biology and "behavior" of the disease to institute the best possible therapy for any given patient.

Much like other areas within oncology, recent years have seen a marked improvement in diagnostic modalities, understanding of disease biology, and availability of therapeutic options for prostate cancer.[7] This has resulted in several years' improvement in the median survival even for patients with metastatic disease at presentation.[8] The availability of multiple treatment options with comparable efficacy in any given disease state has made it mandatory for clinicians to be aware and current on their knowledge of risk benefit profiles of each agent.

Another major phenomenon in prostate cancer is stage migration due to the advent and clinical adoption of novel diagnostic modalities like prostate-specific membrane antigen (PSMA) PET/CT scans.[9] A growing proportion of patients with localized disease based on conventional imaging (CT and nuclear medicine [NM] bone scans) are now upstaged to nodal or distant metastatic disease with these more sensitive imaging studies. In our experience, such patients are increasingly referred to medical oncology clinics to help determine the best course of action. This is likely to substantially alter treatment patterns and survival outcomes for prostate cancer patients in the next decade.

In this chapter, we will review three cases, each representing a unique disease state within prostate cancer to provide insights into the decision-making process for this common malignancy.

CASE SUMMARIES

Case 14.1: Localized Prostate Cancer

A 70-year-old man with well-controlled hypertension (HTN) and type 2 diabetes mellitus presented to his primary care provider (PCP) for an annual follow-up visit. He expressed interest in getting screened for prostate cancer. A serum prostate-specific antigen (PSA) test resulted at 5.68 ng/mL

(upper limit of normal = 4 ng/mL). The patient did not have any urinary or prostatic enlargement symptoms and a repeat PSA level done 2 weeks later remained abnormally elevated at 5.92 ng/mL. He was referred to a urologist for management of suspected prostate cancer. The urologist found an enlarged, hard, and irregular prostate on a digital rectal exam (DRE) and recommended a transrectal ultrasound (TRUS)-guided prostate biopsy. The remainder of his physical exam was normal. Family history is positive for his mother's diagnosis of unilateral breast cancer in her 50s.

How Is a Diagnosis Established?

- Abnormally elevated serum PSA with or without an abnormal DRE can be used as screening tools to detect prostate cancer; however, these are imperfect for diagnosis.[10]
- Imaging (either TRUS or MRI fusion) guided prostate biopsy is the gold standard for obtaining a tissue diagnosis of prostate cancer.[11]
- NM bone scan, most commonly using Technitium-99m (Tc99m) radioisotope, is the preferred imaging modality to detect osteoblastic bony metastases.
- CT abdomen and pelvis with and without contrast is recommended to evaluate for local disease extension, as well as nodal and distant metastases. If the patient has locally advanced or metastatic disease on these scans, a CT of the chest with contrast is also recommended to evaluate for pulmonary metastatic disease.

Patient's Diagnosis

- *PSA is abnormally elevated at 5.92 ng/mL with an abnormal DRE as above.*
- *TRUS prostate biopsy showed acinar adenocarcinoma of the prostate, Gleason grade 4 + 3 = 7 involving 40% to 60% of two cores in the left half of the gland. The other 10 of 12 sampled cores bilaterally were negative for a malignancy. No evidence of perineural invasion, high-grade prostate intraepithelial neoplasia (HG-PIN), or extracapsular extension is seen.*
- *NM bone scan did not show any abnormal uptake concerning for metastatic disease.*
- *CT of the abdomen and prostate with and without intravenous (IV) contrast only showed a mildly enlarged, heterogeneous-appearing prostate gland with no evidence for extraprostatic or nodal spread.*

What Further Molecular or Genomic Testing Is Required?

- The National Comprehensive Cancer Network (NCCN) guidelines[5] recommend germline genetic testing for patients with prostate cancer if they also have any of the following:
  - A positive family history
  - High-risk, very-high risk, regional, or metastatic prostate cancer, regardless of family history
  - Ashkenazi Jewish ancestry
  - A personal history of breast cancer

Patient's Molecular and Genomic Testing

- *Positive for germline biallelic BRCA2 deleterious mutation. Patient was referred for genetic counseling and advised on the possibly increased risk of disease recurrence despite curative-intent therapies.[12]*

How Is This Tumor Staged?

- Clinical decision-making involves staging the tumor using the American Joint Committee on Cancer (AJCC) eighth edition cancer staging manual (Table 14.1)[13] and risk-stratifying the disease using either American Urological Association (AUA)[14] or NCCN[5]-risk classifications.

- AJCC staging factors in the tumor extent, regional lymph node (LN) involvement, and distant metastatic spread, with increasing overall stage signifying a progressively lower likelihood of cure.[13]
- AUA-risk classification factors in the Gleason score, PSA, and AJCC T-stage. Treatment options can change significantly depending on whether the patient is AUA-very-low, low-, favorable-intermediate, unfavorable-intermediate, or high-risk (Table 14.1).[14]

Patient's Clinical Stage

- AJCC stage II (T2 N0 M0); AUA-unfavorable-intermediate risk based on Gleason score of 4 + 3 = 7 (grade group 3), clinical stage T2a, and PSA less than 10.

What Are Appropriate Treatment Options?

- The primary treatment options for localized, unfavorable-intermediate risk prostate cancer include radical prostatectomy (RP) with pelvic lymph node dissection (PLND), external beam radiation therapy (EBRT) with or without brachytherapy and androgen deprivation therapy (ADT), or observation (if life expectancy is less than 10 years).[5,14]
- For a majority of patients with life expectancy over 10 years, surgery and radiation have comparable efficacy, but differing side effect profiles.[15,16]
- A multidisciplinary consultation is recommended for patients with localized prostate cancer.
- Neoadjuvant systemic therapy has not been shown to improve overall survival (OS) in prostate cancer, but remains an option for a select subgroup of patients who may not be able to promptly undergo curative intent treatments.[17–22]

Recommended Treatment Plan for This Patient

- Our patient opted to pursue robotic nerve-sparing RP with PLND with a curative intent. He tolerated the surgery and recovered well. The surgical specimen showed no adverse features or LN metastases, and hence adjuvant radiation therapy (RT) was not recommended. At the 1-month follow-up visit, his urinary incontinence was moderate and improving, and sexual function was intact. His first postoperative PSA level was less than 0.001 ng/mL (undetectable).

Table 14.1 American Joint Committee on Cancer (AJCC) Eighth Edition Metastatic Prostate Cancer Staging Manual

Stage	Simplified Description
1	Tumor is confined to the prostate and there is no regional LN involvement or distant metastasis. PSA is less than 10 and Gleason grade group is 1.
2	Tumor is confined to the prostate and there is no regional LN involvement or distant metastasis. PSA is less than 20 and Gleason grade group is 1 to 4.
3	Tumor confined to prostate with PSA ≥20 and Gleason grade group 1 to 4, OR tumor not confined to prostate with any PSA and Gleason grade group 1 to 4, OR any T-stage and PSA associated with a Gleason grade group 5. Regional LN involvement or distant metastases are not allowed.
4	Any T stage, PSA, and Gleason group with regional LN involvement or distant metastasis.

LN, lymph node; PSA, prostate-specific antigen.

Source: Data from Amin MB, Edge SB, Greene FL, et al, eds. *AJCC Cancer Staging Manual.* 8th ed. Springer Nature; 2017.

What Are the Toxicities Associated With Radical Prostatectomy?

- Apart from the standard risk of perioperative complications including infection, bleeding, and injury to surrounding structures, some specific concerns associated with RP are urinary incontinence due to damage to the urinary sphincter and erectile dysfunction due to damage to the neurovascular bundles that innervate the penis. Complete urinary incontinence is rare, but most men suffer from some degree of urinary incontinence—typically stress incontinence—after RP. While most patients do seem to recover urinary function, the data on rate and extent of recovery remains mixed.[23]
- Estimates of post-RP erectile dysfunction vary significantly based on the surgical center, patient population, and use of nerve-sparing approach. For example, 59% of men in a study of 603 patients reported moderate or worse erectile dysfunction at 2 months after surgery.[23] The likelihood of regaining potency decreases with increasing age at surgery.[24] Because penile sensation and ability to have an orgasm are generally preserved, use of medications (oral phosphodiesterase 5 inhibitors like sildenafil) or vacuum-assisted erection devices effectively improve erectile dysfunction in most patients after an RP.

What Are Other Treatment Considerations?

Minimally Invasive Versus Open Surgery

- RP can be done using minimally invasive (robotic or laparoscopic) or open approaches. The robotic approach now constitutes a majority of RP in the United States, Europe, and Australia.[25]
- Both approaches have similar cancer control and continence and sexual outcomes, but minimally invasive surgery results in lesser perioperative blood loss and shorter time to recovery.[14]

What Is Required for This Patient's Follow-Up and Survivorship?

- After initial definitive therapy, patients are placed on surveillance with PSA every 6 to 12 months for the first 5 years, and then every year. A DRE can be offered yearly.
- Repeat imaging should be based on clinical suspicion of recurrence.
- Most prostate cancer recurrences are associated with an increase in PSA as a leading indicator, but a small subset of patients can have PSA-negative recurrence, typically due to the emergence of neuroendocrine phenotype.

Case 14.2: Biochemically Recurrent Prostate Cancer

A 74-year-old man was diagnosed with AUA-high-risk prostate adenocarcinoma in 2019 on workup for nocturia, urinary hesitancy, and intermittency. His PSA level was elevated to 9.2 ng/mL. He underwent a robotic nerve-sparing RP with PLND that showed a pT2, Gleason 4 + 5 = 9 acinar adenocarcinoma involving 60% of the prostate gland without any extracapsular extension, seminal vesicle invasion, or lymph nodal metastasis. He was offered but declined adjuvant RT and was on surveillance with serial PSA checks every 6 months. His PSA remained less than 0.001 ng/mL (undetectable) until 18 months after the surgery. At the 24-month follow-up visit, his PSA has now become detectable at 0.20 ng/mL. He has no clinical evidence of disease recurrence. Chief comorbidities include morbid obesity, coronary artery disease with history of percutaneous coronary intervention 6 months ago, and uncontrolled type 2 diabetes mellitus.

How Is a Diagnosis Established?

- PSA recurrence is defined as a PSA that was undetectable after RP and has become detectable and rising on two or more checks.[5]

- NM bone scan and CT abdomen and pelvis with contrast are essential for evaluating the extent of disease since 15% to 20% of recurrences are localized (prostatic fossa) and another 25% to 30% are distant/metastatic.[26]
- More sensitive imaging modalities including PET/CT scans using F18 fluciclovine, Ga68 PSMA-11, or F18-piflufolastat PSMA radiotracers have increasingly garnered adoption in this setting and can detect micrometastatic disease. Prognostic and therapeutic significance of these findings is currently unknown.[26,27]

Patient's Diagnosis

- *The second PSA remained elevated at 0.21 ng/mL 2 weeks later.*
- *NM bone scan and CT of the abdomen and pelvis with contrast did not show any evidence of malignancy.*
- *Ga68 PSMA-11 PET/CT scan showed a suspicious focus of uptake (standardized uptake value [SUV] max of 3.8) in a right external iliac LN measuring 0.9 cm.*

What Further Molecular or Genomic Testing Is Required?

- None

How Is This Tumor Staged?

- Biochemically recurrent prostate cancer does not have any additional designation within the AJCC tumor, lymph node, metastasis (TNM) staging system (Table 14.1).
- PSA doubling time (PSADT) is an important predictor of the likelihood of developing metastatic disease in patients with biochemically recurrent prostate cancer.[28]
- The Memorial Sloan Kettering Cancer Center (MSKCC) PSADT calculator tool[29] based on the study that evaluated the prognostic value of PSADT[30] is our preferred choice for PSADT calculation. Note that PSA less than 0.20 ng/mL are not allowed for this calculation because the original nomogram was derived from patients with a minimum detectable PSA level of 0.20 ng/mL.
- Additionally, because of considerable variability between serial PSA measurements in a given patient as well as between different labs,[31] it is recommended to use all available PSA values from a single lab within the preceding year to improve the accuracy of PSADT measurement.

Patient's Clinical Stage

- *Based on conventional imaging, the patient had no evidence of nodal involvement, and meets criteria for AJCC stage II (pT2 N0 M0; Gleason grade 5; PSA less than 10 ng/mL).*
- *However, based on the suspicious PET/CT finding of a regional LN, his AJCC stage is IV (pT2 N1 M0).*
- *This case is a good example of stage migration due to increased use of a more sensitive diagnostic modality in clinical practice.*
- *His PSADT was 12.6 months and serum testosterone level was 261 ng/dL.*

What Are Appropriate Treatment Options?

- If imaging studies are negative for distant metastasis, EBRT +/- ADT is recommended.
- Observation is a reasonable alternative if life expectancy is limited or if expected risks from EBRT exceed the likely benefits.
- In patients with serum testosterone greater than 50 ng/dL, systemic therapy with ADT can be offered in addition to EBRT. Mechanistically, ADT synergizes with RT due to the AR's role in promoting DNA damage response and repair.[32,33]

- We recommend choosing single-agent ADT instead of combined androgen blockage using AR antagonists or other antiandrogen therapies such as abiraterone for biochemically recurrent prostate cancer.
- ADT includes gonadotropin-releasing hormone (GnRH) antagonists such as degarelix, or agonists such as leuprolide or goserelin. Intermittent ADT is preferred due to lack of survival advantage and the inferior adverse event (AE) profile of continuous ADT.[5]

Recommended Treatment Plan for This Patient

- *After a multidisciplinary consultation, the patient opted for salvage RT. He was given a total of 70 Gy EBRT (in 2 Gy fractions) to the prostatic bed and pelvic LNs.*
- *Given the patient's medical comorbidities, it was decided to hold off on ADT.*

What Are the Toxicities Associated With Salvage Radiation Therapy?

- Data from prospective clinical trials[34] and retrospective studies[35,36] of salvage RT suggest that urinary (urgency, incontinence) and bowel symptoms (predominantly blood in stool in ~20% to 25% of patients; bowel incontinence in 5% of patients) were dominant side effects of this treatment. Some studies suggest a worsening of sexual function with salvage radiation, but a causal association is difficult to establish due to the presence of preexisting sexual dysfunction in this patient population.

What Is Required for This Patient's Follow-Up and Survivorship?

- *The patient will resume periodic PSA monitoring and imaging as needed.*

Case 14.3: Metastatic Hormone-Sensitive Prostate Cancer

A 51-year-old male presents with acute mid-lower back pain without any precipitating cause. He denied any radiculopathy, trauma, features of infection, or urinary symptoms. His medical history includes hypercholesterolemia, HTN, obstructive sleep apnea, and a history of kidney stones. He denied having ever used nicotine or illicit drugs but does drink 5 to 10 alcoholic beverages a week. A workup showed elevated PSA of 89.25 ng/mL and urinalysis was negative for infection or hematuria. A lumbar spine x-ray showed multiple sclerotic bone lesions in the lumbar spine.

How Is a Diagnosis Established?

- Significantly elevated PSA with sclerotic bone lesions on imaging strongly suggest a diagnosis of metastatic prostate cancer.
- Imaging-guided biopsy of the prostate gland or a suspected metastatic site is the gold standard for obtaining a tissue diagnosis of prostate cancer.
- Osteosclerotic bone metastases can be challenging to biopsy due to low yield (as low as 30% sensitivity).[37] Strategies to overcome these limitations include choosing a lytic or a mixed lytic-sclerotic lesion, sampling a soft-tissue component of a bony lesion that has disrupted cortical continuity, and obtaining multiple cores.
- Additionally, modified processing techniques that do not degrade nucleic acids during decalcification must be used to maximize feasibility of a complete workup including next-generation sequencing (NGS).
- Staging workup should include a CT of the chest, abdomen, and pelvis with and without IV contrast and NM bone scan. Advanced imaging modalities such as a PET/CT scan may be used if available.

Patient's Diagnosis

- After consultation with interventional radiology and urology, a decision was made to proceed with prostate biopsy. The TRUS-guided biopsy revealed adenocarcinoma and a Gleason score 4 + 5 = 9 involving 80% to 100% of all cores.
- CT of the abdomen and pelvis showed bilateral pelvic lymphadenopathy (short axis measurements of 13 mm in the left external iliac chain, 25 mm in the left pelvic sidewall, and 14 mm in the right upper pelvis) and prostatomegaly (moderately enlarged prostate with mild haziness of periphery of the prostate).
- Conventional bone scan revealed at least seven bone metastases involving the axial and appendicular skeleton (left posterior iliac crest superiorly, the upper sacrum, the T6 to T8 vertebrae, the right inferior lateral body of the sternum, C7 vertebral body, right parietal skull, and left posterior 8th rib).

What Further Molecular or Genomic Testing Is Required?[5]

- Approximately 10% to 15% of patients with metastatic prostate cancer have an inherited cancer syndrome, most commonly of genes involved in DNA damage response and repair.[38]
- Germline testing is recommended if the patient has a first- to third-degree relative with Lynch or *BRCA* cancer syndromes. These include relatives with breast cancer, colorectal cancer, or endometrial cancer at a young age (considered 50 years or younger).
- Exocrine pancreatic cancer, ovarian cancer, very high risk or high risk regional, or metastatic prostate cancer or male breast cancer are also associated with these cancer syndromes. These carry a very high risk and any patient with a first- to third-degree relative with any of these cancers at any age should be offered genetic testing.

Patient's Molecular and Genomic Testing

- Testing was negative for inherited cancer syndromes. A variant of unknown significance was identified in the tp53 gene but no further workup was recommended by the genetic counselor based on available clinical data.

How Is This Tumor Staged?

- The AJCC TNM staging is used for metastatic prostate cancer staging (Table 14.1).
- In addition, for metastatic hormone-sensitive prostate cancer, it is critical to classify the patient into a risk category. Two classification schemas are widely used—CHAARTED criteria[39] that classify patients into high- versus low-<u>volume</u> disease; and LATITUDE criteria[40] that classify patients into high- versus low-<u>risk</u> disease.
- In CHAARTED criteria, high-volume disease is defined as the presence of visceral metastasis or 4+ bone metastasis, with at least one being past the pelvis and lumbar vertebral column.
- In LATITUDE criteria, high-risk disease is defined as meeting at least two of three criteria: (a) Gleason score of 8 or greater, (b) presence of 3 or more lesions on bone scan, and/or (c) presence of measurable visceral lesions.

Patient's Clinical Stage

- This patient met the criteria for de novo metastatic (stage IVb), CHAARTED-high-volume, hormone-sensitive prostate cancer (mHSPC).

What Are Appropriate Treatment Options?[9]

- NCCN guidelines recommend combination therapy with ADT backbone for patients with mHSPC unless they have comorbidities or other patient-specific factors that prohibit such an approach.
- Options include one of the following with continuous ADT until disease progression or treatment intolerance:
  - Docetaxel (taxane chemotherapy) for up to 6 cycles
  - Abiraterone (17 alpha hydroxylase inhibitor) given with prednisone orally every day
  - Enzalutamide (AR antagonist) orally every day
  - Apalutamide (AR antagonist) orally every day
- Palliative RT can be offered for bone or visceral metastasis causing pain or leading to an imminent risk of life-threatening complications including a pathological bone fracture.

Recommended Treatment Plan for This Patient

- *Given the patient's young age and preference for a finite duration of combination agent, we opted for docetaxel with ADT. The patient received 6 cycles at 100% dose intensity of 75 mg/m² /cycle and tolerated it very well except for grade 2 fatigue, myelosuppression (self-resolving), and alopecia. He continues to be on ADT with leuprolide 22.5 mg subcutaneously every 3 months.*

What Are the Toxicities Associated With Chemohormonal Therapy?

GnRH Agonists/Antagonists[41,42]

- Common side effects (greater than 20%) include hot flashes, weight gain, low libido and erectile dysfunction, and gynecomastia.
- Long-term effects include weight gain, metabolic abnormalities such as worsening of diabetes, and increased risk of osteoporosis.
- GnRH agonists cause a temporary increase in testosterone which can cause an increase in tumor activity and worsening of tumor-related symptoms. This is particularly worrisome in patients with extensive bone metastasis to the spine. It is important that these patients are started on an AR antagonist first if there is a concern for tumor flare.

Docetaxel

- Single-agent docetaxel is generally well tolerated. In the CHAARTED study of docetaxel and ADT, grade 3 or worse AEs occurred in 29.6% of patients.[39] Notable among these are infusion reaction (2.1%), fatigue (4.1%), diarrhea (1%), stomatitis (0.5%), neuropathy (1%), thromboembolism (0.8%), anemia (1.3%), thrombocytopenia (0.3%), neutropenia (12.1%), and febrile neutropenia (6.1%).
- Other common side effects include dysgeusia, dyspnea, constipation, anorexia, nail disorders, fluid retention, alopecia, skin reactions, and myalgia.

What Are Other Treatment Considerations?

Follow-Up and Survivorship Plan

- *History and physical exam with serum PSA level every 3 to 6 months*
- *Periodic re-staging CT of the chest, abdomen, and pelvis with contrast and NM bone scans should be strongly considered to monitor treatment response.*

1. A 65-year-old male with suboptimally controlled epileptic disorder was being treated for metastatic hormone-sensitive prostate cancer (mHSPC) with bony metastasis with androgen deprivation therapy (ADT) alone for the past 2 years. His prostate-specific antigen (PSA) has risen to 20 ng/mL from 1 ng/mL on prior check 3 months earlier. The total testosterone level is less than 50 ng/dL. Re-staging CT of the chest, abdomen, and pelvis with contrast revealed new sites of bone metastasis. Which of the following is the preferred treatment of choice?
   A. Apalutamide
   B. Darolutamide
   C. Enzalutamide
   D. Abiraterone + prednisone

2. A 70-year-old male who received docetaxel with androgen deprivation therapy (ADT) for metastatic hormone-sensitive prostate cancer (mHSPC) has been on abiraterone plus prednisone for the last 10 months. Prostate-specific antigen (PSA) levels are stable at 2 ng/mL. On a follow-up visit, he complains of fatigue, weight loss, increased back pain, and hematuria. A repeat PSA is unchanged at 2 ng/mL. Re-staging CT of the chest, abdomen, and pelvis with contrast shows a new pelvic mass compressing on the ureter and causing right-sided hydronephrosis and new metastasis in the lumbar spine. What is the next best step?
   A. Supportive care and repeat PSA in 1 month
   B. Switch treatment to cabazitaxel
   C. Switch treatment to enzalutamide
   D. Biopsy of the pelvic mass

3. A 67-year-old male with a history of American Urological Association (AUA)-intermediate-favorable localized prostate cancer which was treated with external beam radiation therapy (EBRT) alone 8 years ago presents for a follow-up visit. His most recent prostate-specific antigen (PSA) was undetectable 4 years ago but he was lost to follow-up due to a lack of insurance. He has been experiencing pain in the low back for the last 4 weeks, which was not getting better with stretching or exercise. An MRI of the lumbar spine with contrast shows multiple sclerotic bone lesions suspicious for metastases. Repeat PSA was elevated at 223 ng/mL. A CT-guided L3 vertebral metastasis biopsy revealed adenocarcinoma of prostate origin. He was started on bicalutamide followed by androgen deprivation therapy (ADT) with a plan to add docetaxel. A dual-energy x-ray absorptiometry (DEXA) scan revealed that the patient's T score was −2 at L-spine. What's the next best therapeutic step?
   A. Repeat monthly DEXA scans
   B. Start vitamin D, calcium supplements, and dental evaluation
   C. Take part in fall risk evaluation and counseling
   D. Perform a skeletal survey

4. A 57-year-old male with metastatic castration-resistant prostate cancer (mCRPC) is currently on enzalutamide. His mother had breast cancer at 42 years of age and his sister had ovarian cancer at 50 years of age. He declined genetic testing but was willing to undergo targeted tumor next-generation sequencing (NGS). This showed a deleterious

alteration in the *FANCA* gene. Which is the most appropriate treatment upon progression on enzalutamide?

A. Abiraterone
B. Docetaxel
C. Olaparib
D. Rucaparib

5. A 66-year-old male presented with subacute-onset, asymmetric, bilateral lower extremity weakness paresthesia and urinary retention. Evaluation showed a prostate-specific antigen (PSA) level of 115 ng/mL with a serum testosterone level of 38 ng/dL. An MRI lumbar spine with contrast showed multifocal osseous sclerotic lesions with partial spinal cord compression at the L1 level. A CT of the chest, abdomen, and pelvis with contrast showed bulky retroperitoneal lymphadenopathy. Intravenous (IV) dexamethasone was started and the patient was advised to undergo an emergency corpectomy and spinal decompression. However, he wants to be sure this is cancer before undergoing a major surgery. Assuming that biopsy of any metastatic lesion is feasible, what will be your recommended biopsy site?

A. 5-cm osseous L1 vertebral met
B. 6.3-cm retroperitoneal lymph node (LN) conglomerate
C. 1.2-cm right lower lobe lung nodule
D. 0.8-cm segment 7 liver nodule

6. A 70-year-old male is diagnosed with de novo metastatic hormone-sensitive prostate cancer (mHSPC) after having a positive prostate-specific antigen (PSA) screening. Biopsy was consistent with Gleason 4 + 5 = 9. He has no family history of cancer. Which of the following is true regarding germline genetic testing?

A. No genetic testing is indicated given family history
B. Genetic testing is indicated
C. No genetic testing is indicated given he only has bone disease
D. Further imaging of the brain is required before deciding

7. A 74-year-old male is diagnosed with locally advanced prostate cancer. He undergoes a radical prostatectomy (RP) followed by adjuvant radiation. A year later, he is noted to have a rising prostate-specific antigen (PSA). Imaging is concerning for new metastatic bone lesions. Which of the following is true regarding genetic testing?

A. Genetic testing is recommended
B. No genetic testing is needed because he was only locally advanced at initial diagnosis
C. Further family history needs to be obtained before determination
D. The guidelines are not clear so this should be a consideration between patient and doctor.

8. A 58-year-old male was found to have a prostate-specific antigen (PSA) of 24 ng/mL on a routine evaluation. A subsequent PSA checked 4 weeks later is 42 ng/mL. He has no family history of prostate cancers. He has a past medical history (PMH) of bipolar depression, recurrent urinary tract infections (UTIs), and benign prostatic hyperplasia (BPH). Which of the following is the best next step?

A. Send to Urology for radical robotic prostatectomy and pathology
B. Send patient for transrectal ultrasound (TRUS)-guided prostate biopsy
C. Nothing; elevation is due to BPH
D. Nothing; elevation is due to recurrent UTIs

9. A 62-year-old male with a history of American Urological Association (AUA)-high-risk localized prostate cancer is found to have biochemically recurrent disease. Conventional imaging is negative for any metastatic disease. He is started on androgen deprivation therapy (ADT). What is the goal testosterone level?
   A. Undetectable testosterone
   B. Less than 50 ng/dL
   C. Less than 100 ng/dL
   D. Less than 20 ng/dL

10. A 64-year-old male with Crohn's disease is found to have de novo metastatic hormone-sensitive prostate cancer (mHSPC). Conventional imaging showed two metastases, both in the lumbar spine. He was started on androgen deprivation therapy (ADT) 2 weeks ago. Which of the following treatments should he get in addition to the ADT?
   A. Abiraterone plus prednisone
   B. Docetaxel
   C. Radiation to his prostate
   D. He should continue ADT only

ANSWERS AND RATIONALES

1. **D. Abiraterone + prednisone**. The patient has metastatic castration-resistant prostate cancer (mCRPC) with biochemical and radiographic disease progression. Out of the choices, abiraterone or enzalutamide can be used for this patient. Enzalutamide has a small but definite risk of seizure disorders and is not the best option for this patient with suboptimally controlled epileptic disorder. Darolutamide and apalutamide are not approved for first-line mCRPC.

2. **D. Biopsy of the pelvic mass**. Although the PSA levels are stable, development of new cancer-related symptoms and the new lesions on the CT are highly concerning for a neuroendocrine transformation or emergence of a non-androgen receptor (AR) driven phenotype.

3. **B. Start vitamin D, calcium supplements, and dental evaluation**. Patients treated with ADT are at increased risk of fall and fractures. According to the National Osteoporosis Foundation guidelines,[43] all prostate cancer patients over the age of 50 need a baseline DEXA scan to check for bone density and initiate calcium and vitamin D supplementation and treatment with a bisphosphonate or denosumab. Dental evaluation is recommended before initiating bisphosphonate/denosumab due to the increased risk of osteonecrosis of the jaw.

4. **C. Olaparib**. In patients with mCRPC harboring homologous recombination repair gene defects (for example, *FANCA*) who had progressed on abiraterone or enzalutamide, olaparib was shown to have superior radiographic progression-free survival (PFS) and overall survival (OS) compared with standard-of-care.[44]

5. **B. 6.3-cm retroperitoneal lymph node (LN) conglomerate**. Between these lesions, the LN sampling is likely to have a significantly higher yield with lowest risk of procedural complications as previously discussed.

6. **B. Genetic testing is indicated**. Any patient with metastatic prostate cancer is recommended to get genetic testing even in the absence of a family history of cancer. Commonly tested germline genes include *BRCA1/2*, *PALB2*, *ATM*, *MLH1*, *MSH2*, *MSH6*, *CHEK2*, *PMS2*, and *EPCAM*.

7. **A. Genetic testing is recommended**. Any patient with metastatic prostate cancer is recommended to get genetic testing. Every patient needs genetic testing once they become metastatic regardless of the original M stage.

8. **B. Send patient for transrectal ultrasound (TRUS)-guided prostate biopsy**. BPH and recurrent UTIs can cause an elevated PSA, but a persistently high PSA warrants a urology referral and prostate biopsy.

9. **B. Less than 50 ng/dL**. For patients who have a high or normal initial testosterone level, the goal of chemical castration (with ADT) is to keep testosterone at less than 50 ng/dL.

10. **A. Abiraterone plus prednisone**. Based on the information provided, this patient meets the CHAARTED-low volume criteria for mHSPC. Of these options, abiraterone plus prednisone has shown a survival advantage compared with ADT alone in patients with mHSPC irrespective of their CHAARTED or LATITUDE-risk status.[40]

REFERENCES

1. Sung H, Ferlay J, Siegel RL, et al. Global cancer statistics 2020: GLOBOCAN estimates of incidence and mortality worldwide for 36 cancers in 185 countries. *CA Cancer J Clin.* 2021;71:209–249. doi:10.3322/caac.21660
2. Robinson D, Van Allen EM, Wu Y-M, et al. Integrative clinical genomics of advanced prostate cancer. *Cell.* 2015;161:1215–1228. doi:10.1016/j.cell.2015.05.001
3. Fraser M, Sabelnykova VY, Yamaguchi TN, et al. Genomic hallmarks of localized, non-indolent prostate cancer. *Nature.* 2017;541:359–364. doi:10.1038/nature20788
4. Abida W, Cyrta J, Heller G, et al. Genomic correlates of clinical outcome in advanced prostate cancer. *PNAS.* 2019;116:11428–11436. doi:10.1073/pnas.1902651116
5. Mohler JL, Antonarakis ES, Armstrong AJ, et al. Prostate cancer, Version 2.2019, NCCN clinical practice guidelines in oncology. *J Natl Compr Canc Netw.* 2019;17:479–505. doi:10.6004/jnccn.2019.0023
6. Bastos DA, Antonarakis ES. AR-V7 and treatment selection in advanced prostate cancer: are we there yet? *Precis Cancer Med.* 2018;1:13. doi:10.21037/pcm.2018.09.01
7. Sagaram S, Rao A. Rapidly evolving treatment paradigm and considerations for sequencing therapies in metastatic prostate cancer—a narrative review. *Transl Androl Urol.* 2021;10:3188–3198. doi:10.21037/tau-20-1383
8. Siegel RL, Miller KD, Fuchs HE, Jemal A. Cancer statistics. *CA Cancer J Clin.* 2021;71:7–33. doi:10.3322/caac.21654
9. Sundahl N, Gillessen S, Sweeney C, Ost P. When what you see is not always what you get: raising the bar of evidence for new diagnostic imaging modalities. *Eur Urol.* 2021;79:565–567. doi:10.1016/j.eururo.2020.07.029
10. Tian J-Y, Guo F-J, Zheng G-Y, Ahmad A. Prostate cancer: updates on current strategies for screening, diagnosis and clinical implications of treatment modalities. *Carcinogenesis.* 2018;39:307–317. doi:10.1093/carcin/bgx141
11. Sarkar S, Das SA. Review of imaging methods for prostate cancer detection. *Biomed Eng Comput Biol.* 2016;7(suppl 1):1–15. doi:10.4137/BECB.S34255
12. Taylor RA, Fraser M, Rebello RJ, et al. The influence of BRCA2 mutation on localized prostate cancer. *Nat Rev Urol.* 2019;16:281–290. doi:10.1038/s41585-019-0164-8
13. Buyyounouski MK, Choyke PL, McKenney JK, et al. Prostate cancer—major changes in the American Joint Committee on Cancer eighth edition cancer staging manual. *CA Cancer J Clin.* 2017;67:245–253. doi:10.3322/caac.2139
14. Sanda MG, Chen RC, Crispiano T. Clinically localized prostate cancer: AUA/ASTRO/SUO guideline. American Urological Association. http://www.auanet.org/guidelines/clinically-localized-prostate-cancer-new-(aua/astro/suo-guideline-2017)
15. Wallis CJ, Saskin R, Choo R, et al. Surgery versus radiotherapy for clinically-localized prostate cancer: a systematic review and meta-analysis. *Eur Urol.* 2016;70:21–30. doi:10.1016/j.eururo.2015.11.010
16. Spahn M, Dal Pra A, Aebersold D, Tombal B. Radiation therapy versus radical prostatectomy: a never-ending discussion. *Eur Urol.* 2016;70:31–32. doi:10.1016/j.eururo.2016.01.049
17. Fair WR, Aprikian AG, Cohen D, et al. Use of neoadjuvant androgen deprivation therapy in clinically localized prostate cancer. *Clin Invest Med.* 1993;16:516–522.
18. Debruyne FM, Witjes WP, Schulman CC, et al. Multicentre trial of combined neoadjuvant androgen blockade with zoladex and flutamide prior to radical prostatectomy in prostate cancer. The European Study Group on Neoadjuvant Treatment. *Eur Urol.* 1994;26(suppl 1):4. doi:10.1159/000475423
19. Labrie F, Dupont A, Cusan L, et al. Downstaging of localized prostate cancer by neoadjuvant therapy with flutamide and lupron: the first controlled and randomized trial. *Clin Invest Med.* 1993;16:499–509.
20. Taplin M-E, Montgomery B, Logothetis CJ, et al. Intense androgen-deprivation therapy with abiraterone acetate plus leuprolide acetate in patients with localized high-risk prostate cancer: results of a randomized phase II neoadjuvant study. *J Clin Oncol.* 2014;32:3705–3715. doi:10.1200/JCO.2013.53.4578
21. Eastham JA, Heller G, Halabi S, et al. Cancer and leukemia Group B 90203 (Alliance): radical prostatectomy with or without neoadjuvant chemohormonal therapy in localized, high-risk prostate cancer. *J Clin Oncol.* 2020;38(26):3042–3050. doi:10.1200/JCO.20.00315
22. Patel R, Oza E, Dave CN, Kim ED. Neoadjuvant androgen deprivation therapy in prostate cancer. Medscape. Published online November 20, 2017. Updated December 28, 2020. Accessed June 17, 2022. https://emedicine.medscape.com/article/455994-overview
23. Sanda MG, Dunn RL, Michalski J, et al. Quality of life and satisfaction with outcome among prostate-cancer survivors. *N Engl J Med.* 2008;358:1250–1261. doi:10.1056/NEJMoa074311
24. Kundu SD, Roehl KA, Eggener SE, et al. Potency, continence and complications in 3,477 consecutive radical retropubic prostatectomies. *J Urol.* 2004;172:2227–2231. doi:10.1097/01.ju.0000145222.94455.73
25. Sooriakumaran P, Srivastava A, Shariat SF, et al. A multinational, multi-institutional study comparing positive surgical margin rates among 22393 open, laparoscopic, and robot-assisted radical prostatectomy patients. *Eur Urol.* 2014;66:450–456. doi:10.1016/j.eururo.2013.11.018

26. Barbosa FG, Queiroz MA, Nunes RF, et al. Revisiting prostate cancer recurrence with PSMA PET: atlas of typical and atypical patterns of spread. *Radiographics*. 2019;39:186–212. doi:10.1148/rg.2019180079

27. Rao A, Vapiwala N, Schaeffer EM, Ryan CJ. Oligometastatic prostate cancer: a shrinking subset or an opportunity for cure? *Am Soc Clin Oncol Educ Book*. 2019:309–320. doi:10.1200/EDBK_239041

28. Roberts SG, Blute ML, Bergstralh EJ, et al. PSA doubling time as a predictor of clinical progression after biochemical failure following radical prostatectomy for prostate cancer. *Mayo Clin Proc*. 2001;76:576–581. doi:10.4065/76.6.576

29. Memorial Sloan Kettering Cancer Center. PSA doubling time. https://www.mskcc.org/nomograms/prostate/psa_doubling_time

30. Pound CR, Partin AW, Eisenberger MA, et al. Natural history of progression after PSA elevation following radical prostatectomy. *JAMA*. 1999;281:1591–1597. doi:10.1001/jama.281.17.1591

31. Filella X, Albaladejo MD, Allué JA, et al. Prostate cancer screening: guidelines review and laboratory issues. *Clin Chem Lab Med*. 2019; 57:1474–1487. doi:10.1515/cclm-2018-1252

32. Polkinghorn WR, Zelefsky MJ. Improving outcomes in high-risk prostate cancer with radiotherapy. *Rep Pract Oncol Radiother*. 2013;18:333–337. doi:10.1016/j.rpor.2013.10.006

33. Spina CS. Androgen deprivation therapy and radiation therapy for prostate cancer: the mechanism underlying therapeutic synergy. *Transl Cancer Res*. 2018;7(suppl 6):S695–S703. doi:10.21037/tcr.2018.05.42

34. Vale CL, Fisher D, Kneebone A, et al. Adjuvant or early salvage radiotherapy for the treatment of localised and locally advanced prostate cancer: a prospectively planned systematic review and meta-analysis of aggregate data. *Lancet*. 2020;396:1422–1431. doi:10.1016/S0140-6736(20)31952-8

35. Alsadius D, Olsson C, Pettersson N, et al. Patient-reported gastrointestinal symptoms among long-term survivors after radiation therapy for prostate cancer. *Radiother Oncol*. 2014;112:237–243. doi:10.1016/j.radonc.2014.08.008

36. Braide K, Kindblom J, Lindencrona U, et al. A comparison of side-effects and quality-of-life in patients operated on for prostate cancer with and without salvage radiation therapy. *Scand J Urol*. 2020;54:393–400. doi:10.1080/21681805.2020.1782980

37. McKay RR, Zukotynski KA, Werner L, et al. Imaging, procedural and clinical variables associated with tumor yield on bone biopsy in metastatic castration-resistant prostate cancer. *Prostate Cancer Prostatic Dis*. 2014;17:325–331. doi:10.1038/pcan.2014.28

38. Robinson DR, Wu Y-M, Lonigro RJ, et al. Integrative clinical genomics of metastatic cancer. *Nature*. 2017;548:297–303. doi:10.1038/nature23306

39. Sweeney CJ, Chen Y-H, Carducci M, et al. Chemohormonal therapy in metastatic hormone-sensitive prostate cancer. *N Engl J Med*. 2015;373:737–746. doi:10.1056/NEJMoa1503747

40. Fizazi K, Tran N, Fein L, et al. Abiraterone plus prednisone in metastatic, castration-sensitive prostate cancer. *N Engl J Med*. 2017;377:352–360. doi:10.1056/NEJMoa1704174

41. Taylor LG, Canfield SE, Du XL. Review of major adverse effects of androgen-deprivation therapy in men with prostate cancer. *Cancer*. 2009;115:2388–2399. doi:10.1002/cncr.24283

42. Bhatia N, Santos M, Jones LW, et al. Cardiovascular effects of androgen deprivation therapy for the treatment of prostate cancer: ABCDE steps to reduce cardiovascular disease in patients with prostate cancer. *Circulation*. 2016;133:537–541. doi:10.1161/CIRCULATIONAHA.115.012519

43. Cosman F, de Beur SJ, LeBoff MS, et al. Clinician's guide to prevention and treatment of osteoporosis. *Osteoporos Int*. 2014;25:2359–2381. doi:10.1007/s00198-014-2794-2

44. AstraZeneca. *A randomised, double-blind, placebo-controlled, multicentre phase III study of olaparib plus abiraterone relative to placebo plus abiraterone as first-line therapy in men with metastatic castration-resistant prostate cancer (PROpel Study)*. November 7, 2018. Updated April 5, 2022. https://clinicaltrials.gov/ct2/show/NCT03732820.

CHAPTER 15

Testicular Cancer

Thomas C. Westbrook, Eric B. Schwartz, and Zachery R. Reichert

INTRODUCTION

Testicular germ cell tumors represent a unique treatment paradigm within the field of solid oncology. Since the introduction of cisplatin-based chemotherapy, outcomes for men with testicular cancer have improved markedly. This remains one of the few solid tumors that is highly curable in the metastatic setting.

Germ cell testicular cancers represent approximately 0.5% of all new cancers annually, with a peak incidence in men aged 20 to 35. Outcomes are highly favorable with 5-year overall survival (OS) of 95%. In addition, more than 70% of men with metastatic disease experience long-term survival and cure.[1] The high rate of cure is achieved via multimodal treatment with surgery and combination chemotherapy being key components. In contemporary care, radiation therapy (RT) is rarely used due to higher late toxicities. While outcomes remain extremely good, treatments for testicular cancer carry significant comorbidities. Therefore, a key focus is to minimize long-term toxicities such as neuropathy, hearing loss, pulmonary dysfunction, and erectile dysfunction while maintaining a high rate of cure.

Histologically, germ cell tumors are divided into seminoma and nonseminoma, with each having a unique treatment approach. Seminoma tumors make up 30% to 60% of testicular cancer and have more favorable outcomes. Nonseminoma tumors encompass several different histological subtypes and a large number of tumors present with a mixed histology.[2]

The following cases will take you through the workup and management of testicular cancer. These cases are broken down into localized seminoma, advanced seminoma, localized nonseminoma, and advanced nonseminoma. Each of these disease states has a unique treatment approach, and the key considerations are detailed in the text that follows (Table 15.1).

CASE SUMMARIES

Case 15.1: Localized Testicular Cancer—Seminoma

A 25-year-old male with a history of gastroesophageal reflux disease (GERD) presents with 2 weeks of nonpainful left testicular swelling. He has had no cough, hemoptysis, chest pain, nausea, or weight loss. Physical exam reveals no lymphadenopathy but a firm mass is palpated in the left testicle. Testicular ultrasound (US) is performed and shows a 2-cm hypoechoic lesion.

Table 15.1 Risk Stratification for Metastatic Disease

Risk	Seminoma	Nonseminoma
Good risk	Any primary site No nonpulmonary mets Normal AFP Any beta-hCG and LDH	Testicular or RP primary No nonpulmonary mets *Post-orchiectomy markers:* AFP <1000 ng/mL beta-hCG <5000 IU/L LDH <1.5 × ULN
Intermediate risk	Any primary AND Nonpulmonary visceral mets AND Normal AFP Any LDH and beta-hCG	Testicular or RP primary No nonpulmonary visceral mets *Post-orchiectomy markers:* AFP 1000–10,000 ng/mL beta-hCG 5000 – 50,000 IU/L LDH 1.5–10 × ULN
Poor risk	None	Medistinal primary OR Nonpulmonary mets OR *Post-orchiectomy markers:* AFP >10,000 ng/mL beta-hCG >50,000 IU/L LDH >10 × ULN

AFP, alpha-fetoprotein; beta-hCG, beta human chorionic gonadotropin; LDH, lactate dehydrogenase; RP, retroperitoneal; ULN, upper limit of normal.

What Are the Initial Steps In Diagnosis of Testicular Cancer?

- Evaluation of a testicular mass should include physical exam, testicular US, and assessment of tumor markers: beta-human chorionic gonadotropin (beta-hCG), alpha-fetoprotein (AFP), and lactate dehydrogenase (LDH).
- Patients with suspicious findings should not be biopsied and instead proceed directly to radical orchiectomy.
- Histology separates seminoma from nonseminoma germ cell tumors. Seminoma must be 100%; even 1% of another histology alters the diagnosis to nonseminoma.
- CT of the abdomen and pelvis is performed; chest x-ray and CT of the chest performed only if abnormal abdominal/pelvic CT or positive chest x-ray.
- MRI of the brain is used if there are neurological symptoms, nonpulmonary visceral metastasis, or extensive visceral metastasis. This is also performed with choriocarcinoma (nonseminoma histology) if the patient is metastatic.
- Repeat LDH, beta-hCG, AFP, and LDH after orchiectomy until normalization.
- Give consideration to sperm banking if indicated.

Patient's Diagnosis

- *Right radical orchiectomy is performed and shows 100% seminoma. The tumor is limited to the testis but lymphovascular invasion (LVI) is present.*
- *LDH, beta-hCG, and AFP are all within normal limits before and after surgery.*
- *Abdominal/pelvic CT and chest x-ray are negative for signs of metastatic disease.*

How Is Testicular Cancer Staged?

- The American Joint Committee on Cancer (AJCC) eighth edition staging system is used to stage testicular cancer.[3]

- Disease is staged by size; degree of invasion of surrounding structures (T); size and number of lymph nodes (N); presence and type of metastatic lesions (M); and serum markers (S).
- Stages IA, IB, and IS have no nodal or metastatic involvement.
- Stages IIA, IIB, and IIC have differing nodal involvement and serum markers.
- Stages IIIA, IIIB, and IIIC have differing metastatic involvement and serum markers.
- There is no stage IV testicular cancer because of the potential for cure even in advanced cases.

Patient's Clinical Stage
- *The patient's stage is pT2, N0, M0, S0 (stage IB).*

What Are Treatment Options for Stage I Seminoma?

- Surveillance preferred for pT1 to pT3[4]
- Single-agent carboplatin (area under the curve [AUC] = 7 × 1 or × 2 cycles)[5]
- Radiotherapy 20 Gy or 25.5 Gy[6]
- Stage IS is very rare in seminoma; patients should be referred to high-volume centers.

What Are Side Effects Associated With These Treatment Regimens?

- Carboplatin is generally well tolerated: most common acute side effects include thrombocytopenia, nausea, and vomiting.
- RT short-term side effects include fatigue, gastrointestinal (GI) side effects, and myelosuppression. Long-term risks include the risk of second malignancies, cardiovascular disease, and impaired fertility.
- Greater than 85% of men will not recur with no adjuvant treatment, and those that do recur can be cured with subsequent therapy. It is preferable to avoid side effects associated with chemotherapy or radiation with surveillance.

What Is the Recommended Surveillance Regimen?

- For men who undergo surveillance, history and physical (H&P) every 3 to 6 months for the first year, CT of the abdomen and pelvis occurs at months 3, 6, and 12 in the first year with subsequent decreasing frequency per guidelines through year 5. Testing of tumor markers is optional.
- For men who receive chemotherapy or radiation, follow-up can be less frequent: H&P every 6 to 12 months and annual CT in the first year with subsequent decreasing frequency.
- For patients who are unable/unwilling to be compliant with surveillance upfront, adjuvant therapies may be preferable.

Patient's Treatment
- *Tumor markers remained within normal limits following orchiectomy. He went on surveillance and continues on recommended follow-up.*

Case 15.2: Advanced Testicular Cancer—Seminoma

A 34-year-old male with a history of tobacco use presents with 3 weeks of a growing left testicular mass. He has had a mild increase in chronic cough but no hemoptysis. He has lost 5 lbs unintentionally in the last month. No lymphadenopathy is found on exam. A large, firm mass is appreciated in the left testicle. Testicular US shows a 4-cm hypoechoic left-sided lesion. Serum markers include AFP less than 5 ng/mL, beta-hCG 30 IU/L, and LDH 547 U/L. Left radical orchiectomy reveals 100% seminoma invading the scrotum, with margins negative. CT of the abdomen and pelvis reveals numerous retroperitoneal masses up to 2.5 cm in diameter. CT of the chest shows numerous lung masses up to 1.5 cm in size. Post-orchiectomy markers returned with an AFP less than 5 ng/mL, beat-hCG of 12 IU/L and LDH 700 U/L. He is diagnosed with stage IIIB testicular cancer (pT4, cN2, M1a, S2).

What Are the Treatment Options for Stage II Seminoma?

- Recommended treatments for stage IIA seminoma are RT (30 Gy) to include para-aortic and ipsilateral lymph nodes (LNs) or bleomycin + etoposide + cisplatin (BEP) × 3 cycles or etoposide/cisplatin (EP) × 4 cycles.
- Stage IIB can also be treated with BEP × 3 cycles or EP × 4 cycles or RT to the same areas with a different total dose, in this case to 36 Gy.
- Stage IIC is treated like stage III depending on risk classification.

What Are the Risk Categories in Metastatic Seminoma?

- All stage IIC to III seminomas are good risk unless there are nonpulmonary visceral metastases present (for example, brain, bone, liver), in which case it is intermediate risk.

What Are the Treatment Options for Stage III (and IIC) Seminoma?

- Good-risk stage IIC to IIIC seminoma are treated with BEP × 3 cycles[7] or EP × 4 cycles, similar to stage IIB-C disease. Radiotherapy is not an option.
- Intermediate-risk stage IIC to IIIC seminoma can be treated with BEP × 4 cycles or etoposide + ifosfamide + cisplatin (VIP) × 4 cycles.

What Are Side Effects Associated With Initial Chemotherapy Used in Advanced Seminoma?

- All regimens contain cisplatin and etoposide: Side effects include myelosuppression, nausea, fatigue, hair loss, hearing loss, renal toxicity, and peripheral neuropathy.
- Bleomycin rarely causes pulmonary fibrosis, which can be fatal. It occurs more frequently with older patients and those with underlying lung disease. Guidelines recommend avoiding bleomycin in patients older than 50 years of age, patients with underlying lung disease, or active smokers. Bleomycin also frequently causes a rash (often on palmar and plantar surfaces).

Patient's Diagnosis and Treatment

- *The patient is diagnosed with good-risk stage IIIB seminoma. Because he is a smoker, he is treated with etoposide/cisplatin × 4 cycles.*

What Is Done After Primary Treatment With Chemotherapy in Advanced Seminoma?

- Tumor markers are rechecked, and CT of the abdomen and pelvis is performed.
- If there is no residual mass or the mass is less than 3 cm, and AFP and beta-hCG are both normal, begin surveillance.
- If there is a residual mass greater than 3 cm with normal AFP/beta-hCG, surveillance or fluorodeoxyglucose (FDG) PET/CT can be considered.

- If PET/CT is positive at the mass, resection or biopsy can be considered. If complete resection is achieved showing seminoma, ×2 cycles of adjuvant chemotherapy is recommended. Options include EP, paclitaxel, ifosfamide, and cisplatin (TIP), VIP, or vinblastine, ifosfamide, and cisplatin (VeIP). If no active disease, begin surveillance. If complete resection cannot be done with active disease/PET, move on to second-line therapy.
- If disease is growing on post-treatment CT or tumor markers are rising, move to second-line therapy.

Patient's Post-Treatment Follow-Up
- *Post-treatment CT shows no signs of residual disease and tumor markers normalize. He enters surveillance.*

What Does Surveillance Entail in Advance Seminoma?

- The surveillance schedule for IIA-B nonbulky seminoma is very similar to stage I after orchiectomy alone, although chest x-rays are recommended every 6 months for the first 6 months.
- Bulky stage IIA-B, stage IIC, and all stage III require intensive follow-up strategies, which include H&P and chest x-ray every 2 months for the first year and every 3 months in the second year with subsequent decreasing frequency per guidelines. CT of the abdomen and pelvis should be performed every 4 months in the first year with decreasing frequency.

Patient's Post-Treatment Surveillance
- *A 9-month post-treatment CT of the abdomen and pelvis shows a suspicious 1.5-cm mass in the retroperitoneum. Tumor markers remain within normal limits. He is asymptomatic. The mass is biopsied and reveals 100% seminoma.*

What Are Options in Second-Line Therapy for Seminoma?

1. Surgical salvage is recommended if recurrence is greater than 2 years after completion of primary treatment and may be considered in solitary lesions if recurrence is less than 2 years from primary treatment completion.
2. Conventional dose chemotherapy with VeIP or TIP are common salvage regimens.
3. High-dose chemotherapy with stem cell rescue is another option. Common regimens include carboplatin/etoposide or paclitaxel/ifosfamide/carboplatin/etoposide.

There is an ongoing trial to better answer whether conventional chemotherapy or a regimen which requires autologous stem cell transplant high-dose chemotherapy is preferred in the line of therapy.[8] An early trial suggested a high-dose regimen containing carboplatin may be superior to conventional dose chemotherapy.[9]

Patient's Second-Line Therapy and Follow-Up
The patient receives TIP × 4 cycles with post-treatment CT showing complete response. He re-enters surveillance.

What Are Third-Line Options in Seminoma?

- High-dose chemotherapy with stem-cell rescue is preferred (if not already received); otherwise multiple alternate standard dose combination regimens remain options.
- The tumor should be tested for microsatellite instability (MSI) and tumor mutational burden (TMB). High levels of each (MSI-H and TMB-H) are eligible for pembrolizumab.

Case 15.3: Locally Advanced Nonseminoma Testicular Cancer

A 30-year-old male with no prior medical history presents to a urologist for swelling of his left testicle. He first noticed the mass 1 month ago and thinks it has enlarged. An US confirms a solid mass concerning for malignancy. Tumor markers are obtained and show AFP of 50 ng/mL, beta-HCG of 15 IU/L, and LDH of 172 U/L. An orchiectomy is performed and pathology reveals a mixed germ cell tumor with 80% embryonal, 10% yolk sac, and 10% seminoma components. Lymphovascular invasion (LVI) is seen. There is no invasion of the spermatic cord or scrotum. Repeat tumor markers 4 weeks later show normalization of AFP and beta-hCG. CT of the chest, abdomen, and pelvis reveal no additional suspicious lesions.

Patient's Workup

- *Given the suspicious findings, he underwent a radical orchiectomy.*
- *Postoperatively, he underwent appropriate staging with imaging and tumor markers.*

What Are the Subtypes of Nonseminomatous Germ Cell Tumor?

- There are four primary nonseminoma histologies with some typical marker patterns:
  - Embryonal: AFP and beta-hCG may be elevated
  - Choriocarcinoma: beta-hCG elevated
  - Yolk sac: AFP elevated
  - Teratoma: no marker elevation
  - All tumor types can have LDH elevation.
- A large percentage of germ cell tumors are mixed type.

How Would This Patient's Disease Be Characterized?

- *Since the seminoma component is not 100%, this patient has a mixed, nonseminoma germ cell testicular tumor.*
- *This patient has a T2N0M0S0 stage IB tumor with no lymph node involvement.*

What Are the Treatment Options for Stage I Nonseminoma?

- Patients with stage I disease and normalization of tumor markers can be divided into high- or low-risk categories.
- High-risk features include LVI, invasion of spermatic cord or scrotum, or embryonal histology.[10]
- Low-risk patients should generally be observed unless unwilling or unable to participate reliably in the surveillance plan.
  - Observation includes periodic clinical exams, tumor markers, and imaging (CT of the abdomen and pelvis and chest x-rays).
    - Goal with observation is to minimize radiation exposure while identifying potential recurrences.
    - Catching recurrence early is less critical as advanced disease is curable.
- Many high-risk patients can also be observed.
  - Retroperitoneal lymph node dissection (RPLND) or chemotherapy can be considered.
    - Surgery can identify occult stage II disease in some patients.
    - Surgery carries notable risks including erectile dysfunction.
  - One cycle of chemotherapy with BEP can reduce recurrence risk from ~30% to a range of 1% to 3%.[11]
  - Survival benefits are minimal with additional therapy as OS with stage I disease is approximately 98%.
    - Advanced testicular cancer is curable, so the benefit of chemotherapy initially versus at relapse is debatable.

Treatment for the Patient
- *Our patient has stage IB disease with high-risk features (LVI).*
- *One cycle of BEP or RPLND could be considered, although observation would also be appropriate.*

What Are the Treatment Options for Stage II Nonseminoma
- The first step is to ensure negative tumor markers.
- Patients with persistent marker elevation should be treated as having advanced disease.
  - Beta-hCG has a shorter half-life than AFP, so it is expected to normalize more rapidly.
- For patients with negative markers, either RPLND or chemotherapy can be considered.[12]
  - Those with multifocal or highly symptomatic disease should typically receive chemotherapy.
  - Chemotherapy options are either BEP × 3 cycles or EP × 4 cycles.
    - Both options are equivalent; determination is based on toxicities.

Treatment Considerations
- *Our patient has no contraindications to either chemotherapy regimen so BEP × 3 cycles or EP × 4 cycles would be appropriate if he had LN involvement.*

How Are Patients Followed After Treatment?
- Following chemotherapy, patients should have repeat staging.
  - If complete response, patients can be observed.
  - Any persistently involved LNs greater than 1 cm should be addressed with RPLND.
- After primary RPLND (implying no chemotherapy prior to surgery), N2 (2 to 5 cm or extranodal extension) or N3 (greater than 5 cm) LN disease should receive treatment.
  - Patients with N2 disease can receive 2 cycles of EP or BEP.
  - Patients with N3 disease should receive BEP × 3 cycles or EP × 4 cycles.
- Follow-up is similar to that of stage I patients.
  - Clinical exam, tumor markers, and imaging (CT of the abdomen and pelvis and chest X-ray)

What Follow-Up Should Our Patient Receive?
- *For stage I disease, the patient should receive tumor markers every 2 months, CT of the abdomen and pelvis every 4 to 6 months, and a chest x-ray at month 4 and 12 during the first year. Follow-up can be spaced out based on National Comprehensive Cancer Network (NCCN) guidelines after this.*

Case 15.4: Metastatic Nonseminoma Testicular Cancer

A 27-year-old male with no prior medical history presents to his primary care doctor with 1 month of right testicular pain and swelling. A testicular US is suspicious for a testicular mass. Tumor markers are obtained, showing LDH of 431 U/L, AFP of 1.7 ng/mL, and beta-hCG of 113,720 IU/L. He undergoes a radical orchiectomy with pathology revealing 70% seminoma and 30% choriocarcinoma. LVI and invasion of the spermatic cord are seen. No scrotal invasion is seen. Repeat tumor markers 4 weeks later are notable for LDH of 714 U/L, AFP of 2.2 ng/mL, and beta-hCG of 206,250 IU/L. CT of the chest, abdomen, and pelvis reveal enlarged retroperitoneal LNs (largest measuring 4 cm) along with pulmonary and hepatic lesions suspicious for metastatic disease.

How Is Metastatic Testicular Cancer Risk Stratified?

- Patients with metastatic germ cell tumors require risk stratification into good, intermediate, and poor-risk categories.
  - Pure seminoma can only be good- or intermediate-risk (predicated on the presence or absence of nonpulmonary metastases).
  - Nonseminoma tumors are stratified based on primary tumor site, metastatic sites, and tumor markers (Table 15.1).
    - Tumor markers for stratification must be *post*-orchiectomy, and the half-lives of each tumor marker may need to be considered.

How Would This Patient's Disease Be Characterized?

- *As this patient does not have a pure seminoma, he should be treated as a nonseminoma germ cell tumor.*
- *His tumor stage is T3N2M1bS3 stage IIIC.*
- *He has poor-risk disease based on beta-hCG level and the presence of nonpulmonary metastases.*

What Are the Treatment Options for Metastatic Testicular Cancer?

- All patients with metastatic disease require platinum-based chemotherapy.
- Patients with good-risk disease can receive either BEP × 3 cycles or EP × 4 cycles.
  - Determination is based on toxicity profile for a given patient.
- Patients with intermediate- or poor-risk disease require 4 cycles of chemotherapy.
  - BEP is the preferred regimen for these patients.
  - If bleomycin is contraindicated, the recommended regimen is VeIP × 4 cycles.

What Treatment Should Our Patient Receive?

- *Given his poor-risk disease, he should receive BEP × 4 cycles.*
- *If contraindications to bleomycin are identified, VeIP would be an alternative treatment.*

What Follow-Up Is Needed After Treatment?

- If patients have a complete response *and* normalization of tumor markers, they can transition to surveillance.
- Patients with residual disease and resolving markers should undergo surgical resection of all masses if possible.
  - Teratoma is particularly insensitive to chemotherapy, so this post-chemotherapy surgery removes any residual disease. If living nonteratoma disease is found, further chemotherapy is warranted.
  - The risk of leaving residual mature teratoma is that the teratoma cells may become malignant themselves (for example, a teratoma consisting of mature intestinal cells develops colonic adenocarcinoma).
- If a patient has rising tumor markers or progressive disease, they should undergo second-line treatment for refractory disease.

How Are Brain Metastasis Managed?

- Neurological imaging should be performed as part of initial staging for patients at significant risk of brain metastases.
  - Central nervous system (CNS) risk features include choriocarcinoma histology, beta-hCG greater than 5,000 IU/L, AFP greater than 10,000 ng/mL, or nonpulmonary visceral metastases.

- ○ Patients with any symptomatic or clinical neurological findings should undergo brain imaging.
- Between 10% and 15% of patients with advanced disease are found to have brain metastases.
  - ○ These patients have a worse prognosis.[13]
- Patients should receive chemotherapy for poor-risk disease.
  - ○ Four cycles of BEP or VIP are needed if bleomycin ineligible.
- Neurosurgical resection or radiation can be considered, although it is unclear if these approaches improve survival.[14]

Should This Patient Undergo Central Nervous System Imaging?
- *This patient should undergo MRI of the brain because he is at increased risk of CNS metastases.*
- *High-risk features include elevated AFP and beta-hCG as well as extrapulmonary visceral disease.*

What Are Options for Treatment of Relapsed or Refractory Disease?
- Patients who are candidates for autologous stem cell transplant should receive high-dose chemotherapy with autologous transplant for 2 to 3 cycles.
  - ○ High-dose chemotherapy regimens:
    - Carboplatin and etoposide
    - Paclitaxel, ifosfamide, carboplatin, and etoposide
- Patients who cannot receive high-dose chemotherapy should receive conventional chemotherapy.
  - ○ Conventional dose chemotherapy regimens:
    - TIP
    - VeIP
- Patients are considered curable in the second-line setting.
  - ○ These patients should undergo resection of any residual masses if they have partial response and declining tumor markers.

What Is Required for Follow-Up and Survivorship?
- Patients should undergo surveillance for a minimum of 5 years after treatment.
- Patients require monitoring for long-term sequela of chemotherapy.
  - ○ Long-term risks of BEP treatment include pulmonary fibrosis, neuropathy, hearing loss, and risk of secondary leukemia.

If This Patient Has a Complete Response to Treatment, What Follow-Up Should He Receive?
- *This patient has a treated stage III nonseminoma.*
- *He should receive clinical exam and tumor markers every 2 months; CT of the abdomen and pelvis every 6 months; and chest x-ray every 6 months for the first year.*
- *Ongoing surveillance at increasing intervals should continue for a minimum of 5 years.*

REVIEW QUESTIONS

1. A 20-year-old man presents to the ED with abdominal pain after a motor vehicle accident. CT of the chest, abdomen, and pelvis reveals no acute abnormality but a 3-cm heterogenous right testicular mass and suspicious retroperitoneal lymph nodes (LNs) up to 1.5 cm are incidentally discovered. He has been entirely asymptomatic. Which of the following is not required to complete staging for testicular cancer for this patient?
   A. Alpha-fetoprotein (AFP)
   B. Lactate dehydrogenase (LDH)
   C. Beta-human chorionic gonadotropin (beta-hCG)
   D. Right orchiectomy
   E. MRI of the brain

2. A 22-year-old man presents with 4 weeks of left testicular swelling and testicular mass. Scrotal ultrasound (US) shows a 2-cm echodense mass in the left testicle concerning for malignancy. Left radical orchiectomy shows 100% seminoma histology with invasion of the spermatic cord. CT of the abdomen and pelvis and chest x-ray show multiple enlarged lymph nodes (LNs) in the pelvis. Which of the following additional findings would change your chemotherapy management choice?
   A. Lactate dehydrogenase (LDH) greater than 2000
   B. LN greater than 6 cm
   C. Multiple pulmonary metastases
   D. Liver metastasis

3. A 26-year-old man presents with 2 weeks of a rapidly growing left testicular mass. He has not had other symptoms. Ultrasound (US) reveals a 3-cm intratesticular lesion. Alpha-fetoprotein (AFP) is less than 5 ng/mL, beta-human chorionic gonadotropin (beta-hCG) is 14 IU/L, and lactate dehydrogenase (LDH) is 270 ng/mL. Left radical orchiectomy is performed and shows 100% seminoma. Post-orchiectomy AFP is less than 5 ng/mL, beta-hCG is 10 ng/mL, and LDH is 254 ng/mL. CT of the abdomen and pelvis show retroperitoneal lymph nodes (LNs) up to 3 cm in size. CT of the chest shows scattered masses bilaterally up to 1.5 cm in size. Which of the following is the most appropriate treatment plan?
   A. Bleomycin, etoposide, and cisplatin (BEP) × 3 cycles
   B. BEP × 3 cycles followed by fluorodeoxyglucose (FDG)-PET imaging and surgical resection of any FDG-avid lesions
   C. BEP × 4 cycles
   D. BEP × 4 cycles followed by FDG-PET imaging and surgical resection of any FDG-avid lesions

4. A 19-year-old man presents with 4 weeks of painless testicular swelling. Scrotal ultrasound (US) shows a 1.5-cm echodense mass in the left testicle. Left orchiectomy is performed and shows 100% seminoma limited to the testis but with lymphovascular involvement. Post-orchiectomy serum tumor markers are within normal limits. CT of the abdomen and pelvis reveal no suspicious lesions. All of the following are reasonable next steps except:
   A. Begin surveillance
   B. Single-agent carboplatin × 1 cycle
   C. Radiation therapy (RT) 20 Gy
   D. Nerve-sparing retroperitoneal lymph node dissection (RPLND)

5. A 54-year-old man presents with 6 weeks of scrotal swelling and fullness. He has had a 10-lb unintentional weight loss over the past 3 months and some nausea/vomiting. He has

a history of hypertension and right hip arthritis but no known heart, lung, liver, or kidney disease. His Eastern Cooperative Oncology Group (ECOG) performance status is 0. Scrotal ultrasound (US) shows a 5-cm mass involving the right testis with extension to the scrotum. Right radical orchiectomy is performed, and pathology shows 100% seminoma involving the scrotum. CT of the chest, abdomen, and pelvis show retroperitoneal lesions up to 4.5 cm in size, multiple suspicious liver lesions, and scattered lung lesions up to 2 cm. MRI of the brain shows 2 subcentimeter lesions suspicious for metastatic disease. Which of the following is the best choice for further treatment?

A. Bleomycin, etoposide, and cisplatin (BEP) × 3 cycles
B. BEP × 4 cycles
C. Etoposide and cisplatin (EP) × 4 cycles
D. Etoposide, ifosfamide, and cisplatin (VIP) × 4 cycles
E. Vinblastine, ifosfamide, and cisplatin (VeIP) × 4 cycles

6. A 25-year-old male presents to his primary care doctor for a testicular mass. An ultrasound (US) is concerning for malignancy. Labs are obtained and reveal lactate dehydrogenase (LDH) of 200 U/L, alpha-fetoprotein (AFP) of 400 ng/mL, and beta-human chorionic gonadotropin (beta-hCG) of 10 IU/L. He undergoes an orchiectomy, which reveals a mixed germ cell tumor with 20% seminoma, 50% embryonal, and 30% yolk sac. Lymphovascular invasion (LVI) is seen. There is no involvement of the spermatic cord or scrotum. Staging CT of the chest, abdomen, and pelvis show no enlarged retroperitoneal lymph nodes (LNs) and no other abnormalities. Tumor markers normalize 4 weeks later. Which of the following is the most appropriate next step?

A. Adjuvant bleomycin, etoposide, and cisplatin (BEP) × 3 cycles
B. Etoposide and cisplatin (EP) × 4 cycles
C. Clinical observation
D. BEP × 1 cycle followed by retroperitoneal LN dissection (RPLND)

7. A 29-year-old male with no prior medical history undergoes a radical orchiectomy for a suspicious testicular mass, which reveals a mixed germ cell tumor with embryonal, teratoma, and yolk sac components. Staging CT scans show several enlarged retroperitoneal lymph nodes (LNs), with the largest measuring 4 cm. Tumor markers prior to surgery are: lactate dehydrogenase (LDH) of 300 U/L, alpha-fetoprotein (AFP) of 250 ng/mL, and beta-human chorionic gonadotropin (beta-hCG) less than 5 IU/L. Four weeks after surgery, LDH has normalized and AFP is 30 ng/mL. Which of the following would be the most appropriate treatment?

A. Recheck tumor markers in 1 month and observe if normalized
B. Bleomycin, etoposide, and cisplatin (BEP) × 3 cycles
C. Retroperitoneal LN dissection (RPLND) followed by BEP × 1 cycle
D. Stereotactic radiation to retroperitoneal LNs

8. A 27-year-old male undergoes a radical orchiectomy for a suspicious testicular mass, which reveals a mixed germ cell tumor with embryonal, teratoma, and yolk sac components. He has no prior medical history but smokes one pack of cigarettes per day. Staging CT scans show several enlarged retroperitoneal lymph nodes (LNs), with the largest measuring 3.5 cm. Tumor markers prior to surgery are: lactate dehydrogenase (LDH) of 280 U/L, alpha-fetoprotein (AFP) of 300 ng/mL, and beta-human chorionic gonadotropin (beta-hCG) less than 5. Four weeks after surgery, LDH has normalized and AFP is 35 ng/mL. Which of the following would be the most appropriate treatment?

A. Bleomycin, etoposide, and cisplatin (BEP) × 3 cycles
B. Etoposide, ifosfamide, and cisplatin (VIP) × 4 cycles

C. Etoposide and cisplatin (EP) × 4 cycles

D. Recheck tumor markers in 1 month and observe if normalized

9. A 31-year-old male previously underwent treatment with bleomycin, etoposide, and cisplatin (BEP) × 4 cycles for a mixed germ cell tumor with metastases to lung, retroperitoneal lymph nodes (LNs), and liver. He had normalization of tumor markers and complete radiological response. However, 6 months later, his alpha-fetoprotein (AFP) reaches 200 ng/mL and repeat CT imaging shows numerous new pulmonary lesions and enlarging retroperitoneal LNs concerning for recurrence. He otherwise feels well and has no other medical conditions. Which of the following is most appropriate?

A. High-dose carboplatin and etoposide followed by autologous stem cell transplant

B. Additional BEP × 4 cycles

C. Paclitaxel, ifosfamide, and cisplatin (TIP) × 4 cycles

D. Pembrolizumab 200 mg every 3 weeks

10. A 34-year-old male with a history of chronic back pain and intermittent sciatic nerve pain undergoes a right radical orchiectomy for suspected testicular mass on ultrasound (US). Pathology reveals a mixed germ cell tumor with seminoma, yolk sac, and choriocarcinoma components. Tumor markers 4 weeks later are lactate dehydrogenase (LDH) of 400 U/L, alpha-fetoprotein (AFP) of 5000 ng/mL, and beta-human chorionic gonadotropin (beta-hCG) of 60,000 IU/L. CT imaging shows six suspicious pulmonary nodules and two enlarged retroperitoneal lymph nodes (LNs). MRI of the brain is negative. Which of the following is the most appropriate treatment?

A. Surgical resection of all sites of disease

B. Bleomycin, etoposide, and cisplatin (BEP) × 4 cycles

C. Carboplatin and etoposide × 4 cycles

D. Bleomycin and etoposide × 4 cycles

ANSWERS AND RATIONALES

1. **E. MRI of the brain.** Only patients who have neurological symptoms, nonpulmonary metastasis, or extensive pulmonary/lymphadenopathy metastasis require MRI of the brain. All of the other items are required to complete staging.

2. **D. Liver metastasis.** This patient has at least stage II seminoma. Bleomycin + etoposide + cisplatin × 3 cycles or etoposide + cisplatin × 4 cycles are the treatments of choice for good-risk stage II to III seminoma. LDH, LN bulk, or presence of pulmonary metastasis may change the stage but do not alter risk stratification. Presence of nonpulmonary metastasis (liver) would change the risk category to intermediate and alter treatment recommendation.

3. **A. Bleomycin, etoposide, and cisplatin (BEP) × 3 cycles.** This patient has good-risk stage IIIA seminoma. BEP × 3 cycles is a treatment of choice for seminoma stage IIA, IIB and good-risk IIC to IIIC. CT and, to a lesser extent, tumor markers are used post-treatment to assess response in seminoma. FDG-PET/CT can be considered if partial response is found on CT and residual masses are greater than 3 cm.

4. **D. Nerve-sparing retroperitoneal lymph node dissection (RPLND).** This patient has stage IB (pT2, cN0, M0, S0) seminoma. Choices A to C are reasonable options, although surveillance is preferred. RPLND currently has no role in seminoma, though it is an option in a variety of nonseminoma scenarios.

5. **D. Etoposide, ifosfamide, and cisplatin (VIP) × 4 cycles.** This patient has intermediate-risk stage IIIC seminoma. BEP × 4 cycles is an option for patients with intermediate-risk stage IIC to IIIC seminoma and is often preferred to VIP but is generally not used in patients older than 50 or those with underlying lung disease because of increased risk of pulmonary fibrosis. BEP × 3 cycles can be used in stage IIA, IIB, and good-risk IIC to IIIC disease. VeIP is generally reserved for second-line or salvage chemotherapy.

6. **C. Clinical observation.** This patient was diagnosed with a stage I nonseminoma germ cell tumor. He does have high-risk features, including LVI and embryonal component. Therefore, additional treatment with either a retroperitoneal LN dissection or 1 cycle of chemotherapy with BEP could be considered. These treatments may lower his risk of recurrence but are unlikely to improve his survival. Additional cycles of chemotherapy should not be given for stage 1 disease so answers A and B are incorrect. Combined chemotherapy and RPLND are too aggressive, so answer D is incorrect.

7. **B. Bleomycin, etoposide, and cisplatin (BEP) × 3 cycles.** This patient has a stage IIB nonseminoma germ cell tumor. He therefore requires additional treatment, even with improving tumor markers, so answer A is incorrect. Appropriate options would be RPLND or chemotherapy with either BEP × 3 cycles or etoposide and cisplatin (EP) × 4 cycles. If surgery is performed, adjuvant chemotherapy is based on pathological LN size, but 1 cycle would never be appropriate, so answer C is incorrect. Radiation therapy (RT) does not play a role in this patient's treatment, so answer D is incorrect.

8. **C. Etoposide and cisplatin (EP) × 4 cycles.** This patient has a stage IIB nonseminoma germ cell tumor. He therefore requires additional treatment, so answer D is incorrect. Either BEP × 3 cycles or EP × 4 cycles are appropriate for patients with stage II disease. However, given his smoking history, bleomycin should be avoided, so answer A is incorrect. VIP is used for patients with metastatic disease who cannot receive bleomycin but would be unnecessary in this patient, so answer B is incorrect.

9. **A. High-dose carboplatin and etoposide followed by autologous stem cell transplant.** This patient had stage III disease with an initial response to appropriate first-line chemotherapy, but a quick relapse 6 months later. He appears to be a candidate for stem cell transplant, so he should undergo high-dose chemotherapy with stem cell rescue. Repeating BEP × 4 cycles would not be appropriate. TIP chemotherapy could be considered if he is not transplant eligible, but high-dose chemotherapy is preferred. Pembrolizumab is not a standard therapy in testicular cancer, so answer D is incorrect.

10. **B. Bleomycin, etoposide, and cisplatin (BEP) × 4 cycles.** This patient has a metastatic germ cell tumor. Based on his post-orchiectomy tumor markers, he has intermediate-risk disease and requires systemic treatment. Although he has underlying nerve damage, cisplatin is a key component of treatment with curative intent in testicular cancer so should not be withheld in his case. The alternative systemic regimens listed would not be adequate. Surgical resection of residual disease is considered after chemotherapy, but this patient requires systemic treatment, so answer A is incorrect.

REFERENCES

1. Surveillance, Epidemiology, and End Results Program. *Cancer stat facts: testicular cancer.* National Cancer Institute. 2021. https://seer.cancer.gov/statfacts/html/testis.html
2. Milose JC, Filson CP, Weizer AZ, et al. Role of biochemical markers in testicular cancer: diagnosis, staging, and surveillance. *Open Access J Urol.* 2011;4:1–8. doi:10.2147/OAJU.S15063
3. Edge SB. *American Joint Committee on Cancer. AJCC Cancer Staging Manual.* 8th ed. Springer, 2017.
4. National Comprehensive Cancer Network. *Testicular Cancer* Version 1.2022. http://www.nccn.org/professionals/physician_gls/pdf/bone.pdf
5. Oliver RT, Mead GM, Rustin GJ, et al. Randomized trial of carboplatin versus radiotherapy for stage I seminoma: mature results on relapse and contralateral testis cancer rates in MRC TE19/EORTC 30982 study (ISRCTN27163214). *J Clin Oncol.* 2011;29(8):957–962. doi:10.1200/JCO.2009.26.4655
6. Einhorn LH, Williams SD, Loehrer PJ, et al. Evaluation of optimal duration of chemotherapy in favorable-prognosis disseminated germ cell tumors: a southeastern cancer study group protocol. *J Clin Oncol.* 1989;7(3):387–391. doi:10.1200/JCO.1989.7.3.387
7. Mead GM, Fossa SD, Oliver RT, et al. Randomized trials in 2466 patients with stage I seminoma: patterns of relapse and follow-up. *J Natl Cancer Inst.* 2011;103(3):241–249. doi:10.1093/jnci/djq525
8. Ongoing Clinical Trials in Testicular Cancer: The TIGER trial. *Oncol Res Treat.* 2016;39(9):553–556. doi:10.1159/000448868
9. Lorch A, Bascoul-Mollevi C, Kramar A, et al. Conventional-dose versus high-dose chemotherapy as first salvage treatment in male patients with metastatic germ cell tumors: evidence from a large international database. *J Clin Oncol.* 2011;29(16):2178–2184. doi:10.1200/JCO.2010.32.6678
10. de Wit R, Fizazi K. Controversies in the management of clinical stage I testis cancer. *J Clin Oncol.* 2006;24(35):5482–5492. doi:10.1200/JCO.2006.07.9434
11. Tandstad T, Ståhl O, Håkansson U, et al. One course of adjuvant BEP in clinical stage I nonseminoma mature and expanded results from the SWENOTECA group. *Ann Oncol.* 2014;25:2167–2172. doi:10.1093/annonc/mdu375
12. Weissbach L, Bussar-Maatz R, Flechtner H, et al. RPLND or primary chemotherapy in clinical stage IIA/B nonseminomatous germ cell tumors? Results of a prospective multicenter trial including quality of life assessment. *Eur Urol.* 2000;37:582–594. doi:10.1159/000020197
13. Bokemeyer C, Nowak P, Haupt A, et al. Treatment of brain metastases in patients with testicular cancer. *J Clin Oncol.* 1997;15:1449–1454. doi:10.1200/JCO.1997.15.4.1449
14. Feldman DR, Lorch A, Kramar A, et al. Brain metastases in patients with germ cell tumors: prognostic factors and treatment options—an analysis from the global germ cell cancer group. *J Clin Oncol.* 2016;34:345–351. doi:10.1200/JCO.2015.62.7000

CHAPTER 16

Renal Cancer

Eric Granowicz and Mamta Parikh

INTRODUCTION

Renal cell carcinoma (RCC) is the ninth most common cause of cancer in the United States.[1] Numerous histological subtypes are seen, with clear cell being the most common (about 75% of cases) and the most extensively studied, while the remaining variants are collectively referred to as non-clear cell. Cancers that occur near the renal pelvis often have urothelial histology, similar to bladder cancer. This chapter will largely focus on the clear cell variety, which has different prognosis and treatment recommendations when compared to other variants.

RCC is more common in the developed world, with an incidence of about 14.9/100,000 in the United States in 2016, almost twice as high as the incidence reported in the 1970s. RCC is almost twice as common in men than women. The median age at diagnosis is 64. Smoking remains an important modifiable risk factor, while family history represents an important unmodifiable risk factor often associated with a hereditary RCC syndrome.[1]

Most cases of RCC are asymptomatic at diagnosis with a renal mass incidentally noted on imaging of the abdomen. The classic clinical presentation is flank pain, a renal mass, and hematuria, although this is only seen in about 9% of cases.[2] Various paraneoplastic phenomena have been seen with RCC including polycythemia, thrombocytosis, hypercalcemia, transaminitis (Stauffer's syndrome), and Cushing's disease. Early-stage RCCs are typically managed by a urologist, with lesions less than 4 cm sometimes followed with routine surveillance, and larger lesions managed with partial or radical nephrectomy. The medical oncologist largely plays a role in managing more advanced locoregional or metastatic disease. The remainder of this chapter will focus on these clinical scenarios.

CASE SUMMARIES

Case 16.1: Early-Stage Renal Cell Carcinoma

A 58-year-old woman with no past medical history (PMH) presents with 2 weeks of painless hematuria. This was first noted 1 month ago and has become more persistent over the last week, with passage of small clots. She denies any dysuria, urgency, frequency, or pain with urination, but has experienced some discomfort in her right flank region. Physical examination reveals a 5-cm palpable mass in the right flank region.

How Is a Diagnosis Established?

- Although the clinical presentation of painless hematuria with flank pain and a palpable kidney mass is classic for RCC, it is also rare, with only 9% of cases associated with all three findings.[2]
- Early-stage RCC can usually be diagnosed clinically with a CT scan of the abdomen with intravenous (IV) contrast or renal ultrasound (US) based off of its distinct radiographic features.
- MRI of the abdomen can be considered in cases where other imaging modalities are equivocal.
- Staging evaluation should be completed with CT of the abdomen and pelvis with IV contrast and chest x-ray or CT of the chest to assess for metastatic disease. Patients with bone pain or neurological symptoms can also be assessed with bone scan or MRI of the brain, respectively.
- Percutaneous biopsy of a renal mass with imaging findings consistent with RCC is generally not warranted unless the mass is less than 4 cm and a nonsurgical treatment approach is being considered.

Patient's Diagnosis

- Renal US shows a 7.3-cm mass in the right kidney concerning for RCC.
- CT of the abdomen and pelvis with IV contrast confirms a 7.4-cm mass in the right renal parenchyma consistent with RCC without any locoregional lymphadenopathy or distant metastases.
- CT of the chest does not reveal any distant metastases.

What Further Molecular or Genomic Testing Is Required?

- No genetic testing is required for early-stage RCC, but a thorough family history and physical exam should be performed to assess for the possibility of hereditary RCC that would warrant genetic counseling and appropriate testing (Table 16.1).

How Is This Tumor Staged?

- RCC is staged using the eighth edition of the American Joint Committee on Cancer/Union for International Cancer Control (AJCC/UICC) tumor, node, and metastasis (TNM) staging system published in 2017.
- Stage IV disease requires distant metastases or invasion of the primary tumor beyond Gerota's fascia into the ipsilateral adrenal gland (T4 and/or M1).
- Stage I to III is localized to the kidney and local lymph nodes (LNs). Stage I tumors are 7 cm or less (T1N0). Stage II disease requires a T2 tumor, which is greater than 7 cm (T2a) or greater than 10 cm (T2b). Stage III disease requires invasion of major veins or perinephric tissues (not beyond Gerota's fascia) and/or regional LN involvement (T3 and/or N1).

Patient's Clinical Stage

- Stage II (cT2N0M0)

What Are Appropriate Treatment Options?

- For surgical candidates with cT1b and larger tumors, partial nephrectomy or radical nephrectomy is recommended with greater than 80% to 90% of patients achieving long-term survival.[3-4]

Table 16.1 Hereditary Renal Cell Carcinoma Syndromes

Syndrome	Gene	Histology	Clinical Features	Other Malignancies
von Hippel-Lindau (VHL)	VHL	Clear cell	Pancreatic cysts	Hemangioblastomas, pheochromocytomas, paragangliomas
Tuberous sclerosis complex (TSC)	TSC1/TSC2	Clear cell, angiomyolipoma	Hypomelanotic macules, retinal hamartomas, Shagreen patch	Cardiac rhabdomyoma, angiofibroma, lyphangioleiomyomatosis, subependymal giant cell
BAP1 tumor predisposition syndrome (TPDS)	BAP1	Clear cell, chromophobe	Atypical Spitz tumors	Melanoma, uveal melanoma, mesothelioma
Hereditary paragangliomas/pheochromocytoma syndrome	SDHA/B/C/D	Clear cell, chormophobe, oncocytoma, papillary		Paragangliomas, pheochromocytomas
PTEN hamartoma syndrome (PHTS)	PTEN	Clear cell	Macrocephaly, mucocutaneous lesions, gastrointestinal hamartomas	Breast cancer, endometrial cancer, follicular thyroid cancer
Familial clear cell renal carcinoma with chromosome 3 translocation	Translocation Chr 3	Clear cell		
Hereditary papillary renal carcinoma (HPRC)	MET	Papillary		
Birt-Hogg-Dubé syndrome (BHDS)	FLCN	Chormophobe, oncocytic, papillary	Fibrofolliculoma, pulmonary cysts, spontaneous pneumothorax	
Hereditary leiomyomatosis and renal cell carcinoma	HLRCC/FH	Papillary		Cutaneous leiomyomas, uterine leiomyomas

- Patients with or at risk for developing kidney disease can also be managed with partial nephrectomy with similar results if all disease is felt to be surgically resectable with partial nephrectomy.[5]
- For some frail patients, T1b tumors may be followed with active surveillance.

Recommended Treatment Plan for This Patient
- *Radical nephrectomy is performed, with pathology showing a 8-cm RCC, clear cell type, with tumor extending into the renal vein but not beyond Gerota's fascia. No LNs are involved and margins are negative. Final staging is stage III (pT3N0M0).*

What Are Other Treatment Considerations?

- Patients with stage II disease should undergo surveillance, but there is no adjuvant therapy available for this patient population.
- One year of pembrolizumab can be offered to those with stage III disease treated with nephrectomy. In the KEYNOTE-564 trial, high-risk (stage III or worse) clear cell RCC patients who were treated with nephrectomy (and metastatectomy for oligometastatic disease) were randomized to adjuvant pembrolizumab or placebo for up to 17 cycles. Pembrolizumab demonstrated improved 2-year disease-free survival (DFS; 77.3% vs. 68.1%) without a clear overall survival (OS) advantage at this point in follow-up. Grade 3 or greater toxicity occurred in 32.4% of patients.[6]
- Sunitinib is also approved in the stage III setting with improvement in DFS, although toxicity (hypertension, hand–foot syndrome, rash, fatigue) limits its use. In a randomized, double-blind, Phase 3 trial, patients with locoregional, high-risk clear cell RCC were randomized to sunitinib (4 weeks on, 2 weeks off) or placebo for up to 1 year. The median duration of DFS was improved with sunitinib (6.8 vs. 5.6 years) without an OS benefit and a grade 3 or greater toxicity rate of almost 50%.[7]
- There are no clear adjuvant treatments for patients with variant histology; thus, these patients should be followed with surveillance after nephrectomy.

Patient Adjuvant Treatment
- *One year of pembrolizumab*

What Is Required for This Patient's Follow-Up and Survivorship?

- Follow-up for stage II/III disease is the same, regardless of whether or not adjuvant therapy is provided.
- Patients should be seen every 3 to 6 months for 3 years, and then annually until year 5.
- Each visit should include a comprehensive metabolic panel (CMP), and a CT of the chest, abdomen, and pelvis.
- MRI can also substitute for CT of the abdomen and pelvis to help minimize radiation exposure.
- Further surveillance beyond year 5 is not required and can be performed as clinically indicated.

Case 16.2: Metastatic Renal Cell Carcinoma

A 65-year-old man presents for evaluation of new right hip pain. The pain started about 2 months ago and has become increasingly severe and persistent. He is unable to walk more than a few steps and wakes up several times during the night due to his hip pain. He notes a 30-lb weight loss over the past 3 months and has become progressively more weak and fatigued. He has a PMH of hypertension and was a former smoker for 30 years. Physical examination reveals a thin, frail male with tenderness to palpation over the right trochanter.

Radiograph of the right hip demonstrates a 2.5-cm lytic lesion in the right trochanter. A CT of the chest, abdomen, and pelvis is performed demonstrating a solid 6-cm right renal mass with widespread osseous lesions throughout the axial skeleton. Laboratory evaluation demonstrates mild polycythemia and hypercalemia.

How Is a Diagnosis Established?

- In the setting of possible metastatic disease, tissue biopsy of a metastatic site is necessary to assess for the histological subtype in cases of suspected RCC.
- Clear cell carcinoma is the most common subtype of RCC, present in 75% to 85% of cases. The remaining cases are classified as either non-clear cell (papillary, chromophobe, oncocytic, collecting duct, translocating) or unclassifiable.[8] Treatment options differ depending on the histological subtype.
- CT of the abdomen and pelvis with/without IV contrast and CT of the chest or chest x-ray are used for staging. Bone scan and MRI brain are warranted if there are clinical signs suggestive of bone disease or brain involvement.

Patient's Diagnosis
- *Biopsy of the trochanter lesion demonstrates RCC, clear cell subtype, confirming stage IV (T1N0M1) disease.*

What Are Other Prognostic Factors?

- Additional clinical characteristics can be used to aid in prognostication and treatment planning for patients with stage IV disease.
- The International Metastatic Renal Cell Carcinoma Database Consortium (IMDC) criteria consists of prognostic factors that were found to be important in patients being treated with anti-angiogenesis agents. Although the relevance of these criteria is unknown in the setting of more modern therapies, they continue to be used to help risk-stratify patients.
- Patients receive one point for Karnofsky Performance Status (KPS) less than 80, time from original diagnosis to initiation of therapy less than 1 year, hemoglobin (hgb) less than the upper limit of normal (ULN), absolute neutrophil count (ANC) greater than ULN, platelet count greater than ULN, and serum calcium greater than ULN. Favorable, intermediate, and high-risk groups are defined by 0, 1 to 2, and 3 or more risk factors, respectively.
- The Memorial Sloan Kettering Cancer Center (MSKCC) prognostic model is an older score that was developed in the interferon-alpha era that was used for many clinical trials, but is no longer used to make treatment decisions. Patients receive one point if the interval from diagnosis to treatment was less than 1 year, KPS is less than 80%, lactate dehydrogenase (LDH) is greater than 1.5x ULN, serum calcium is greater than ULN, or hgb is less than the lower limit of normal (LLN). Low-, intermediate-, and high-risk groups have no, one or two, or three or more risk factors.

Patient's Prognostic Group
- *IMDC high-risk*

Table 16.2 Combination Therapy Data

Regimen	Trial	ORR	CRR	OS	Median PFS
Pembrolizumab plus axitinib	KEYNOTE-426	59%	6%	2-year 74%	15.4 months
Nivolumab plus cabozantinib	CheckMate-9ER	56%	8%	1-year 86%	17 months
Pembrolizumab plus lenvatinib	CLEAR	71%	16%	2-year 79.2%	24 months
Nivolumab plus ipilmumab*	CheckMate-214	39%	11%	4-year 53%	11.6 months

*For intermediate-poor risk only.

CRR, complete response rate; ORR, objective response rate; OS, overall survival; PFS, progression-free survival.

What Are Appropriate Treatment Options?

- Numerous immunotherapies and anti-angiogenesis tyrosine kinase inhibitors (TKIs) are approved for metastatic RCC. The most appropriate regimen will depend on the risk-stratification and disease/symptom burden.
- Patients with favorable-, intermediate-, and poor-risk disease can be managed with combination regimens involving immunotherapy with an angiogenesis inhibitor. Pembrolizumab/lenvatinib, pembrolizumab/axitinib, and nivolumab/cabozantinib are the most commonly employed regimens due to their improved OS, progression-free survival (PFS), objective response rate (ORR), and complete response rate (CRR) in comparison to sunitinib.[9–11]
- Combination immunotherapy with nivolumab/ipilimumab is an additional option for intermediate/poor-risk disease patients, with improvement in OS, ORR, and CRR in comparison to sunitinib in this patient population.[12] This strategy may not be preferred in those with high disease burden or symptoms since responses are quicker with TKI combination therapy.
- Patients who cannot tolerate immunotherapy can be treated with TKI monotherapy. Sunitinib, pazopanib, and cabozantinib can be tried, with the latter being preferred in intermediate-poor risk patients given its PFS advantage over sunitinib (Table 16.2).[13–15]

Recommended Treatment Plan for This Patient
- Combination therapy with nivolumab/cabozanitinb.

What Are the Toxicities Associated With Systemic Therapy?

- Checkpoint inhibitor immunotherapies are associated with immune-related adverse events (irAEs). These can involve almost any organ, with the most common presentations being dermatitis, pneumonitis, hepatitis, and endocrinopathies.[9–11,13] This occurs more frequently in patients treated with combination immunotherapy. About 22% of patients treated with nivolumab/ipilimumab had to discontinue therapy, with 35% having to receive high-dose steroids (greater than 40 mg prednisone/day or equivalent) at some point to reverse toxicity.
- Anti-angiogenesis TKIs are associated with several adverse events as a class, including hypertension, hemorrhage, thromboembolic disease, hand–foot syndrome, delayed wound healing, nausea/vomiting, diarrhea, hepatotoxicity, proteinuria, and thyroid dysfunction. When compared to sunitinib alone, treatment discontinuation rates were higher for combination therapy as follows: 37.2% versus 14.4% for pembrolizumab/lenvatinib, 30.5% versus 13.3% for pembrolizumab/axitinib, and 19.7% versus 16.9% for nivolumab/cabozantinib.[9–11]

Case 16.3: Oligometastatic Disease

A 63-year-old man is referred for evaluation of a new renal mass. He was recently in a motor vehicle accident, after which the renal mass was incidentally discovered on a CT scan as a part of his evaluation in the ED. The mass involves the left renal parenchyma, measuring about 6.5 cm, suspicious for RCC. A CT of the chest is ordered to complete his staging evaluation, which demonstrates a 3-cm mass in the right lower lobe without any other signs of metastatic disease. He reports no symptoms aside from lower back pain that is improving after the accident. Physical examination, CMP, and complete blood count (CBC) do not show any abnormalities.

How Is a Diagnosis Established?

- A biopsy of the pulmonary lesion should be performed for histological confirmation of metastatic disease.

Patient's Diagnosis

- *An endobronchial US-guided biopsy of the pulmonary lesions demonstrates RCC, with insufficient tissue to determine the histological subtype.*

What Is the Patient's Stage and Prognostic Group?

- Evaluation is consistent with stage IV (T2N0M1) disease.
- The IMDC prognostic group is intermediate-risk given the time from diagnosis to initiation of treatment is less than 1 year.

What Are Appropriate Treatment Options?

- Systemic therapy is typically indicated for stage IV disease. However, patients with a surgically resectable primary and oligometastatic disease can be considered for surgical resection of all involved sites. A subset of these patients will experience a long disease-free interval with a chance for cure.[16]
- In oligometastatic disease presentations where all sites of disease are not amenable to surgical resection or the patient is not considered a surgical candidate, a cytoreductive nephrectomy can still be considered in addition to systemic therapy. The SWOG 8949 trial evaluated cytoreductive nephrectomy prior to treatment with interferon alfa versus interferon alfa alone, which demonstrated a benefit in median OS (mOS; 11 vs. 8 months). This benefit was more pronounced in patients with an Eastern Cooperative Oncology Group (ECOG) score of 0 (17 vs. 7 months) and in those with lung only metastases (14 vs. 10 months).[17] In the setting of modern therapies, the benefit is less clear. The CARMENA trial evaluated cytoreductive nephrectomy plus sunitinib versus sunitinib alone in patients with MSKCC intermediate/poor prognosis metastatic RCC, with noninferior outcomes in the sunitinib arm when compared to the nephrectomy arm (mOS 18.4 vs. 13.9 months, respectively).[18] The trial was slow to accrue and a smaller number of patients were enrolled than expected, which reduced the statistical power of the study. There are no prospective trials that specifically assess nephrectomy in the setting of newer TKIs, immune checkpoint inhibition, and combination therapies that are currently used today. A retrospective analysis of 391 patients from the U.S. national cancer database demonstrated an OS benefit in patients who were treated with cytoreductive nephrectomy plus a checkpoint inhibitor when compared to those that received a checkpoint inhibitor alone.[19] Additionally, most patients enrolled in trials studying checkpoint inhibitors had already received a cytoreductive nephrectomy (92% in CheckMate-214, 70% in CheckMate-9ER, 83% in KEYNOTE-426, 73.3% in CLEAR trial).[9–11,13]

- The timing of cytoreductive nephrectomy depends on the overall clinical presentation. Patients with ECOG less than 2 and low disease burden are often considered for upfront nephrectomy prior to initiation of systemic therapy, while patients with higher disease burden are typically treated with systemic therapy first, and offered nephrectomy if they are clearly benefiting from therapy at some point in their treatment course.
- The intent of nephrectomy is important when making such decisions. The previous discussion is specifically applicable to cytoreductive nephrectomy. However, patients are sometimes considered for palliative nephrectomy if significant symptoms are caused by the primary tumor.

Patient's Treatment
- *Radical nephrectomy with right lower lobectomy was offered.*
- *Final pathology demonstrated RCC, clear cell subtype.*

What Are Other Treatment Considerations?

- One year of pembrolizumab can be offered to those with oligometastatic disease treated with surgical resection of all involved sites. In the KEYNOTE-564 trial, high-risk (stage III or worse) clear cell RCC patients who were treated with nephrectomy were randomized to adjuvant pembrolizumab or placebo for up to 17 cycles. Pembrolizumab demonstrated improved 2-year DFS (77.3% vs. 68.1%) without a clear OS advantage at this point in follow-up. A small percentage of patients in this study (5.8%) also had M1 involvement with no evidence of disease after complete surgical resection of all involved areas. This DFS benefit was maintained in this subgroup, with a hazard ratio (HR) for death of 0.29 (95% confidence interval [CI] 0.12 to 0.69). Grade 3 or greater toxicity occurred in 32.4% of patients.[6]

Patient's Adjuvant Treatment
- *One year of pembrolizumab*

What Is Required for This Patient's Follow-Up and Survivorship?

- Follow-up for oligometastatic disease after definitive surgical resection is the same as stage II/III disease.
- Patients should be seen every 3 to 6 months for 3 years, and then annually until year 5.
- Each visit should include a CMP, as well as CT of the chest, abdomen, and pelvis.
- MRI can also substitute for CT of the abdomen and pelvis to help minimize radiation exposure.
- Further surveillance beyond year 5 is not required, and can be performed as clinically indicated.

REVIEW QUESTIONS

1. A 78-year-old man presents with 2 months of worsening flank pain. Physical examination reveals a blood pressure of 165/95 and palpable mass in the right flank. CT of the abdomen and pelvis demonstrated an 8-cm mass in the right kidney suspicious for renal cell carcinoma (RCC). After staging evaluation does not reveal any metastatic disease, he undergoes a right nephrectomy, with pathology demonstrating RCC, clear cell type, with invasion into the renal vein and no lymph node (LN) involvement. What is the next best step in management?
   A. Surveillance
   B. Adjuvant sunitinib
   C. Adjuvant pembrolizumab
   D. Adjuvant atezolizumab

2. A 28-year-old woman presents to the ED with shortness of breath after running a half marathon and is found to have a right spontaneous pneumothorax. CT scan incidentally notes bilateral masses in the kidneys measuring 2 cm, which is concerning for renal cell carcinoma (RCC). Family history is notable for spontaneous pneumothorax and RCC in her mother, and fibrofolliculoma-like tumors in her sister. After she recovers from her pneumothorax, a biopsy is performed of the right renal lesion demonstrating RCC, chromophobe subtype. She is referred for genetic counseling where genetic testing is performed. A mutation in which of the following genes is most likely to be detected?
   A. FCLN1
   B. TSC2
   C. VHL
   D. SDHA

3. A 68-year-old man with a past medical history (PMH) of stage II renal cell carcinoma (RCC), clear cell type, presents for follow-up 2 years after right nephrectomy. He reports new low back pain that has been waking him up at night. Physical examination demonstrates tenderness to palpation in the midline in the lumbar region, with 5/5 strength in the extremities. CT of the chest, abdomen, and pelvis demonstrates multiple pulmonary nodules measuring up to 2 cm and a 3-cm lytic lesion in the L4 vertebrae. Laboratory evaluation demonstrates no abnormalities on comprehensive metabolic panel (CMP) or complete blood count (CBC) and his Karnofsky Performance Status is 90. He completes palliative radiation therapy to the L4 lesion. Which of the following is the most appropriate systemic treatment option?
   A. Nivolumab plus cabozantinib
   B. Pembrolizumab
   C. Cabozantinib
   D. Nivolumab

4. A 65-year-old woman presents with progressive fatigue and a 30-lb weight loss over the last month. She has had right hip pain that has prevented her from being able to walk. CT of the chest, abdomen, and pelvis demonstrates a 6-cm mass in the left kidney, a 3-cm lytic lesion in the right femoral head, and six lesions in the liver measuring up to 2 cm in greatest dimension. Biopsy of a liver lesion demonstrates renal cell carcinoma (RCC), clear cell type. Laboratory evaluation demonstrates a platelet count of 621 × 10⁹/L and an otherwise normal complete blood count (CBC) and comprehensive metabolic panel

(CMP). She undergoes palliative radiation therapy (RT) to the femoral head lesion. What is the most appropriate systemic treatment option?

A. Nivolumab
B. Pembrolizumab plus lenvatinib
C. Lenvatinib
D. Axitinib

5. A 58-year-old man with a history of dermatomyositis presents for a new diagnosis of metastatic renal cell carcinoma (RCC), clear cell type, with widespread osseous disease involving the axial skeleton. He was diagnosed with dermatomyositis when he presented with proximal muscle weakness and a facial rash 6 weeks ago, and has been improving since starting prednisone, though he remains on a 20-mg dose. What is the most appropriate systemic treatment option?

A. Pembrolizumab plus lenvatinib
B. Nivolumab plus cabozantinib
C. Sunitinib
D. Cabozantinib

6. A 59-year-old woman presents with 2 weeks of progressive hematuria and is found to have an 8-cm mass in the left kidney suspicious for renal cell carcinoma (RCC). Staging evaluation demonstrates a 2-cm lesion in the right hepatic lobe with biopsy demonstrating RCC, clear cell type. She has no past medical history (PMH), Eastern Cooperative Oncology Group (ECOG) performance status of 1, and no abnormalities on complete blood count (CBC) or comprehensive metabolic panel (CMP). She undergoes radical nephrectomy and resection of the hepatic metastasis. Which of the following is the best treatment approach?

A. Cabozantinib
B. Nivolumab plus ipilimumab
C. Pembrolizumab plus axitinib
D. Pembrolizumab

7. A 71-year-old man presents with shortness of breath and is found to have a pleural effusion. Cytological evaluation of pleural fluid demonstrates an exudate involved by renal cell carcinoma (RCC), clear cell type. Staging evaluation demonstrates a 5-cm renal mass and widespread osseous disease throughout the axial skeleton. He is started on pembrolizumab plus axitinib and demonstrates a partial response after 3 months of therapy, with resolution of the pleural fluid, and persistence of a 4-cm renal mass. What is the next most appropriate intervention?

A. Continuation of systemic therapy
B. Cytoreductive nephrectomy and continuation of systemic therapy
C. Observation
D. Switch to cabozantinib

8. A 71-year-old man with metastatic renal cell carcinoma (RCC), clear cell type with hepatic involvement, is treated with nivolumab/ipilimumab. Re-staging evaluation after 4 cycles of therapy demonstrates progressive hepatic disease. He is started on pazopanib therapy. Which of the following does not need to be monitored during therapy?

A. Blood pressure
B. Urinalysis
C. Pulmonary function testing
D. Electrocardiogram

9. An 88-year-old woman with a history of type 2 diabetes mellitus, coronary artery disease, and Alzheimer's disease presents for an incidental finding of a renal mass on a CT scan that was performed during a trauma evaluation after she tripped and fell at home. There is a 3-cm mass in the right kidney suspicious for renal cell carcinoma (RCC) without any evidence of metastatic disease on staging evaluation. She uses a walker for ambulation and needs assistance with most of her activities of daily living (ADLs). Over the past year, she has become increasingly forgetful and is alert to only person and place at baseline. What is the most appropriate treatment approach?
   A. Observation
   B. Partial nephrectomy
   C. Radical nephrectomy
   D. Radiofrequency ablation

10. A 69-year-old man with a history of hypertension and tobacco use presents with right flank pain and hematuria and is found to have a 4-cm mass on CT scan. Staging evaluation does not reveal any evidence of distant metastatic disease. He undergoes right partial nephrectomy demonstrating a 5-cm renal cell carcinoma (RCC), clear cell type, without any invasion of major vascular structures or lymph nodes (LNs). What is the next most appropriate step?
   A. Radical nephrectomy
   B. Radiation therapy
   C. Surveillance
   D. Adjuvant pembrolizumab

ANSWERS AND RATIONALES

1. **C. Adjuvant pembrolizumab.** Adjuvant pembrolizumab is indicated in patients with stage III RCC, clear cell type. Sunitinib could also be considered, but would not be preferred in this patient with preexisting hypertension that is not well controlled.

2. **A. *FCLN1*.** This patient's presentation with spontaneous pneumothorax and bilateral RCC, chromophobe type, along with a family history of fibrofolliculoma-like tumors is consistent with Birt-Hogge-Dube syndrome, resulting from a mutation in the *FCLN1* gene.

3. **A. Nivolumab plus cabozantinib.** This patient has International Metastatic Renal Cell Carcinoma Database Consortium (IMDC) low-risk disease and is a candidate for combination therapy, making nivolumab/cabozantinib the most appropriate treatment option. Cabozantinib could be considered in cases where immunotherapy is contraindicated. Pembrolizumab and nivolumab as single agents are not standard of care options for metastatic RCC.

4. **B. Pembrolizumab plus lenvatinib.** Combination therapy with pembrolizumab and lenvatinib is approved for high-risk metastatic RCC, clear cell subtype. The other options do not have good data as single agents in the first-line setting.

5. **D. Cabozantinib.** Single-agent tyrosine kinase inhibitor (TKI) therapy is appropriate in this patient who is not a candidate for immunotherapy given his ongoing prednisone requirement. Cabozantinib is preferred over sunitinib per the CABOSUN trial given that this patient has intermediate-risk disease.

6. **D. Pembrolizumab.** This patient presents with oligometastatic disease that is amenable to surgical resection of all involved areas. Pembrolizumab is the only approved adjuvant treatment of the options listed in the question and would be indicated in this case.

7. **B. Cytoreductive nephrectomy and continuation of systemic therapy.** This patient presented with high disease burden on presentation with partial response after several cycles of therapy. Cytoreductive nephrectomy is appropriate in this situation along with continuation of his current systemic therapy regimen.

8. **C. Pulmonary function testing.** Pazopanib is associated with hypertension, proteinuria, and QTc prolongation, which all need to be monitored during therapy. Although pulmonary complications such as interstitial lung disease (ILD) can rarely be seen with pazopanib, routine pulmonary function tests (PFTs) are not indicated during therapy.

9. **A. Observation.** In patients with a limited life expectancy due to other medical comorbidities, observation is an appropriate option for early-stage RCC given the frequently indolent nature of this neoplasm.

10. **C. Surveillance.** This patient has stage I (pT1bN0) disease, which does not require adjuvant therapy. He should undergo routine surveillance for 5 years.

REFERENCES

1. Padala SA, Barsouk A, Thandra KC, et al. Epidemiology of renal cell carcinoma. *World J Oncol.* 2020;11(3):79–87. doi:10.14740/wjon1279
2. Skinner DG, Colvin RB, Vermillion CD, et al. Diagnosis and management of renal cell carcinoma. a clinical and pathologic study of 309 cases. *Cancer.* 1971;28(5):1165–1177. doi:10.1002/1097-0142(1971)28:5<1165::aid-cncr2820280513>3.0.co;2-g
3. Colombo JR Jr, Haber GP, Jelovsek JE, et al. Seven years after laparoscopic radical nephrectomy: oncologic and renal functional outcomes. *Urol.* 2008;71(6):1149–1154. doi:10.1016/j.urology.2007.11.081
4. Van Poppel H, Da Pozzo L, Albrecht W, et al. A prospective, randomised EORTC intergroup phase 3 study comparing the oncologic outcome of elective nephron-sparing surgery and radical nephrectomy for low-stage renal cell carcinoma. *Eur Urol.* 2011;59(4):543–552. doi:10.1016/j.eururo.2010.12.013
5. Mir MC, Derweesh I, Porpiglia F, et al. Partial nephrectomy versus radical nephrectomy for clinical T1b and T2 renal tumors: a systematic review and meta-analysis of comparative studies. *Eur Urol.* 2017;71(4):606–617. doi:10.1016/j.eururo.2016.08.060
6. Choueiri TK, Tomczak P, Park SH, et al. Adjuvant pembrolizumab after nephrectomy in renal-cell carcinoma. *N Engl J Med.* 2021;385(8):683–694. doi:10.1056/NEJMoa2106391
7. Ravaud A, Motzer RJ, Pandha HS, et al. Adjuvant sunitinib in high-risk renal-cell carcinoma after nephrectomy. *N Engl J Med.* 2016;375(23):2246–2254. doi:10.1056/NEJMoa1611406
8. Störkel S, van den Berg E. Morphological classification of renal cancer. *World J Urol.* 1995;13(3):153–158. doi:10.1007/BF00184870
9. Powles T, Plimack ER, Soulières D, et al. Pembrolizumab plus axitinib versus sunitinib monotherapy as first-line treatment of advanced renal cell carcinoma (KEYNOTE-426): extended follow-up from a randomised, open-label, phase 3 trial [published correction appears in *Lancet Oncol.* 2020;21(12):e553]. *Lancet Oncol.* 2020;21(12):1563–1573. doi:10.1016/S1470-2045(20)30436-8
10. Choueiri TK, Powles T, Burotto M, et al. Nivolumab plus cabozantinib versus sunitinib for advanced renal-cell carcinoma. *N Engl J Med.* 2021;384(9):829–841. doi:10.1056/NEJMoa2026982
11. Motzer R, Alekseev B, Rha SY, et al. Lenvatinib plus pembrolizumab or everolimus for advanced renal cell carcinoma. *N Engl J Med.* 2021;384(14):1289–1300. doi:10.1056/NEJMoa2035716
12. Motzer RJ, Rini BI, McDermott DF, et al. Nivolumab plus ipilimumab versus sunitinib in first-line treatment for advanced renal cell carcinoma: extended follow-up of efficacy and safety results from a randomised, controlled, phase 3 trial [published correction appears in *Lancet Oncol.* 2019;20(10):e559] [published correction appears in *Lancet Oncol.* 2020;21(6):e304] [published correction appears in *Lancet Oncol.* 2020;21(11):e518]. *Lancet Oncol.* 2019;20(10):1370–1385. doi:10.1016/S1470-2045(19)30413-9
13. Choueiri TK, Hessel C, Halabi S, et al. Cabozantinib versus sunitinib as initial therapy for metastatic renal cell carcinoma of intermediate or poor risk (Alliance A031203 CABOSUN randomised trial): progression-free survival by independent review and overall survival update [published correction appears in *Eur J Cancer.* 2018;103:287]. *Eur J Cancer.* 2018;94:115–125. doi:10.1016/j.ejca.2018.02.012
14. Motzer RJ, Hutson TE, Tomczak P, et al. Sunitinib versus interferon alfa in metastatic renal-cell carcinoma. *N Engl J Med.* 2007;356(2):115–124. doi:10.1056/NEJMoa065044
15. Motzer RJ, Hutson TE, Cella D, et al. Pazopanib versus sunitinib in metastatic renal-cell carcinoma. *N Engl J Med.* 2013;369(8):722–731. doi:10.1056/NEJMoa1303989
16. Kavolius JP, Mastorakos DP, Pavlovich C, et al. Resection of metastatic renal cell carcinoma. *J Clin Oncol.* 1998;16(6):2261–2266. doi:10.1200/JCO.1998.16.6.2261
17. Flanigan RC, Salmon SE, Blumenstein BA, et al. Nephrectomy followed by interferon alfa-2b compared with interferon alfa-2b alone for metastatic renal-cell cancer. *N Engl J Med.* 2001;345(23):1655–1659. doi:10.1056/NEJMoa003013
18. Méjean A, Ravaud A, Thezenas S, et al. Sunitinib alone or after nephrectomy in metastatic renal-cell carcinoma. *N Engl J Med.* 2018;379(5):417–427. doi:10.1056/NEJMoa1803675
19. Singla N, Hutchinson RC, Ghandour RA, et al. Improved survival after cytoreductive nephrectomy for metastatic renal cell carcinoma in the contemporary immunotherapy era: an analysis of the national cancer database. *Urol Oncol.* 2020;38(6):604.e9–604.e17. doi:10.1016/j.urolonc.2020.02.029

CHAPTER 17

Bladder Cancer

Eric Granowicz and Mamta Parikh

INTRODUCTION

Bladder cancer is the 10th most common cancer in the world, and the sixth most common cancer in the United States.[1] There are numerous histological subtypes of bladder cancer that vary in frequency depending on geographic location and exposure to environmental factors. The most common subtype in the United States and other Western nations is urothelial carcinoma, originating from the urothelial cells that line the bladder. These cells are uniquely able to allow for stretching of the bladder wall as it fills with urine. Squamous cell carcinoma (SCC) and adenocarcinoma can also be seen, the former often in association with *Schistosoma haematobium* infection while the latter is often associated with a remnant of the urachus. This chapter will focus on urothelial carcinoma of the bladder rather than these rarer histologies, which have different prognoses and treatment recommendations.

An estimated 80,500 cases of bladder cancer were reported in the United States in 2019.[2] The incidence initially rose to reach a peak in the 1980s and has now declined to 18.1/100,000 per a 2016 report. Bladder cancer is about four times more common in men than women, and typically occurs in those who are 65 years of age and older. The greatest risk factor is a history of smoking, which is implicated in greater than 50% of cases.[1]

Bladder cancer often presents with painless hematuria. Early-stage bladder cancer that does not invade into the muscularis propria is typically managed by a urologist. Transurethral resection of bladder tumor (TURBT) and intravesical Bacillus Calmette-Guerin (BCG) or chemotherapy are used in many cases depending on various risk factors. The medical oncologist plays a larger role in the treatment of localized bladder cancer that is refractory to these treatments, has invaded into or beyond the muscle layer, or has spread to locoregional lymph nodes (LNs) and/or more distant sites. This chapter will focus on these clinical scenarios.

CASE SUMMARIES

Case 17.1: Muscle-Invasive Bladder Cancer in a Surgical Candidate

A 69-year-old man presents for evaluation of painless, gross hematuria. His symptoms started 2 months ago. At first his hematuria was intermittent, but has become more persistent with passage of small clots. He denies any pain, weight loss, or other urinary symptoms. His past medical history (PMH) includes chronic obstructive pulmonary disease (COPD) that is well-controlled on medical therapy and an extensive smoking history. He is otherwise fit. He was diagnosed with a urinary tract infection (UTI) and treated with a course of bactrim without any improvement in his symptoms. He was referred to urology where a cystoscopy was performed demonstrating a 3.5-cm hemorrhagic, exophytic lesion occupying the left lateral bladder wall. The remainder of his physical examination, comprehensive metabolic panel (CMP), and complete blood count (CBC) are unremarkable.

How Is a Diagnosis Established?

- A tissue biopsy is required to confirm a diagnosis of bladder cancer and confirm histology.
- Cystoscopy with TURBT is done to obtain a pathological diagnosis and assess the depth of invasion into the submucosa and muscularis propria.
- Urine cytology is often assessed at the time of cystoscopy as well. Evidence of malignant cells without an obvious mass in the bladder is an indication to explore more proximal parts of the urinary tract for extravesicular tumors.
- CT urography of the abdomen and pelvis with CT of the chest or chest x-ray are used to assess for the presence of a bladder mass, lymphadenopathy, and metastatic disease. CT urogram and urine cytology are usually performed prior to referral to a urologist.
- A nuclear medicine (NM) bone scan or MRI of the brain can be performed based on clinical symptoms. PET/CT may be useful in patients who have impaired renal function and cannot therefore undergo a CT scan with contrast to adequately image for LN or metastatic involvement.

Patient's Diagnosis

- *TURBT demonstrates high-grade urothelial carcinoma with invasion into the muscularis propria without involvement of the perivesical soft tissue.*
- *CT scan demonstrates a 2-cm internal iliac LN without any other evidence of metastatic disease.*

How Is This Tumor Staged?

- The eighth edition of the American Joint Committee on Cancer (AJCC) tumor, node, metastasis (TNM) system, published in 2017, is used to stage bladder cancer.
- Stage I disease is limited to the bladder without invasion into the muscularis propria (T1N0). Stage II disease requires invasion into the muscularis propria (T2–4aN0). Stage III disease has evidence of LN involvement in the true pelvis (perivesical, obturator, internal/external iliac, or sacral LNs) and/or common iliac nodes (T1–4N1–3). Stage IV disease requires evidence of distant metastases or direct invasion of the abdominal wall, pelvic wall, or other organs aside from the vagina, prostate, or uterus.
- Clinical staging can be performed with cystoscopy, TURBT, and CT of the chest, abdomen, and pelvis, which suffices for most cases of stage I disease. In order to confirm the diagnosis of stage I disease, however, it is critical that muscularis propria be identified in the TURBT specimen, as patients are otherwise at risk of being understaged.
- True pathological staging requires radical cystectomy for adequate assessment of primary tumor invasion and pelvic LN involvement, although this is only pursued in patients with stage II or III disease or stage I disease that does not respond to or relapses after intravesical BCG.

Patient's Clinical Stage

- *Stage IIIA (cT2N1M0)*

What Are Appropriate Treatment Options?

- Stage II to III urothelial carcinoma of the bladder is treated with curative intent. The most important considerations in determining the appropriate treatment include the patient's surgical candidacy, performance status, and presence of other comorbidities.
- Surgical candidates who are cisplatin-eligible should receive neoadjuvant cisplatin-based chemotherapy followed by radical cystectomy with bilateral pelvic lymphadenectomy.[3] This is based on the SWOG-8710 study, a randomized Phase III trial which enrolled patients who had cT2–4a muscle-invasive bladder cancer to receive either neoadjuvant methotrexate, vinblastine, doxorubicin, and cisplatin (MVAC) followed by radical cystectomy or radical cystectomy alone. Patients receiving neoadjuvant chemotherapy prior to radical cystectomy experienced a longer overall survival (OS) compared to those who underwent radical cystectomy alone.
- Dose-dense MVAC and gemcitabine/cisplatin (GC) given for 3 to 4 cycles are the most commonly utilized neoadjuvant regimens. Neoadjuvant therapy in this setting is associated with improvements in OS, disease-free survival (DFS), and risk of recurrence in comparison to local therapy alone.[3–4]
- Cisplatin-ineligibility is defined by the presence of any of the following:
  - Eastern Cooperative Oncology Group (ECOG) performance status (PS) of 2 or greater or Karnofsky Performance Status (KPS) less than 60% to 70%
  - Creatinine clearance of less than 60 mL/min
  - Grade 2 or greater peripheral neuropathy
  - Hearing loss of 25 dB at two contiguous frequencies
  - New York Heart Association (NYHA) class greater than or equal to III heart failure
- Cisplatin-ineligible surgical candidates should undergo upfront radical cystectomy without neoadjuvant therapy. It is important to note that there is no data supporting carboplatin-based neoadjuvant chemotherapy.
- Patients with variant histology are managed differently than noted in the previous text. For patients with pure squamous or adenocarcinoma of the bladder, there are no data supporting the use of neoadjuvant chemotherapy; thus, radical cystectomy is recommended. Patients with neuroendocrine differentiation or small cell carcinoma of the bladder should receive cisplatin-based neoadjuvant chemotherapy if they are a candidate, prior to undergoing radical cystectomy.

Recommended Treatment Plan for This Patient

- Neoadjuvant cisplatin-based chemotherapy followed by radical cystectomy.
- Final pathological staging was found to be ypT0N1.

What Are Other Treatment Considerations?

- Final pathological staging should be assessed from the radical cystectomy specimen to aid in further prognostication and help determine the need for adjuvant therapy.
- Pathological complete response (pCR) or downstaging after neoadjuvant chemotherapy is associated with improved OS and DFS.[5]
- For patients who have already received neoadjuvant chemotherapy, 1 year of adjuvant nivolumab is an option for those with evidence of persistent high-risk disease (ypT2-T4 and/or ypN1–3) due to improvements in DFS per the CheckMate 274 trial.[5] This Phase III study enrolled patients who had undergone radical cystectomy with pT3, pT4a, or pN+ disease if they had not received neoadjuvant chemotherapy, or ypT2-T4a or ypN+ disease if they had received neoadjuvant cisplatin-based chemotherapy. Patients were randomized to receive adjuvant nivolumab or placebo for 1 year, and the primary endpoint

of the trial was DFS, which was improved in patients receiving nivolumab. Nivolumab has not yet demonstrated an OS benefit.

- For patients who did not receive neoadjuvant chemotherapy, adjuvant therapy should be considered if final pathology demonstrates pT3–T4 and/or pN1–3 disease. Cisplatin-based chemotherapy (similar regimens as previously described) is preferred, as the DFS benefit in the CheckMate-274 trial was more pronounced in those who received neoadjuvant chemotherapy. However, for patients who are not chemotherapy candidates, treatment with adjuvant nivolumab remains an additional option per the CheckMate 274 trial.[5]

Recommended Adjuvant Treatment for This Patient
- *One year of nivolumab*

What Is Required for the Patient's Follow-Up and Survivorship?

- Laboratory evaluation should consist of CMP and CBC every 3 to 6 months for 1 year and then annually until year 5. Urine cytology can also be considered every 6 to 12 months during the first year.
- Imaging should consist of CT urography (CTU) of the abdomen and pelvis and CT of the chest or chest x-ray every 3 to 6 months for 2 years and then annually until year 5.
- Patients treated with bladder-sparing approaches should undergo cystoscopy every 3 months for 2 years, every 6 months until year 4, and then annually until year 10.

Case 17.2: Muscle-Invasive Bladder Cancer in a Nonsurgical Candidate

A 75-year-old woman with a PMH of diabetes mellitus and hypertension presents with 2 months of dysuria, intermittent hematuria, and a sensation of incomplete voiding. During the last week she developed progressive oliguria despite straining during urination. On exam she has suprapubic tenderness and distension. A post-void residual volume is recorded as 1.2L, which was drained after Foley catheter placement. She was referred to urology where cystoscopy demonstrated a 3-cm tumor at the bladder neck. A TURBT is performed, with pathology findings of high-grade urothelial carcinoma with invasion into the lamina propria with no muscularis propria identified.

How Is a Diagnosis Established?

- An important point to keep in mind is that a patient cannot be considered to have non-muscle-invasive bladder cancer in the absence of muscularis propria identified in the tissue sample. Historically, in patients who underwent TURBT without muscularis propria identified, there was a significant risk of understaging that was found when they later underwent cystectomy.[6] Thus, when pathology results indicate urothelial carcinoma without muscularis propria identified, it is recommended that patients undergo repeat TURBT.

What Further Molecular or Genomic Testing Is Required?

- While there are evolving treatment options for urothelial carcinoma, currently for patients with muscle-invasive bladder cancer, there are no recommended molecular or genomic tests.

Patient's Further Testing
- *The patient underwent repeat TURBT with pathology findings of high-grade urothelial carcinoma with muscularis propria identified and involved with cancer.*
- *CT of the chest and CTU of the abdomen and pelvis did not demonstrate any evidence of metastatic disease.*

Case Continued

- *The patient meets with medical oncology and urology. After discussion about the benefits and risks of radical cystectomy, she does not wish to proceed with surgery and would prefer a bladder-sparing treatment approach.*

What Are Appropriate Treatment Options?

- Many patients are not suitable candidates for radical cystectomy or simply prefer a bladder-sparing approach.
- Combined modality therapy with maximal TURBT followed by concurrent chemoradiation is the most aggressive approach, with improved locoregional control in comparison to radiation therapy alone and disease-specific survival rates that are comparable to cystectomy. This was shown in a Phase III trial in which muscle-invasive bladder cancer patients were randomized to receive fluorouracil (FU) 500 mg/m^2 and mitomycin 12 mg/m^2 with concurrent bladder radiotherapy or bladder radiotherapy alone. Two-year locoregional DFS was improved in the chemoradiotherapy arm (67% vs. 54%), with a hazard ratio (HR) in the chemoradiotherapy group of 0.68 after a median follow-up of 69.9 months.[7]
- 5-FU/mitomycin, 5-FU/cisplatin, and cisplatin/paclitaxel are the most commonly employed regimens for chemoradiotherapy.[7–10]
- Radiation after TURBT is another option for patients who are not fit enough to tolerate or have medical comorbidities that would preclude them from receiving concurrent chemotherapy.[7]

What Are the Toxicities Associated With Treatment?

- Radiation administered to the pelvis is associated with several adverse effects (AEs). Genitourinary (GU) problems include sexual dysfunction and cystitis, which can present with urgency, dysuria, hematuria, and pelvic pain. Gastrointestinal (GI) problems result from colitis and proctitis often presenting with diarrhea, abdominal pain, and tenesmus.
- Acute gastrointestinal symptoms are more common with chemoradiotherapy than with radiotherapy alone, while delayed GI and GU toxicity rates are similar for both.[5]

What Is Required for This Patient's Follow-Up and Survivorship?

- Similar to patients who were treated with cystectomy, laboratory evaluation should consist of CMP and CBC every 3 to 6 months for 1 year and then annually until year 5. Urine cytology can also be considered every 6 to 12 months during the first year.
- Imaging should consist of CTU of the abdomen and pelvis and CT of the chest or chest x-ray every 3 to 6 months for 2 years and then annually until year 5.
- Patients treated with bladder-sparing approaches should undergo cystoscopy every 3 months for 2 years, every 6 months for until year 4, and then annually until year 10.

Case 17.3: Metastatic Bladder Cancer

A 68-year-old woman with a history of hyperlipidemia and hypertension presents for 1 month of progressive abdominal discomfort and bloating. Physical examination reveals a distended abdomen with generalized tenderness, fluid wave, and shifting dullness. An abdominal ultrasound (US) is performed demonstrating evidence of moderate ascites. A paracentesis is performed with drainage of 4L of straw-colored ascitic fluid. Cytological analysis demonstrates evidence of urothelial carcinoma.

How Is a Diagnosis Established?

- Tissue biopsy of a metastatic lesion is always needed to confirm a case of disseminated urothelial carcinoma. In this case, ascitic fluid cytology is sufficient.
- CT of the chest, abdomen, and pelvis is used to complete the staging evaluation.
- NM bone scan and/or MRI of the brain can be considered in patients with clinical concern for bone and central nervous sytem (CNS) involvement, respectively, to complete staging, but is not otherwise required.

Patient's Diagnosis

- *CT scan demonstrates a 5-cm mass in the bladder along with extensive peritoneal involvement, bulky pelvic lymphadenopathy, and moderate ascites.*

What Further Molecular or Genomic Testing Is Required?

- Next-generation sequencing (NGS) is recommended, though it does not influence immediate treatment for metastatic urothelial carcinoma.
- Programmed death-ligand 1 (PD-L1) immunohistochemical (IHC) staining can be useful in guiding treatment in patients who are not eligible to receive cisplatin.
- CMP and CBC should be obtained to help determine candidacy for chemotherapy.

Patient's Molecular and Genomic Testing

- *NGS does not reveal any mutations.*
- *IHC reveals PD-L1 staining in 30% of tumor-infiltrating immune cells.*
- *CMP and CBC findings are both within normal limits.*

What Are Appropriate Treatment Options?

- First-line treatment in cisplatin-eligible patients is cisplatin-based chemotherapy. Recommended regimens include dose dense methotrexate, vinblastine, doxorubicin, and cisplatin (dd-MVAC) and GC, with similar overall response rates (ORRs) of 46% and 49%, respectively.[11–12]
- Cisplatin ineligibility is defined by the presence of any of the following:
  - ECOG PS of 2 or greater or KPS less than 60% to 70%
  - Creatinine clearance less than 60 mL/min
  - Grade 2 or greater peripheral neuropathy
  - Hearing loss of 25 dB at two contiguous frequencies
  - NYHA class of III heart failure or greater
- Patients who are cisplatin-ineligible but candidates for chemotherapy can be treated with GC or atezolizumab if PD-L1–positive (tumor-infiltrating immune cells covering 5% or more of the tumor).[13–14]
- Patients who are not candidates for platinum-based chemotherapy can be treated with pembrolizumab or atezolizumab, regardless of PD-L1 expression.[14–15] Atezolizumab demonstrated an ORR of 23% with median PFS and OS of 2.7 and 15.9 months, respectively, in a single-arm, multicenter, Phase 2 study involving locally advanced or metastatic urothelial cancer patients ineligible for cisplatin. Responses were seen across all PD-L1 and poor prognostic factor subgroups.[14] In the same clinical setting with pembrolizumab, the ORR was 24%.[15]

Patient's Treatment

- *GC is chosen as initial therapy in this cisplatin-eligible patient.*
- *After completion of therapy, a re-staging CT scan demonstrates a partial response.*

What Are the Toxicities Associated With This Regimen?

- Hematological toxicity is universal for cisplatin-based chemotherapy regimens, with around 50% of patients suffering from grade 3 or greater toxicity.
- Other important toxicities include cardiac disease (typically congestive heart failure [CHF] exacerbations associated with the intravenous [IV] fluid requirement), nephropathy, neuropathy, and nausea/vomiting.

What Is Required for This Patient's Follow-Up and Survivorship?

- In patients who achieve stable disease or better after completion of platinum-based chemotherapy, maintenance avelumab is indicated per the JAVELIN Bladder 100 trial. This Phase III randomized controlled trial compared maintenance avelumab to best supportive care in patients with locally advanced or metastatic disease that did not progress after completing platinum-based chemotherapy. Avelumab resulted in higher 1-year OS (71.3% vs. 58.4%), median OS (21.4 vs. 14.3 months), and median PFS (3.7 vs. 2.0 months).[16]

Patient's Ongoing Treatment
- *Maintenance avelumab is offered.*

Case 17.4: Platinum-Refractory Metastatic Bladder Cancer

A 59-year-old man with no significant PMH presented with a 2-month history of hematuria and abdominal pain. Physical examination revealed a palpable suprapubic mass. CT scan demonstrated a 7-cm bladder mass with invasion of the anterior abdominal wall and bulky pelvic lymphadenopathy. Biopsy of the mass via cystoscopy demonstrated high-grade urothelial carcinoma, with clinical stage IVA (T4bN2M0). He was treated with 4 cycles of gemcitabine plus cisplatin before a re-staging CT scan demonstrated progression of his primary lesion, with a new 2-cm lesion in the right lower lobe of the lung that was consistent with urothelial carcinoma on biopsy.

What Further Molecular or Genomic Testing Is Required?

- NGS should be performed if it was not already done on presentation.

Patient's Molecular and Genomic Testing
- *NGS reveals a CDKN2A mutation, without any other abnormalities.*

What Are Appropriate Treatment Options?

- Several systemic therapies are available in patients who are either refractory to or unable to tolerate platinum-based chemotherapy.
- Two checkpoint inhibitors, pembrolizumab and nivolumab, are approved in this setting. When compared to the investigator's choice of chemotherapy (paclitaxel, docetaxel, or vinflunine), pembrolizumab improved median 1-year-OS (44.2% vs. 29.8%), 2-year OS (26.9% vs. 14.3%), and ORR (21.1% vs. 11%) with lower rates of treatment-related adverse events in the KEYNOTE-045 trial.[17] Nivolumab has shown ORRs in the platinum-refractory setting of 19.6% to 24.4% in Phase I to II trials, although an OS benefit over second-line chemotherapy has yet to be proven.[18–19]
- In patients with targetable mutations in *FGFR2* or *FGFR3* on NGS that are not candidates for immunotherapy, the *FGFR* inhibitor, erdafitinib, can be offered. ORR was

reported as 40% in a Phase II trial involving patients who progressed after platinum-based chemotherapy (some patients had also received previous immunotherapy).[20]

- In patients who are unable to tolerate immunotherapy without a targetable *FGFR* mutation on NGS, enfortumab vedotin can be considered. This is an anti-nectin-4 monoclonal antibody drug conjugate that delivers a dose of the microtubule inhibitor, monomethyl auristatin E (MMAE), to urothelial cancer cells, which highly express nectin-4. It has technically only been approved for two patient populations: those who have progressed on both platinum-based chemotherapy and a PD-1/PD-L1 inhibitor and those who have progressed on a PD-1/PD-L1 inhibitor alone if cisplatin-ineligible. A Phase III trial comparing the first population to investigator-chosen chemotherapy (paclitaxel, docetaxel, or vinflunine) was able to demonstrate an OS advantage for enfortumab vedotin (median OS 12.88 vs. 8.97 months).[21] Single-arm Phase II trials demonstrated ORRs of 44% and 52% for the former and latter populations, respectively.[22-23]

Recommended Treatment Plan for This Patient
- *Pembrolizumab*

What Are the Toxicities Associated With Treatment?

- Like other checkpoint inhibitors, pembrolizumab and nivolumab are associated with various immune-related adverse events (irAEs), which can involve almost any organ. Dermatitis is the most frequent presentation, with pneumonitis, hepatitis, colitis, and endocrinopathies being other commonly seen toxicities.[17-19]
- The most common toxicities associated with erdafitinib include hyperphosphatemia, diarrhea, stomatitis, dry mouth, and hand–foot syndrome. Detachment of the retinal pigment epithelium is an important side effect that should be considered in any patient with visual changes during therapy.[20]
- Notable adverse events associated with enfortumab vedotin include peripheral neuropathy, hyperglycemia, corneal toxicity, dermatologic toxicity (including Stevens-Johnson syndrome/toxic epidermal necrolysis), and pneumonitis.[21-23]

REVIEW QUESTIONS

1. A 68-year-old woman presents with 1 week of progressive oliguria and straining during urination, which was proceeded by 1 month of painless hematuria. Renal ultrasound (US) reveals bilateral hydronephrosis, and complete metabolic evaluation reveals a creatinine level of 2.1 mg/dL with a growth factor receptor (GFR) of 22 mL/min/1.73 m^2. Cystoscopy reveals a 4-cm tumor in the neck of the bladder leading to bladder outlet obstruction. A transurethral resection of bladder tumor (TURBT) is performed with pathological evaluation demonstrating high-grade urothelial carcinoma with invasion into the muscularis propria. After a CT of the chest, abdomen, and pelvis shows no evidence of metastatic disease, a radical cystectomy is performed, with final pathological staging consistent with stage IIIA (T3aN0) disease. Four weeks after cystectomy her creatinine and GFR have normalized and she has excellent performance status with no other major medical comorbidities. What is the next best step in management?
   A. Routine surveillance
   B. Offer adjuvant gemcitabine plus carboplatin
   C. Offer adjuvant gemcitabine plus cisplatin
   D. Offer adjuvant nivolumab

2. A 58-year-old man presents with 1 month of painless hematuria and is subsequently found to have a 3-cm tumor in the right lateral wall of the bladder. Pathology report after a transurethral resection of bladder tumor (TURBT) demonstrates urothelial carcinoma with invasion into the muscularis propria. CT of the chest, abdomen, and pelvis reveals no evidence of metastatic disease or lymphadenopathy. He is deemed to be a good surgical candidate by urology and is willing to proceed with cystectomy if necessary. Complete metabolic evaluation reveals no abnormalities and his Eastern Cooperative Oncology Group (ECOG) performance status is 1. He has a history of heart failure with reduced ejection fraction that is well controlled with medical management. What is the next best step in management?
   A. Offer neoadjuvant dose dense methotrexate, vinblastine, doxorubicin, and cisplatin (dd-MVAC) followed by radical cystectomy
   B. Offer neoadjuvant gemcitabine plus carboplatin followed by radical cystectomy
   C. Offer upfront radical cystectomy
   D. Offer definitive chemoradiotherapy

3. A 76-year-old woman with a history of type 2 diabetes mellitus complicated by coronary artery disease and grade 2 peripheral sensory neuropathy presents with 2 weeks of intermittent hematuria. She is ultimately found to have clinical stage IIIA (T3aN0) urothelial carcinoma of the bladder. She is not considered to be a surgical candidate due to her cardiac history. Her Eastern Cooperative Oncology Group (ECOG) performance status is 1. What is the most appropriate treatment?
   A. Dose dense methotrexate, vinblastine, doxorubicin, and cisplatin (dd-MVAC)
   B. Concurrent chemoradiotherapy with 5-FU/mitomycin
   C. Concurrent chemoradiotherapy with 5-FU/cisplatin
   D. Definitive radiation therapy (RT)

4. A 62-year-old man is diagnosed with clinical stage II (T2N1) urothelial carcinoma of the bladder. He undergoes neoadjuvant gemcitabine/cisplatin (GC) followed by radical cystectomy. Final pathological evaluation demonstrates ypT0N1 disease. What is the next best step in management?
   A. Surveillance
   B. Adjuvant dose dense methotrexate, vinblastine, doxorubicin, and cisplatin (dd-MVAC)
   C. Adjuvant radiation therapy
   D. Adjuvant nivolumab

5. A 56-year-old man with a history of tobacco abuse presents with 1 month of worsening fatigue, weight loss, and swelling in the right side of the neck. Physical examination reveals a nontender, 2-cm cervical lymph node (LN). Biopsy demonstrates urothelial carcinoma, and complete staging evaluation reveals cervical, mediastinal, and intra-abdominal lymphadenopathy with a 5-cm mass in the bladder. Laboratory evaluation reveals normal kidney function and his Eastern Cooperative Oncology Group (ECOG) performance status is 1. What is the most appropriate treatment?
   A. Pembrolizumab
   B. Dose dense methotrexate, vinblastine, doxorubicin, and cisplatin (dd-MVAC)
   C. Gemcitabine plus carboplatin
   D. Enfortumab vedotin

6. A 78-year-old woman with a history of myelodysplastic syndrome (MDS), hypertension, and stage III chronic kidney disease (CKD) presented with right shoulder pain and arm weakness and was found to have metastatic urothelial carcinoma of the bladder involving the right humerus leading to pathological fracture along with three liver lesions measuring up to 3 cm. Her baseline laboratory evaluation demonstrates the following:
   White blood cell (WBC) count $2.7 \times 10^9/L$
   Hemoglobin (Hgb)   7.2 g/dL
   Platelets   78,000 $10^9/L$
   Creatinine   2.1 g/dL
   Growth factor receptor (GFR)   20 mL/min/1.73 m^2
   Diagnosis was confirmed with a core needle biopsy of liver lesion. Next-generation sequencing (NGS) does not reveal any mutations and programmed death-ligand 1 (PD-L1) staining was positive in 1% of infiltrating tumor immune cells. What is the best treatment recommendation?
   A. Dose dense methotrexate, vinblastine, doxorubicin, and cisplatin (dd-MVAC)
   B. Gemcitabine plus carboplatin
   C. Erdafitinib
   D. Pembrolizumab

7. A 72-year-old woman is diagnosed with metastatic urothelial carcinoma of the bladder after presenting with abdominal distension secondary to malignant ascites. She is started on dose dense methotrexate, vinblastine, doxorubicin, and cisplatin (dd-MVAC), but progresses after 3 cycles with evidence of new liver lesions. Next-generation sequencing (NGS) reveals an *ERCC1* mutation and programmed death-ligand 1 (PD-L1) staining is positive in 40% of infiltrating tumor immune cells. What is the next best line of therapy?
   A. Pembrolizumab
   B. Erdafitinib
   C. Enfortumab vedotin
   D. Atezolizumab

8. A 62-year-old woman with a history of hypertension is diagnosed with metastatic urothelial carcinoma of the bladder with involvement of the lung and pelvic lymph nodes (LNs) after she presented with cough and abdominal pain. She is treated with gemcitabine plus cisplatin and progresses 1 month after completion of therapy with new lesions in the lung. Next-generation sequencing (NGS) reveals an *FGFR2* mutation and she is considered for erdafitinib therapy. Which of the following is required prior to initiation therapy?
   A. Ophthalmologic exam
   B. Echocardiogram
   C. Pulmonary function tests
   D. Thyroid function tests

9. A 71-year-old man with a history of hypertension and stage IV chronic kidney disease (CKD) presented with painless hematuria and abdominal pain and was found to have a 7-cm mass in the bladder with invasion into the anterior abdominal wall. Biopsy demonstrates urothelial carcinoma with programmed death-ligand 1 (PD-L1) staining 70% of infiltrating tumor immune cells. He is started on atezolizumab and subsequently progresses after completing 3 cycles, with enlargement of his primary mass. His Eastern Cooperative Oncology Group (ECOG) performance status is 2 and next-generation sequencing (NGS) on repeat biopsy does not reveal any mutations. What is the next best line of treatment?
   A. Dose dense methotrexate, vinblastine, doxorubicin, and cisplatin (dd-MVAC)
   B. Enfortumab vedotin
   C. Erdafitinib
   D. Gemcitabine plus cisplatin

10. A 73-year-old man presented with headaches and ataxia and was ultimately found to have a 3-cm lesion in the right cerebellar hemisphere on MRI of the brain. CT of the chest, abdomen, and pelvis reveals a 3-cm mass in the dome of the bladder, pelvic, and intra-abdominal lymphadenopathy. Lymph node (LN) biopsy revealed urothelial carcinoma of the bladder. He was treated with 6 cycles of gemcitabine plus carboplatin after completing stereotactic radiotherapy for his brain metastasis. Re-staging evaluation after completion of chemotherapy reveals a partial response. What is the next best step?
   A. Surveillance
   B. Additional cycles of gemcitabine/carboplatin
   C. Avelumab
   D. Nivolumab

ANSWERS AND RATIONALES

1. **C. Offer adjuvant gemcitabine plus cisplatin.** Patients with stage II to III disease that did not receive neoadjuvant chemotherapy and have T3 and/or N1 or worse findings on final pathological evaluation should be offered adjuvant therapy. This patient is a candidate for cisplatin-based chemotherapy, which is the preferred treatment, while 1 year of nivolumab can be offered to those who are not cisplatin-eligible.

2. **A. Offer neoadjuvant dose dense methotrexate, vinblastine, doxorubicin, and cisplatin (dd-MVAC) followed by radical cystectomy.** This patient is eligible for cisplatin-based neoadjuvant therapy, which should be offered to patients prior to radical cystectomy. Carboplatin is not used in the neoadjuvant setting. Definitive chemoradiotherapy can be offered to patients who are not candidates for surgery or who prefer a bladder-sparing approach.

3. **B. Concurrent chemoradiotherapy with 5-FU/mitomycin.** Concurrent chemoradiotherapy is an acceptable treatment option for patients with otherwise good performance status who are not candidates for cystectomy. She is not a candidate for cisplatin due to her neuropathy, so 5-FU/mitomycin should be offered. Definitive RT can be considered in patients with an inadequate performance status for chemoradiotherapy.

4. **D. Adjuvant nivolumab.** Patients who have received neoadjuvant therapy are candidates for 1 year of adjuvant nivolumab if final pathological staging reveals at least ypT2 and/or pN1 or worse. There are no other adjuvant treatment options available.

5. **B. Dose dense methotrexate, vinblastine, doxorubicin, and cisplatin (dd-MVAC).** Newly diagnosed metastatic bladder cancer patients should be offered cisplatin-based chemotherapy when eligible. Carboplatin can be used as an alternative in those who are not cisplatin-eligible, while pembrolizumab can be considered in patients who are not candidates for any platinum-based chemotherapy.

6. **D. Pembrolizumab.** First-line treatment for metastatic bladder cancer is platinum-based chemotherapy. However, this patient is not a cisplatin candidate due to her CKD, nor is she a chemotherapy candidate given her baseline cytopenias. Pembrolizumab is approved for patients who are not candidates for platinum-based chemotherapy, regardless of PD-L1 expression, and could be recommended here.

7. **A. Pembrolizumab.** Second-line therapy in patients who have progressed on platinum-based therapy is typically immunotherapy, with pembrolizumab and nivolumab both being approved in this setting. Erdafitinib can be considered only in those with *FGFR2/3* mutations and enfortumab vedotin can be tried in those who have progressed on or are not candidates for immunotherapy.

8. **A. Ophthalmologic exam.** Erdafitinib is associated with ocular toxicity including retinal detachment that requires an ophthalmologic exam at baseline, monthly for 4 months, and then every 3 months.

9. **B. Enfortumab vedotin.** This patient is cisplatin-ineligible due to stage IV CKD and has progressed on atezolizumab, making him a candidate for enfortumab vedotin. He is not a candidate for erdafitinib without a *FGFR2/3* mutation.

10. **C. Avelumab.** Maintenance therapy with avelumab is indicated in metastatic bladder cancer patients who have at least stable disease or better after completion of platinum-based chemotherapy.

REFERENCES

1. Saginala K, Barsouk A, Aluru JS, et al. Epidemiology of bladder cancer. *Med Sci (Basel)*. 2020;8(1):15. Published 2020 March 13. doi:10.3390/medsci8010015

2. Siegel RL, Miller KD, Jemal A. Cancer statistics, 2020. *CA Cancer J Clin*. 2020;70(1):7–30. doi:10.3322/caac.21590

3. Grossman HB, Natale RB, Tangen CM, et al. Neoadjuvant chemotherapy plus cystectomy compared with cystectomy alone for locally advanced bladder cancer. *N Engl J Med*. 2003;349(9):859–866. doi:10.1056/NEJMoa022148

4. Vale C. Advanced bladder cancer meta-analysis collaboration. Neoadjuvant chemotherapy in invasive bladder cancer: a systematic review and meta-analysis. *Lancet*. 2003;361(9373):1927–1934. doi:10.1016/s0140-6736(03)13580-5

5. Bajorin DF, Witjes JA, Gschwend JE, et al. Adjuvant nivolumab versus placebo in muscle-invasive urothelial carcinoma. *N Engl J Med*. 2021;384(22):2102–2114. doi:10.1056/NEJMoa2034442

6. Dutta SC, Smith JA Jr, Shappell SB, et al. Clinical under staging of high risk nonmuscle invasive urothelial carcinoma treated with radical cystectomy. *J Urol*. 2001;166(2):490–493. doi:10.1016/S0022-5347(05)65969-1

7. James ND, Hussain SA, Hall E, et al. Radiotherapy with or without chemotherapy in muscle-invasive bladder cancer. *N Engl J Med*. 2012;366(16):1477–1488. doi:10.1056/NEJMoa1106106

8. Mak RH, Hunt D, Shipley WU, et al. Long-term outcomes in patients with muscle-invasive bladder cancer after selective bladder-preserving combined-modality therapy: a pooled analysis of radiation therapy oncology group protocols 8802, 8903, 9506, 9706, 9906, and 0233 [published correction appears in *J Clin Oncol*. 2015;33(7):814]. *J Clin Oncol*. 2014;32(34):3801–3809. doi:10.1200/JCO.2014.57.5548

9. Hussain MH, Glass TR, Forman J, et al. Combination cisplatin, 5-fluorouracil and radiation therapy for locally advanced unresectable or medically unfit bladder cancer cases: a Southwest Oncology Group study. *J Urol*. 2001;165(1):56–61. doi:10.1097/00005392-200101000-00014

10. Mitin T, Hunt D, Shipley WU, et al. Transurethral surgery and twice-daily radiation plus paclitaxel-cisplatin or fluorouracil-cisplatin with selective bladder preservation and adjuvant chemotherapy for patients with muscle invasive bladder cancer (RTOG 0233): a randomised multicentre phase 2 trial. *Lancet Oncol*. 2013;14(9):863–872. doi:10.1016/S1470-2045(13)70255-9

11. Sternberg CN, de Mulder PH, Schornagel JH, et al. Randomized phase III trial of high-dose-intensity methotrexate, vinblastine, doxorubicin, and cisplatin (MVAC) chemotherapy and recombinant human granulocyte colony-stimulating factor versus classic MVAC in advanced urothelial tract tumors: European Organization for Research and Treatment of Cancer Protocol no. 30924. *J Clin Oncol*. 2001;19(10):2638–2646. doi:10.1200/JCO.2001.19.10.2638

12. von der Maase H, Hansen SW, Roberts JT, et al. Gemcitabine and cisplatin versus methotrexate, vinblastine, doxorubicin, and cisplatin in advanced or metastatic bladder cancer: results of a large, randomized, multinational, multicenter, phase III study. *J Clin Oncol*. 2000;18(17):3068–3077. doi:10.1200/JCO.2000.18.17.3068

13. De Santis M, Bellmunt J, Mead G, et al. Randomized phase II/III trial assessing gemcitabine/carboplatin and methotrexate/carboplatin/vinblastine in patients with advanced urothelial cancer who are unfit for cisplatin-based chemotherapy: EORTC study 30986. *J Clin Oncol*. 2012;30(2):191–199. doi:10.1200/JCO.2011.37.3571

14. Balar AV, Galsky MD, Rosenberg JE, et al. Atezolizumab as first-line treatment in cisplatin-ineligible patients with locally advanced and metastatic urothelial carcinoma: a single-arm, multicentre, phase 2 trial [published correction appears in Lancet. 2017;390(10097):848]. *Lancet*. 2017;389(10064):67–76. doi:10.1016/S0140-6736(16)32455-2

15. Balar AV, Castellano D, O'Donnell PH, et al. First-line pembrolizumab in cisplatin-ineligible patients with locally advanced and unresectable or metastatic urothelial cancer (KEYNOTE-052): a multicentre, single-arm, phase 2 study. *Lancet Oncol*. 2017;18(11):1483–1492. doi:10.1016/S1470-2045(17)30616-2

16. Powles T, Park SH, Voog E, et al. Avelumab maintenance therapy for advanced or metastatic urothelial carcinoma. *N Engl J Med*. 2020;383(13):1218–1230. doi:10.1056/NEJMoa2002788

17. Fradet Y, Bellmunt J, Vaughn DJ, et al. Randomized phase III KEYNOTE-045 trial of pembrolizumab versus paclitaxel, docetaxel, or vinflunine in recurrent advanced urothelial cancer: results of > 2 years of follow-up. *Ann Oncol*. 2019;30(6):970–976. doi:10.1093/annonc/mdz127

18. Sharma P, Callahan MK, Bono P, et al. Nivolumab monotherapy in recurrent metastatic urothelial carcinoma (CheckMate 032): a multicentre, open-label, two-stage, multi-arm, phase 1/2 trial [published correction appears in *Lancet Oncol*. 2019;20(2):e71]. *Lancet Oncol*. 2016;17(11):1590–1598. doi:10.1016/S1470-2045(16)30496-X

19. Sharma P, Retz M, Siefker-Radtke A, et al. Nivolumab in metastatic urothelial carcinoma after platinum therapy (CheckMate 275): a multicentre, single-arm, phase 2 trial. *Lancet Oncol*. 2017;18(3):312–322. doi:10.1016/S1470-2045(17)30065-7

20. Loriot Y, Necchi A, Park SH, et al. Erdafitinib in locally advanced or metastatic urothelial carcinoma. *N Engl J Med*. 2019;381(4):338–348. doi:10.1056/NEJMoa1817323

21. Powles T, Rosenberg JE, Sonpavde GP, et al. Enfortumab vedotin in previously treated advanced urothelial carcinoma. *N Engl J Med.* 2021;384(12):1125–1135. doi:10.1056/NEJMoa2035807

22. Rosenberg JE, O'Donnell PH, Balar AV, et al. Pivotal trial of enfortumab vedotin in urothelial carcinoma after platinum and anti-programmed death 1/programmed death ligand 1 therapy. *J Clin Oncol.* 2019;37(29):2592–2600. doi:10.1200/JCO.19.01140

23. Yu EY, Petrylak DP, O'Donnell PH, et al. Enfortumab vedotin after PD-1 or PD-L1 inhibitors in cisplatin-ineligible patients with advanced urothelial carcinoma (EV-201): a multicentre, single-arm, phase 2 trial [published correction appears in *Lancet Oncol.* 2021;22(6):e239]. *Lancet Oncol.* 2021;22(6):872–882. doi:10.1016/S1470-2045(21)00094-2

CHAPTER 18

Cervical Cancer

Alli M. Straubhar and Jean H. Siedel

INTRODUCTION

Epidemiology, Risk Factors, and Pathology

The global incidence of new cervical cancer cases in 2020 was 604,127 with 341,831 deaths, making it the fourth-most common cancer among women.[1] In the United States in 2021, there were an estimated 14,480 new cases and 4,290 deaths.[2] Most cases are from the histological subtype squamous cell carcinoma (SCC) and are associated with high-risk human papillomavirus (HPV) infections.[3] Invasive SCC and adenocarcinoma both can be associated with HPV infections, with strains 16, 18, 31, 33, 45, 52, and 58 accounting for almost 70% of cases. In recent years, there has been a rise in the proportion of cases of adenocarcinoma. This is likely due to improved public health screening programs that have led to early detection of the precursors of SCC and increased uptake of HPV vaccinations.[4] Invasive adenocarcinoma now accounts for 25% of annual cervical cancer cases.[4,5] Neuroendocrine carcinoma, including small cell carcinoma, accounts for approximately 2% of cervical cancer cases. These are more aggressive tumors that can present at more advanced stages due to early lymphatic spread.[6]

Additional risk factors for cervical cancer include low socioeconomic status (likely due to limited access to preventative screening), early onset of sexual activity, multiple sexual partners, use of oral contraceptive pills, cigarette smoking, immunosuppression including HIV, and history of vulvar or vaginal squamous neoplasia or cancer.

Natural History and Prognosis

In the absence of preventative screening, the diagnosis of cervical cancer often occurs at advanced stages when symptoms arise. The most common symptom is abnormal bleeding which can be postcoital bleeding, but also intermenstrual bleeding or postmenopausal bleeding. Patients may complain of abnormal vaginal discharge that is malodorous. At more advanced stages, patients may have pelvic pressure and/or pain, leg pain, flank pain, changes to bowel habits, or passage of urine or feces from the vagina.[7]

Symptoms and signs are a result of the pattern of spread of cervical cancer: direct invasion to the cervical stroma and surrounding structures (vagina, parametria, rectum, bladder), lymphatic permeation, and hematologic dissemination.[7] The most important prognostic factor for local disease is lymph node (LN) status as LN involvement is correlated with poorer overall survival (OS). Additional prognostic factors include histological subtype and tumor size.[7]

CASE SUMMARIES

Case 18.1: Early Cervical Cancer

A 36-year-old female presents to her gynecologist for a 5-month history of abnormal vaginal bleeding with intermenstrual bleeding. This originally was postcoital bleeding, but it has worsened to being every few days. She denies pelvic pain with the bleeding. She has a history of a normal Pap smear 6 years ago during her last pregnancy. She is otherwise healthy but a current smoker with a 10 pack-year history. On speculum exam, she has a 1.2 × 1.5 cm friable mass on the posterior lip of the cervix. On bimanual exam, there is no vaginal or parametrial involvement. Her Eastern Cooperative Oncology Group (ECOG) performance status (PS) is 0 and hemoglobin (Hgb) is 10.2 g/dL.

How Is a Diagnosis Established?

- A biopsy of the cervical mass can be obtained in the office.
- All cervical cancers should be evaluated for HPV.
- The clinician should strongly consider HIV testing at the time of diagnosis.

Patient's Diagnosis
- *A biopsy of the mass demonstrates an SCC of the cervix.*

How Is This Tumor Staged?

- Cervical cancer is staged clinically based upon physical exam and imaging studies (Table 18.1).
- MRI can be used to assess the extent of tumor size, disease spread including vaginal and parametrial involvement, and LN metastases.[8-10]
- PET can be used to evaluate for metastatic disease, particularly for nodal disease that cannot be detected by conventional CT. PET has a pooled sensitivity for para-aortic LN metastases of 84% (95% confidence interval [CI], 68 to 94) and specificity of 95% (95% CI, 89 to 98).[11]
- If a more advanced stage is suspected or there is a large, bulky tumor, an exam under anesthesia with cystoscopy and proctoscopy may be considered.
- In 2018, the FIGO (Fédération Internationale de Gynécologie et d'Obstétrique) staging was updated to subdivide stage IB into three groups based upon size of the tumor. Additionally, imaging or pathology findings may be used to reflect pelvic and para-aortic LN involvement (stage IIIC1, IIIC2),[12] whereas prior to the staging update, LN involvement did not affect staging.

Patient's Clinical Stage
- *An MRI of the pelvis confirms the diagnosis of a mass confined to the cervix without parametrial or vaginal extension.*
- *PET/CT shows a hypermetabolic mass on the posterior cervix without LN involvement.*
- *The patient's stage is FIGO stage IB1.*

What Management Strategies Are Available for Early-Stage Cervical Cancer (Stage IA2, IB1, IB2, and IIA)?

- Patients with early-stage cervical cancer can be cured with either surgery or radiation therapy (RT) with 5-year OS of 83% and progression-free survival (PFS) of 74% for either treatment modality. The combination of surgery followed by adjuvant RT is associated with worse morbidity including risk of urological complications.[13] As such, the

Table 18.1 International Federation of Gynecology and Obstetrics (FIGO) Surgical Staging of Cervical Cancer (2018)

Stage			Description
I			The carcinoma is strictly confined to the cervix.
	IA		Invasive carcinoma that can be diagnosed only by microscopy with maximum depth of invasion ≤5 mm
		IA1	Measured stromal invasion ≤3 mm in depth
		IA2	Measured stromal invasion >3 mm and ≤5 mm in depth
	IB		Invasive carcinoma with measured deepest invasion >5 mm (greater than stage IA); lesion limited to the cervix with size measured by maximum tumor diameter
		IB1	Invasive carcinoma >5 mm depth of stromal invasion and ≤2 cm in greatest dimension
		IB2	Invasive carcinoma >2 cm and ≤4 cm in greatest dimension
		IB3	Invasive carcinoma >4 cm in greatest dimension
II			The cervical carcinoma invades beyond the uterus, but has not extended onto the lower third of the vagina or to the pelvic wall.
	IIA		Involvement limited to the upper two-thirds of the vagina without parametrial involvement
		IIA1	Invasive carcinoma ≤4 cm in greatest dimension
		IIA2	Invasive carcinoma >4 cm in greatest dimension
	IIB		With parametrial involvement but not up to the pelvic wall
III			The carcinoma involves the lower third of the vagina and/or extends to the pelvic wall and/or causes hydronephrosis or nonfunctioning kidney and/or involves pelvic and/or para-aortic LNs.
	IIIA		Carcinoma involves the lower third of the vagina, with no extension to the pelvic wall
	IIIB		Extension to the pelvic wall and/or hydronephrosis or nonfunctioning kidney (unless known to be due to another cause)
	IIIC		Involvement of pelvic and/or para-aortic LNs (including micrometastases), irrespective of tumor size and extent (with radiological and pathological notations)
		IIIC1	Pelvic LN metastasis only
		IIIC2	Para-aortic LN metastasis
IV			The carcinoma has extended beyond the true pelvis or has involved (biopsy proven) the mucosa of the bladder or rectum.
	IVA		Spread of growth to adjacent pelvic organs
	IVB		Spread to distant organs

LN, lymph node.
Source: Data from Bhatla N, Berek JS, Cuello Fredes M, et al. Revised FIGO staging for carcinoma of the cervix uteri. *Int J Gynaecol Obstet.* 2019 Apr;145(1):129–135. doi:10.1002/ijgo.12749. Epub 2019 Jan 17. Erratum in: *Int J Gynaecol Obstet.* 2019 Nov;147(2):279–280. PMID: 30656645.

preferred treatment for smaller tumors (stage IA2, IB1, IB2) is radical hysterectomy, whereas large, bulky tumors (stage IB3, IIA2) are treated with pelvic radiation with concurrent cisplatin.
• Smoking cessation counseling should be offered.

What Route of Surgery Is Recommended for Early-Stage Cervical Cancer?

- For patients who are medically fit for surgery and whose tumors are less than 4 cm in size, an exploratory laparotomy with radical hysterectomy, bilateral salpingectomy +/- oophorectomy, and pelvic LN evaluation should be performed. A minimally invasive approach is not recommended due to lower rates of disease-free survival (DFS) and OS with this approach, compared to an open approach.[14-16]
- Sentinel LN mapping and biopsies can be considered instead of pelvic lymphadenectomy as this has been shown to have a sensitivity of 92% with a negative predictive value (NPV) of 98% in early-stage cervical cancer.[17]
- Ovarian preservation is an option for young patients with SCCs and early-stage adenocarcinomas without lymphovascular space invasion (LVSI) or large tumors.[18,19]

Following Surgery, Who Should Receive Adjuvant Therapy?

- In patients who were treated with surgery, adjuvant therapy may be indicated based upon final pathological results to decrease risk of recurrence. Pathological risk factors are stratified between intermediate and high risk.

Intermediate Risk Factors and Management

- The Sedlis criteria are used to determine the need for adjuvant therapy based upon the primary tumor following surgery.[20] In a randomized controlled trial, patients who met any of the following four criteria were randomized after surgery to receive adjuvant pelvic radiation or no further treatment:
  - LVSI + deep one-third stromal invasion and any tumor size
  - LVSI + middle one-third stromal invasion and tumor greater than 2 cm
  - LVSI + superficial one-third stromal invasion and tumor greater than 5 cm
  - No LVSI but middle to deep stromal invasion and tumor greater than 4 cm
- 15% of the patients in the adjuvant radiation group experienced disease recurrence, versus 28% of patients in the no further treatment group, reflecting a significant decrease in recurrence risk in patients who received adjuvant radiation. As such, patients who meet these criteria are recommended to undergo adjuvant external beam RT.[21]

High-Risk Factors and Management

- In a randomized controlled trial, patients with high-risk features including positive margins, and/or positive pelvic LNs, and/or microscopic involvement of the parametria by tumor in the surgical specimen were randomized to receive external beam RT with or without concurrent chemotherapy. These high-risk features are associated with a 40% risk of recurrence and 50% risk of death. Patients randomized to the chemotherapy arm received cisplatin 70 mg/m² and 5-fluorouracil 1,000 mg/m²/d over 96 hours every 3 weeks for 4 cycles.[22] Subsequent studies have demonstrated superior outcomes and reduced toxicity with cisplatin regimens. Single-agent cisplatin was found to be as efficacious as dual regimens and is the current standard of care dosed at 40 mg/m² weekly.
- The addition of chemotherapy was associated with improved PFS and OS. As such, patients who have high-risk features including positive surgical margins, positive pelvic LNs, or parametrial involvement should be treated with the combination of radiation and chemotherapy. This is typically administered as concurrent chemoradiation using cisplatin as a radiosensitizer.

Who Is a Candidate for Fertility Sparing Surgery?

- Patients should desire to preserve fertility and be of reproductive age (typically less than 40 years old).
- Other candidates are patients who have undergone a diagnostic workup with imaging to evaluate for nodal or distant metastases. Additionally, they should have pathological findings consistent with low risk of recurrent disease (lesions of 2 cm or less, at least 1 centimeter distance from the tumor to the internal cervical os on MRI, no suspicious LNs on imaging, and low-risk histology). Patients with neuroendocrine tumors, gastric type adenocarcinoma, or adenoma malignum are not candidates for fertility preservation due to their aggressive nature with higher risk of occult nodal disease and disease recurrence.
- Therefore, patients with stage IAI with LVSI, stage IA2, stage IB1 SCC, adenocarcinoma, or adenosquamous carcinoma may be candidates for fertility sparing management with radical trachelectomy and pelvic lymphadenectomy.[23]
- Radical trachelectomy involves removing the cervix, vaginal margin, and parametria while leaving the body and fundus of the uterus intact. The proximal vagina and lower uterine segment are reapproximated intraoperatively.

What Is the Management for Patients Who Are Not Surgical Candidates?

- Definitive RT is an option for patients who are not surgical candidates due to medical comorbidities or functional status. External beam RT with brachytherapy has equivalent OS compared to surgery in prospective, randomized trials. The total dose of radiation to the cervix should be 80 to 85 Gy.[13]

How Should Patients Be Surveilled Following Completion of Treatment?

- Most recurrences occur within the first 2 years. As such, patients with low-risk disease treated with surgery alone should undergo pelvic exams every 6 months for 2 years and then annually. Patients with high-risk disease who received adjuvant therapy after surgery should undergo pelvic exams every 3 months for 2 years, and then every 6 months until 5 years after completion of treatment.[24]
- Annual cytology with Pap smears may be helpful to detect recurrent dysplasia or cancer. Any visible lesions identified should be biopsied.

Case 18.2: Locally Advanced Cervical Cancer

A 51-year-old female presents with malodorous vaginal discharge, pelvic pressure, and left flank pain. On exam, the cervix is firm, lobulated, and approximately 8 cm in size with extension to the left pelvic sidewall. A cervical biopsy is obtained and demonstrates invasive moderate to poorly differentiated keratinizing SCC.

The patient's clinical stage is FIGO stage IIIB.

What Management Strategies Are Available for Locally Advanced Cervical Cancer (Stage IB3 to IVA)?

- Large, randomized trials have demonstrated that concurrent chemoradiation offers a curative management strategy and this is the standard of care.
- Several chemotherapy regimens have been investigated in these randomized trials.

○ Patients with locally advanced disease were randomized to radiation alone versus radiation with concurrent cisplatin and 5-fluorouracil. Patients treated with radiation alone had a 5-year DFS of 40% compared to 67% in the chemoradiation arm (*P* less than 0.001). The rates of locoregional recurrence and distant failure were significantly higher in the radiation-only group.[25]

○ In patients with negative para-aortic LNs, hydroxyurea alone (3 g/m^2 orally twice weekly) was compared to weekly cisplatin alone (40 mg/m^2 weekly) or cisplatin (50 mg/m^2 day 1 and 29) with hydroxyurea (2 g/m^2 orally twice weekly) and 5-fluorouracil (4 g/m^2 as a 96h infusion, day 1 and 29). The platinum-containing arms had improved PFS and OS compared to hydroxyurea alone. Cisplatin alone became the treatment of choice as this was better tolerated than the three-drug regimen.[26,27]

- Patients are commonly treated with daily external beam radiation with a total dose of 45 Gy and concurrent cisplatin 40 mg/m^2 weekly. The primary tumor then receives an additional 30 to 40 Gy using brachytherapy.[23]

- As an alternative to cisplatin, patients who are older (older than 60 years), who have impaired renal function or underlying renal disease (creatinine clearance of greater than 40 mL/min, or those who have a poor PS (ECOG PS of 2 or greater), can be treated with carboplatin 100 mg/m^2 weekly. A Phase II trial demonstrated similar efficacy and survival of carboplatin and radiation compared to a historical cohort treated with cisplatin and radiation.[28]

What Is the Management of Para-Aortic Lymph Node Metastases?

- Patients who have para-aortic nodal disease (either biopsy proven or seen on imaging) have a worse prognosis with a 5-year survival of 40%.[29] These patients were excluded from several of the aforementioned studies.

- Patients with positive para-aortic nodes are treated with extended field radiation to cover the para-aortic region, in combination with weekly cisplatin. This is associated with a high rate of grade 3 to 4 gastrointestinal (19%) and hematologic (15.1%) toxicities.[30]

How Should Patients With Locally Advanced Disease Be Surveilled Following Completion of Treatment?

- A PET/CT scan should be obtained 3 to 4 months after completion of chemoradiation to assess for treatment response.

- Most recurrences occur within the first 2 years. As such, patients should be seen for symptom evaluation and pelvic exam every 3 months for 2 years and then every 6 months until 5 years.[24]

- Annual cytology with Pap smears may be helpful to detect recurrent dysplasia or cancer. Any visible lesions identified should be biopsied.

- Patients should be educated on symptoms associated with recurrence: vaginal bleeding, abnormal vaginal discharge, abdominal or pelvic pain, or changes to urinary or bowel habits.

Case 18.3: Distant Metastatic and Recurrent Cervical Cancer

A 65-year-old female presents to the ED with new-onset shortness of breath and fatigue in the setting of a 1-year history of vaginal bleeding. She reports a history of a normal Pap smear 15 years ago but stopped screening after she went through menopause. Pelvic exam shows a 6-cm friable mass that fills the upper third of the vaginal canal with extension to the pelvic sidewall bilaterally. A CT of the chest, abdomen, and pelvis demonstrates a 6.5-cm pelvic mass completely obliterating the cervix with extension into the vagina, retroperitoneal lymphadenopathy, and several pulmonary nodules 1 to 2 cm in size. A biopsy of a lung nodule is consistent with metastatic SCC of the cervix. She is noted to be severely anemic with an Hgb of 6.1 g/dL. Her PS is ECOG 1.

What Management Options Are Available for Metastatic Cervical Cancer?

Systemic Chemotherapy

- The role of chemotherapy in patients with metastatic cervical cancer is palliative. The 5-year OS rates in this patient population are less than 10%.
- Several prospective randomized trials evaluated systemic treatment options in metastatic or recurrent cervical cancer. Cisplatin was compared to cisplatin plus paclitaxel and the combination therapy was found to have a better response rate and PFS.[31]
- GOG 240 evaluated the addition of bevacizumab 15 mg/kg to cisplatin 50 mg/m² and paclitaxel 135 or 175 mg/m² or topotecan 0.75 mg/m² on days 1 to 3, plus paclitaxel 175 mg/m². The topotecan-paclitaxel combination was not found to be superior to cisplatin-paclitaxel. The addition of bevacizumab to combination therapy resulted in improvement in OS by 3.7 months and higher response rates overall (48% vs. 36%). Bevacizumab resulted in increased hypertension (25% vs. 2%), thromboembolic events (8% vs. 1%), and gastrointestinal fistulas (3% vs. 0%) when compared to chemotherapy alone.[32] As such, bevacizumab should be used with chemotherapy for treatment of metastatic or recurrent cervical cancer in all patients unless there is a medical contraindication such as poorly controlled hypertension, untreated venous thromboembolism, risk of acute hemorrhage, or perforated viscus.
- Cisplatin 50 mg/m² and paclitaxel 135 mg/m² were compared to carboplatin area under the curve (AUC) 5 mg/mL/min and paclitaxel 175 mg/m² in patients with recurrent or metastatic cervical cancer. The combination of carboplatin and paclitaxel was noninferior to cisplatin and paclitaxel and was associated with less hematologic toxicities. In patients who had not been previously treated with a platinum agent, cisplatin was favored with a hazard ratio (HR) of 1.57 (95% CI 1.06 to 2.32).[33] Based upon this study, it is recommended that patients who have not received prior cisplatin as a radiosensitizer should receive cisplatin as part of their systemic chemotherapy regimen, but patients who have received cisplatin previously may receive carboplatin with equivalent outcomes and less toxicity.
- In patients who have not received prior chemotherapy, pembrolizumab (a monoclonal antibody to programmed death-ligand 1 [PD-L1]) may be used as a first-line agent. See the following section on immunotherapy.

What Prognostic Factors May Indicate a Poor Response to Systemic Chemotherapy?

- The Moore criteria are a set of prognostic factors that identify patients who are likely to benefit from the addition of bevacizumab to chemotherapy. These factors were identified using pooled data from three prospective randomized trials. Clinical prognostic factors include African American race, PS greater than 0, pelvic disease, prior platinum chemotherapy, and time from diagnosis to recurrence less than 1 year. Patients are then stratified based upon the number of factors: low risk (0 to 1 factor), medium risk (2 to 3 factors), and high risk (4 to 5 factors). Patients who were classified as low risk did not benefit from the addition of bevacizumab to chemotherapy (OS 21.8 vs. 22.9 months, HR 1.119 [95% CI 0.558 to 2.244]), whereas high-risk patients had a significant survival benefit if they received bevacizumab (OS 6.3 vs. 12.1 months, HR 0.377 [95% CI 0.201 to 0.701]).[34,35]

Immunotherapy

- In HPV-induced cancers, the PD-L1 pathway is unregulated. Pembrolizumab is a highly selective antibody to PD-1.
- In cervical cancer, PD-L1 expression is measured by a combined positive score (CPS), which is the ratio of PD-L1–positive cells (lymphocytes, macrophages, and tumor cells) to the total number of tumor cells. Positivity is defined as a CPS score of 1 or greater.
- In 2018, the U.S. Food and Drug Administration (FDA) approved pembrolizumab for treatment of PD-L1–positive advanced cervical cancer with progression after chemotherapy.

Pembrolizumab as First-Line Therapy

- In a Phase III trial (KEYNOTE-826), 617 patients were randomized 1:1 to receive pembrolizumab or placebo plus platinum-based chemotherapy with or without bevacizumab as first-line therapy for persistent, recurrent, or metastatic cervical cancer. The OS at 2 years was 53% in patients who received pembrolizumab versus 41.7% in the placebo group (HR 0.67, 95% CI 0.54 to 0.84).[36] Patients with CPS scores of 1 or greater appeared to benefit more from the addition of pembrolizumab than patients with CPS scores of 0.

Pembrolizumab as a Second-Line Therapy

- KEYNOTE-028 was a Phase Ib basket trial that assessed the safety and efficacy of pembrolizumab in 24 patients with heavily pretreated cervical cancer whose tumors were PD-L1–positive. The overall response rate (ORR) was 17% with a median duration of response of 5.4 months in those who achieved a partial response.[37]
- In KEYNOTE-158, a Phase II basket study, 98 patients with cervical cancer were treated with pembrolizumab 200 mg every 3 weeks for 2 years or until progression or intolerable toxicity. In PD-L1–positive tumors, the ORR was 14.6%.[38] Although the ORR was low, in patients who did respond to treatment, the median duration of response was not reached.

Immunotherapy Adverse Events

- The most common adverse events (AEs) from anti-PD-1/PD-L1 therapies are rash, pruritis, and fatigue. Less common AEs are thyroid dysfunction, hepatotoxicity, colitis, and pneumonitis. Cardiac toxicities (myocarditis, pericarditis, arrhythmias, cardiomyopathies), rheumatologic toxicities (myalgias or arthralgias), renal dysfunction, and ocular toxicities are all rare.[39] Management of these toxicities is dependent upon the grade of the AE. This may include supportive care with continuation of the treatment drug. Treatment delays or drug cessation and administration of glucocorticoids are required for grade 3 or 4 toxicities.

Surgery

- Patients who have oligometastatic recurrent disease confined to a central location in the pelvis without sidewall extension or LN involvement may be candidates for an exenterative procedure. Pelvic exenteration involves an en bloc resection of all pelvic viscera which may include removal of the distal colon, rectum, bladder, ureters, uterus, cervix, and adnexal structures. This is accompanied by reconstructive procedures to divert the urine and stool, and occasionally vaginal reconstruction. Patients should be well counseled about the associated morbidity with this procedure. The goal of an exenterative procedure is curative.

REVIEW QUESTIONS

1. A 33-year-old nulligravid female underwent a preconception workup including a Pap smear that resulted as high-grade squamous intraepithelial lesion (HSIL) and human papillomavirus (HPV) 16-positive. She then had a colposcopy with biopsy at 11 o'clock due to acetowhite changes and atypical vessels. The biopsy demonstrated at least HSIL for which a loop electrosurgical excision procedure (LEEP) was performed. This specimen showed a well-differentiated squamous cell carcinoma (SCC) with a depth of invasion of 4 mm without lymphovascular space invasion (LVSI) and negative margins. What treatment option would you offer to her?
   A. Radical hysterectomy with pelvic lymphadenectomy
   B. Systemic therapy with cisplatin, paclitaxel, and bevacizumab
   C. Radical trachelectomy with pelvic lymphadenectomy
   D. Serial Pap smears

2. A 55-year-old patient has been diagnosed with a stage IIB adenocarcinoma of the cervix. She has a past medical history (PMH) significant for chronic kidney disease (CKD) with a creatinine clearance of 44 mL/min. She has an Eastern Cooperative Oncology Group (ECOG) performance status (PS) of 2. Which of the following agents would you recommend for chemosensitization with external beam radiation?
   A. Cisplatin
   B. Gemcitabine
   C. Fluorouracil
   D. Carboplatin

3. A 44-year-old patient has a preoperative diagnosis of a moderately differentiated squamous cell carcinoma (SCC) confined to the cervix that is 1.8 cm in diameter. She has undergone an exploratory laparotomy, radical hysterectomy with bilateral salpingectomy, and pelvic lymphadenectomy. On her final pathology report, her tumor is 2.2 cm in size, and there is lymphovascular space invasion (LVSI) and stromal invasion of the middle third. What would you recommend next for her?
   A. External beam radiation therapy (RT)
   B. Systemic therapy with cisplatin, paclitaxel, and bevacizumab
   C. Systemic therapy with 5-fluorouracil and cisplatin
   D. Serial Pap smears

4. A 47-year-old patient presents to the ED with foul-smelling vaginal discharge and right-sided flank pain. She is noted to have a bulky cervical mass extending to the pelvic sidewall causing hydronephrosis. Biopsy shows a squamous cell carcinoma (SCC) of the cervix, and she is noted to be stage IIIB. Which of the following single agents is NOT used for chemoradiation in cervical cancer?
   A. Cisplatin
   B. Gemcitabine
   C. 5-Fluorouracil
   D. Carboplatin

5. A 61-year-old patient has been diagnosed with a stage IB3 adenocarcinoma of the cervix. She has a past medical history (PMH) significant for chronic kidney disease (CKD) and has a 40-year pack per day smoking history. She has an Eastern Cooperative Oncology Group (ECOG) performance status (PS) of 1. She is undergoing concurrent chemotherapy and radiation with cisplatin 40 mg/m² weekly. On her pretreatment labs, she is noted to

have a hemoglobin (Hgb) of 7.8 g/dL. What would be your next step in management for this patient?

A. Erythropoietin infusion

B. Iron supplementation

C. Packed red blood cell transfusion

D. Filgrastim infusion

6. A 48-year-old patient who has a history significant for stage IIB squamous cell carcinoma (SCC) of the cervix is presenting with new-onset vaginal bleeding and pelvic pain. She completed concurrent chemoradiation with cisplatin 2 years ago. Imaging shows a new 2-cm enhancing mass within the cervix without evidence of nodal or distant metastases. Biopsy confirms a recurrence of her SCC. Her Eastern Cooperative Oncology Group (ECOG) performance status (PS) is 0. What treatment strategy would you offer to her?

A. Total pelvic exenteration

B. Pembrolizumab

C. External beam radiation therapy (RT) with brachytherapy

D. Cisplatin and paclitaxel

7. A 66-year-old patient with a history of stage IIIC1 squamous cell carcinoma (SCC) of the cervix is presenting with new-onset shortness of breath. CT of the chest shows concerns for a new pleural effusion and multiple new 1- to 2-cm pulmonary nodules. She completed concurrent chemoradiation with cisplatin 40 mg/m^2 13 months ago. Her Eastern Cooperative Oncology Group (ECOG) performance status (PS) is 1. What would be your next treatment recommendation for her?

A. Cisplatin and gemcitabine

B. Pembrolizumab

C. Cisplatin and paclitaxel

D. Carboplatin, paclitaxel, and bevacizumab

E. Stereotactic body radiation therapy (RT) to the pulmonary lesions

8. A 66-year-old patient presents to the clinic for evaluation for cycle 3 of pembrolizumab 200 mg intravenous (IV) for her recurrent cervical cancer. Three days prior, she presented to the ED with a diffuse, itchy rash on her lower extremities. She was started on a topical steroid cream which she has been using daily. On exam, her rash appears to be slightly improved. What is your next step in management?

A. Proceed with cycle 3 of pembrolizumab but dosed at 100 mg this cycle

B. Increase the potency of her topical steroid and delay this cycle by 2 weeks

C. Proceed with cycle 3 of pembrolizumab at 200 mg IV with weekly clinic visits to evaluate her

D. Stop this regimen and change to nivolumab

9. A 34-year-old female is 15 weeks' pregnant. A Pap smear was obtained during her prenatal visit, and this was concerning for squamous cell carcinoma (SCC). Diagnostic workup with biopsy and imaging shows she has a stage IA1 SCC without lymphovascular space invasion (LVSI), and this is a desired pregnancy. What is your next step in management of this during pregnancy?

A. External beam radiation

B. Conization

C. Neoadjuvant chemotherapy

D. Radical hysterectomy

10. A 57-year-old patient with stage IIB squamous cell carcinoma (SCC) of the cervix has completed her concurrent chemoradiation with a total dose of 45 Gy. On exam, there is no residual tumor visualized on the cervix. What is your next step in management?

A. Surveillance

B. Radical hysterectomy

C. Conization

D. Brachytherapy

1. **C. Radical trachelectomy with pelvic lymphadenectomy.** As a patient with stage IA2 SCC desiring future fertility, she would be a candidate for fertility preservation with a radical trachelectomy with pelvic lymphadenectomy. If she did not desire future fertility, A would be an option for her.

2. **D. Carboplatin.** Patients who are older, who have a poorer PS, or who have impaired kidney function can be treated with carboplatin 100 mg/m^2 with similar results as compared to cisplatin.

3. **A. External beam radiation therapy (RT).** This patient meets the Sedlis criteria and would be recommended adjuvant external beam RT to reduce the risk of recurrence.

4. **C. 5-Fluorouracil.** Fluorouracil alone is not recommended for primary chemoradiation as this has not been shown to be better than radiation therapy alone in locally advanced cervical cancer.[40] Single-agent paclitaxel has been studied in locally advanced or recurrent cervical cancer but had significant toxicities associated including grade 3 gastrointestinal (GI) toxicities.[41] As such, it is not recommended for use. In patients with stage IIIB cervical cancer and obstructive uropathy with renal dysfunction, gemcitabine 300 mg/m^2 weekly has been shown to be an option for chemoradiation.[42] Several studies support using cisplatin alone for chemoradiation, and this is the standard of care.

5. **C. Packed red blood cell transfusion.** Anemia in this patient population is common and generally multifactorial due to vaginal bleeding, anemia of chronic disease, and concurrent chemotherapy. It is theorized that adequate oxygenation of tumors leads to increased radiosensitization by facilitating the formation of reactive oxygen species resulting in permanent DNA damage and cell death. Correcting for anemia is hypothesized to improve oxygenation to the tumors, making them more sensitive to radiation. In the International Delphi Consensus study in 2020, gynecologic radiation oncologists suggest a target Hgb of 9 g/dL while being judicious, as this is a scarce resource.[43] Erythropoietin infusion is not recommended due to an increased risk of venous thromboembolic events.

6. **A. Total pelvic exenteration.** She is a candidate for exenteration due to the central location of her recurrence, lack of metastatic disease, relatively long treatment-free interval, and good PS. Exenterations should be offered with curative intent. As she has already undergone definitive chemoradiation, additional radiation cannot be given without significant side effects. Systemic therapy may be indicated for patients who are not medically fit to undergo an exenteration or who have multiple sites of disease. These patients would be treated with cisplatin or carboplatin, paclitaxel, or bevacizumab.

7. **D. Carboplatin, paclitaxel, and bevacizumab.** In patients who have recurrent cervical cancer who have not had prior platinum, management would be systemic therapy with cisplatin, paclitaxel, and bevacizumab. In patients who have had prior platinum therapy, the combination of carboplatin, paclitaxel, and bevacizumab is recommended as this has the same oncological outcomes but less toxicity.[33]

8. **C. Proceed with cycle 3 of pembrolizumab at 200 mg IV with weekly clinic visits to evaluate her.** Dermatologic changes are some of the most common adverse events (AEs) associated with anti-programmed death-ligand 1 (PD-L1)/PD-L1 therapies. This patient has a grade 2 skin rash (defined as a rash that covers 10% to 30% of body surface area).

The management entails applying topical steroids to the affected area; proceed with treatment on schedule, and evaluate weekly for improvement. If the rash covers more than 30% of the body surface area (grade 3 and greater), treatment includes initiation of systemic steroids and to hold or stop treatment. Once symptoms have improved to grade 1 to 2, treatment can be resumed.[39]

9. **B. Conization.** Cervical cancer is one of the most common cancers diagnosed in pregnancy. Approximately 3% of cervical cancer cases are diagnosed during the antepartum or postpartum period. Management depends upon the stage of disease and gestational age. As this patient's gestational age is less than 22 weeks, intervention with conization is reasonable during pregnancy with definitive treatment to follow postpartum.

10. **D. Brachytherapy.** Brachytherapy is a critical component of definitive treatment and is used to boost the radiation dose to the primary tumor by 30 to 40 Gy, bringing the total dose of radiation to 85 Gy or greater.

REFERENCES

1. Sung H, Ferlay J, Siegel RL, et al. Global cancer statistics 2020: GLOBOCAN estimates of incidence and mortality worldwide for 36 cancers in 185 countries. *CA Cancer J Clin.* 2021;71(3):209–249. doi:10.3322/caac.21660

2. Siegel RL, Miller KD, Fuchs HF, Jemal A. Cancer statistics, 2021. *CA Cancer J Clin.* 2021;71(1):7–33. doi:10.3322/caac.21654

3. Park KJ. Cervical adenocarcinoma: integration of HPV status, pattern of invasion, morphology and molecular markers into classification. *Histopathol.* 2020;76(1):112–127. doi:10.1111/his.13995

4. Stolnicu S, Barsan I, Hoang L, et al. International Endocervical Adenocarcinoma Criteria and Classification (IECC): a new pathogenetic classification for invasive adenocarcinomas of the endocervix. *Am J Surg Pathol.* 2018;42(2):214–226. doi:10.1097/PAS.0000000000000986

5. Smith HO, Tiffany MF, Qualls CR, Key CR. The rising incidence of adenocarcinoma relative to squamous cell carcinoma of the uterine cervix in the United States—a 24-year population-based study. *Gynecol Oncol.* 2000;78(2):97–105. doi:10.1006/gyno.2000.5826

6. Gardner GJ, Reidy-Lagunes D, Gehrig PA. Neuroendocrine tumors of the gynecologic tract: a Society of Gynecologic Oncology (SGO) clinical document. *Gynecol Oncol.* 2011;122(1):190–198. doi:10.1016/j.ygyno.2011.04.011

7. Berek JS, Hacker NF. *Berek and Hacker's Gynecologic Oncology.* 7th ed. Wolters Kluwer; 2021.

8. Subak LL, Hricak H, Powell CB, et al. Cervical carcinoma: computed tomography and magnetic resonance imaging for preoperative staging. *Obstet Gynecol.* 1995;86(1):43–50. doi:10.1016/0029-7844(95)00109-5

9. Narayan K, McKenzie A, Fisher R, et al. Estimation of tumor volume in cervical cancer by magnetic resonance imaging. *Am J Clin Oncol.* 2003;26(5):e163–e168. doi:10.1097/01.coc.0000091358.78047.b5

10. Scheidler J, Hricak H, Yu KK, et al. Radiological evaluation of lymph node metastases in patients with cervical cancer. A meta-analysis. *JAMA.* 1997;278(13):1096–1101. doi:10.1001/jama.1997.03550130070040

11. Havrilesky LJ, Kulasingam SL, Matchar DB, Myers ER. FDG-PET for management of cervical and ovarian cancer. *Gynecol Oncol.* 2005;97(1):183–191. doi:10.1016/j.ygyno.2004.12.007

12. Bhatla N, Berek JS, Cuello Fredes M, et al. Revised FIGO staging for carcinoma of the cervix uteri. *Int J Gynaecol Obstet.* 2019;145(1):129–135. doi:10.1002/ijgo.12749

13. Landoni F, Maneo A, Colombo A, et al. Randomised study of radical surgery versus radiotherapy for stage Ib-IIa cervical cancer. *Lancet.* 1997;350(9077):535–540. doi:10.1016/S0140-6736(97)02250-2

14. Ramirez PT, Frumovitz M, Pareja R, et al. Minimally invasive versus abdominal radical hysterectomy for cervical cancer. *N Engl J Med.* 2018;379(20):1895–1904. doi:10.1056/NEJMoa1806395

15. Melamed A, Margul DJ, Chen L, et al. Survival after minimally invasive radical hysterectomy for early-stage cervical cancer. *N Engl J Med.* 2018;379(20):1905–1914. doi:10.1056/NEJMoa1804923

16. Uppal S, Gehrig PA, Peng K, et al. Recurrence rates in patients with cervical cancer treated with abdominal versus minimally invasive radical hysterectomy: a multi-institutional retrospective review study. *J Clin Oncol.* 2020;38(10):1030–1040. doi:10.1200/JCO.19.03012

17. Lécuru F, Mathevet P, Querleu D, et al. Bilateral negative sentinel nodes accurately predict absence of lymph node metastasis in early cervical cancer: results of the SENTICOL study. *J Clin Oncol.* 2011;29(13):1686–1691. doi:10.1200/JCO.2010.32.0432

18. McCall ML, Keaty EC, Thompson JD. Conservation of ovarian tissue in the treatment of carcinoma of the cervix with radical surgery. *Am J Obstet Gynecol.* 1958;75(3):590–600; discussion 600–605. doi:10.1016/0002-9378(58)90614-8

19. Touhami O, Plante M. Should ovaries be removed or not in (early-stage) adenocarcinoma of the uterine cervix: a review. *Gynecol Oncol.* 2015;136(2):384–388. doi:10.1016/j.ygyno.2014.12.011

20. Sedlis A, Bundy BN, Rotman MZ, et al. A randomized trial of pelvic radiation therapy versus no further therapy in selected patients with stage IB carcinoma of the cervix after radical hysterectomy and pelvic lymphadenectomy: a Gynecologic Oncology Group study. *Gynecol Oncol.* 1999;73(2):177–183. doi:10.1006/gyno.1999.5387

21. Rotman M, Sedlis A, Piedmonte MR, et al. A phase III randomized trial of postoperative pelvic irradiation in Stage IB cervical carcinoma with poor prognostic features: follow-up of a Gynecologic Oncology Group study. *Int J Radiat Oncol Biol Phys.* 2006;65(1):169–176. doi:10.1016/j.ijrobp.2005.10.019

22. Peters WA 3rd, Liu PY, Barrett RJ 2nd, et al. Concurrent chemotherapy and pelvic radiation therapy compared with pelvic radiation therapy alone as adjuvant therapy after radical surgery in high-risk early-stage cancer of the cervix. *J Clin Oncol.* 2000;18(8):1606–1613. doi:10.1200/JCO.2000.18.8.1606

23. National Comprehensive Cancer Network. NCCN Guidelines. Cervical Cancer. Version 1.2021 https://www.nccn.org/professionals/physician_gls/pdf/cervical.pdf

24. Salani R, Khanna N, Frimer M, et al. An update on post-treatment surveillance and diagnosis of recurrence in women with gynecologic malignancies: Society of Gynecologic Oncology (SGO) recommendations. *Gynecol Oncol.* 2017;146(1):3–10. doi:10.1016/j.ygyno.2017.03.022

25. Morris M, Eifel PJ, Lu J, et al. Pelvic radiation with concurrent chemotherapy compared with pelvic and para-aortic radiation for high-risk cervical cancer. *N Engl J Med.* 1999;340(15):1137–1143. doi:10.1056/NEJM199904153401501

26. Rose PG, Bundy BN, Watkins EB, et al. Concurrent cisplatin-based radiotherapy and chemotherapy for locally advanced cervical cancer. *N Engl J Med.* 1999;340(15):1144–1153. doi:10.1056/NEJM199904153401502

27. Rose PG, Ali S, Watkins E, et al. Long-term follow-up of a randomized trial comparing concurrent single agent cisplatin, cisplatin-based combination chemotherapy, or hydroxyurea during pelvic irradiation for locally advanced cervical cancer: a Gynecologic Oncology Group study. *J Clin Oncol.* 2007;25(19):2804–2810. doi:10.1200/JCO.2006.09.4532

28. Nam EJ, Lee M, Yim GW, et al. Comparison of carboplatin- and cisplatin-based concurrent chemoradiotherapy in locally advanced cervical cancer patients with morbidity risks. *Oncologist.* 2013;18(7):843–849. doi:10.1634/theoncologist.2012-0455

29. Macdonald OK, Chen J, Dodson M, et al. Prognostic significance of histology and positive lymph node involvement following radical hysterectomy in carcinoma of the cervix. *Am J Clin Oncol.* 2009;32(4):411–416. doi:10.1097/COC.0b013e31819142dc

30. Varia MA, Bundy BN, Deppe G, et al. Cervical carcinoma metastatic to para-aortic nodes: extended field radiation therapy with concomitant 5-fluorouracil and cisplatin chemotherapy: a Gynecologic Oncology Group study. *Int J Radiat Oncol Biol Phys.* 1998;42(5):1015–1023. doi:10.1016/s0360-3016(98)00267-3

31. Moore DH, Blessing JA, McQuellon RP, et al. Phase III study of cisplatin with or without paclitaxel in stage IVB, recurrent, or persistent squamous cell carcinoma of the cervix: a Gynecologic Oncology Group study. *J Clin Oncol.* 2004;22(15):3113–3119. doi:10.1200/JCO.2004.04.170

32. Tewari KS, Sill MW, Long HJ, et al. Improved survival with bevacizumab in advanced cervical cancer. *N Engl J Med.* 2014;370(8):734–743. 10.1056/NEJMoa1309748

33. Kitagawa R, Katsumata N, Shibata T, et al. Paclitaxel plus carboplatin versus paclitaxel plus cisplatin in metastatic or recurrent cervical cancer: the open-label randomized phase III Trial JCOG0505. *J Clin Oncol.* 2015;33(19):2129–2135. doi:10.1200/JCO.2014.58.4391

34. Moore DH, Tian C, Monk BJ, et al. Prognostic factors for response to cisplatin-based chemotherapy in advanced cervical carcinoma: a Gynecologic Oncology Group study. *Gynecol Oncol.* 2010;116(1):44–49. doi:10.1016/j.ygyno.2009.09.006

35. Tewari KS, Sill MW, Monk BJ, et al. Prospective validation of pooled prognostic factors in women with advanced cervical cancer treated with chemotherapy with/without bevacizumab: NRG Oncology/GOG study. *Clin Cancer Res.* 2015;21(24):5480–5487. doi:10.1158/1078-0432.CCR-15-1346

36. Colombo N, Dubot C, Lorusso D, et al. Pembrolizumab for persistent, recurrent, or metastatic cervical cancer. *N Engl J Med.* 2021;385(20):1856–1867. doi:10.1056/NEJMoa2112435

37. Frenel J-S, Le Tourneau C, O'Neil B, et al. Safety and efficacy of pembrolizumab in advanced, programmed death ligand 1-positive cervical cancer: results from the phase Ib KEYNOTE-028 trial. *J Clin Oncol.* 2017;35(36):4035–4041. doi: 0.1200/JCO.2017.74.5471

38. Chung HC, Ros W, Delord J-P, et al. Efficacy and safety of pembrolizumab in previously treated advanced cervical cancer: results from the phase II KEYNOTE-158 study. *J Clin Oncol.* 2019;37(17):1470–1478. doi:10.1200/JCO.18.01265

39. Haanen JBAG, Carbonnel F, Robert C, et al. Management of toxicities from immunotherapy: ESMO clinical practice guidelines for diagnosis, treatment and follow-up. *Ann Oncol.* 2017;28(suppl_4):iv119–iv142. doi:10.1093/annonc/mdx225

40. Thomas G, Dembo A, Ackerman I, et al. A randomized trial of standard versus partially hyperfractionated radiation with or without concurrent 5-fluorouracil in locally advanced cervical cancer. *Gynecol Oncol.* 1998;69(2):137–145. doi:10.1006/gyno.1998.4990
41. Cerrotta A, Gardan G, Cavina R, et al. Concurrent radiotherapy and weekly paclitaxel for locally advanced or recurrent squamous cell carcinoma of the uterine cervix. A pilot study with intensification of dose. *Eur J Gynaecol Oncol.* 2002;23(2):115–119. https://www.imrpress.com/journal/EJGO/23/2/pii/2002125
42. Cetina L, Rivera L, Candelaria M, et al. Chemoradiation with gemcitabine for cervical cancer in patients with renal failure. *Anticancer Drugs.* 2004;15(8):761–766. doi:10.1097/00001813-200409000-00004
43. Zayed S, Nguyen TK, Lin C, et al. Red blood cell transfusion practices for patients with cervical cancer undergoing radiotherapy. *JAMA Netw Open.* 2021;4(4):e213531. doi:10.1001/jamanetworkopen.2021.3531

CHAPTER 19

Uterine Cancer

Claire Hoppenot

INTRODUCTION

In 2021, over 66,000 new cases of uterine cancer were diagnosed, which made up 3.5% of all new cancers in the United States. Uterine cancer includes cancers of the endometrium as well as rare histologies such as sarcomas.

Endometrial cancer is the most common gynecologic cancer. Over 85% of women with endometrial cancer present with abnormal vaginal bleeding or discharge. Other symptoms include abdominal pain or glandular cells on a Pap smear. Many have a precursor lesion (endometrial intraepithelial neoplasia [EIN] or complex atypical hyperplasia). Major risk factors include increased estrogen and genetic predisposition. Obesity is by far the strongest risk factor and the risk of endometrial cancer increases exponentially with increasing body mass index (BMI). Other risk factors include tamoxifen use, nulliparity, early menarche, and late menopause. Genetic syndromes associated with endometrial cancer include loss of mismatch repair (MMR) proteins (hereditary non-polyposis colorectal cancer syndromes [HNPCC]) and loss of PTEN (Cowden's syndrome).

Endometrial cancers have classically been divided by histology (endometrioid, serous, clear cell). However, The Cancer Genome Atlas (TCGA) developed classifications for endometrial cancer based on genomic expression and prognosis. The molecular groupings from best to worst prognosis are polymerase epsilon (POLE) ultramutated, copy number low (generally low-grade endometrioid cancers), microsatellite instability (MSI)/hypermutated, and copy number high (with high $p53$ expression). While these classifications are not yet used clinically, they are guiding research and individualized treatment decisions.

Sarcomas are much less common, and frequently present with bulk symptoms or abnormal vaginal bleeding. These include leiomyosarcomas, which are aggressive and carry a poor prognosis, as well as endometrial stromal sarcomas, which tend to be more indolent. These are not associated with the typical endometrial cancer risk factors.

CASE SUMMARIES

Case 19.1: Type 1 Endometrial Cancer

SF is a 56-year-old with a past medical history (PMH) of diabetes, hypertension, and obesity. She went through menopause at age 52 and mentioned intermittent vaginal bleeding over the past 6 months at her annual primary care visit. She was referred to her gynecologist for further evaluation. On exam, she is overall well appearing, no palpable cervical or inguinal lymphadenopathy, there is a small amount of dark blood in the vaginal vault, and her uterus is small, mobile, and nontender.

How Is a Diagnosis Established?

- The workup for postmenopausal bleeding includes a pelvic ultrasound (US) to evaluate the endometrial stripe and/or an endometrial biopsy.
- Women with postmenopausal bleeding and an endometrial stripe less than 4 to 5 mm in thickness have a less than 1% chance of cancer or hyperplasia.[1]
- An endometrial biopsy is indicated for women with an endometrial stripe over 4 mm or with ongoing bleeding. If an endometrial biopsy cannot be achieved in the office, the patient can be taken to the operating room for a dilation and curettage (D&C).

Patient's Diagnosis

- *A pelvic US revealed an endometrial stripe of 11 mm.*
- *An endometrial biopsy revealed grade 2 endometrial cancer.*
- *A CT scan was unremarkable except for a slightly thickened endometrial stripe. No lymphadenopathy or distant disease was appreciated.*

What Further Molecular or Genomic Testing Is Required?

- MMR protein immunohistochemistry (IHC) will show loss of MMR protein expression in about 40% of endometrial cancers. Loss of *MLH1* should prompt evaluation for *MLH1* promoter hypermethylation, which is a somatic mutation affecting *MLH1* expression and is the most common reason for loss of MMR expression. Loss of any other MMR protein or loss of *MLH1* in the absence of promoter hypermethylation should prompt genetic testing.

Patient's Molecular and Genomic Testing

- *SF's pathology shows loss of MLH1, and MLH1 promoter hypermethylation is present.*

How Is This Tumor Staged?

- Endometrial cancer is staged surgically. Patients who are surgical candidates undergo hysterectomy, bilateral salpingo-oophorectomy, and sentinel or complete pelvic lymph node (LN) dissection. Patients with grade 3 endometrioid, serous, or clear cell histology on endometrial biopsy also undergo an omental biopsy.
- Sentinel LNs are detected by injecting Indocyanine Green (ICG) into the cervix; the first draining LN is removed and has been shown to have a 99% negative predictive value and 97% sensitivity for positive pelvic LNs. In the absence of a sentinel LN, the entire pelvic basin is resected.[2]
- Patients who are not surgical candidates or desire fertility-sparing treatments can be staged with imaging including CT, MRI, and/or PET scans.
- Stage I cancers are confined to the uterus. Stage II cancers involve the cervical stroma, and stage III cancers have spread outside the uterus. Pelvic LNs are stage IIIC1 and para-aortic LNs are consistent with stage IIIC2. Stage IV disease is either local involvement (IVA) or distant metastases such as to the omentum, liver, lung, or inguinal LNs (IVB).

Patient's Clinical Stage

- *SF undergoes a laparoscopic hysterectomy, bilateral salpingo-oophorectomy, and bilateral sentinel pelvic LN dissection. There is no evidence of disease in the abdomen or enlarged retroperitoneal LNs. The postoperative pathology shows grade 2 endometrial cancer with 30% myometrial invasion and positive lymphovascular space invasion. Sentinel LNs are negative.*

What Are Appropriate Treatment Options?

- SF has stage IA grade 2 endometrial cancer based on less than 50% myometrial invasion with uterus-confined disease.
- SF is high-intermediate risk, defined by age group and the following risk factors: lympho-vascular space invasion, grade 2 or 3, and more than 50% myometrial invasion. Women aged 50 to 70 with two risk factors are considered high-intermediate risk; younger women require all three risk factors and older women require only one.
- The risk of vaginal cuff recurrence is decreased with vaginal cuff brachytherapy, which is the standard of care for high-intermediate risk endometrial cancer.[3]

Recommended Treatment Plan for This Patient
- SF underwent vaginal cuff brachytherapy for a total of 21 Gy in three high-dose rate (HDR) fractions.

What Are the Toxicities Associated With the Treatment?

- Vaginal cuff brachytherapy has a low rate of complications. Radiation does not affect the bowel or bladder but can cause mild vaginal scarring.

Associated Toxicities for This Patient
- SF tolerated the radiation well with some vaginal dryness but no long-term side effects.

What Are Other Treatment Considerations?

- Studies are underway to evaluate the use of immunotherapy with radiation treatments for high-intermediate risk endometrial cancer and MMR deficiency.
- GOG 249 compared pelvic radiation to vaginal cuff brachytherapy with chemotherapy and did not find any difference in outcomes for high-intermediate risk patients.[4] Additionally, PORTEC II compared pelvic radiation to vaginal cuff brachytherapy alone for high-intermediate risk patients, and did not find a difference in survival.[5]
- Fertility-preserving treatments with hormone therapy can be an option for stage IA grade 1 endometrial cancer. About 60% of stage IA grade 1 endometrial cancers respond to hormone treatments; however, many will recur after cessation of treatments. Fertility rates after fertility-sparing surgery are about 50%, many of which require assisted reproductive therapies.[6,7]
- Young women with early endometrial cancer may benefit from ovarian preservation to avoid early menopause. A retrospective study showed similar cancer-related outcomes for young women regardless of oophorectomy. Leaving ovaries improves menopause-related symptoms as well as cardiovascular health.

What Is Required for This Patient's Follow-Up and Survivorship?
- Symptoms and physical exam with speculum exam, pelvic exam, and rectovaginal exam performed every 3 months for 2 years, then every 6 months until 5 years after diagnosis, then yearly.
- Clinically indicated imaging (usually CT scan) is based on symptoms and physical exam.
- Cytology (Pap smears) have not been shown to improve detection rates for vaginal cuff recurrence.
- The major risk factor for endometrial cancer is obesity. Mortality is more likely from cardiovascular disease than cancer-related mortality due to early endometrial cancer. Follow-up with primary care, control of chronic disease such as hypertension and diabetes, and weight loss have important roles to play in the survivorship of women with early endometrial cancer.

- *In premenopausal women, it is important to monitor for symptoms of menopause. There is insufficient evidence regarding the safety of estrogen supplementation for women with a history of early endometrial cancer, which is almost always estrogen receptor-positive. However, other options for control of menopausal symptoms can be discussed.*

Case 19.2: Advanced Type 2 Endometrial Cancer

KM is a 72-year-old with no PMH coming in with abnormal uterine bleeding. She started having intermittent vaginal bleeding 9 months previously and thought nothing of it until it became more frequent and accompanied by cramping. She is now bleeding daily and changing one to two soaked pads daily. On exam she is well appearing, has no palpable cervical or inguinal lymphadenopathy, and has a slightly enlarged 10-week size uterus.

How Is a Diagnosis Established?

- A pelvic US is the best way to evaluate the size of the endometrium. Women with postmenopausal bleeding and an endometrial stripe less than 4 to 5 mm in thickness have a less than 1% chance of cancer or hyperplasia.[1] Any woman with a thicker endometrium should undergo an endometrial biopsy.
- An endometrial biopsy can be done in the office prior to imaging based on the suspicion for a neoplastic or preneoplastic process.
- If an endometrial biopsy is unsuccessful or benign despite a high level of suspicion for cancer, a D&C can be done as an office procedure with anesthesia or (more commonly) in the operating room.
- CT of the chest, abdomen, and pelvis is used to evaluate for evidence of extrauterine disease.
- A Ca125 level can be done, particularly for type 2 endometrial cancers such as high-grade serous, clear cell, and grade 3 endometrial cancers on biopsy, since up to 16% of them will have an elevated CA125 and peritoneal spread.

Patient's Diagnosis
- *Endometrial biopsy shows serous uterine cancer.*
- *CT scan shows a slightly enlarged uterus with a 3-cm endometrial mass, with no evidence of extrauterine disease.*
- *CA125 is slightly elevated at 52.*

What Further Molecular or Genomic Testing Is Required?

- *HER2* testing IHC with reflex to in situ hybridization for equivocal IHC is performed for advanced or recurrent serous uterine cancers to evaluate for possible improved outcome with trastuzumab.[9,10]
- MMR protein IHC is performed for all endometrial cancers.
- Consider estrogen receptor (ER) testing, as well a *p53* expression and POLE.

Patient's Molecular and Genomic Testing
- *KM's pathology reveals p53 aberrant expression consistent with serous uterine cancer.*
- *MMR proteins have normal expression.*
- *HER2/neu testing shows overexpression.*

How Is This Tumor Staged?

- Patients who are surgical candidates are staged surgically with a hysterectomy and bilateral salpingo-oophorectomy. The LNs must be assessed with a full pelvic and (potentially) para-aortic LN dissection or sentinel LN evaluation after ICG injection.[8] Type 2 endometrial cancers also undergo omental biopsy and biopsy or removal of all other suspicious areas.
- Patients who are not surgical candidates can be staged radiologically with a CT scan, MRI, and/or a PET scan.
- Stage I cancers are confined to the uterus. Stage II cancers involve the cervical stroma, and stage III cancers have spread outside the uterus. Pelvic LNs are stage IIIC1 and para-aortic LNs are consistent with stage IIIC2. Stage IV disease is either local involvement (IVA) or distant metastases such as to the omentum, liver, lung, or inguinal lymph nodes (IVB).

Patient's Clinical Stage

- *KM undergoes a laparoscopic hysterectomy, bilateral salpingo-oophorectomy, bilateral sentinel pelvic LN dissection, and omental biopsy. There is no evidence of disease in the abdomen during the procedure. The pathology shows a 3-cm serous uterine cancer, invading 10/11 cm of the myometrium with lymphovascular space invasion; after ultrastaging, two of the three pelvic sentinel LNs are positive for serous uterine cancer. Her final stage was stage IIIC1 serous endometrial adenocarcinoma.*

What Are Appropriate Treatment Options?

- KM is stage IIIC1 based on her positive pelvic LNs. She will need adjuvant treatments involving chemotherapy and/or external beam pelvic radiation with or without vaginal cuff brachytherapy.
- There is some debate about the best treatment for stage III type 2 endometrial cancer. PORTEC3 studied high-risk endometrial cancers (high-risk stage I histologies such as serous or clear cell, stage II or stage III endometrial cancers). Patients were randomized to pelvic external beam radiation therapy (EBRT) followed by carboplatin and paclitaxel versus pelvic EBRT alone. Progression-free survival (PFS) and overall survival (OS) were improved with the addition of chemotherapy, particularly for stage III patients and patients with serous histology.[11]
- GOG258 randomized optimally debulked advanced-stage endometrial cancer (most of which were endometrioid) to cisplatin with pelvic EBRT followed by 4 cycles of carboplatin and paclitaxel versus 6 cycles of carboplatin and paclitaxel without radiation. There was no difference in PFS. The patients who received radiation and chemotherapy had more distant recurrences but fewer locoregional recurrences. All subgroups, including serous histology (17% of the cohort), were noted to have similar outcomes between the two treatment groups. The OS data is not yet mature.[12]
- PORTEC3 and GOG258 show the importance of systemic treatments for advanced-stage and high-risk endometrial cancers due to the risk for distant relapse. Chemotherapy alone or in combination with external beam pelvic radiation would be appropriate treatments for her.[11,12]
- Research presented at the Society of Gynecologic Oncologists in 2020 suggests that patients with HER2-positive advanced uterine serous cancer (about 25% to 30% of serous cancers) have prolonged PFS (13 months versus 8 months) and OS (29 months versus 24 months) with trastuzumab in conjunction with carboplatin and paclitaxel, particularly for those who had not had previous treatments.[9,10]

Recommended Treatment Plan for This Patient

- *KM underwent 6 cycles of carboplatin area under the curve (AUC) 5 and paclitaxel 175 mg/m^2 with trastuzumab 8 mg/kg for the first dose then 6 mg/kg every 3 weeks followed by trastuzumab maintenance as adjuvant treatment.*

What Are the Toxicities Associated With the Treatment?

- Chemotherapy with carboplatin and paclitaxel commonly cause fatigue, alopecia, neuropathy, nausea, neutropenia, anemia, thrombocytopenia, and allergic reactions. Patients can also have extravasation reactions and may consider a port placement to protect their veins and skin. Severe reactions such as febrile neutropenia and sepsis can be life-threatening.
- Trastuzumab can be associated with an increase in anemia and hypertension. Echocardiograms are also required to evaluate for cardiac toxicity.

Treatment Toxicities for This Patient

- *KM tolerated the chemotherapy well, with grade 2 fatigue, grade 1 nausea, hair loss, and grade 2 anemia that led to a dose reduction for the last cycle. Her echocardiogram prior to starting showed no evidence of cardiac dysfunction, making her eligible for the trastuzumab.*

What Are Other Treatment Considerations?

- Patients who are not surgical candidates can consider definitive treatment with a combination of chemotherapy and radiation with brachytherapy.
- Ongoing studies are evaluating the role of immunotherapy in conjunction with chemotherapy for advanced endometrial cancer.
- Women with imaging suggestive of unresectable endometrial cancer can be treated with neoadjuvant chemotherapy.
- Immunotherapy is incorporated in second-line treatment for stage IV or recurrent endometrial cancer. Women with MSI are candidates for single-agent pembrolizumab, while for women with microsatellite stable endometrial cancers, responses are enhanced with the addition of lenvatinib.[13,14]

What Is Required for Patient's Follow-Up and Survivorship?[15]

- *Symptoms and physical exam with speculum exam, pelvic exam, and rectovaginal exam should be performed every 3 months for 2 years, then every 6 months up to 5 years after diagnosis, then yearly.*
- *Clinically indicated imaging (usually CT scan) based on symptoms and physical exam is recommended.*
- *Cytology (Pap smears) has not been shown to improve detection rates for vaginal cuff recurrences.*
- *CA125 levels can be followed for high-risk disease, especially if it was elevated at the time of diagnosis.*

Case 19.3: Leiomyosarcoma

LC is a 58-year-old with abnormal uterine bleeding and pelvic pressure. She comes into the ED because of heavy vaginal bleeding for the past 2 weeks. She is found to have a hemoglobin (Hgb) of 6. A pelvic US shows an enlarged uterus with a dominant 19-cm fibroid. She has no medical history and no family history of cancer.

What Preoperative Evaluations Are Necessary?

- It is very difficult to differentiate a leiomyoma from a leiomyosarcoma. Rapid growth, particularly after menopause, increases the risk of leiomyosarcoma but can be found in leiomyomas as well. An MRI can be considered; features more suggestive of leiomyosarcoma on MRI include nodular borders, intralesional hemorrhage, T2 dark areas, and central unenhanced areas.[16,17]
- An endometrial biopsy will have about a 30% to 50% sensitivity for leiomyosarcoma and is more likely to be beneficial in women with postmenopausal bleeding. It can be considered in select cases; however, a negative biopsy does not rule out leiomyosarcoma.[18]
- Patients with evidence of disease outside of the uterus for whom neoadjuvant chemotherapy is being considered can have a transcutaneous biopsy of the leiomyosarcoma or metastasis for diagnosis.
- Considerations in terms of surgical procedures depend on the patient's age and the level of suspicion for leiomyosarcoma. Resection of the fibroid only (myomectomy) is not appropriate for leiomyosarcoma and has a high rate of recurrence. A completion hysterectomy should be recommended if a leiomyosarcoma is found on pathology after a myomectomy.
- For uterus-confined leiomyosarcoma without enlarged LNs on imaging, there is minimal risk of lymphatic involvement with leiomyosarcoma. In retrospective studies, all LNs involved were in patients with extrauterine disease.
- Metastasis to the ovaries is rare (less than 5%). Oophorectomy has not been proven to be associated with improved survival. Oophorectomy can be individualized and ovarian preservation can be appropriate in select patients prior to menopause who wish to decrease their risks of early menopause.

Patient's Surgery

- LC was taken to the operating room for a total abdominal hysterectomy, bilateral salpingo-oophorectomy, and partial omentectomy due to adhesions to the omentum. She recovered well from surgery.

How Is a Diagnosis Established?

- Diagnosis is established with pathology after removal of the uterine mass. In order to limit the chance of intraperitoneal spread, specimens concerning for leiomyosarcoma should not be morcellated. If necessary, morcellation contained within a bag can be considered.
- Pathological diagnosis is based on the presence of spindle cells with blunt-ended nuclei, greater than 10 mitoses per 10 high power fields (HPFs), atypical forms, nuclear polymorphism, hypercellularity, coagulative necrosis, and infiltrative surrounding myometrium. Leiomyosarcoma is not graded. It can be difficult to diagnose as some of these features may not be present and it can look similar to smooth muscle tumors of uncertain malignant potential (STUMP), bizarre leiomyoma, and endometrial stromal sarcomas.

Patient's Diagnosis

- The mass was sent for an intraoperative pathologic evaluation and areas of necrosis and atypia were seen. A definitive diagnosis of leiomyosarcoma was made at the final pathology due to greater than 10 mitoses per 10 HPF with atypical nuclei and coagulative necrosis.

What Further Molecular or Genomic Testing Is Required?

- There is no immediate molecular or genetic testing done for leiomyosarcoma.
- Somatic genetic testing can be useful in the setting of advanced disease to determine eligibility for targeted therapies.
- Hereditary leiomyomatosis and renal cell carcinoma (HLRCC) syndrome, a germline mutation of fumarate hydratase gene, does increase the risk of leiomyoma as well as leiomyosarcoma. It is rare and is not routinely tested for.

Patient's Molecular and Genomic Testing
- *No further testing done.*

How Is This Tumor Staged?

- Uterine leiomyosarcoma is staged surgically, as well as with imaging, to evaluate for distant disease after diagnosis. CT scan is usually adequate for evaluation for distant disease, although a PET scan can also be considered.
- Staging is different than for endometrial cancer. Stage I is determined by size, with stage IA for tumors less than 5 cm and stage IB for those more than 5 cm.
- Stage II describes local pelvic involvement, whether the adnexae (IIA) or other pelvic tissues (IIB).
- Stage III involves the abdominal tissues, and stage IV is locally advanced with invasion of the bladder or rectum, or distant metastases such as lung or liver.

Patient's Clinical Stage
- *LC had stage IB disease with a tumor more than 5 cm in size. A postoperative CT scan showed no evidence of disease.*

What Are Appropriate Treatment Options?

- Leiomyosarcoma is an aggressive cancer even in its early stages. However, the role for adjuvant chemotherapy has not been well established and is controversial. GOG277, designed to study randomizing women with early-stage leiomyosarcoma to chemotherapy (gemcitabine/docetaxel followed by doxorubicin) versus observation, was unable to recruit.
- First-line adjuvant treatment, if used, is doxorubicin or gemcitabine/docetaxel. A recent study in unresected or metastatic soft-tissue sarcomas (GeDDIS) randomizing patients to doxorubicin versus gemcitabine/docetaxel showed equivalent outcomes between the two, with decreased tolerance for gemcitabine/docetaxel. A subgroup analysis of uterine leiomyosarcomas was consistent with the primary findings.[19]

Recommended Treatment Plan for This Patient
- *The patient discussed the possibility of adjuvant treatment with chemotherapy with her physician. Due to the absence of evidence suggesting improved outcomes with chemotherapy, she agreed to proceed with surveillance.*

What Are Other Treatment Considerations?

- Radiation therapy may be used in select cases, such as for palliation. However, a large European study of stage I and II uterine leiomyosarcomas randomized to pelvic radiation versus observation after surgery showed no improvement in local recurrence, distant recurrence, or overall survival between the two.[20]

- For symptomatic patients with progressive uterine leiomyosarcoma, adding ifosfamide to doxorubicin can improve PFS and tumor response, allowing for relief of symptoms. However, OS is unchanged and the regimen is associated with increased toxicity.
- In the metastatic setting, bevacizumab has not been shown to improve outcomes.[21]

What Is Required for This Patient's Follow-Up and Survivorship?

- *Symptoms and physical exam with speculum exam, pelvic exam, and rectovaginal exam is performed every 3 months for 2 years, then every 6 months up to 5 years after diagnosis, then yearly.*
- *National Comprehensive Cancer Network (NCCN) guidelines recommend routine CT scans every 3 to 6 months for the first 3 years, then every 6 to 12 months for the next 2 years. Based on risk, imaging can be continued 1 to 2 times per year for up to another 5 years.*
- *Cytology (Pap smears) have not been shown to improve detection rates for vaginal cuff recurrences.*

REVIEW QUESTIONS

1. The most common presenting symptom for endometrial cancer is:
    A. Postmenopausal bleeding
    B. Abdominal pain
    C. Bloating
    D. Asymptomatic

2. In addition to age, all these tumor-related factors define high-intermediate risk endometrial cancer, except:
    A. Tumor size
    B. Depth of myometrial invasion
    C. Presence of lymphovascular space invasion
    D. Tumor grade

3. Who should have somatic mismatch repair (MMR) protein immunohistochemistry (IHC) testing?
    A. Women under the age of 60 with endometrial cancer
    B. Women under the age of 50 with endometrial cancer
    C. Women with endometrial cancer and a family history of endometrial or colon cancer
    D. All women with endometrial cancer

4. What is the standard of care treatment for women with high-intermediate risk endometrial cancer?
    A. Pelvic radiation
    B. Vaginal cuff radiation
    C. Chemotherapy
    D. Surveillance

5. In addition to mismatch repair (MMR) testing, women with serous endometrial cancer are recommended to undergo somatic testing for:
    A. *BRCA* mutation
    B. *ARID1A*
    C. *HER2* amplification
    D. Programmed death-ligand 1 (PD-L1)

6. Based on PORTEC 3 and GOG 258, what is the backbone of treatment for stage III endometrial cancer?
    A. Radiation
    B. Chemotherapy
    C. Immunotherapy
    D. Surgery

7. What additional staging procedures are recommended for high-risk endometrial cancers?
    A. Omental biopsy
    B. Peritoneal biopsies
    C. Peritoneal washings
    D. None

8. The feature of a uterine mass most commonly associated with leiomyosarcoma on imaging is:
   A. Rapid growth
   B. Necrosis
   C. Size more than 8 cm
   D. Fundal location

9. What adjuvant treatment has been shown to decrease the chance of recurrence for stage I leiomyosarcoma?
   A. Chemotherapy with Adriamycin and ifosfamide
   B. Pelvic radiation
   C. Chemotherapy with bevacizumab
   D. None

10. Which of the following is part of routine surveillance for leiomyosarcoma?
    A. Pap smear
    B. PET scan
    C. Dual-energy x-ray absorptiometry (DEXA) scan
    D. CT scan

ANSWERS AND RATIONALES

1. **A. Postmenopausal bleeding.** Most endometrial cancers can be caught early at the time of workup for abnormal vaginal bleeding, most frequently postmenopausal, as the average age for the diagnosis of endometrial cancer is over 60 years of age.

2. **A. Tumor size.** High-intermediate risk is defined by age group and the following risk factors: lymphovascular space invasion, grade 2 or 3, and more than 50% myometrial invasion. Women aged 50 to 70 with two risk factors are considered high-intermediate risk; younger women require all three risk factors and older women require only one.

3. **D. All women with endometrial cancer.** Because of the treatment and genetic implications of somatic loss of MMR expression, the National Comprehensive Cancer Network (NCCN) guidelines recommend testing for all women with endometrial cancer.

4. **B. Vaginal cuff radiation.** Based on PORTEC I, there is benefit to radiation for high-intermediate risk endometrial cancer. However, PORTEC 2 and GOG 249 suggest that vaginal cuff brachytherapy is sufficient to decrease the rate of vaginal cuff recurrences in these patients.

5. **C. *HER2* amplification.** About 25% to 30% of serous endometrial cancers have an *HER2* amplification. It is clinically relevant, as studies have shown improved survival with the addition of trastuzumab to adjuvant chemotherapy for women with an *HER2* amplification.

6. **B. Chemotherapy.** PORTEC3 and GOG 258 both showed activity of chemotherapy with carboplatin and paclitaxel for high-risk and stage III endometrial cancer. PORTEC3 compared radiation alone with chemotherapy in conjunction with pelvic radiation, and GOG258 compared chemotherapy to the combination of chemotherapy with radiation, and both showed equivalent overall survival (OS) between groups.

7. **A. Omental biopsy.** High-risk endometrial cancers such as serous and clear cell histologies, as well as grade 3 endometrial cancer, should undergo omental biopsy as part of the staging procedure. This can be conducted laparoscopically at the time of the hysterectomy.

8. **B. Necrosis.** While rapid growth and large size are also associated with malignancy, the feature most suggestive of leiomyosarcoma at the time of imaging is necrosis.

9. **D. None.** No adjuvant treatment has been shown to be of benefit in the setting of stage I leiomyosarcoma. The National Comprehensive Cancer Network (NCCN) does not recommend adjuvant treatment although it can be discussed with the patient in the appropriate setting.

10. **D. CT scan.** Routine CT scans are done every 3 to 6 months for 3 years after diagnosis with leiomyosarcoma, then every 6 to 12 months for another 2 years.

REFERENCES

1. Karlsson B, Granberg S, Wikland M, et al. Transvaginal ultrasonography of the endometrium in women with postmenopausal bleeding—a nordic multicenter study. *Am J Obstet Gynecol.* 1995;172(5):1488–1494. doi:10.1016/0002-9378(95)90483-2
2. Rossi EC, Kowalski LD, Scalici J, et al. A comparison of sentinel lymph node biopsy to lymphadenectomy for endometrial cancer staging (FIRES trial): a multicentre, prospective, cohort study. *Lancet Oncol.* 2017;18(3):384–392. doi:10.1016/S1470-2045(17)30068-2

3. Creutzberg CL, van Putten WL, Koper PC, et al. Surgery and post-operative radiotherapy versus surgery alone for patients with stage-1 endometrial carcinoma: multicentre randomised trial. *Lancet*. 2000;355:1404–1411. doi:10.1016/s0140-6736(00)02139-5

4. Randall ME, Filiaci V, McMeekin DS, et al. Phase III trial: adjuvant pelvic radiation therapy versus vaginal brachytherapy plus paclitaxel/carboplatin in high-intermediate and high-risk early-stage endometrial cancer. *J Clin Oncol*. 2019;37(21):1810–1818. doi:10.1200/JCO.18.01575

5. Nout RA, Smit VTHBM, Putter H, et al. Vaginal brachytherapy versus pelvic external beam radiotherapy for patients with endometrial cancer of high-intermediate risk (PORTEC II): an open-label, non-inferiority, randomized trial. *Lancet*. 2010;375(9717):816–823. doi:10.1016/S0140-6736(09)62163-2

6. Eskander RN, Randall LM, Berman ML, et al. Fertility preserving options in patients with gynecologic malignancies. *Am J Obstet Gyneco*. 2011;205(2):103–110. doi:10.1016/j.ajog.2011.01.025

7. Laurelli G, Falcone F, Gallo MS, et al. Long-term oncologic and reproductive outcomes in young women with early endometrial cancer conservatively treated: a prospective study and literature update. *Int J Gynecol Cancer*. 2016;26(9):1650–1657. doi:10.1097/IGC.0000000000000825

8. Soliman PT, Westin SN, Dioun S, et al. A prospective validation study of sentinel lymph node mapping for high-risk endometrial cancer. *Gynecol Oncol*. 2017;146(2):234–239. doi:10.1016/j.ygyno.2017.05.016

9. Fader AN, Roque DM, Siegel ER, et al. Randomized phase II trial of carboplatin-paclitaxel compared to carboplatin-paclitaxel-trastuzumab in advanced (stage III–IV) or recurrent uterine serous carcinomas that overexpress HER2/neu (NCT01367002): updated overall survival analysis. *Clin Cancer Res*. 2020;26(15):3928–3935. doi:10.1158/1078-0432.CCR-20-0953

10. Fader AN, Roque DM, Siegel E, et al. Randomized phase II trial of carboplatin-paclitaxel versus carboplatin-paclitaxel-trastuzumab in uterine serous carcinomas that overexpress human epidermal growth factor receptor 2/neu. *J Clin Oncol*. 2018;36(20):2044–2051. doi:10.1200/JCO.2017.76.5966

11. de Boer SM, Powell ME, Mileshkin L, et al. Adjuvant chemoradiotherapy versus radiotherapy alone in women with high risk endometrial cancer (PORTEC-3): patterns of recurrence and post-hoc survival analysis of a randomized phase 3 trial. *Lancet*. 2019;20(9):1273–1285. doi:10.1016/S1470-2045(19)30395-X

12. Matei D, Filiaci V, Randall ME, et al. Adjuvant chemotherapy plus radiation for locally advanced endometrial cancer. *N Engl J Med*. 2019;380:2317–2326. doi:10.1056/NEJMoa1813181

13. Makker V, Rasco D, Vogelzang NJ, et al. Lenvatinib plus pembrolizumab in patients with advanced endometrial cancer: an interim analysis of a multicenter, open-label, single-arm, phase 2 trial. *Lancet*. 2019;20(5):711–718. doi:10.1016/S1470-2045(19)30020-8

14. Makker V, Colombo N, Casado Herráez A, et al. A multicenter, open-label, randomized phase 3 study to compare the efficacy and safety of lenvatinib in combination with pembrolizumab vs treatment of physician's choice in patients with advanced endometrial cancer. *Gynecol Oncol*. 2021;162(suppl 1):S4. doi:10.1016/S0090-8258(21)00657-0

15. Salani R, Khanna N, Frimer M, et al. An update on post-treatment surveillance and diagnosis of recurrence in women with gynecologic malignancies: Society of Gynecologic Oncology (SGO) recommendations. *Gynecol Oncol*. 2017;146:3–10. doi:10.1016/j.ygyno.2017.03.022

16. Lakhman Y, Veeraraghavan H, Chaim J, et al. Differentiation of uterine leiomyosarcoma from atypical leiomyoma: diagnostic accuracy of qualitative mr imaging features and feasibility of texture analysis. *Eur Radiol*. 2017;27:2903–2915. doi:10.1007/s00330-016-4623-9

17. Roberts ME, Aynard JT, Chu CS. Uterine leiomyosarcoma: a review of the literature and update on management options. *Gynecol Oncol*. 2018;151:562–572. doi:10.1016/j.ygyno.2018.09.010

18. Hinchcliff EM, Esselen KM, Watkins JK, et al. The role of endometrial biopsy in the preoperative detection of uterine leiomyosarcoma. *J Minim Invasive Gynecol*. 2016;23(4):567–572. doi:10.1016/j.jmig.2016.01.022

19. Seddon B, Strauss S, Whelan J, et al. Gemcitabine and docetaxel versus doxorubicin as first-line treatment for previously untreated advanced unresectable or metastatic soft tissue sarcoma (GeDDIS): a randomized controlled phase 3 trial. *Lancet*. 2017;18(10):1397–1410. doi:10.1016/S1470-2045(17)30622-8

20. Reed NS, Mangioni C, Malmström H, et al. Phase III randomised study to evaluate the role of adjuvant pelvic radiotherapy in the treatment of uterine sarcomas stages I and II: an European Organisation for Research and Treatment of Cancer Gynaecological Cancer Group study (protocol 55874). *Eur. J. Cancer*. 2008;44(6):808–818. doi:10.1016/j.ejca.2008.01.019

21. Hensley ML, Miller A, O'Malley DM, et al. Randomized phase III trial of gemcitabine plus docetaxel plus bevacizumab or placebo as first-line treatment for metastatic uterine leiomyosarcoma: an NRG Oncology/Gynecologic Oncology Group study. *J Clin Oncol*. 2015;33(10):1180–1185. doi:10.1200/JCO.2014.58.3781

CHAPTER 20

Ovarian Cancer

Katelyn Tondo-Steele and Jean H. Siedel

INTRODUCTION

Ovarian cancer is the most lethal gynecologic malignancy and the fifth leading cause of cancer death in women in the United States. It is estimated that there will be 21,500 new cases of ovarian cancer in 2021 in the United States with a 5-year relative survival rate of 49.1%.[1] It is the second most common gynecologic malignancy in the United States behind endometrial cancer.[1]

The average lifetime risk of developing ovarian cancer is 1 in 78.[1] Early menarche, late menopause, and nulliparity are among the reproductive risk factors for ovarian cancer. Family history of ovarian cancer carries the largest risk in developing ovarian cancer. Patients with one first degree relative with ovarian cancer have approximately a 5% lifetime risk of developing ovarian cancer, as opposed to 1.3% in the general population.[2] Approximately 14% to 15% of all epithelial ovarian cancers are associated with hereditary breast-ovarian cancer syndrome (HBOC) and 3% are associated with mismatch repair (MMR) mutations including heredi-tary nonpolyposis colorectal cancer (HNPCC) syndrome, also known as Lynch syndrome.[3] HBOC syndrome occurs due to pathogenic variants in *BRCA1* or *BRCA2* tumor suppressor genes. *BRCA1* and *BRCA2* are mediators in the homologous recombination pathway, which is essential to the repair of double-stranded DNA breaks. Homologous recombination deficient (HRD) tumors are unable to repair DNA damage via a high-fidelity repair pathway. When these tumors are treated with poly adenosine diphosphate-ribose polymerase (PARP) inhibitors, cell death occurs due to dysfunction in multiple DNA repair pathways by a principle known as synthetic lethality.[3] Patients with *BRCA1* pathogenic variants have a 35% to 46% lifetime risk of developing ovarian cancer, while patients with *BRCA2* pathogenic variants have a 13% to 23% lifetime risk.[4,5] Lynch syndrome results from a pathogenic variant in DNA MMR genes including *MLH1, MSH2, MSH6, PMS2,* and *EPCAM.* Lynch syndrome is associated with an increased risk of several cancers, the most common being colorectal and endometrial cancer, but is also associated with an increased lifetime risk of ovarian cancer. The lifetime risk of ovarian cancer is approximately 11% to 17% in patients with Lynch syndrome, depending on the affected gene.[6]

There are also factors associated with a reduced risk of epithelial ovarian cancer. These factors include use of oral contraceptives, increased parity, and breastfeeding.[7] Most serous ovarian cancer precursor lesions arise in the distal fallopian tube; therefore, opportunistic salpingectomy has been shown to decrease the risk of ovarian cancer.[8] Risk-reducing surgery is an option for those with both *BRCA1/2* and Lynch syndrome. For *BRCA* mutation carriers, risk-reducing bilateral salpingo-oophorectomy is recommended. *BRCA1* patients are recom-mended for risk-reducing surgery at 35 to 40 years old and *BRCA2* at 40 to 45 years old.[9] For

Lynch syndrome, hysterectomy and bilateral salpingo-oophorectomy can be considered and decisions should be individualized based on gene mutation and risks.[10]

Ovarian cancer is categorized into epithelial and nonepithelial tumors. Epithelial ovarian cancers make up approximately 90% of all ovarian cancer and the most common subtype is high-grade serous carcinoma. The term "ovarian cancer" also encompasses tumors arising in the fallopian tube and peritoneum. Nonepithelial ovarian cancer includes malignancies arising in germ cells, sex cord and stromal cells, and other rare ovarian cancers including carcinosarcomas.

The majority of ovarian cancers are diagnosed at an advanced stage due to the inability to detect early ovarian cancer and nonspecific presenting symptoms. Symptoms can include abdominal or pelvic pain, bloating, gastrointestinal, and urinary symptoms. There is no reliable method of screening. If ovarian cancer is suspected, initial workup includes pelvic exam, tumor markers, and imaging. Diagnosis is made with histological evaluation. Ovarian cancer is surgically staged, and the surgical stage then determines subsequent treatment. The staging system is defined by the International Federation of Gynecology and Obstetrics (Fédération Internationale de Gynécologie et d'Obstétrique; FIGO; see Table 20.1).

CASE SUMMARIES

Case 20.1: Early Ovarian Cancer

A 52-year-old female presents for an annual gynecologic exam. She complains of abdominal pain and bloating. She is noted to have right-sided fullness on bimanual exam. A transvaginal ultrasound (US) was performed which demonstrated a 4-cm cystic and solid mass with papillary excrescences. A CT of the chest, abdomen, and pelvis shows no evidence of metastatic disease.

What Is the Utility of Tumor Markers?

- Tumor markers are not recommended for ovarian cancer screening but may be used to determine treatment effect when followed over time in patients with known ovarian cancer. CA-125 is frequently elevated in epithelial ovarian cancer but can also be elevated in benign conditions including liver disease, heart failure, pancreatitis, diverticulitis, pneumonia, endometriosis, pregnancy, pelvic inflammatory disease, and others.[11,12] In postmenopausal patients, CA-125 should be 35 U/mL or less.[13] The sensitivity is lower in premenopausal patients as several of the benign conditions that raise CA-125 occur in premenopausal patients and the overall incidence of epithelial ovarian cancer is higher in postmenopausal patients. Although an elevated CA-125 has less value in predicting ovarian malignancy in premenopausal patients, elevated values should raise suspicion for malignancy and warrant further investigation. Obtaining tumor markers in the preoperative setting can be helpful for monitoring postoperatively with treatment and/or surveillance.

Patient's Result
- *CA-125 is elevated at 578 U/mL and carcinoembryonic antigen (CEA) is 0.2 ng/mL.*

What Is the Standard of Care Treatment for Early-Stage Ovarian Cancer?

- For patients with ovarian cancer that appears to be confined to one or both ovaries, with no gross evidence of metastatic disease, surgical staging is the standard of care. This includes aspiration of ascites or peritoneal lavage for cytological evaluation, inspection of the entire abdomen, hysterectomy, bilateral salpingo-oophorectomy, omentectomy, bilateral pelvic and para-aortic lymph node dissection, and peritoneal biopsies from the pelvis, paracolic gutters, and diaphragm.[14] Fertility-sparing surgery can be considered in premenopausal patients with select early-stage epithelial tumors, borderline tumors,

Table 20.1 FIGO Staging System for Ovarian, Fallopian Tube, and Primary Peritoneal Cancer (8th ed., 2017).

FIGO Stage	Criteria
I	Tumor limited to ovaries (one or both) or fallopian tube(s)
IA	Tumor limited to one ovary (capsule intact) or fallopian tube, no tumor on ovarian or fallopian tube surface; no malignant cells in ascites or peritoneal washings
IB	Tumor limited to both ovaries (capsules intact) or fallopian tubes; no tumor on ovarian or fallopian tube surface; no malignant cells in ascites or peritoneal washings
IC	Tumor limited to one or both ovaries or fallopian tubes, with any of the following:
IC1	Surgical spill
IC2	Capsule ruptured before surgery or tumor on ovarian or fallopian tube surface
IC3	Malignant cells in ascites or peritoneal washings
II	Tumor involves one or both ovaries or fallopian tubes with pelvic extension below pelvic brim or primary peritoneal cancer
IIA	Extension and/or implants on the uterus and/or fallopian tube(s) and/or ovaries
IIB	Extension to and/or implants on other pelvic tissues
III	Tumor involves one or both ovaries or fallopian tubes, or primary peritoneal cancer, with microscopically confirmed peritoneal metastasis outside the pelvis and/or metastasis to the retroperitoneal (pelvic and/or para-aortic) lymph nodes
IIIA1	Positive retroperitoneal lymph nodes only (histologically confirmed)
IIIA1i	Metastasis up to and including 10 mm in greatest dimension
IIIA1ii	Metastasis more than 10 mm in greatest dimension
IIIA2	Microscopic extrapelvic (above the pelvic brim) peritoneal involvement with or without positive retroperitoneal lymph nodes
IIIB	Macroscopic peritoneal metastasis beyond pelvis 2 cm or less in greatest dimension with or without metastasis to the retroperitoneal lymph nodes
IIIC	Macroscopic peritoneal metastasis beyond the pelvis more than 2 cm in greatest dimension with or without metastasis to the retroperitoneal lymph nodes (includes extension of tumor to capsule of liver and spleen without parenchymal involvement of either organ)
IV	Distant metastasis, including pleural effusion with positive cytology; liver or splenic parenchymal metastasis; metastasis to extra-abdominal organs (including inguinal lymph nodes and lymph nodes outside the abdominal cavity); and transmural involvement of intestine
IVA	Pleural effusion with positive cytology
IVB	Liver or splenic parenchymal metastases; metastases to extra-abdominal organs (including inguinal lymph nodes and lymph nodes outside the abdominal cavity); transmural involvement of intestine

FIGO, International Federation of Gynecology and Obstetrics.

Source: Data from Buamah P. Benign conditions associated with raised serum CA-125 concentration. *J Surg Oncol.* 2000;75(4):264–265. doi:10.1002/1096-9098(200012)75:4<264::aid-jso7>3.0.co;2-q; International Federation of Gynecology and Obstetrics (FIGO) and American Joint Committee on Cancer (AJCC). *AJCC Cancer Staging Manual.* 8th ed. Springer; 2017.

malignant germ cell tumors, or malignant sex cord-stromal tumors. Fertility-sparing surgery includes unilateral salpingo-oophorectomy with preservation of the uterus and contralateral ovary or bilateral salpingo-oophorectomy with uterine preservation.[14]

Patient's Treatment
- *She is taken to the operating room for resection of the mass. Frozen section demonstrates high-grade serous carcinoma. She has no obvious disease on surveillance of the abdomen. She undergoes a staging procedure to include hysterectomy, bilateral salpingo-oophorectomy, omentectomy, bilateral pelvic and para-aortic lymphadenectomy, peritoneal washings, and peritoneal biopsies. Final pathology reveals stage IC3 high-grade serous carcinoma of the ovary.*

Which Patients Need Adjuvant Treatment?

- Adjuvant treatment should be considered in all patients with high-risk early-stage disease including stage I high-grade serous, clear cell, carcinosarcoma and grade 2 to 3 endometrioid carcinoma, stage IC grade 1 endometrioid, mucinous, and low-grade serous carcinoma, and all stage II disease.[14] This is based on the European Organization for Research and Treatment of Cancer (EORTC) ACTION trial and International Collaborative Ovarian Neoplasm (ICON1) trial. A combined analysis of the two parallel randomized clinical trials demonstrated improved overall survival (OS) and disease-free survival (DFS) in women receiving adjuvant platinum-based chemotherapy.[15]
- Carboplatin and paclitaxel were established as standard of care in 2003 by GOG 158 which demonstrated carboplatin and paclitaxel resulted in less toxicity, easier administration, and were not inferior in terms of progression-free survival (PFS) and OS, when compared with cisplatin plus paclitaxel.[16] The number of cycles necessary for treatment was addressed in GOG 157, which concluded that 3 cycles of carboplatin and paclitaxel are non-inferior to 6 cycles after complete surgical staging for women with early-stage ovarian cancer.[17] An exploratory analysis of GOG 157 demonstrated that those with high-grade serous tumors had a lower risk of recurrence after 6 versus 3 cycles of chemotherapy. Therefore, all stages of high-grade serous carcinoma require 6 cycles of chemotherapy.[18] For other histologies with stage II to IV disease, 6 cycles of chemotherapy are recommended.[11]

Recommended Treatment Plan for This Patient
- *Six cycles carboplatin/paclitaxel and a referral for genetic testing*

Case 20.2: Borderline Ovarian Tumor

A 41-year-old female presents to her gynecologist with pelvic pain. On bimanual exam, she was noted to have a left-sided pelvic mass. An US was performed that revealed a complex left ovarian mass measuring 7 cm that was suspicious for an endometrioma versus hemorrhagic cyst. She was taken to the operating room (OR) for a left salpingo-oophorectomy.

What Are the Different Histologies of Borderline Ovarian Tumor?

- Borderline epithelial neoplasms are noninvasive neoplasms that exhibit atypical epithelial proliferation. Borderline ovarian tumors (BOTs) can be divided according to their histology and the majority are serous (50%) or mucinous (46%).[19]
- Extraovarian spread is found in approximately 35% of cases in the form of peritoneal implants. These implants can be divided into noninvasive (papillary structure similar to that of the BOT) or invasive (a similar structure to that of low-grade serous carcinoma). Invasive peritoneal implants are associated with a poor prognosis.[20]

Patient's Final Pathology
- *Serous borderline tumor involving the ovary without surface involvement*

How Are Borderline Tumors Staged?

- Borderline tumors are staged according to the FIGO ovarian cancer staging. The majority of borderline tumors are stage I at the time of diagnosis. Although lymphadenectomy may upstage patients, lymphadenectomy can be omitted for borderline ovarian tumors as it does not affect recurrence or survival.[19,21,22]

Patient's Stage
- *At least stage IA, incompletely staged*

What Is the Role of Fertility-Sparing Surgery in Patients With Borderline Tumors?

- Premenopausal patients who desire fertility preservation may be managed with fertility-sparing surgery. This includes a unilateral salpingo-oophorectomy, thorough inspection of the abdomen, peritoneal washings, infracolic omentectomy, removal of all suspicious lesions, and peritoneal biopsies. The National Comprehensive Cancer Network (NCCN) advises consideration of completion surgery upon completion of childbearing for patients with a remaining ovary.[11]

How Are Invasive Implants Treated?

- Invasive implants have a 31% chance of developing invasive disease over a 5-year period, compared to noninvasive implants which have a 2% risk.[19] Radical surgery, including hysterectomy, bilateral salpingo-oophorectomy, omentectomy, and peritoneal biopsies, should be considered in patients with invasive implants. Borderline tumors with invasive implants can be treated as low-grade serous carcinoma with observation in stage IA or IB and consideration of systemic therapy in all other stages.[11]

Should Patients With Borderline Tumors Receive Adjuvant Chemotherapy Postoperatively?

- Surgically staged BOTs do not benefit from adjuvant therapy.[20]

Recommended Treatment Plan for This Patient
- *Surveillance*

What Is the Prognosis? What Is the Risk of Recurrence for a BOT After an Oophorectomy? After an Ovarian Cystectomy?

- Borderline tumors have an excellent prognosis with OS estimated at 90% to 95% at 10 years.[20,21] The risk of recurrence after an ovarian cystectomy is between 12% and 58%.[19] Therefore, cystectomy alone is not recommended unless the tumor is bilateral or the patient only has one remaining ovary.[19,23] The risk of recurrence is approximately 15% to 20% after unilateral oophorectomy.[20,24] The recurrence rate after radical surgery, which includes hysterectomy and bilateral salpingo-oophorectomy, is between 2.5% and 5.7%.[19]

- After surgery, surveillance visits are recommended every 3 to 6 months for 5 years, then annual visits are recommended. These visits should include a physical exam and CA-125. Imaging and other labs are only ordered if clinically indicated. For women who have undergone fertility-preserving surgery, recommendations include serial pelvic USs to monitor the remaining ovary or ovaries.[25] NCCN does not distinguish between surveillance for invasive ovarian cancer and borderline tumors, but typical practice is to employ a less rigorous surveillance schedule for patients with borderline tumors.[11]

Case 20.3: Primary Treatment: Neoadjuvant Treatment Versus Primary Cytoreductive Surgery

A 78-year-old female presents to the ED with nausea and abdominal pain. For the past 2 months, she has noticed her abdomen getting larger and attributed this to weight gain. She has a past medical history (PMH) of obesity, coronary artery disease, uncontrolled type 2 diabetes, and hypertension. Her past surgical history includes an appendectomy and cholecystectomy. She undergoes a CT scan which reveals peritoneal carcinomatosis with tumor plaques involving the bowel, involvement of the liver capsule, and a 5-cm pelvic mass. An omental biopsy reveals high-grade serous carcinoma.

Which Patients Should Undergo Primary Cytoreductive Surgery and Which Should Receive Neoadjuvant Chemotherapy?

- Women with a low likelihood of achieving cytoreduction to less than 1 cm should receive neoadjuvant chemotherapy (NACT). This includes women who have evidence of disease in the lungs or mediastinum, unresectable liver metastasis, bulky periportal lymph nodes, or nonresectable extra-abdominal lymph nodes. Several factors should be considered to evaluate perioperative risk including advanced age or frailty, multiple chronic conditions, poor nutritional status, low albumin, and newly diagnosed venous thromboembolism. These have been shown to increase the risk of morbidity associated with primary cytoreductive surgery; women with a high perioperative risk should receive NACT. All others should undergo primary debulking surgery (PDS).[26]
- There are several studies that compare the outcomes of PDS versus NACT. EORTC 55971 was a noninferiority randomized controlled trial that compared NACT to PDS in patients with stage IIIC to IV ovarian cancer. It demonstrated that NACT followed by interval debulking was associated with noninferior PFS and OS compared to PDS followed by chemotherapy. Furthermore, a larger proportion of patients in the NACT group achieved optimal or complete gross resection. This study emphasized the importance of complete tumor resection as the strongest predictor of OS.[27] The CHORUS trial, also a noninferiority randomized controlled trial, demonstrated similar outcomes. These trials have been criticized due to limitations, namely, relatively short median operative times possibly reflecting insufficient surgical effort, and relatively short PFS and OS compared to contemporary studies.[28]
- The SCORPION trial also showed that NACT and PDS have similar efficacy.[29] The SCORPION trial was limited to patients with a high tumor burden. Although PFS was similar, patients in the primary surgery arm had significantly more complications (46.4% vs. 9.5%).[29] This suggests that in patients with high tumor burden, NACT may be preferable, as it leads to significantly fewer postoperative complications without compromising PFS.
- The TRUST trial (Trial on Radical Upfront Surgical Therapy in Advanced Ovarian Cancer; NCT02828618) is currently enrolling patients. The two arms in this trial are PDS followed by 6 cycles of chemotherapy versus 3 cycles of NACT followed by interval

debulking surgery followed by 3 more cycles (for a total of 6) of standard chemotherapy with a primary outcome of OS. By limiting this study to high volume debulking centers, which removes the question of surgical quality, the TRUST trial hopes to answer the question of optimal timing of debulking surgery.[30]

Patient's Clinical Decision

- *You believe the patient is an appropriate candidate for NACT.*

What Chemotherapy Regimen Would You Recommend for a Patient Receiving Neoadjuvant Chemotherapy? Does This Differ From Patients Who Undergo Primary Debulking Surgery Followed by Adjuvant Chemotherapy?

- NACT includes 3 cycles of intravenous paclitaxel (175 mg/m^2) combined with intravenous carboplatin (area under the curve [AUC] of 5 to 6) every 3 weeks.[28,29,31]
- Intraperitoneal (IP) chemotherapy can be considered in patients with stage II to IV epithelial ovarian tumors that have been optimally debulked. Patients who had a suboptimal debulking surgery are not candidates for IP chemotherapy due to limited penetration into tumors. GOG 172 compared 6 cycles of IV cisplatin/paclitaxel to IV paclitaxel followed by IP cisplatin/paclitaxel. This trial showed improvement in PFS and OS in the IP chemotherapy group.[32] More recently, GOG 252 studied patients with optimally cytoreduced stage II to III ovarian cancer who were randomly assigned to a treatment arm with bevacizumab plus one of the following: dose-dense IV paclitaxel with IV carboplatin, dose-dense IV paclitaxel with IP carboplatin, or IV paclitaxel with IP cisplatin and paclitaxel. PFS and OS were similar in all three arms.[33] The results of this study led to decreased utilization of IP chemotherapy in the United States; currently, carboplatin and paclitaxel IV every 3 weeks is the preferred regimen.[11]
- Two clinical trials have demonstrated improvement in PFS with the addition of bevacizumab to upfront chemotherapy followed by single-agent bevacizumab maintenance. ICON7 and GOG 218 demonstrated an additional 4 months PFS with the addition of bevacizumab to chemotherapy.[34,35] These trials established that patients with inoperable stage III disease, stage III disease with suboptimal debulking, and stage IV disease are candidates for bevacizumab concurrently with primary chemotherapy.[34,35] Other patients who demonstrated benefit from the addition of bevacizumab are patients with ascites and high-risk groups with poor performance status, high-grade serous histology, and high pretreatment CA-125.[34,35]

Patient's Recommended Treatment

- *This patient will receive 3 cycles of carboplatin and paclitaxel followed by CT imaging for consideration of interval debulking surgery at that time.*

Is There a Role for Maintenance Therapy After Completion of Primary Treatment of Ovarian Cancer?

- Certain patients can benefit from maintenance therapy with PARP inhibitors. A Phase III trial, SOLO1, demonstrated after complete or partial response to primary platinum-based chemotherapy, patients with germline or somatic *BRCA* mutations had prolonged PFS when treated with olaparib as compared to placebo.[36] This effect continued for 5 years at which point approximately 48% of patients on olaparib were disease free, as compared to 20% of patients in the placebo group.[37] Olaparib is also approved in combination with bevacizumab as frontline maintenance. A Phase III trial, PAOLA-1, reported a prolonged PFS in patients who received olaparib and bevacizumab as compared to bevacizumab alone following complete or partial response to primary platinum-based chemotherapy.[38] The greatest benefit was noted in *BRCA*-mutated patients or HRD tumors, as assessed by somatic tumor testing measuring the degree of genomic instability in the tumor. Similar to SOLO1, a Phase III trial, PRIMA, established niraparib as maintenance treatment after primary chemotherapy. Although the use of niraparib demonstrated significant improvement in patients who were HRD-positive, all patients had significantly longer PFS than the placebo arm regardless of HRD status.[39]

Patient Scenario

- *This patient should have germline genetic testing performed, ideally, prior to her surgery. After her surgery, regardless of her germline testing, she will receive three more cycles of carboplatin/paclitaxel. If she is BRCA-positive and has a complete or partial response to chemotherapy, she would qualify for PARP inhibitor maintenance following adjuvant chemotherapy. If her germline testing is negative, we would then send somatic tumor testing to measure the degree of genomic instability in the tumor from her surgical specimen. If she is HRD-positive and has a complete or partial response to chemotherapy, she would qualify for PARP inhibitor maintenance.*

Case 20.4: Recurrent Ovarian Cancer

A 51-year-old female with stage IIIC ovarian cancer presents for a surveillance visit. She underwent optimal cytoreduction followed by adjuvant carboplatin and paclitaxel with complete response and completed therapy 19 months ago. She complains of flank pain. Her physical exam is unremarkable. You obtain a CA-125 and a CT of the chest, abdomen, and pelvis. Her CA-125 is 44 U/mL and her CT reveals mild right hydronephrosis and a 4-cm right pelvic mass. No other evidence of metastatic disease is found.

What Are the Definitions of Platinum-Sensitive and Platinum-Resistant Ovarian Cancer? How Does This Impact Treatment Recommendations?

- Platinum-resistant ovarian cancer is defined as disease recurrence within 6 months of completion of first-line platinum-based chemotherapy. A subset of platinum-resistant ovarian cancer is platinum-refractory ovarian cancer, which is disease that progresses during first-line platinum-based therapy. Platinum-sensitive disease is defined as disease recurrence 6 months or greater after completion of first-line platinum-based chemotherapy.
- In patients with advanced-stage disease, approximately 80% will recur.[40]
- Patients with platinum-sensitive cancer can continue to receive further platinum-based therapy with recurrences. Patients with platinum-resistant ovarian cancer can no longer be treated with platinum-based therapy. The response rates to second-line chemotherapy in platinum-resistant patients is approximately 10% to 30%.[36]

What Are the Appropriate Treatment Options for This Patient?

- Secondary cytoreduction has been shown to have benefit in select patients with platinum-sensitive recurrences. Several randomized studies have evaluated the benefit of secondary cytoreduction, each using a different method to determine eligibility for surgery.
- The AGO (Arbeitsgemeinschaft Gynaekologische Onkologie) score was proposed to predict the success of complete cytoreduction in recurrent ovarian cancer. A positive AGO score includes patients with Eastern Cooperative Oncology Group (ECOG) performance status of 0, ascites less than 500 mL, and complete resection at initial surgery.[38] In DESKTOP III, this scoring system was evaluated in patients with platinum-sensitive

recurrent ovarian cancer who were randomized to undergo secondary cytoreduction followed by chemotherapy versus chemotherapy alone. This trial demonstrated an OS benefit in the secondary cytoreduction group versus those who had chemotherapy alone, provided that a complete resection was achieved.[38]

- GOG 213 was a randomized Phase III trial including patients with platinum-sensitive recurrent ovarian cancer and randomly assigned patients to secondary cytoreduction followed by chemotherapy versus chemotherapy alone.[41] This also included the use of bevacizumab at the discretion of the gynecologic oncologist. In contrast to DESKTOP III, this trial did not demonstrate improved survival outcomes in the group that underwent secondary cytoreduction.[41]

- SOC-1 was a Phase III trial performed in China that used the iMODEL score and PET imaging to predict the success of surgical cytoreduction.[31,42] The investigators aimed to assess the efficacy of secondary cytoreduction followed by chemotherapy versus chemotherapy alone, using the iMODEL score to stratify patients prior to surgery. The iMODEL score uses six variables: FIGO stage, residual disease after primary surgery, platinum-free interval, ECOG performance status, CA-125 level, and presence of ascites. A score of 4.7 or less predicted a successful complete cytoreduction. This trial found that secondary cytoreduction followed by chemotherapy was associated with significantly longer PFS than chemotherapy alone.[31,42]

- Carboplatin and pegylated liposomal doxorubicin can be considered in place of carboplatin and paclitaxel. The CAeLYx in Platinum Sensitive Ovarian Patients (CALYPSO) trial demonstrated improved PFS and no difference in OS in patients who received carboplatin and pegylated liposomal doxorubicin compared to carboplatin and paclitaxel.[42] This regimen may be helpful for patients who had unacceptable or persistent side effects from paclitaxel.

Patient's Treatment

- *This patient is considered platinum-sensitive and therefore she may be a candidate for a secondary cytoreductive surgery.*
- *Following secondary cytoreduction, or, in place of secondary cytoreduction if the patient is deemed not to be a candidate, platinum-sensitive patients should receive platinum-based chemotherapy.*

Case 20.5: Malignant Germ Cell Tumor

A 20-year-old female presents to the ED with a history of increasing pelvic pain over the past few months. She also admits to frequent constipation but denies other pertinent symptoms. She has no PMH. Surgical history includes a prior appendectomy. The ED orders a pregnancy test and pelvic US. Her pregnancy test is negative. US reveals a 6-cm highly vascularized, solid adnexal mass with septations. You order tumor markers which are notable for a lactate dehydrogenase (LDH) of 5,000 U/L.

What in This Patient's History Makes You Suspicious of a Germ Cell Tumor?

- Germ cell tumors present at an average age of 16 to 20 years old. Germ cell tumor markers include LDH, alpha-fetoprotein (AFP), and beta-human chorionic gonadotropin (hCG). Dysgerminomas primarily produce LDH. Yolk sac tumors and embryonal tumors produce AFP. Choriocarcinoma, embryonal tumors, and some dysgerminomas produce beta-HCG. A CA-125 should also be obtained when exam or imaging findings are suspicious for ovarian malignancy.

Patient Scenario

- *The patient's age and concerning features of adnexal mass on US make you suspicious for a germ cell tumor. Her LDH level is also suspicious for a dysgerminoma.*

A Dysgerminoma Is Suspected. What Are the Initial Steps in Management?

- Two-thirds of malignant ovarian germ cell tumors will be confined to one ovary.[43]
- The complete staging procedure for a malignant germ cell tumor is the same for epithelial ovarian cancer. This includes total hysterectomy, bilateral salpingo-oophorectomy, omentectomy, bilateral pelvic and para-aortic lymphadenectomy, and peritoneal biopsies.[43] In cases where disease is not confined to one ovary, debulking of all visible tumor should be performed where feasible.
- Around 28% of women with dysgerminomas have positive lymph nodes; therefore, lymph node dissection is important for staging and prognostic information.[43]

Patient Scenario

- The initial management for this patient with apparent ovarian-confined disease includes surgery for histological diagnosis and staging. The extent of surgical staging depends on whether or not the patient desires fertility. Since this tumor typically presents in adolescents and young adults, it can be important to preserve ovarian function. Fertility-sparing surgery can be safely performed in all stages of disease due to the high chemosensitivity of these tumors.[44] This includes a unilateral salpingo-oophorectomy, peritoneal cytology, omentectomy, lymphadenectomy, and peritoneal biopsies with preservation of the uterus and contralateral ovary.

Which Patients With Malignant Germ Cell Tumors Require Postoperative Adjuvant Therapy? What Is the Recommended Adjuvant Therapy?

- Patients with FIGO stage IA or IB dysgerminoma and stage IA grade 1 immature teratoma may be safely observed postoperatively without chemotherapy.[23] In patients with stage IA dysgerminoma, postsurgical clinical surveillance will result in 80% to 85% cure in the absence of adjuvant chemotherapy. All other germ cell tumors should receive adjuvant chemotherapy.[43]
- Either 3 or 4 cycles of adjuvant bleomycin, etoposide, and cisplatin (BEP) is the recommended regimen for adjuvant chemotherapy. This regimen leads to cure in most germ cell tumors.[43] Patients should be risk stratified with 3 cycles of BEP for completely resected disease and 4 cycles for those with residual disease.[43]

What Is the Most Worrisome Toxicity of the Chemotherapy Regimen?

- Bleomycin is associated with an increased risk of pulmonary fibrosis.[45] Risk of pulmonary toxicity ranges from 6% to 11% based on patient characteristics and dose of bleomycin.[43,46–48] Toxicity spans hypersensitivity pneumonitis, interstitial pneumonitis pulmonary fibrosis, and fatal pulmonary toxicity. The risk of pulmonary fibrosis increases in patients receiving more than 400 units cumulative lifetime dose, and an attempt should be made to keep cumulative doses less than 270 units.[43,45,46] Prior to each cycle, patients need lung auscultation, chest x-ray, and pulmonary function testing. If the diffusion capacity of the lung for carbon monoxide (DLCO) decreases by 30%, bleomycin must be removed from the treatment regimen.[43] Early discontinuation of bleomycin after an asymptomatic decrease in DLCO leads to decreased risk of bleomycin toxicity without compromising cancer outcomes.[49]

What Is the Prognosis for Germ Cell Tumors?

- Malignant germ cell tumors have an excellent prognosis. The 5-year OS rate is 95.6% in stage I tumors and 73.2% in advanced stages.[50]

REVIEW QUESTIONS

1. A 40-year-old female with an elevated CA-125 and pelvic mass undergoes a comprehensive staging procedure consisting of a hysterectomy, bilateral salpingo-oophorectomy, bilateral pelvic and para-aortic lymphadenectomy, staging biopsies, and omentectomy. Intraoperatively, the mass was ruptured. Intraoperative frozen section of the pelvic mass demonstrates high-grade serous carcinoma. Final pathology reveals high-grade serous ovarian cancer in bilateral ovaries and negative washings. All remaining specimens were negative for carcinoma. What would be the optimal next step for this patient?
   A. Observation
   B. 6 cycles intravenous (IV) carboplatin/paclitaxel
   C. 6 cycles intraperitoneal (IP) carboplatin/docetaxel
   D. 3 cycles IV carboplatin/paclitaxel
   E. Immune checkpoint inhibitor

2. A 65-year-old female with stage IIIB ovarian cancer presents to your office complaining of right lower abdominal fullness. She completed adjuvant carboplatin/paclitaxel 4 months ago. Her CA-125 is elevated and CT reveals a 2-cm mass abutting the rectum and multiple enlarged pelvic lymph nodes (LNs). Interventional radiology (IR) biopsy of the mass is positive for recurrence of high-grade serous ovarian carcinoma. What is the next step in management?
   A. Secondary cytoreduction
   B. Intravenous (IV) carboplatin/paclitaxel for 3 to 6 cycles
   C. Poly adenosine diphosphate-ribose polymerase (PARP) inhibitor
   D. Single-agent paclitaxel with bevacizumab
   E. Immune checkpoint inhibitor

3. A 54-year-old female with a history of stage IIIC high-grade serous ovarian cancer presents to your office with pelvic pain. Her initial surgery was 5 years ago and she had a complete cytoreduction to R0. She completed platinum-based adjuvant therapy over 4 years ago. She states the pain has been occurring for about 1 month now. Her Eastern Cooperative Oncology Group (ECOG) performance status (PS) is 0. On physical exam, you note slight pain on bimanual exam in the right lower quadrant. You order a CA-125 which is within normal limits and a CT scan which reveals a 3-cm nodule in the right pelvis and no other metastatic disease. What is the next best step to offer this patient which would yield the longest progression-free survival (PFS)?
   A. Surveillance with serial imaging
   B. Secondary cytoreduction followed by platinum-based combination chemotherapy
   C. Intravenous (IV) single-agent chemotherapy only
   D. IV platinum-based combination chemotherapy only
   E. Poly adenosine diphosphate-ribose polymerase (PARP) inhibitor

4. A 63-year-old female with germline pathogenic variant in *BRCA1* and stage IIIC high-grade serous ovarian cancer presents to your office after complete cytoreduction with no gross residual disease. She is here to discuss the next steps in her cancer treatment. Which of the following is the next best therapy option for her?
   A. Surveillance
   B. Intravenous (IV) carboplatin/paclitaxel alone
   C. IV/intraperitoneal (IP) chemotherapy

    D. IV carboplatin/paclitaxel followed by poly adenosine diphosphate-ribose polymerase (PARP) inhibitor maintenance

    E. Bevacizumab alone

5. A 28-year-old female presents to her gynecologist's office for a postoperative appointment. She underwent a right ovarian cystectomy for ovarian torsion and final pathology revealed a serous borderline tumor. She strongly desires fertility. What is the next best step for this patient?

    A. Surveillance

    B. Referral to gynecologic oncology for completion of staging surgery including bilateral salpingo-oophorectomy, hysterectomy, thorough inspection of the abdomen, peritoneal washings, infracolic omentectomy, and pelvic and para-aortic lymph node dissection

    C. Referral to gynecologic oncology for fertility-sparing surgical staging including unilateral salpingo-oophorectomy, thorough inspection of the abdomen, peritoneal washings, infracolic omentectomy, and removal of all suspicious lesions and peritoneal biopsies

    D. Between 3 and 6 cycles of intravenous (IV) carboplatin/paclitaxel

    E. Between 3 and 6 cycles of IV/intraperitoneal (IP) cisplatin/paclitaxel

6. A 21-year-old female had an ovarian cystectomy for a torsed 7-cm ovarian mass. Final pathology revealed a malignant dysgerminoma. You take her back to the operating room (OR) for fertility-sparing surgery including a unilateral salpingo-oophorectomy, bilateral pelvic and para-aortic lymphadenectomy, omentectomy, peritoneal biopsies, and washings as well as removal of a plaque on the uterus. Final pathology reveals negative biopsies, but the uterine plaque was positive for metastatic dysgerminoma. The patient has a stage II dysgerminoma. She does desire future fertility. What do you recommend next?

    A. Surveillance

    B. Hysterectomy and removal of contralateral ovary

    C. Carboplatin/paclitaxel

    D. Bleomycin, etoposide, and cisplatin

    E. Vincristine, dactinomycin, and cyclophosphamide

7. An 80-year-old female presents to the ED with abdominal pain, bloating, and weight loss. She states the pain continues to get worse each day. A CT is performed which shows a 15-cm complex pelvic mass with possible internal hemorrhage versus necrosis. Her CA-125 was 222 U/mL. She is taken to the operating room (OR) for an exploratory laparotomy and removal of pelvic mass. Frozen section notes possible carcinosarcoma. What are the next best steps?

    A. Completion of debulking surgery with placement of an intraperitoneal (IP) port for IP chemotherapy

    B. Completion of debulking surgery; no further treatment

    C. Completion of debulking surgery, followed by intravenous (IV) platinum-based chemotherapy

    D. Discontinue the surgery, followed by IV platinum-based chemotherapy

    E. Hyperthermic IP chemotherapy

8. A 65-year-old female with stage III high-grade serous ovarian cancer presents to your office for a second opinion. Her gynecologist oncologist performed a primary debulking surgery (PDS) with greater than 1 cm residual disease. She is concerned that not all of the

cancer was able to be removed. What therapy will give this patient the longest progression-free survival (PFS)?

A. Intravenous/intraperitoneal (IV/IP) carboplatin/paclitaxel
B. IV carboplatin/paclitaxel
C. IV carboplatin/paclitaxel/bevacizumab followed by bevacizumab maintenance
D. IV carboplatin/paclitaxel plus poly adenosine diphosphate-ribose polymerase (PARP) inhibitor
E. Repeat surgical excision

9. A 50-year-old female comes to your office for a second opinion. She has stage III ovarian cancer and recently underwent an optimal debulking surgery to R0 (no gross residual disease). Her Eastern Cooperative Oncology Group (ECOG) status is 0 and she has no other medical problems. She wants to know which adjuvant treatment will give her the best overall survival (OS). You recommend:

A. Observation
B. Intarvenous (IV) cisplatin/paclitaxel
C. IV cisplatin/paclitaxel, and gemcitabine
D. Intraperitoneal (IP) cisplatin
E. IP cisplatin/paclitaxel, and IV paclitaxel

10. A 61 year-old female undergoes comprehensive surgical staging for a newly diagnosed ovarian cancer. Her surgical procedure included hysterectomy, bilateral salpingo-oophorectomy, bilateral pelvic and para-aortic lymphadenectomy, omentectomy, washings, and peritoneal biopsies. Pathology demonstrates a grade 1 endometrioid carcinoma limited to the left ovary with all other specimens negative for malignancy. What is the next best step?

A. Surveillance
B. Between 3 and 6 cycles intravenous (IV) carboplatin/paclitaxel
C. Between 3 and 6 cycles IV carboplatin/doxorubicin
D. 3 cycles IV carboplatin/gemcitabine
E. Intraperitoneal (IP) cisplatin/paclitaxel

ANSWERS AND RATIONALES

1. **B. 6 cycles intravenous (IV) carboplatin/paclitaxel.** This patient has stage IC1 high-grade serous carcinoma due to intraoperative rupture. Based on a subset analysis of GOG 157, all stages of high-grade serous ovarian cancer should receive 6 rather than 3 cycles of chemotherapy.[18] The 5-year recurrence-free survival was improved in patients who received 6 cycles of carboplatin and paclitaxel.[18]

2. **D. Single-agent paclitaxel with bevacizumab.** To answer this question, you must understand platinum-resistant versus platinum-sensitive disease. This patient has platinum-resistant ovarian cancer. If clinical trials are available, these patients should first be recommended for a clinical trial. Other treatment options for platinum-resistant disease include single-agent chemotherapy. Several chemotherapy agents have been studied for platinum-resistant disease including paclitaxel, liposomal doxorubicin, topotecan, and gemcitabine. These single-agent therapies in the platinum-resistant setting have low response rates. To improve treatment options for these patients, the Phase III AURELIA trial randomized patients to receive single-agent chemotherapy (paclitaxel, topotecan, or pegylated liposomal doxorubicin) with or without bevacizumab.[51] AURELIA demonstrated improved progression-free survival (PFS) in patients who received bevacizumab plus chemotherapy as compared to those who received chemotherapy alone (6.7 vs. 3.4 months).[51]

3. **B. Secondary cytoreduction followed by platinum-based combination chemotherapy.** This question requires you to identify whether this patient has platinum-resistant or platinum-sensitive disease. This patient has platinum-sensitive disease (recurrence greater than 6 months from completion of prior platinum-based chemotherapy). She would be a candidate for a secondary cytoreduction based on a positive Arbeitsgemeinschaft Gynaekologische Onkologie (AGO) score which includes patients with ECOG PS of 0, ascites less than 500 mL, and complete resection at initial surgery.[38] It is important to be able to achieve a complete cytoreduction, as survival benefit is only seen in patients who had no residual disease after secondary cytoreduction.[31,38] Surgery would be followed by platinum-based chemotherapy.[42,52]

4. **D. IV carboplatin/paclitaxel followed by poly adenosine diphosphate-ribose polymerase (PARP) inhibitor maintenance.** This patient had a complete cytoreduction of stage III ovarian cancer and is now a candidate for adjuvant therapy. This would consist of carboplatin/paclitaxel followed by PARP inhibitor maintenance. PARP inhibitors block the repair of DNA single-strand breaks. *BRCA*-mutated tumors are unable to repair double-stranded DNA breaks. Inhibiting PARP in *BRCA*-mutated cells causes an accumulation of DNA lesions which are inadequately repaired, leading to apoptosis. This concept is called synthetic lethality. PARP inhibitors, including olaparib, niraparib, and rucaparib, have been well studied in patients with ovarian cancer who have *BRCA* mutations. SOLO1 demonstrated that patients with germline or somatic *BRCA* mutations had prolonged progression-free survival (PFS) when treated with olaparib as maintenance therapy, as compared to placebo, following complete or partial response to platinum-based chemotherapy in the frontline setting.[53] This effect continued to 5 years, at which point approximately 48% of patients on olaparib were disease free, as compared to 20% of patients in the placebo group.[37] Olaparib has also been established as maintenance treatment with bevacizumab in PAOLA-1, noting a prolonged PFS in patients with advanced ovarian cancer as compared to bevacizumab alone.[54] The greatest benefit was noted in *BRCA*-mutated patients or homologous recombination deficient (HRD) tumors. Niraparib has also been established as

maintenance treatment. The Phase III clinical trial, PRIMA, demonstrated all patients had significantly longer PFS with niraparib than the placebo arm regardless of HRD status.[39]

5. **C. Referral to gynecologic oncology for fertility-sparing surgical staging including unilateral salpingo-oophorectomy, thorough inspection of the abdomen, peritoneal washings, infracolic omentectomy, and removal of all suspicious lesions and peritoneal biopsies.** All patients with borderline ovarian tumors should be referred to a gynecologic oncologist. This patient strongly desires fertility and therefore should undergo a fertility-sparing staging procedure which includes unilateral salpingo-oophorectomy, thorough inspection of the abdomen, peritoneal washings, infracolic omentectomy, and removal of all suspicious lesions and peritoneal biopsies.

6. **D. Bleomycin, etoposide, and cisplatin.** Patients with International Federation of Gynecology and Obstetrics (FIGO) stage IA and IB dysgerminoma and stage IA grade 1 immature teratoma may be safely observed postoperatively without chemotherapy.[55] All other patients, including the previously noted patient, should receive adjuvant chemotherapy.[43] This includes 3 to 4 cycles of adjuvant bleomycin, etoposide, and cisplatin (BEP). This regimen leads to cure in most germ cell tumors.[43] Although it is an option, it is not necessary to delay chemotherapy for oocyte harvesting or reproductive endocrinology referral prior to chemotherapy. Chemotherapy-induced infertility has been reported to occur in 18% or less of patients who have received BEP.[43]

7. **C. Completion of debulking surgery, followed by intravenous (IV) platinum-based chemotherapy.** Ovarian carcinosarcomas, previously known as malignant mixed mullerian tumors (MMMTs) of the ovary, have a poor prognosis with an overall 5-year survival of less than 30%.[56] Due to their rarity, there are few randomized trials on which to base treatment decisions. Up to 90% of ovarian carcinosarcomas will have disease that has spread beyond the ovary.[56] Ovarian carcinosarcomas use the same staging system as epithelial ovarian cancer. Like epithelial ovarian cancer, the standard treatment is maximum cytoreductive surgical effort followed by platinum-based chemotherapy, usually carboplatin and paclitaxel. This is based off of GOG 261, which found carboplatin and paclitaxel were not inferior to ifosfomide and paclitaxel.[57] Patients with all stages of ovarian carcinosarcoma should receive postoperative chemotherapy.

8. **C. IV carboplatin/paclitaxel/bevacizumab followed by bevacizumab maintenance.** In patients who have had a suboptimal debulking surgery, two trials have shown that the addition of bevacizumab to chemotherapy improved PFS but not overall survival (OS). ICON7 and GOG 218 demonstrated an improvement in PFS by approximately 4 months when bevacizumab was added to chemotherapy and continued as maintenance.[34,35] These trials established that patients with stage III disease, with residual disease after surgery, and stage IV disease are candidates for bevacizumab concurrently with primary chemotherapy followed by bevacizumab maintenance.[34,35] Patients who are suboptimally debulked (residual disease of greater than 1 cm) are not candidates for IP chemotherapy. Based on GOG 152, a second debulking attempt does not provide a statistically significant difference in PFS or OS if the first attempt at cytoreduction was performed by a gynecologic oncologist.[58,59]

9. **E. IP cisplatin/paclitaxel, and IV paclitaxel.** Several studies have demonstrated an increase in survival with IP as compared to IV chemotherapy in optimally debulked patients. GOG 172 compared 6 cycles of IV cisplatin/paclitaxel to IV paclitaxel followed by IP cisplatin/paclitaxel. This trial showed improvement in progression-free survival (PFS; 18 months vs. 23.8 months) and OS (49.7 months vs. 65.6 months) in the IP chemotherapy group.[32]

10. **A. Surveillance**. Clear cell and endometrioid ovarian carcinomas are two less common types of epithelial ovarian cancer and tend to present at an early stage. Both clear cell and endometrioid histologies can be associated with endometriosis. Unlike endometrioid histology, clear cell is considered a high-grade tumor and chemotherapy is recommended for all stages of disease. Endometrioid tumors are typically low grade. Endometrioid ovarian tumors can be associated with endometrioid endometrial cancer in approximately 20% of cases.[40] In a retrospective cohort study, patients with stage IA and IB endometrioid ovarian cancers had no survival benefit with the use of chemotherapy and therefore do not require adjuvant therapy after comprehensive surgical staging.[60]

REFERENCES

1. American Cancer Society. Key statistics for ovarian cancer. 2021. https://www.cancer.org/cancer/ovarian-cancer/about/key-statistics.html
2. National Cancer Institure Surveillance, Epidemiology, and End Results Program. Cancer stat facts: ovarian cancer. October 30, 2021. https://seer.cancer.gov/statfacts/html/ovary.html
3. Konstantinopoulos PA, Ceccaldi R, Shapiro GI, D'Andrea AD. Homologous recombination deficiency: exploiting the fundamental vulnerability of ovarian cancer. *Cancer Discov.* 2015;5(11):1137–1154. doi:10.1158/2159-8290.CD-15-0714
4. King M-C, Marks JH, Mandell JB. Breast and ovarian cancer risks due to inherited mutations in *BRCA1* and *BRCA2*. *Sci.* 2003;302(5645):643–646. doi:10.1126/science.1088759
5. Zhang S, Royer R, Li S, et al. Frequencies of *BRCA1* and *BRCA2* mutations among 1,342 unselected patients with invasive ovarian cancer. *Gynecol Oncol.* 2011;121(2):353–357. doi:10.1016/j.ygyno.2011.01.020
6. Hampel H, Bennett RL, Buchanan A, et al. A practice guideline from the American College of Medical Genetics and Genomics and the National Society of Genetic Counselors: referral indications for cancer predisposition assessment. *Genet Med.* 2015;17(1):70–87. doi:10.1038/gim.2014.147
7. Sueblinvong T, Carney ME. Current understanding of risk factors for ovarian cancer. *Curr Treat Options Oncol.* 2009;10(1–2):67–81. doi:10.1007/s11864-009-0108-2
8. Falconer H, Yin L, Grönberg H, Altman D. Ovarian cancer risk after salpingectomy: a nationwide population-based study. *J Natl Cancer Inst.* 2015;107(2):dju410. doi:10.1093/jnci/dju410
9. National Comprehensive Cancer Network. *Genetic/Familial High Risk Assessment: Breast, Ovarian, and Pancreatic.* Version 1.2022. 2021. https://www.nccn.org/guidelines/guidelines-detail?category=2&id=1503
10. National Comprehensive Cancer Network. *Genetic/Familial High Risk Assessment: Colorectal.* Version 1.2021. 2021. https://www.nccn.org/guidelines/guidelines-detail?category=2&id=1436
11. Miralles C, Orea M, España P, et al. Cancer antigen 125 associated with multiple benign and malignant pathologies. *Ann Surg Oncol.* 2003;10(2):150–154. doi:10.1245/ASO.2003.05.015
12. Buamah P. Benign conditions associated with raised serum CA-125 concentration. *J Surg Oncol.* 2000;75(4):264–265. doi:10.1002/1096-9098(200012)75:4<264::aid-jso7>3.0.co;2-q
13. Sölétormos G, Duffy MJ, Hassan SOA, et al. Clinical use of cancer biomarkers in epithelial ovarian cancer: updated guidelines from the European Group on Tumor Markers. *Int J Gynecol Cancer.* 2016;26(1):43–51. doi:10.1097/IGC.0000000000000586
14. National Comprehensive Cancer Network. *Ovarian Cancer Including Fallopian Tube Cancer and Primary Peritoneal Cancer.* Version 3.2021. 2021. https://www.nccn.org/guidelines/guidelines-detail?category=1&id=1453
15. Trimbos JB, Mahesh P, Ignace V, et al. International Collaborative Ovarian Neoplasm trial 1 and adjuvant chemotherapy in ovarian neoplasm trial: two parallel randomized phase III trials of adjuvant chemotherapy in patients with early-stage ovarian carcinoma. *J Natl Cancer Inst.* 2003;95(2):105–112. doi:10.1093/jnci/95.2.105
16. Ozols RF, Bundy BN, Greer BE, et al. Phase III trial of carboplatin and paclitaxel compared with cisplatin and paclitaxel in patients with optimally resected stage III ovarian cancer: a Gynecologic Oncology Group study. *J Clin Oncol.* 2003;21(17):3194–3200. doi: 10.1200/JCO.2003.02.153
17. Bell J, Brady MF, Young RC, et al. Randomized phase III trial of three versus six cycles of adjuvant carboplatin and paclitaxel in early stage epithelial ovarian carcinoma: a Gynecologic Oncology Group study. *Gynecol Oncol.* 2006;102(3):432–439. doi:10.1016/j.ygyno.2006.06.013
18. Chan JK, Tian C, Fleming GF, et al. The potential benefit of 6 vs. 3 cycles of chemotherapy in subsets of women with early-stage high-risk epithelial ovarian cancer: an exploratory analysis of a Gynecologic Oncology Group study. *Gynecol Oncol.* 2010;116(3):301–306. doi:10.1016/j.ygyno.2009.10.073
19. Cadron I, Leunen K, Van Gorp T, et al. Management of borderline ovarian neoplasms. *J Clin Oncol.* 2007;25(20):2928–2937. doi:10.1200/JCO.2007.10.8076

20. Rao GG, Skinner E, Gehrig PA, et al. Surgical staging of ovarian low malignant potential tumors. *Obstet Gynecol*. 2004;104(2):261–266. doi:10.1097/01.AOG.0000133484.92629.88

21. Lesieur B, Kane A, Duvillard P, et al. Prognostic value of lymph node involvement in ovarian serous borderline tumors. *Am J Obstet Gynecol*. 2011;204(5):438.e1–438.e7. doi:10.1016/j.ajog.2010.12.055

22. Seidman JD, Kurman RJ. Ovarian serous borderline tumors: a critical review of the literature with emphasis on prognostic indicators. *Hum Pathol*. 2000;31(5):539–557. doi:10.1053/hp.2000.8048

23. Coumbos A, Sehouli J, Chekerov R, et al. Clinical management of borderline tumours of the ovary: results of a multicentre survey of 323 clinics in Germany. *Br J Cancer*. 2009;100(11):1731–1738. doi:10.1038/sj.bjc.6605065

24. Morice P, Camatte S, El Hassan J, et al. Clinical outcomes and fertility after conservative treatment of ovarian borderline tumors. *Fertil Steril*. 2001;75(1):92–96. doi:10.1016/s0015-0282(00)01633-2

25. Salani R, Khanna N, Frimer M, et al. An update on post-treatment surveillance and diagnosis of recurrence in women with gynecologic malignancies: Society of Gynecologic Oncology (SGO) recommendations. *Gynecol Oncol*. 2017;146(1):3–10. doi:10.1016/j.ygyno.2017.03.022

26. Wright AA, Bohlke K, Armstrong DK, et al. Neoadjuvant chemotherapy for newly diagnosed, advanced ovarian cancer: Society of Gynecologic Oncology and American Society of Clinical Oncology clinical practice guideline. *Gynecol Oncol*. 2016;143(1):3–15. doi:10.1016/j.ygyno.2016.05.022

27. Vergote I, Tropé CG, Amant F, et al. Neoadjuvant chemotherapy or primary surgery in stage IIIC or IV ovarian cancer. *N Engl J Med*. 2010;363(10):943–953. doi:10.1056/NEJMoa0908806

28. Kehoe S, Hook J, Nankivell M, et al. Primary chemotherapy versus primary surgery for newly diagnosed advanced ovarian cancer (CHORUS): an open-label, randomised, controlled, non-inferiority trial. *Lancet*. 2015;386(9990):249–257. doi:10.1016/S0140-6736(14)62223-6

29. Fagotti A, Ferrandina MG, Vizzielli G, et al. Randomized trial of primary debulking surgery versus neoadjuvant chemotherapy for advanced epithelial ovarian cancer (SCORPION-NCT01461850). *Int J Gynecol Cancer*. 2020;30(11):1657–1664. doi:10.1136/ijgc-2020-001640

30. Reuss A, du Bois A, Harter P, et al. TRUST: Trial of Radical Upfront Surgical Therapy in advanced ovarian cancer (ENGOT ov33/AGO-OVAR OP7). *Int J Gynecol Cancer*. 2019;29(8):1327–1331. doi:10.1136/ijgc-2019-000682

31. Shi T, Zhu J, Feng Y, et al. Secondary cytoreduction followed by chemotherapy versus chemotherapy alone in platinum-sensitive relapsed ovarian cancer (SOC-1): a multicentre, open-label, randomised, phase 3 trial. *Lancet Oncol*. 2021;22(4):439–449. doi:10.1016/S1470-2045(21)00006-1

32. Armstrong DK, Bundy B, Wenzel L, et al. Intraperitoneal cisplatin and paclitaxel in ovarian cancer. *N Engl J Med*. 2006;354(1):34–43. doi:10.1056/NEJMoa052985

33. Walker JL, Brady MF, Wenzel L, et al. Randomized trial of intravenous versus intraperitoneal chemotherapy plus bevacizumab in advanced ovarian carcinoma: an NRG Oncology/Gynecologic Oncology Group study. *J Clin Oncol*. 2019;37(16):1380–1390. doi:10.1200/JCO.18.01568

34. Burger RA, Brady MF, Bookman MA, et al. Incorporation of bevacizumab in the primary treatment of ovarian cancer. *N Engl J Med*. 2011;365(26):2473–2483. doi:10.1056/NEJMoa1104390

35. Perren TJ, Swart AM, Pfisterer J, et al. A phase 3 trial of bevacizumab in ovarian cancer. *N Engl J Med*. 2011;365(26):2484–2496. doi:10.1056/NEJMoa1103799

36. González-Martín A, Pothuri B, Vergote I, et al. Niraparib in patients with newly diagnosed advanced ovarian cancer. *N Engl J Med*. 2019;381(25):2391–2402. doi: 10.1056/NEJMoa1910962

37. Berek JS, Hacker NF. *Berek & Hacker's Gynecologic Oncology*. 7th ed. Wolters Kluwer; 2021.

38. Harter P, du Bois A, Hahmann M, et al. Surgery in recurrent ovarian cancer: the Arbeitsgemeinschaft Gynaekologische Onkologie (AGO) DESKTOP OVAR trial. *Ann Surg Oncol*. 2006;13(12):1702–1710. doi:10.1245/s10434-006-9058-0

39. Banerjee S, Moore KN, Colombo N, et al. 811MO maintenance olaparib for patients (pts) with newly diagnosed, advanced ovarian cancer (OC) and a *BRCA* mutation (*BRCAm*): 5-year (y) follow-up (f/u) from SOLO1. *Ann Oncol*. 2020;31(suppl 4):S613. doi:10.1016/j.annonc.2020.08.950

40. Chi D, Berchuck A, Dizon DS, Yashar CM. *Principles and Practice of Gynecologic Oncology*. 7th ed. Lippincott Williams & Wilkins; 2017.

41. Coleman RL, Brady MF, Herzog TJ, et al. Bevacizumab and paclitaxel-carboplatin chemotherapy and secondary cytoreduction in recurrent, platinum-sensitive ovarian cancer (NRG Oncology/Gynecologic Oncology Group study GOG-0213): a multicentre, open-label, randomised, phase 3 trial. *Lancet Oncol*. 2017;18(6):779–791. doi:10.1016/S1470-2045(17)30279-6

42. Pujade-Lauraine E, Wagner U, Aavall-Lundqvist E, et al. Pegylated liposomal doxorubicin and carboplatin compared with paclitaxel and carboplatin for patients with platinum-sensitive ovarian cancer in late relapse. *J Clin Oncol*. 2010;28(20):3323–3329. doi:10.1200/JCO.2009.25.7519

43. Brown J, Friedlander M, Backes FJ, et al. Gynecologic Cancer Intergroup (GCIG) consensus review for ovarian germ cell tumors. *Int J Gynecol Cancer*. 2014;24(9 suppl 3):S48–S54. doi:10.1097/IGC.0000000000000223

44. Vasta FM, Dellino M, Bergamini A, et al. Reproductive outcomes and fertility preservation strategies in women with malignant ovarian germ cell tumors after fertility sparing surgery. *Biomedicines*. 2020;8(12):554. doi:10.3390/biomedicines8120554

45. Sleijfer S. Bleomycin-induced pneumonitis. *Chest*. 2001;120(2):617–624. doi:10.1378/chest.120.2.617

46. O'Sullivan JM, Huddart RA, Norman AR, et al. Predicting the risk of bleomycin lung toxicity in patients with germ-cell tumours. *Ann Oncol*. 2003;14(1):91–96. doi:10.1093/annonc/mdg020

47. Delanoy N, Pécuchet N, Fabre E, et al. Bleomycin-induced pneumonitis in the treatment of ovarian sex cord-stromal tumors: a systematic review and meta-analysis. *Int J Gynecol Cancer*. 2015;25(9):1593–1598. doi:10.1097/IGC.0000000000000530

48. Necchi A, Miceli R, Oualla K, et al. Effect of bleomycin administration on the development of pulmonary toxicity in patients with metastatic germ cell tumors receiving first-line chemotherapy: a meta-analysis of randomized studies. *Clin Genitourin Cancer*. 2017;15(2):213–220.e5. doi:10.1016/j.clgc.2016.08.021

49. Lauritsen J, Kier MGG, Bandak M, et al. Pulmonary function in patients with germ cell cancer treated with bleomycin, etoposide, and cisplatin. *J Clin Oncol*. 2016;34(13):1492–1499. doi:10.1200/JCO.2015.64.8451

50. Mangili G, Sigismondi C, Gadducci A, et al. Outcome and risk factors for recurrence in malignant ovarian germ cell tumors: a MITO-9 retrospective study. *Int J Gynecol Cancer*. 2011;21(8):1414–1421. doi:10.1097/IGC.0b013e3182236582

51. Pujade-Lauraine E, Hilpert F, Weber B, et al. Bevacizumab combined with chemotherapy for platinum-resistant recurrent ovarian cancer: the AURELIA open-label randomized phase III trial. *J Clin Oncol*. 2014;32(13):1302–1308. doi:10.1200/JCO.2013.51.4489

52. Parmar MK, Ledermann JA, Colombo N, et al. Paclitaxel plus platinum-based chemotherapy versus conventional platinum-based chemotherapy in women with relapsed ovarian cancer: the ICON4/AGO-OVAR-2.2 trial. *Lancet*. 2003;361(9375):2099–2106. doi:10.1016/s0140-6736(03)13718-x

53. Moore K, Colombo N, Scambia G, et al. Maintenance olaparib in patients with newly diagnosed advanced ovarian cancer. *N Engl J Med*. 2018;379(26):2495–2505. doi:10.1056/NEJMoa1810858

54. Ray-Coquard I, Pautier P, Pignata S, et al. Olaparib plus bevacizumab as first-line maintenance in ovarian cancer. *N Engl J Med*. 2019;381(25):2416–2428. doi:10.1056/NEJMoa1911361

55. Colombo N, Peiretti M, Castiglione M. Non-epithelial ovarian cancer: ESMO clinical recommendations for diagnosis, treatment and follow-up. *Ann Oncol*. 2009;20(suppl 4):IV24–IV26. doi:10.1093/annonc/mdp118

56. Berton-Rigaud D, Devouassoux-Shisheboran M, Ledermann JA, et al. Gynecologic Cancer InterGroup (GCIG) consensus review for uterine and ovarian carcinosarcoma. *Int J Gynecol Cancer*. 2014;24(9 suppl 3):S55–S60. doi:10.1097/IGC.0000000000000228

57. Powell MA, Filiaci VL, Hensley ML, et al. A randomized phase 3 trial of paclitaxel (P) plus carboplatin (C) versus paclitaxel plus ifosfamide (I) in chemotherapy-naive patients with stage I-IV, persistent or recurrent carcinosarcoma of the uterus or ovary: an NRG Oncology trial. *J Clin Oncol*. 2019;37(15 suppl):5500. doi:10.1200/JCO.2019.37.15_suppl.5500

58. Vergote I, van Gorp T, Amant F, et al. Neoadjuvant chemotherapy for ovarian cancer. *Oncology (Williston Park)*. 2005;19(12):1615–1622. https://www.cancernetwork.com/view/neoadjuvant-chemotherapy-ovarian-cancer

59. Rose PG, Nerenstone S, Brady MF, et al. Secondary surgical cytoreduction for advanced ovarian carcinoma. *N Engl J Med*. 2004;351(24):2489–2497. doi:10.1056/NEJMoa041125

60. Oseledchyk A, Leitao MM Jr, Konner J, et al. Adjuvant chemotherapy in patients with stage I endometrioid or clear cell ovarian cancer in the platinum era: a Surveillance, Epidemiology, and End Results Cohort Study, 2000–2013. *Ann Oncol*. 2017;28(12):2985–2993. doi:10.1093/annonc/mdx525

CHAPTER 21

Melanoma

Vincent T. Ma, Luke T. Fraley, and Leslie A. Fecher

INTRODUCTION

Melanoma is one of the most aggressive types of skin cancer. It is the fifth most common cancer in men and women in the United States and its incidence continues to increase worldwide.[1,2] While melanoma most often originates from the skin, it can also arise from the mucous membranes or the uveal tract of the eye. An association between sun or UV exposure and cutaneous melanoma exists; however, it appears more strongly associated with intermittent exposure compared with non-melanoma skin cancers, which correlates with total cumulative sun exposure.

Histological subtypes of cutaneous melanoma include superficial spreading, nodular, and lentigo maligna, as well as other less common subtypes. Activating mutations are found in melanoma with *BRAF* and *NRAS* being altered in about approximately 50% and 15% of cutaneous cases, respectively.[3,4] In subtypes of melanomas that are associated with minimal UV exposure, such as mucosal and acral melanomas, a *KIT* mutation may be present.[5]

The management of early-stage melanoma involves wide local excision (WLE) of the primary tumor with sentinel lymph node (SLN) mapping and biopsy based on histological features. The Multicenter Selective Lymphadenectomy Trial-I (MSLT-I) established the prognostic value of lymphatic mapping with SLN biopsy and found that SLN assessment was associated with improved disease-specific survival in a subgroup of patients.[6] Subsequently, MSLT-II found that immediate complete lymph node dissection (CLND) compared with nodal observation in SLN-positive patients improved regional disease control but did not improve melanoma-specific survival.[7] Patients with a positive SLN may be offered surveillance with serial ultrasounds (US) of the lymph node (LN) basin instead of CLND.

Systemic treatment with immune checkpoint inhibitors has revolutionized the care of advanced-stage melanoma and non-melanoma skin cancers. Immunotherapy and molecularly targeted therapies were initially U.S. Food and Drug Administration (FDA)-approved in unresectable stage III and stage IV melanoma, where melanoma tumors that harbor a *BRAF* V600 mutation have the option to be treated with combined *BRAF* and *MEK* inhibitors. These treatments have led to a decrease in melanoma mortality between 2014 to 2018.[8] Some of these agents have also demonstrated intracranial response in patients with brain metastases.[9,10]

In patients with resected stage II, III, and IV melanoma, adjuvant systemic therapy may be considered after weighing the risk of recurrence, potential benefits of treatments, and potential toxicities. Interferon alfa, ipilimumab, dabrafenib with trametinib, pembrolizumab, and nivolumab are FDA approved in various adjuvant settings. All agents have shown a relapse-free survival benefit with known, possible, unknown, or no impact on overall survival (OS) depending on the agent and clinical trial.[11-17] Overall, the therapeutic landscape of melanoma has dramatically changed over the last decade and the current role of immunotherapy and targeted therapy continues to evolve. In non-melanoma skin cancers, such as Merkel cell carcinoma (MCC), immunotherapy is FDA approved in the advanced, unresectable setting.

CASE SUMMARIES

Case 21.1: Stage I to II Disease

A 19-year-old woman with no significant past medical history (PMH) noted a changing skin lesion on her left abdomen. It started as a flesh-colored raised spot that turned pink and increased in size over a period of months. It was not painful or itchy. She has no family history of melanoma or other cancers. No palpable lymphadenopathy was detected on exam. She was referred to and seen by a dermatologist who performed a deep shave biopsy which revealed a superficial spreading melanoma extending to the deep margin.

How Does One Evaluate a Suspicious Skin Lesion?

- For clinical lesions concerning for melanoma, use the acronym ABCDE: asymmetry, border irregularity, color variegation, diameter greater than 6 mm, and evolving (with respect to size, shape, color(s), features, or symptoms).[18]
- The first step in diagnosis is biopsy; full-thickness skin biopsy is preferred to avoid compromising assessment of tumor thickness. Options include punch biopsy, shave biopsy with deep saucerization technique, or excisional or incisional biopsy. Wide margins should not be taken before a diagnosis is established. Pathology reports should note Breslow thickness, presence or absence of ulceration, presence or absence microsatellites, margin (deep and peripheral) status, mitotic rate, lymphovascular invasion, and histological subtype.[18]
- Breslow depth and ulceration status are considered the two most important prognostic factors for patients with localized melanoma.[19]
- All patients should have a full skin exam to evaluate for other concerning lesions.
- Routine labs or imaging are not indicated in stage I or II disease in the absence of concerning signs or symptoms.
- Phenotypic risk factors for melanoma include lighter skin, lighter hair (red, blond, light brown), lighter eyes (green, hazel, blue), dense freckling, higher number of melanocytic nevi, and atypical melanocytic nevi.[20]
- Additional risk factors for melanoma include history of skin cancer, history of melanoma, UV light exposure (including sun and indoor tanning), sunburn, xeroderma pigmentosum, *BRCA2* germline mutation, and family history of melanoma.[20]
- Most melanomas are sporadic with rare germline mutations.

When Is Further Molecular or Genomic Testing Required?

- *BRAF* testing is not recommended for stage I or II disease. It is a predictive marker of *BRAF/MEK* inhibitor therapy, which is only FDA-approved for stage III and IV disease.
- In the setting of three or more relatives with melanoma, referral to a cancer genetics clinic for testing may be considered.

What Are Appropriate Treatment Options?

- Surgery (performed by an experienced melanoma surgeon) is the standard of care.
- Cryotherapy, cautery, and local destruction are not used to treat primary melanomas.
- Patients should undergo WLE of the primary melanoma with at least 0.5- to 2-cm margins based on Breslow depth. For any invasive melanoma up to 1.99 mm in thickness, a clinical margin of at least 1 cm is recommended. Clinical surgical margins of 2 cm are recommended for a Breslow depth of 2.0 mm or greater. For melanoma in situ lesions, a surgical margin of 0.5 cm is recommended.
- SLN mapping and biopsy should be considered for patients with clinically negative nodes when a primary melanoma has any of the following features: 1 mm or more thick or less than 0.8 mm thick but with other aggressive features such as ulceration, greater than 1 mitosis/mm^2, positive deep margin, or lymphovascular invasion. Primary melanomas that are 0.8- to 1-mm thick require a risk and benefit discussion of SLN mapping and biopsy.
- For any clinically detected LN on physical exam or imaging, biopsy of the LN(s) is recommended to confirm malignancy. Definitive management in this scenario involves wide excision of the primary tumor and a therapeutic LN dissection.

Recommended Treatment Plan for This Patient

- *Follow-up WLE with SLN biopsy revealed residual melanoma with negative margins and negative SLNs.*

What Are Other Treatment Considerations?

- SLN mapping and biopsy require general anesthesia.
- SLN mapping and biopsy require special training.

What Are the Principles of Staging?

- The American Joint Committee on Cancer (AJCC) eighth edition staging system was updated in 2017.[21]
- Tumors are staged using pathology and clinical exam.
- Stage 0 is melanoma in situ.
- Stage IA is thickness of less than 0.8 mm without ulceration (pT1a).
- Stage IB includes thickness of less than 0.8 mm with ulceration or thickness of 0.8 to 1.0 with or without ulceration (pT1b), or greater than 1.0 to 2.0 mm without ulceration (pT2a).
- Stage IIA includes thickness greater than 1.0 to 2.0 mm with ulceration (pT2b) or greater than 2.0 to 4.0 mm without ulceration (pT3a).
- Stage IIB includes thickness greater than 2.0 to 4.0 mm with ulceration (pT3b) and greater than 4.0 mm without ulceration (pT4a).
- Stage IIC includes thickness greater than 4.0 mm with ulceration (pT4b).
- Any LN involvement by melanoma is considered at least stage III disease.
- A separate focus of melanoma within the cutaneous or subcutaneous tissues near the primary lesion is known as a satellite (within 2 cm from the primary) or in-transit (more than 2 cm from the primary) disease. Satellites can be microscopic or macroscopic. All are thought to be intralymphatic extensions of the primary melanoma and meet criteria for stage III disease regardless of nodal metastases. Satellite and in-transit lesions should be completely resected at the time of primary tumor excision, as feasible.

Patient's Clinical Stage
- *Stage Ib (pT2a, pN0, cM0)*

What Follow-up Is Appropriate?

- Patients with surgically resected stage I or II melanoma should be followed by dermatology every 3 to 6 months with a focus on skin and LN examinations for at least the first 2 years and then spaced out to every 3 to 12 months until year 5 depending on risk/stage.
- Patients may continue to follow for skin exams, with dermatology or primary care, annually for life given the risk of recurrence as well as for additional primary melanomas.
- Patients should be instructed on regular skin and LN self-examination and should be educated on sun and UV light safety.
- No routine laboratory or imaging studies are indicated in the absence of concerning signs or symptoms.
- First-degree relatives are recommended to have annual full skin exams.

What Is the Role for Systemic Therapy?

- Outside of clinical trials, adjuvant *BRAF*-targeted systemic therapy is not recommended for patients with stage I or IIA melanoma. High-dose interferon alfa is approved for primary tumors greater than 4 mm in thickness but is not typically recommended.[16] Pembrolizumab was FDA approved in December 2021 as adjuvant therapy in resected stage IIB and IIC melanoma based on improvement in recurrence-free survival compared with placebo.[17]
- The role of adjuvant systemic therapy in high-risk stage II melanoma continues to be investigated.

Case 21.2: Locally Advanced Stage III With Positive Sentinel Node

A 36-year-old man noted a changing pigmented skin lesion on his right upper back. He reported a long history of a nevus that began to increase in size, itch, and bleed over a few months. He presented to his primary care physician (PCP) for further evaluation. His PMH is significant for Crohn's disease that is well managed with maintenance vedolizumab. He has no family history of melanoma or other cancers. Physical examination was remarkable for an approximately 8-mm raised, irregularly bordered, darkly pigmented, ulcerated lesion on the right upper back. No clinically detected lymphadenopathy or satellite/in-transit disease was noted on exam. He was referred to a dermatologist and an excisional biopsy was performed and interpreted as a superficial spreading-type melanoma, Breslow depth of 5.6 mm, ulcerated with a focus of angiolymphatic invasion. The patient underwent a WLE with 2-cm margins and sentinel node mapping and biopsy. Three SLNs were identified in the right axilla and one was positive for melanoma with the largest deposit measuring 0.8 mm. No extracapsular extension was seen.

What Staging Workup Is Considered for Stage III Melanoma?

- Cross-sectional imaging studies include CT of the chest, abdomen, and pelvis (and neck if clinically indicated) and/or whole-body fluorodeoxyglucose (FDG) PET/CT.
- MRI of the brain is generally recommended to evaluate for brain metastases (particularly for stage IIIB/C/D).
- Scans should be performed with intravenous (IV) contrast unless contraindicated.

Staging Workup
- *A CT scan of the chest, abdomen, and pelvis and an MRI of the brain were negative for distant metastatic disease.*
- *The patient is staged as stage IIIC (T4b N1a(sn) M0) per the AJCC eighth edition.*

What Are the Management Options for a Positive Sentinel Lymph Node?

- See Figure 21.1.
- If there is evidence of LN involvement on the SLN biopsy, options for surgical management are US surveillance of the involved LN basin or immediate CLND depending on disease and patient characteristics, patient preference, and capacity for nodal US surveillance.
- Disease-free survival is improved with immediate CLND, but there is no significant difference in melanoma-specific survival with either approach.[7]
- Surveillance US of the LN basin should occur every 4 months during the first 2 years, then every 6 months during years 3 through 5, and then annually according to MSLT-2.
- Follow-up for patients who receive or do not receive adjuvant systemic therapy for stage III melanoma includes a history and physical examination (with an emphasis on LNs and skin) every 3 to 6 months for 2 years, then every 3 to 12 months for 3 years, then annually as clinically indicated. Consider systemic imaging (PET/CT, CT, and/or MRI) every 3 to 12 months for 2 years, then every 6 to 12 months for another 3 years, with additional imaging as clinically indicated.

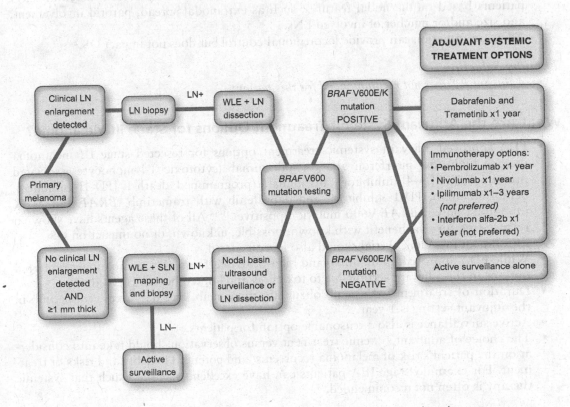

Figure 21.1 Management options for a positive sentinel lymph node

LN, lymph node; SLN, sentinel lymph node; WLE, wide local excision.

Postoperative Planning
- *The patient elects for surveillance US of the right axillary LN bed.*
- *He will continue to follow with his dermatologist and surgical oncologist for surveillance examinations.*

What Further Molecular or Genomic Testing Is Required?

- All patients with newly diagnosed stage III and IV melanoma should undergo testing for *BRAF* V600 mutation. *BRAF* V600 mutations occur in approximately 40% to 50% of all new melanoma diagnoses.[3]
- Primary tumor or core LN biopsy provides sufficient pathological material for *BRAF* mutation testing.
- *BRAF* V600 is a predictive biomarker for response to combined *BRAF* and *MEK* targeted therapies.
- Other molecular alterations like *NRAS* and *KIT* mutations may be found, but currently have no prognostic or therapeutic implications in the resected stage III setting.

Patient's Molecular and Genomic Testing
- *The patient's tumor tested positive for BRAF V600E mutation.*

What Is the Role for Adjuvant Radiation Therapy?

- Adjuvant radiation therapy (RT) to a nodal dissection bed may be considered in select patients based on the nodal features, such as extranodal spread, parotid involvement, and size and/or number of involved LNs.
- Adjuvant radiation can provide locoregional control but does not impact OS.[22]

Therapy Selection
- *Adjuvant RT was not recommended for this patient.*

What Are the Adjuvant Systemic Treatment Options for Stage III Melanoma?

- FDA-approved adjuvant systemic treatment options for resected stage III melanoma include high-dose interferon alfa-2b; ipilimumab (cytotoxic T-lymphocyte-associated protein 4 [CTLA-4] inhibitor), nivolumab (programmed death-1 [PD-1] inhibitor), pembrolizumab (PD-1 inhibitor), and dabrafenib with trametinib (*BRAF* and *MEK* inhibitors; only if *BRAF* V600 mutation-positive).[11-16] All of these agents have shown a relapse-free survival benefit with known, possible, unknown, or no impact on OS.
- Enrollment in a clinical trial should also be considered.
- While FDA approved, ipilimumab and high-dose interferon alfa are no longer preferred options in the adjuvant setting due to toxicities and limited benefit (IFN-alfa).
- Duration of treatment with pembrolizumab, nivolumab, and dabrafenib/trametinib in the adjuvant setting is 1 year.
- Active surveillance is also a reasonable option for patients.
- The choice of adjuvant systemic treatment versus observation should take into consideration the patient's risk of melanoma recurrence and potential benefits and risks of treatment. For example, stage IIIA patients can have excellent outcomes such that systemic therapy is often not recommended.[21]

Therapy Selection
- *Due to the patient's history of Crohn's disease, the decision was to pursue adjuvant dabrafenib 150 mg oral twice daily and trametinib 2 mg oral daily for 1 year.*

What Are the Potential Toxicities Associated With Adjuvant Systemic Therapy?

- Immunotherapy with checkpoint inhibitors such as pembrolizumab and nivolumab can cause unpredictable and potentially severe immune-mediated toxicities that can impact various organs, termed "immune-related adverse events" (irAEs). A relative contraindication to use of immunotherapy is the presence of preexisting autoimmune conditions, as they may be exacerbated by therapy and there may be a higher risk of irAEs overall.[23]
- Examples of irAEs from immunotherapy include dermatitis, arthritis, hypophysitis, thyroiditis, enterocolitis, hepatitis, pancreatitis, pneumonitis, myocarditis, and nephritis, as well as others.
- The most common side effect associated with dabrafenib and trametinib is fevers and/or chills, which can occur in up to 63% of cases and can be managed by dose interruption with or without dose reduction.[11] Other potential side effects include rashes, fatigue, nausea, diarrhea, peripheral edema, arthralgias, QT prolongation, change in cardiac ejection fraction, secondary skin malignancies (squamous cell carcinoma [SCC], basal cell carcinoma, and melanoma), and potential ocular toxicities. EKG and echocardiogram monitoring and skin surveillance are frequently recommended during the course of therapy.

Treatment Outcome

- *The patient tolerates dabrafenib and trametinib well. He did experience a fever up to 103°F after 3 weeks of therapy. Following symptomatic management with acetaminophen and dose interruption of both dabrafenib and trametinib for 2 days, he was able to resume treatment at the original doses.*
- *He completes 1 year of adjuvant therapy with no other treatment-limiting toxicities.*
- *He had no evidence of disease recurrence with serial US monitoring, CT imaging, and skin/LN examination during his 1-year course of treatment.*

Case 21.3: Metastatic *BRAF* V600 Mutation-Positive Disease

A 48-year-old woman with a history of systemic lupus erythematosus and no prior history of melanoma noted insidious onset of cognitive difficulties. She noticed decreased depth perception and began having difficulty typing and texting. She has no family history of melanoma or other cancers. No palpable lymphadenopathy or suspicious skin lesions were detected on exam. She was evaluated by her PCP and a CT of the head revealed multiple intracranial lesions. Follow-up MRI of the brain revealed right frontal subinsular, left lateral occipital, left cerebellar, and a large right parietal lobe intraparenchymal hemorrhage with mild patchy postcontrast enhancement concerning for hemorrhagic metastasis. PET/CT revealed intracranial abnormalities as well as a left upper lung nodule and left hilar LN. She then developed acutely worsened headache and repeat CT of the head revealed leftward midline shift and tumoral hemorrhage and required urgent craniotomy and tumor resection. Pathology revealed tissue necrosis and metastatic melanoma with cells positive for melan-A and HMB45. Bronchoscopy with hilar LN biopsy confirmed malignant melanoma.

How Is the Diagnosis Established?

- Diagnosis is suggested by symptoms, physical exam, or imaging findings and confirmed with biopsy.
- All patients with metastatic melanoma should have baseline imaging for staging and evaluation of specific symptoms.

- Baseline imaging modalities include contrast-enhanced MRI of the brain and contrast-enhanced CT of the chest, abdomen, and pelvis or whole-body FDG PET/CT. Staging scans may include CT of the neck or other imaging based on sites of metastases.
- Choice of biopsy site should consider which tumor would establish the most advanced disease as well as accessibility and safety. Tissue is preferred over cytology for mutational analysis.
- Melanoma can metastasize to almost any organ of the body, including the central nervous system (CNS). The most common site of metastasis from uveal melanoma is the liver.
- Stage III or IV melanomas should be tested for *BRAF* V600E and V600K mutations (not found in uveal melanomas). Additional mutational analysis, such as *KIT* (found in about 15% of acral lentiginous and mucosal melanomas), can be considered.

Patient's Diagnosis
- *Genetic testing on the hilar LN biopsy revealed BRAF V600E mutation.*

How Is This Tumor Staged?

- The AJCC eighth edition staging system is used to stage melanomas.[21]
- Evidence of distant metastasis (M1) establishes stage IV disease.
- Anatomic site of metastasis is further divided into M1a (skin, soft tissue, and nonregional LN), M1b (lung), M1c (non-CNS visceral sites), and M1d (CNS, new to AJCC eighth edition).
- Lactate dehydrogenase (LDH) is prognostic and incorporated into staging criteria: M1(0) indicates normal LDH at the time of staging while M1(1) indicates elevated LDH.[21]

Patient's Clinical Stage
- *Stage IV [Tx, Nx, M1d(1)].*

What Are Appropriate Treatment Options?

- Systemic therapy options for advanced, unresectable, or metastatic melanoma include single-agent checkpoint inhibitor therapy (ipilimumab, nivolumab, or pembrolizumab);[24-26] combination checkpoint inhibitor therapy (ipilimumab with nivolumab or nivolumab with relatlimab)[27,28]; combination *BRAF/MEK* targeted therapy (dabrafenib with trametinib, encorafenib with binimetinib, or vemurafenib with cobimetinib) for tumors harboring a *BRAF* V600-activating mutation[29-31]; combination *BRAF/MEK* targeted therapy with checkpoint inhibitor therapy (vemurafenib and cobimetinib with atezolizumab)[32]; high-dose interleukin-2[33]; chemotherapy (dacarbazine); and clinical trials.
- Immunotherapy is typically favored if no contraindications.
- Distant metastasis can be resected in select patients, such as those with a oligometastatic disease, long disease-free intervals, isolated site(s) of progression after systemic therapy, and/or limited systemic therapy options.[34]

Recommended Treatment Plan for This Patient
- *Patient was started on treatment with dabrafenib/trametinib due to the presence of symptomatic brain metastases with cerebral edema.*[9]

What Are the Toxicities Associated With This Treatment?

- This is also discussed in the stage III case discussion (see Case 21.2).
- Common side effects with combination targeted therapy for *BRAF* V600-activating mutations include partial alopecia, rash, photosensitivity, serous retinal detachment,

fever, nausea/vomiting, diarrhea, non-melanoma skin cancers, hypertension, QT prolongation, and hepatitis.[35]

Treatment Outcome

- *After approximately 2 months of therapy, dabrafenib/trametinib was placed on a 1-week hold due to fevers, chills, and myalgias.*
- *Therapy resumed with a dose reduction and currently is tolerated without significant side effects.*

What Are Other Treatment Considerations?

- Preexisting autoimmune conditions or a higher risk of irAEs may occur with immunotherapy.[23]
- Combination targeted therapy for *BRAF* V600-activating mutations is associated with rapid clinical results, but the duration of treatment response is short (median of 9 to 12 months).[36]
- Ipilimumab in combination with nivolumab demonstrated improved OS compared with dabrafenib with trametinib in the first-line setting for patients with *BRAF* V600E mutant metastatic melanoma.[37]
- Patients with CNS metastasis should have multidisciplinary consultation for consideration of palliative resection and/or RT.
- Ipilimumab with nivolumab as well as dabrafenib and trametinib have shown activity in CNS metastases, but extent of disease as well as hemorrhage and/or cerebral edema should be considered.[9,10]
- Best supportive and palliative care remain important considerations in stage IV melanoma.

What Is Required for This Patient's Follow-Up and Survivorship?

- All patients with stage IV disease typically have lifelong follow-up due to the risk for relapse.
- Follow-up is determined by cancer status and treatment status. Patients should be followed regularly while on active systemic therapy.
- Patients should be evaluated with a history and physical exam at least every 3 to 6 months for 5 years after coming off treatment if cancer status is controlled. Follow-up can be spaced out over time.
- Patients with a good treatment response should also be followed by dermatology for skin examination due to the risk of developing another primary melanoma.
- Imaging may be considered every 3 to 12 months for the first 2 years and then every 6 to 12 months for the next 3 years and then as clinically indicated.
- Patients with CNS metastases should have ongoing monitoring with brain imaging, with contrasted MRI scans preferred.

Case 21.4: Merkel Cell Carcinoma

A 60-year-old man presents for evaluation of a nontender skin lesion on his left anterior thigh. The patient noticed this lesion 3 months ago and it has been steadily growing. He is otherwise healthy and denies any history of prior skin malignancies or autoimmune conditions. On examination, the lesion is 1.0 cm in diameter, red and nodular-appearing, and without any ulceration. The remainder of his skin exam was unremarkable. The patient is referred to dermatology and a punch biopsy of the thigh lesion is interpreted as MCC.

What Is Merkel Cell Carcinoma and How Is It Diagnosed?

- MCC is a rare, aggressive, cutaneous neuroendocrine malignancy that predominantly affects older adults with light complexions and has a high propensity for recurrence.
- Several factors have been associated with the development of MCC including infection with the Merkel cell polyomavirus, UV radiation exposure, and immunosuppression.[38,39]
- On immunohistochemistry (IHC), MCC frequently express both epithelial markers (AE1/AE3, CAM5.2, pan-cytokeratin) and neuroendocrine markers (chromogranin, synaptophysin, CD56). MCC also stains positive for CK20 and negative for CK7 and thyroid transcription factor 1 (TTF-1).[38,39]

What Additional Staging Workup Is Recommended?

- A thorough skin and LN examination is warranted.
- If no clinical evidence of regional LN involvement is detected, SLN mapping and biopsy is recommended at the time of WLE.
- Given the metastatic potential of MCC, full body PET/CT scan and/or CT of the chest, abdomen, and pelvis is recommended for initial workup. MRI of the brain may be obtained if the patient is symptomatic to assess for CNS metastases.

Patient's Staging

- *Physical examination was negative for any lymphadenopathy.*
- *SLN mapping and biopsy from the left inguinal region demonstrate one out of two SLNs positive for MCC.*
- *Full-body PET/CT scan was negative for any metastatic disease.*

What Is the Definitive Management of Locoregional Merkel Cell Carcinoma?

- For LN-negative disease, surgical resection of the primary tumor is indicated with 1- to 2-cm margins. If surgery is not feasible, then definitive RT to the primary tumor and nodal region is an alternative.[39]
- Adjuvant RT to the resected primary tumor site is typically recommended except if the primary tumor is less than 2 cm with appropriate surgical margins.[39]
- For SLN-positive disease, in addition to WLE and/or radiation to the primary site, nodal management should include dissection and/or radiation.

Definitive Treatment

- *The patient undergoes primary tumor resection and left inguinal LN dissection.*
- *Pathology revealed a 1.5-cm tumor with negative margins and no additional LNs involved by MCC.*
- *The patient's final staging is stage IIIA (T1, pN1a, M0) per AJCC eighth edition.[39]*

What Adjuvant Systemic Treatment Is Available for Stage III Merkel Cell Carcinoma?

- As of 2021, there is no FDA-approved adjuvant systemic treatment for stage III MCC. Currently, anti-PD-1/programmed death-ligand 1 (PD-L1) inhibitors are under investigation in clinical trials.
- Participation in a clinical trial, if available, should be offered to patients following completion of surgery with or without RT.

Follow-Up

- *The patient undergoes active surveillance including full skin and LN examination every 3 to 6 months by his dermatologist.*
- *Around 2 years later, he developed new lymphadenopathy involving his right axilla. Staging FDG-PET/CT scan revealed multiple bilateral lung nodules and a 3-cm lesion in his liver. Core biopsy of the liver lesion confirmed metastatic MCC.*

What Are the Treatment Options for Metastatic Merkel Cell Carcinoma?

- Factors to be considered when deciding treatment include site(s) of disease, age, comorbidities, and patient preference.
- Pembrolizumab (anti-PD-1 inhibitor) and avelumab (anti-PD-L1 inhibitor) are FDA-approved treatments for metastatic MCC.[40,41]
- Chemotherapy retains a role in the treatment of patients who do not respond to or relapse after immunotherapy or in those patients in whom immunotherapy is contraindicated. Chemotherapy regimen options include carboplatin with etoposide and cyclophosphamide/doxorubicin/vincristine as well as others, but durability of response typically is only a few months.[39]
- A clinical trial is recommended whenever possible.

Therapy Selection

- *Given no contraindications for treatment with immune checkpoint therapy, the patient is treated with pembrolizumab. After 3 doses of treatment, he achieves a partial response.*

REVIEW QUESTIONS

1. A 35-year-old man is diagnosed with melanoma located on his right forearm. Initial punch biopsy revealed a superficial spreading melanoma, Breslow depth 0.8 mm, Clark level III, no ulceration, mitotic rate 1 per mm^2, no lymphovascular invasion, no perineural invasion, and no tumor regression. He is due to undergo wide local excision (WLE) without sentinel lymph node (SLN) mapping. Which of the following is considered the most important prognostic variable in a primary melanoma?
   A. Breslow depth
   B. Clark level
   C. Lymphovascular invasion
   D. Mitotic rate
   E. Tumor regression

2. A 50-year-old woman is diagnosed with an ulcerated melanoma arising on the right arm. She underwent wide local excision (WLE) and sentinel lymph node (SLN) biopsy, which detected two positive lymph nodes (LNs). A CT scan of the chest, abdomen, and pelvis show no evidence of metastases. Which of the following studies should be ordered at this time?
   A. Fluorodeoxyglucose (FDG)-PET/CT scan
   B. Ultrasound (US) of right axillary LN basin
   C. MRI of the brain
   D. CT scan of the head without contrast

3. An obese 44-year-old accountant comes to a follow-up visit 2 weeks after completing his second induction dose of ipilimumab with nivolumab for stage IV melanoma. He reports fatigue and headaches. Laboratory findings show sodium of 131 mmol/L (low), potassium of 4.8 mmol/L, thyroid-stimulating hormone (TSH) of 0.2 mIU/L (low), free T4 of 0.54 ng/dL (low), testosterone of 1.31 ng/mL (low), and AM cortisol level of 1.5 mcg/dL (low). On examination, blood pressure is found to be 100/54 mmHg and he looks fatigued. What is the pathophysiology of his endocrine disruption?
   A. Obesity-related hypogonadism
   B. Primary hypothyroidism
   C. Immune-mediated hypophysitis
   D. Addison's disease

4. A 74-year-old woman notes a new pigmented lesion on her shoulder. Pathological examination of a deep shave biopsy specimen reveals a superficial spreading melanoma with a Breslow depth of 0.5 mm and less than 1 mitosis/mm^2. It is not ulcerated. All margins are negative. What is the next appropriate step in management?
   A. Active surveillance
   B. CT of the chest, abdomen, and pelvis to complete staging
   C. Wide local excision (WLE) with a 1-cm margin
   D. WLE with a 2-cm margin
   E. Sentinel lymph node (SLN) mapping and biopsy, followed by WLE with a 2-cm margin
   F. Adjuvant nivolumab or pembrolizumab

5. A 22-year-old lifeguard has a history of stage IIIA melanoma arising on the back, diagnosed 4 years ago. On surveillance imaging, he is found to have multiple new nodules in

the lungs. Biopsy of one of the larger lung nodules shows metastatic melanoma. What genetic testing should be performed on the tumor tissue at this time?

A. C-KIT
B. NRAS
C. EGFR
D. BRAF
E. GNAQ

6. A 62-year-old man is diagnosed with a left eye uveal melanoma after presenting with a 4-month history of progressively worsening vision loss. Staging scans revealed no metastatic disease. Options of management were discussed including plaque radiotherapy or enucleation, and he decides to proceed with enucleation. Genetic expression profiling of his tumor revealed a class 2 gene signature and PReferentially expressed Antigen in MElanoma (PRAME) positivity, which places him at high risk of metastasis. Which of the following is the most common site of metastases in uveal melanoma?

A. Lung
B. Brain
C. Kidneys
D. Liver
E. Skin

7. A 67-year-old man has a history of stage IIIA melanoma arising on the leg. His tumor demonstrates an activating mutation in *BRAF* at the V600 codon. He is offered adjuvant treatment with dabrafenib with trametinib. What is the most common side effect associated with this treatment?

A. Rash
B. Diarrhea
C. Elevated liver enzymes
D. Neutropenia
E. Fevers and/or chills

8. A 50-year-old man with no significant past medical history (PMH) was recently diagnosed with melanoma of his right upper arm. He underwent wide local excision (WLE) and sentinel lymph node biopsy (SLNB) and was found to have a positive SLNB with one of two lymph nodes (LNs) harboring melanoma. Full-body imaging was negative for distant metastases. He has resected stage III disease. Mutation analysis reveals that he has a *BRAF* V600E mutation. Which of the following options is not a U.S. Food and Drug Administration (FDA)-approved adjuvant therapy option for this patient?

A. High-dose interferon alfa
B. Nivolumab
C. Pembrolizumab
D. Ipilimumab
E. Ipilimumab with nivolumab
F. Dabrafenib with trametinib

9. A 69-year-old female is diagnosed with metastatic Merkel cell carcinoma (MCC) involving the lung. She is otherwise healthy and has no major comorbidities. Which of the following is a U.S. Food and Drug Administration (FDA)-approved and recommended treatment option for this patient?

A. Avelumab
B. Atezolizumab

C. Pembrolizumab
D. Carboplatin with etoposide
E. A or C
F. Any of the above

10. A 68-year-old female with *BRAF* V600E-mutated, stage IV melanoma with both lung and liver metastases was started on nivolumab 480 mg every 4 weeks as first-line therapy. After 3 cycles of treatment, a CT scan is done which revealed that all the lesions are stable, except her liver lesion has increased from 2.5 cm to 3.0 cm. She otherwise feels well and has not developed any treatment-related adverse events. What do you recommend for her treatment?

A. Continue therapy
B. Increase the dose of nivolumab
C. Stop nivolumab and switch to ipilimumab
D. Add ipilimumab
E. Add dabrafenib and trametinib
F. Switch to encorafenib and binimetinib

ANSWERS AND RATIONALES

1. **A. Breslow depth.** Breslow depth and ulceration status are considered the two most important prognostic factors for patients with localized melanoma (stage I or II).

2. **C. MRI of the brain.** MRI is a sensitive and specific test for imaging melanoma, particularly in the brain. An MRI of the brain should be included in staging workup to evaluate for brain metastases.

3. **C. Immune-mediated hypophysitis.** The constellation of central hypothyroidism (low TSH and low free T4), adrenal insufficiency (low cortisol and hyponatremia), and hypogonadism (low testosterone level) is suggestive of hypophysitis. Although a relatively rare complication of immune checkpoint therapy, hypophysitis is often manifested by clinical symptoms of fatigue and headache. In addition to abnormal lab findings, the diagnosis of hypophysitis may be supported radiographically by enhancement and swelling of the pituitary gland. If symptomatic hypophysitis, high-dose steroids should be given during the acute phase to reverse the inflammatory process. In most cases, patients require long-term hormone replacement. The adrenal axis should always be replaced prior to initiation of thyroid replacement.

4. **C. Wide local excision (WLE) with a 1-cm margin.** Based on the surgical guidelines, a primary melanoma with a tumor thickness of 1.0 mm or less, a wide excision with a clinical margin of 1.0 cm is recommended (category 1). In this patient case, given a primary tumor depth of less than 0.8 mm with absence of aggressive features (ulceration, greater than 1 mitosis/mm^2, or positive deep margins), a sentinel lymph node (SLN) biopsy is not recommended.

5. **D. *BRAF*.** *BRAF* mutations occur in about 40% to 50% of invasive cutaneous melanoma cases. The presence of this mutation is predictive of response to *BRAF* and *MEK* targeted therapy. *C-KIT* mutations are commonly found in acral and mucosal melanomas and may be predictive of response to *KIT*-inhibitors in the metastatic setting. *GNAQ* is frequently mutated in uveal melanoma.

6. **D. Liver.** The most common sites of metastasis from uveal melanoma include liver (89%), lung (29%), bone (17%), and skin/subcutaneous tissue (12%), whereas lymph node (LN) and brain metastasis are rarer.[42]

7. **E. Fevers and/or chills.** The most common side effect associated with dabrafenib and trametinib is fevers and/or chills, which can occur in up to 63% of cases.[11,35] This side effect can be managed by dose interruption with or without dose reduction. Antipyretics such as nonsteroidal anti-inflammatory drugs (NSAIDs) and acetaminophen are frequently used to manage these symptoms.

8. **E. Ipilimumab with nivolumab.** All other agents listed are approved in the adjuvant setting for resected stage III melanoma. However, combination ipilimumab and nivolumab is only recommended and FDA-approved for unresectable or metastatic melanoma.

9. **E. A or C.** Immune checkpoint therapy is the preferred initial systemic treatment for patients with advanced MCC if there are no absolute contraindications to such therapy. Compared to chemotherapy, immunotherapy has a greater capacity to induce clinically meaningful, durable responses. The U.S. Food and Drug ADministration (FDA) has approved avelumab and pembrolizumab for advanced or metastatic MCC, irrespective of prior therapy.

10. A. Continue therapy. Responses to immunotherapy can be delayed compared with cytotoxic therapy. It is not uncommon for responses to occur after radiological evidence of initial disease progression and caution should be exercised regarding premature stopping of treatment. Pseudoprogression refers to a transient worsening of disease, manifested by progression of known lesions or appearance of new lesions on a scan, but may eventually stabilize or regress with time.[43]

REFERENCES

1. Urban K, Mehrmal S, Uppal P, et al. The global burden of skin cancer: a longitudinal analysis from the global burden of disease study, 1990–2017. *JAAD Int.* 2021;4(2):98–108. doi:10.1016/j.jdin.2020.10.013
2. Siegel RL, Miller KD, Fuchs JE, Jemal A. Cancer statistics, 2021. *CA Cancer J Clin.* 2021;71:7–33. doi:10.3322/caac.21654
3. Davies H, Bignell GR, Cox C, et al. Mutations of the *BRAF* gene in human cancer. *Nature.* 2002;417:949–954. doi:10.1038/nature00766
4. Curtin JA, Frilyand J, Kageshita T, et al. Distinct sets of genetic alterations in melanoma. *N Engl J Med.* 2005;353:2135–2147. doi:10.1056/NEJMoa050092
5. Curtin JA, Busam K, Pinkel D, Bastian BC. Somatic activation of KIT in distinct subtypes of melanoma. *J Clin Oncol.* 2006;24(26):4340–4346. doi:10.1200/JCO.2006.06.2984
6. Morton DL, Thompson JF, Cochran AJ, et al. Final trial report of sentinel-node biopsy versus nodal observation in melanoma. *N Engl J Med.* 2014;370(7):599–609. doi:10.1056/NEJMoa1310460
7. Faries MB, Thompson JF, Cochran AJ, et al. Completion dissection or observation for sentinel-node metastasis in melanoma. *N Engl J Med.* 2017;376(23):2211–2222. doi:10.1056/NEJMoa1613210
8. Islami F, Ward EM, Sung H, et al. Annual report to the nation on the status of cancer, part 1: national cancer statistics. *J Natl Cancer Inst.* 2021;113(12):1648–1669. doi:10.1093/jnci/djab131
9. Davies MA, Saiag P, Robert C, et al. Dabrafenib plus trametinib in patients with *BRAF* V600-mutant melanoma brain metastases (COMBI-MB): a multicentre, multicohort, open-label, phase 2 trial. *Lancet Oncol.* 2017;18(7):863–873. doi:10.1016/S1470-2045(17)30429-1
10. Tawbi HA, Forsyth PA, Algazi A, et al. Combined nivolumab and ipilimumab in melanoma metastatic to the brain. *N Engl J Med.* 2018;379(8):722–730. doi:10.1056/NEJMoa1805453
11. Long GV, Hauschild A, Santinami M, et al. Adjuvant dabrafenib plus trametinib in stage III *BRAF*-mutated melanoma. *N Engl J Med.* 2017;377(19):1813–1823. doi:10.1056/NEJMoa1708539
12. Eggermont AM, Blank CU, Mandalà M, et al. Adjuvant pembrolizumab versus placebo in resected stage III melanoma (EORTC 1325-MG/KEYNOTE-054): distant metastasis-free survival results from a double-blind, randomised, controlled, phase 3 trial. *Lancet Oncol.* 2021;22(5):643–654. doi:10.1016/S1470-2045(21)00065-6
13. Eggermont AM, Chaiarion-Sileni V, Grob J-J, et al. Adjuvant ipilimumab versus placebo after complete resection of high-risk stage III melanoma (EORTC 18071): a randomised, double-blind, phase 3 trial. *Lancet Oncol.* 2015;16(5):522–530. doi:10.1016/S1470-2045(15)70122-1
14. Ascierto PA, Del Vecchio M, Mandalà M, et al. Adjuvant nivolumab versus ipilimumab in resected stage IIIB-C and stage IV melanoma (CheckMate-238): 4-year results from a multicentre, double-blind, randomised, controlled, phase 3 trial. *Lancet Oncol.* 2020;21(11):1465–1477. doi:10.1016/S1470-2045(20)30494-0
15. Tarhini AA, Lee SJ, Hodi FS, et al. Phase III study of adjuvant ipilimumab (3 or 10 mg/kg) versus high-dose interferon alfa-2b for resected high-risk melanoma: North American Intergroup E1609. *J Clin Oncol.* 2020;38(6):567–575. doi:10.1200/JCO.19.01381
16. Kirkwood JM, Strawderman MH, Ernstoff MS, et al. Interferon alfa-2b adjuvant therapy of high risk resected cutaneous melanoma: the Eastern Cooperative Oncology Group Trial EST 1684. *J Clin Oncol.* 1996;14:7–17. doi:10.1200/JCO.1996.14.1.7
17. U.S. Food and Drug Administration. FDA approves pembrolizumab for adjuvant treatment of stage IIB or IIC melanoma. https://www.fda.gov/drugs/resources-information-approved-drugs/fda-approves-pembrolizumab-adjuvant-treatment-stage-iib-or-iic-melanoma
18. Abbasi NR, Shaw HM, Rigel DS, et al. Early diagnosis of cutaneous melanoma: revisiting the ABCD criteria. *JAMA.* 2004;292(22):2771–2776. doi:10.1001/jama.292.22.2771
19. Balch CM, Soong SJ, Gershenwald JE, et al. Prognostic factors analysis of 17,600 melanoma patients: validation of the American Joint Committee on Cancer melanoma staging system. *J Clin Oncol.* 2001;19:3622–3634. doi:10.1200/JCO.2001.19.16.3622
20. O'Neill CH, Scoggins CR. Melanoma. *J Surg Oncol.* 2019;120(5):873–881. doi:10.1002/jso.25604

21. Gershenwald JE, Scolyer RA, Hess KR, et al. Melanoma staging: evidence-based changes in the American Joint Committee on Cancer eighth edition cancer staging manual. *CA Cancer J Clin.* 2017;67(6):472–492. doi:10.3322/caac.21409

22. Henderson MA, Burmeister BH, Ainslie J, et al. Adjuvant lymph-node field radiotherapy versus observation only in patients with melanoma at high risk of further lymph-node field relapse after lymphadenectomy (ANZMTG 01.02/TROG 02.01): 6-year follow up of a phase 3, randomized controlled trial. *Lancet Oncol.* 2015;16(9):1049–1060. doi:10.1016/S1470-2045(15)00187-4

23. Kennedy LC, Bhatia S, Thompson JA, Grivas P. Preexisting autoimmune disease: implications for immune checkpoint inhibitor therapy in solid tumors. *J Natl Compr Canc Netw.* 2019;17(6):750–757. doi:10.6004/jnccn.2019.7310

24. Hodi FS, O'Day SJ, McDermott DF, et al. Improved survival with ipilimumab in patients with metastatic melanoma. *N Engl J Med.* 2010;363(8):711–723. doi:10.1056/NEJMoa1003466

25. Hamid O, Robert C, Daud A, et al. Five-year survival outcomes for patients with advanced melanoma treated with pembrolizumab in KEYNOTE-001. *Ann Oncol.* 2019;30:582–588. doi:10.1093/annonc/mdz011

26. Topalian SL, Hodi FS, Brahmer JR, et al. Five-year survival and correlates among patients with advanced melanoma, renal cell carcinoma, or non-small cell lung cancer treated with nivolumab. *JAMA Oncol.* 2019;5(10):1411–1420. doi:10.1001/jamaoncol.2019.2187

27. Wolchok JD, Chiarion-Sileni V, Gonzalez R, et al. Long-term outcomes with nivolumab plus ipilimumab or nivolumab alone versus ipilimumab in patients with advanced melanoma. *J Clin Oncol.* 2022;40(2):127–137. doi:10.1200/JCO.21.02229

28. Tawbi HA, Schadendorf D, Lipson EJ, et al. Relatlimab and nivolumab versus nivolumab in untreated advanced melanoma. *N Engl J Med.* 2022 Jan 6;386(1):24–34. doi:10.1056/NEJMoa2109970

29. Robert C, Karaszewska B, Schachter J, et al. Improved overall survival in melanoma with combined dabrafenib and trametinib. *N Engl J Med.* 2015;372(1):30–39. doi:10.1056/NEJMoa1412690

30. Larkin J, Ascierto PA, Dréno B, et al. Combined vemurafenib and cobimetinib in *BRAF*-mutated melanoma. *N Engl J Med.* 2014;371(20):1867–1876. doi:10.1056/NEJMoa1408868

31. Dummer R, Ascierto PA, Gogas HJ, et al. Encorafenib plus binimetinib versus vemurafenib or encorafenib in patients with *BRAF*-mutant melanoma (COLUMBUS): a multicentre, open-label, randomised phase 3 trial. *Lancet Oncol.* 2018;19(5):603–615. doi:10.1016/S1470-2045(18)30142-6

32. Gutzmer R, Stroyakovskiy D, Gogas H, et al. Atezolizumab, vemurafenib, and cobimetinib as first-line treatment for unresectable advanced *BRAF* V600 mutation-positive melanoma (IMspire150): primary analysis of the randomised, double-blind, placebo-controlled, phase 3 trial. *Lancet.* 2020;395(10240):1835–1844. doi:10.1016/S0140-6736(20)30934-X

33. Atkins MB, Kunkel L, Sznol M, Rosenberg SA. High-dose recombinant interleukin-2 therapy in patients with metastatic melanoma: long-term survival update. *Cancer J Sci Am.* 2000;6(suppl 1):S11–S14.

34. O'Neill CH, McMasters KM, Egger ME. Role of surgery in stage IV melanoma. *Surg Oncol Clin North Am.* 2020;29(3):485–495. doi:10.1016/j.soc.2020.02.010

35. Heinzerling L, Eigentler TK, Fluck M, et al. Toleratbility of *BRAF/MEK* inhibitor combinations: adverse event evaluation and management. *ESMO Open.* 2019;4(3):e000491. doi:10.1136/esmoopen-2019-000491

36. Sun J, Carr MJ, Khushalani KI. Principles of targeted therapy for melanoma. *Surg Clin North Am.* 2020;100(1):175–188. doi:10.1016/j.suc.2019.09.013

37. Atkins M. Lee SJ, Chmielowski B. DREAMseq (Doublet, Randomized Evaluation in Advanced Melanoma Sequencing): a phase III trial—ECOG-ACRIN EA6134. *J Clin Oncol.* 39;2021(36 suppl):356154. doi:10.1200/JCO.2021.39.36_suppl.356154

38. Harms PW, Harms KL, Moore PS, et al. The biology and treatment of Merkel cell carcinoma: current understanding and research priorities. *Nat Rev Clin Oncol.* 2018;15(12):763–776. doi:10.1038/s41571-018-0103-2

39. National Comprehensive Cancer Network. Merkel cell carcinoma (Version 1.2021). https://www.nccn.org/professionals/physician_gls/pdf/mcc.pdf

40. Nghiem P, Bhatia S, Lipson EJ, et al. Durable tumor regression and overall survival in patients with advanced Merkel cell carcinoma receiving pembrolizumab as first-line therapy. *J Clin Oncol.* 2019;37(9):693–702. doi:10.1200/JCO.18.01896

41. Kaufman HL, Russel JS, Hamid O, et al. Updated efficacy of avelumab in patients with previously treated metastatic Merkel cell carcinoma after ≥1 year follow up: JAVELIN Merkel 200, a phase 2 clinical trial. *J Immunother Cancer.* 2018;6(1):7. doi:10.1186/s40425-017-0310-x

42. Diener-West M, Reynolds SM, Agugliaro DJ, et al. Development of metastatic disease after enrollment in the COMS trials for treatment of choroidal melanoma: Collaborative Ocular Melanoma Study Group report No. 26. *Arch Ophthalmol.* 2005;123(12):1639–1643. doi:10.1001/archopht.123.12.1639

43. Kurra V, Sullivan RJ, Gainor JF, et al. Pseudoprogression in cancer immunotherapy: rates, time course and patient outcomes. *J Clin Oncol.* 2016;34(15_suppl):6580. doi:10.1200/JCO.2016.34.15_suppl.6580

CHAPTER 22

Bone Sarcoma

James Liu and Janai R. Carr-Ascher

INTRODUCTION

Primary bone cancers are a rare group of tumors, making up less than 1% of all cancers diagnosed each year.[1] These tumor types include osteosarcoma, chondrosarcoma, giant cell tumor of bone, and Ewing sarcoma. In adults, metastatic bone lesions as well as benign bone lesions are far more common than primary bone cancers. Interestingly, benign bone lesions such as hemangiomas and osteochondromas can present as lytic lesions, making radiographic diagnosis difficult. For adults (over age 40) with a suspicious radiographically identified bone lesion, it should be assumed this lesion is metastatic and these patients should undergo evaluation to identify the primary tumor. Specifically, these patients should be evaluated for prostate or breast cancer as well as multiple myeloma with a prostate-specific antigen (PSA), mammogram, and serum protein electrophoresis (SPEP)/urine protein electrophoresis (UPEP), respectively. In addition to these studies, imaging of the chest, abdomen, pelvis, and other extremities is recommended.[2] If this workup does not yield additional sites of disease and there is concern for a primary bone lesion, given the rarity of these tumors, the heterogeneous presentation, and potential for associated morbidity, these patients should be evaluated at a specialty care center by a multidisciplinary team. The following cases illustrate the workup, treatment, and staging for the most common bone sarcomas affecting adults.

CASE SUMMARIES

Case 22.1: Osteosarcoma

A 49-year-old had progressively worsening left leg pain with ambulation for the past month. Due to his eventual inability to bear weight, he presented to the local ED. Initial imaging with x-ray of the left tibia revealed a osteolytic lesion at the mid diaphysis with cortical breakthrough and an associated soft-tissue mass. MRI of the lower extremity identified a large destructive osseous mass (9 cm) centered at the mid diaphysis of the tibia with a large posterior extraosseous soft-tissue mass (5 × 3 × 12 cm). A biopsy of the left tibia was consistent with high-grade conventional osteosarcoma. A PET scan redemonstrated the left tibial mass with a standardized uptake value (SUV) of 50.6 and concerning left external inguinal lymph nodes (LNs; 2.1 × 1.4 cm, SUV 4.7). A follow-up biopsy of the left inguinal LN was negative for metastatic osteosarcoma.

How Is a Diagnosis Established?

- The initial evaluation of osteosarcoma includes plain radiographs of the primary tumor. These tumors are commonly identified in the metaphyseal regions of the long bones. Plain radiographs reveal both lucent and sclerotic features due to aggressive bone destruction. The radiographic appearance of new subperiosteal bone formed as the primary tumor lifts the periosteum is classically described as "Codman's triangle."[3] Once plain radiographs raise suspicion for osteosarcoma, an MRI of the bone is performed for surgical planning and staging. This allows for more accurate assessment of tumor size, intramedullary involvement, and surrounding structures. An important consideration is evaluation of skip metastases, which are small foci of discontiguous metastasis within the involved bone which can be better identified with an MRI than plain radiographs.[4]
- Complete staging includes a CT of the chest to identify distant metastasis given that the lungs are the most common site of metastasis for osteosarcoma.[5] Other bony sites should be evaluated by whole body PET scan or technetium bone scan to evaluate distant metastasis. The diagnosis for osteosarcoma is established by either a core needle or open biopsy.

Patient's Diagnosis
- Tibial osteosarcoma

What Is the Staging System for Bone Cancers?

- Current National Comprehensive Cancer Network (NCCN) guidelines adopted the American Joint Committee on Cancer (AJCC) staging system for bone sarcoma, which is based on tumor size, regional node status, presence of distant metastasis, and histological grade. Histological grading is based on three general categories: tumor differentiation, mitotic count, and extent of tumor necrosis.[2]

Patient's Clinical Stage
- Clinical stage IIB (T2N0M0G3)

What Is the Recommended Treatment?

- The addition of chemotherapy has improved outcomes for non-metastatic osteosarcoma, though surgical resection remains the standard of care. Modern chemotherapy is given in a perioperative approach, utilizing both neoadjuvant and adjuvant chemotherapy in patients with resectable osteosarcoma. For patients 40 years old and younger, treatment regimens extrapolated from the pediatric population are used. This consists of high-dose methotrexate, doxorubicin, and cisplatin (MAP regimen).[6] The optimal regimen for older adults is not well established. Typically for those who are older than 40 years old, doxorubicin and cisplatin are used with close attention to dose adjustments based on tolerance. High-dose methotrexate has not shown a clear benefit in this age group.[7] Radiation therapy (RT) has not been shown to improve outcomes in resectable osteosarcoma; however, it can be considered as a surgical alternative for local control in those with unresectable or incompletely resected disease.[8]

Patient's Treatment and Outcome
- The patient underwent 3 cycles of neoadjuvant chemotherapy with doxorubicin and cisplatin followed by surgical resection of the left tibial mass with pathology consistent with a 9-cm, grade 3 osteoblastic osteosarcoma with negative margins (T2NM0, stage IIB). He

then completed 3 additional cycles of adjuvant doxorubicin and cisplatin. At his most recent follow-up 2 years from surgical resection, he remains disease free.

What Are the Common Toxicities of Treatment?

- Side effects of doxorubicin and cisplatin include fatigue, nausea, alopecia, decreased blood counts, and infertility. Therefore, growth factor support should be provided. Doxorubicin as well as other anthracyclines have a risk of cardiac toxicity and secondary malignancy. Side effects that are specific to cisplatin include nephrotoxicity and ototoxicity.

What Is the Recommended Surveillance?

- Evidence for post-treatment surveillance in osteosarcoma is limited. The current recommendations are based on NCCN guidelines. Postoperative baseline imaging can be considered after surgical resection or completion of adjuvant chemotherapy. Patients are evaluated every 3 months by physical exam, imaging of the primary tumor site, and chest imaging for the first 2 years when relapse risk is highest, then less frequently in subsequent years.[9] For patients without evidence of recurrence after 5 years, the likelihood of recurrent disease is low; thus, follow-up should be individualized.[2]

Case 22.2: Ewing Sarcoma

A 31-year-old male who presented for evaluation of pelvic pain and urinary hesitancy was found to have a pelvic mass. A CT of his abdomen and pelvis identified a large 15.7 × 11 × 11.3 cm mass leading to bilateral hydronephrosis. Biopsy of the pelvic lesion was consistent with Ewing sarcoma. Cytogenetic analysis identified an EWSR1 gene rearrangement. A whole-body PET/CT did not show other regions of involvement and an MRI was performed for surgical planning.

How Is a Diagnosis Established and What Is the Recommended Workup?

- The initial workup for Ewing sarcoma consists of plain radiographic imaging. These x-rays can demonstrate bone destruction from the tumor which typically appears as a "moth-eaten pattern" on radiographs. Periosteal reactions from this aggressive disease can also manifest as a laminated ("onionskin") or spiculated ("sunburst") appearance.[10] An MRI of the tumor site should be completed for surgical planning. This typically reveals evidence of marrow replacement, cortical destruction, and an associated soft-tissue mass.[10] A whole-body PET scan can be utilized for staging and evaluation of distant metastasis. Alternatively, CT scans and a bone scan can be considered to evaluate the whole body.
- Biopsy with pathological and cytogenetic evaluation is critical for the diagnosis of Ewing sarcoma. Histology demonstrates small round blue cells with CD99 positivity. The typical cytogenetic aberration of Ewing sarcoma is reciprocal translocation of chromosome 11 and 22 (t[11;22][q24;q12]) resulting in a *EWS-FLI1* fusion transcript. Less common translocations include *EWS-ERG* t(21;22)(q22;q12) and *EWS-ETV1* t(7;22)(p22;q12).[11] Staging of Ewing sarcoma follows the NCCN guidelines for bone cancers, although treatment and prognosis are determined by resectability of the primary tumor or the presence of metastatic lesions.

Patient's Diagnosis and Stage

- *Biopsy reveals Ewing sarcoma, conformed by EWSR1 gene rearrangement.*

What Is the General Course of Treatment?

- Around 80% of patients with localized Ewing sarcoma will develop metastasis if treated with surgery alone. Therefore, this tumor is considered metastatic at diagnosis.[12] The risk of metastasis is decreased by approximately 5% to 30% with chemotherapy, which emphasizes the importance of chemotherapy in the treatment of Ewing sarcoma. For localized disease, perioperative chemotherapy is used. Patients under age 50 should receive compressed dose (every 14 days) vincristine, doxorubicin, and cyclophosphamide (VDC) alternating with ifosfamide and etoposide (IE). Patients typically receive 3 total cycles of VDC/IE (6 treatments), then undergo definitive local control with surgical resection. If surgical resection is not possible or if margins are positive, RT can be considered. Surgical resection should be followed by an additional 4 total cycles of VDC/IE (8 treatments).[13] Ewing sarcoma in patients over the age of 50 is exceedingly rare; therefore, treatment recommendations are not standardized.

Patient's Treatment

- *The patient completed 6 cycles of induction VDC/IE and declined subsequent systemic chemotherapy due to personal preference. He then underwent pelvic RT followed by tumor resection with final pathology revealing a 13.5-cm soft-tissue mass consistent with Ewing sarcoma.*

What Are the Common Toxicities of Treatment?

- Specific side effects related to this regimen include neuropathy caused by vincristine, as well as cardiotoxicity and secondary malignancy from doxorubicin. Cyclophosphamide and ifosfamide can result in hemorrhagic cystitis; therefore, mesna should be included in the regimen. Ifosfamide can cause a neurotoxicity that can be treated with methylene blue.

What Is the Recommended Surveillance?

- Prospective evidence for post-treatment surveillance in Ewing sarcoma is limited and current surveillance recommendations reflect those from NCCN. This entails a history and physical every 3 months as well as imaging of the primary tumor site and chest for the first 2 years. Then, the interval can be increased for the next 3 years. Ongoing imaging after year 5 can be considered.[2]

How Is Metastatic Disease Treated?

- In select patients with metastatic disease, local treatment with curative intent can be considered generally in conjunction with chemotherapy.[14] Systemic treatment options in adults with widely metastatic disease are limited and are extrapolated from the pediatric population for relapsed disease. Chemotherapy options include cyclophosphamide and topotecan,[15] irinotecan and temozolomide,[16] and ICE (Ifosfamide, carboplatin, and etoposide).[17] Palliative radiation in those with symptomatic or bulky disease is a reasonable adjunctive treatment option.

Patient's Outcome

- *A surveillance CT scan of his chest a year after surgical resection of his pelvic mass revealed new lung lesions. These were removed by VATS lobectomy with pathology demonstrating recurrent metastatic Ewing sarcoma. He was treated with 1 cycle of adjuvant topotecan and cyclophosphamide but declined further systemic chemotherapy. He subsequently relapsed with extensive pulmonary metastasis and thereafter declined all systemic treatment and elected for hospice.*

Case 22.3: Chondrosarcoma

A 22-year-old man presented with a femur fracture. He was exercising and had the sudden onset of pain in his upper thigh and became non-ambulatory. Evaluation in the ED identified an 8.1 × 6 cm mass in the femur with associated pathological fracture. A CT of the chest, abdomen, and pelvis did not show any additional sites of disease. He was taken to the operating room (OR) and had resection of the mass as well as repair of the fracture. Pathology demonstrated a grade 2 chondrosarcoma.

How Is a Diagnosis Established and What Is the Recommended Workup for Chondrosarcoma?

- For patients with a suspicious cartilaginous lesion seen on x-ray, CT or MRI should be performed to determine the extent of disease and for surgical planning. A CT of the chest or PET scan can be used to evaluate metastatic disease.[18] Patients should be referred to an orthopedic oncology specialist for biopsy as the biopsy track will need to be completely excised at the time of surgical resection.

How Are Chondrosarcomas Staged?

- Traditional staging systems for chondrosarcoma based on tumor size and nodal involvement have not given accurate prognostic information and are therefore rarely used. The musculoskeletal tumor society (MSTS) staging is often used which distinguishes tumors by grade and presence within or outside of the bone with high-grade, extracompartmental tumors portending a poor prognosis.[19]

Patient's Diagnosis and Stage
- *He is diagnosed with dedifferentiated chondrosarcoma, stage IV.*

What Is the Recommended Treatment of Localized Disease?

- Localized chondrosarcoma is a surgical disease. There is not a role for adjuvant radiation or chemotherapy. Patients with low-grade chondrosarcoma (grade I) have a low risk of recurrence and distant disease while those with high grade (grade III) are at an increased risk of developing metastatic disease. Low-grade chondrosarcomas are often slow growing and recurrent or metastatic disease can often be treated surgically. As with our patient, conventional chondrosarcomas can undergo transformation into dedifferentiated chondrosarcoma.[20]

How Is Metastatic Disease Treated?

- Chemotherapy has shown limited efficacy in chondrosarcoma. In oligometastatic disease or low burden metastatic disease, surgical resection can be considered. In unresectable disease, tyrosine kinase inhibitors (TKIs) such as pazopanib and dasatanib have shown efficacy.[21,22] For those with metastatic conventional or dedifferentiated chondrosarcoma, tumors should be tested for *IDH1* mutations as these are reported in approximately 60% of tumors. Susceptible *IDH1* mutations can be treated with ivosidenib.[23] A subset of dedifferentiated chondrosarcomas have shown high programmed death-ligand 1

(PD-L1) expression yet the clinical significance is not known given the limited number of chondrosarcoma patients included in sarcoma immunotherapy trials.[24-26]

What Are the Common Toxicities of Treatment?

- Side effects of TKIs include fatigue, palmar-plantar erythrodysesthesia, metabolic abnormalities, and nausea. Pazopanib can cause cardiotoxicity and hypertension as well as hypopigmentation of the skin and hair. Dasatinib can cause cytopenias as well as pleural effusions.

Patient Outcome

- *Imaging 3 months after surgery showed a local recurrence in the tumor bed and lung nodules. Repeat biopsy demonstrated dedifferentiated chondrosarcoma without an IDH1 mutation. He started therapy with pazopanib.*

REVIEW QUESTIONS

1. A 23-year-old female presents with right thigh pain. On examination she was found to have a palpable mass in her right thigh. Plain radiographs revealed a spiculated 5-cm lesion on her right femur with an associated soft-tissue component. A PET/CT did not reveal any evidence of distant metastasis. What additional imaging would be helpful in surgical planning for this patient?
   A. Radionucleotide bone scanning with technetium
   B. MRI of the lower extremity
   C. Conventional CT scan of the chest, abdomen, and pelvis
   D. No additional imaging needed

2. A 52-year-old male presented to the hospital after a fall that led to significant right arm pain. He was found to have a 5-cm mass in the right humerus. Further staging workup revealed extensive metastasis in the lung and a pulmonary nodule, which was consistent with metastatic chondrosarcoma. Which genetic mutation is most likely associated with this patient's diagnosis?
   A. *IDH 1/2*
   B. *COL2A1*
   C. *CDKN2A*
   D. *PTCH1*

3. A 24-year-old male presented for evaluation of chest wall pain and swelling and was found to have a 3-cm chest wall mass. Subsequent biopsy was consistent with Ewing sarcoma. Which of the following translocations correctly match the typical chromosomal transloca-tion seen in Ewing sarcoma with the associated genetic mutation?
   A. t(2;13)(q35;q14) resulting in *PAX3-FOXO1A*
   B. t(11;22)(q24;q12) resulting in *EWS-FLI1*
   C. t(7;22)(p22;q12) resulting in *EWS-FLI1*
   D. t(11;22(q24;q12) resulting in *PAX3-FOXO1A*

4. A 42-year-old man had 2 weeks of knee pain and presented to his primary care doctor. X-rays showed a destructive lesion in the distal femur. Further evaluation by MRI raised concern for an aggressive cartilaginous lesion. Biopsy demonstrates a high-grade (grade III) chondrosarcoma. What is the recommended treatment?
   A. Neoadjuvant radiation followed by resection
   B. Surgical resection
   C. Neoadjuvant chemotherapy followed by resection
   D. Neoadjuvant chemotherapy and radiation followed by resection

5. A 62-year-old woman presents after a ground level fall. She is found to have a pathologi-cal fracture of the hip. The fracture is surgically repaired and pathology is pending. CT of the chest, abdomen, and pelvis show several lytic lesions in the pelvis and spine. What additional studies would be recommended?
   A. Lactate dehydrogenase (LDH)
   B. Bone marrow biopsy
   C. Serum protein electrophoresis (SPEP), urine protein electrophoresis (UPEP)
   D. CA-125

6. A 22-year-old man is diagnosed with localized Ewing sarcoma. He undergoes 6 cycles of neoadjuvant chemotherapy with vincristine, doxorubicin, and cyclophosphamide alternating with ifosfamide and etoposide (VDC/IE) and then surgical resection of a proximal humerus mass. The resection results in margins that are microscopically positive (R1) and the surgeon does not think that negative margins can be obtained without damage to the brachial plexus. What should the next step be in the care of this patient?
   A. Radiation therapy (RT)
   B. Chemotherapy with VDC/IE for 8 cycles
   C. Surveillance
   D. Amputation

7. A 56-year-old woman presents with knee pain and is found to have a destructive bone lesion in the femur. Biospy demonstrates osteosarcoma. Staging studies do not show any other sites of involvement. What treatment should be considered?
   A. Neoadjuvant radiation followed by resection
   B. Neoadjuvant chemotherapy followed by resection and adjuvant chemotherapy
   C. Resection followed by adjuvant chemotherapy
   D. Surgical resection

8. A 22-year-old woman was diagnosed with a 14-cm synovial sarcoma of the left thigh. She was admitted to the hospital for cycle 1 of neoadjuvant AIM (doxorubicin and ifosfamide) chemotherapy. On day 3 of treatment, she began to have difficulty ambulating and appeared confused. In addition to holding chemotherapy, what would you recommend?
   A. MRI of the brain
   B. Methylene blue
   C. Mesna
   D. Lumbar puncture

ANSWERS AND RATIONALES

1. **B. MRI of the lower extremity.** MRI of the lower extremity is the imaging modality of choice for surgical planning as it can accurately achieve definition of tumor size, extent of bony involvement, and imaging of local neurovascular structures. Although conventional CT scans can be considered to evaluate for metastatic disease, this patient already has had staging and imaging with PET/CT.

2. **A. *IDH 1/2*.** Mutations in *IDH 1/2* are commonly associated with chondrosarcomas. Mutations in *IDH 1* and 2 result in accumulation of oncometabolite D-2-hydroxyglutarate thought to block osteogenic differentiation leading to development of early cartilaginous tumors. Aberrations in *IDH* are thought to be an early event in oncogenesis of chondrosarcomas.

3. **B. t(11;22)(q24;q12) resulting in *EWS-FLI1*.** The Ewing sarcoma family of tumors (EFT) share a unique pattern of translocation between the *EWS* and *FLI1* gene and are characterized by specific t(11;22)(q24;q12) on cytogenetic analysis. Given the ubiquity of t(11;22) in Ewing sarcoma, identification of the fusion genes can provide diagnostic guidance in challenging cases in which the histological diagnosis is uncertain.

4. **B. Surgical resection.** For localized chondrosarcomas, treatment with surgical resection alone is recommended. Given the refractory nature of the disease, neoadjuvant radiation or chemotherapy is not indicated and does not improve survival or local recurrence rates.

5. **C. Serum protein electrophoresis (SPEP), urine protein electrophoresis (UPEP).** For a new bone lesion in a patient over age 40, this is most likely to be metastatic disease and not a primary bone cancer. In the case of this patient, the CT scans only show lytic bone lesions making metastases from a lung or renal cell carcinoma less likely. The possibility of multiple myeloma should be considered and evaluated by SPEP/UPEP. For a woman, a mammogram should be done as well. For males, prostate-specific antigen (PSA) can be considered.

6. **A. Radiation therapy (RT).** In the case of positive margins and no option for further resection, RT should be considered. This will be followed by another 8 cycles of chemotherapy, but radiation should be considered prior to chemotherapy. Surveillance would not be appropriate for any patient who has only received 6 of the recommended 14 cycles. Amputation has not been associated with improved survival in the case of an R1 resection and should not be considered.

7. **B. Neoadjuvant chemotherapy followed by resection and adjuvant chemotherapy.** Osteosarcomas should be treated with perioperative chemotherapy. In adults over age 40, this should be doxorubicin and cisplatin for 3 cycles followed by surgical resection and 3 additional cycles. In those under age 40, MAP (high-dose methotrexate, doxorubicin, and cisplatin) can be used. High-dose methotrexate in those over 40 results in additional toxicity without a clear benefit.

8. **B. Methylene blue.** Ifosfamide metabolites can cause neurotoxicity. In general, this presents as confusion, somnolence, and cerebellar ataxia. Chemotherapy should be held and methylene blue should be given to counteract this toxicity. Ifosfamide-induced neurotoxicity is a clinical diagnosis. An MRI or lumbar puncture would be normal and, therefore, not helpful. Mesna is given with ifosfamide to protect from hemorrhagic cystitis.

REFERENCES

1. Siegel RL, Miller KD, Fuchs HE, Jemal A. Cancer statistics, 2022. *CA Cancer J Clin.* 2022;72(1):7–33. doi:10.3322/caac.21708

2. Network N.C.C. *Bone Cancer.* Version 4.2.22. https://www.nccn.org/professionals/physician_gls/pdf/bone.pdf

3. Cascella M, Rajnik M, Aleem A, et al. Features, evaluation, and treatment of coronavirus (COVID-19). *StatPearls* [internet]. StatsPearls Publishing; 2022. https://www.ncbi.nlm.nih.gov/books/NBK554776

4. Kager L, Zoubek A, Kastner U, et al. Skip metastases in osteosarcoma: experience of the Cooperative Osteosarcoma Study Group. *J Clin Oncol.* 2006;24(10):1535–1341. doi:10.1200/JCO.2005.04.2978

5. Sheng G, Gao Y, Yang Y, Wu H. Osteosarcoma and metastasis. *Front Oncol.* 2021;11:780264. doi:10.3389/fonc.2021.780264

6. Whelan JS, Bielack SS, Marina N, et al. EURAMOS-1, an international randomised study for osteosarcoma: results from pre-randomisation treatment. *Ann Oncol.* 2015;26(2):407–414. doi:10.1093/annonc/mdu526

7. Wippel B, Gundle KR, Dang T, et al. Safety and efficacy of high-dose methotrexate for osteosarcoma in adolescents compared with young adults. *Cancer Med.* 2019;8(1):111–116. doi:10.1002/cam4.1898

8. DeLaney TF, Park L, Goldberg SI, et al. Radiotherapy for local control of osteosarcoma. *Int J Radiat Oncol Biol Phys.* 2005;61(2):492–498. doi:10.1016/j.ijrobp.2004.05.051

9. Kempf-Bielack B, Bielack SS, Jürgens H, et al. Osteosarcoma relapse after combined modality therapy: an analysis of unselected patients in the Cooperative Osteosarcoma Study Group (COSS). *J Clin Oncol.* 2005;23(3):559–568. doi:10.1200/JCO.2005.04.063

10. Murphey MD, Senchak LT, Mambalam PK, et al. From the radiologic pathology archives: Ewing sarcoma family of tumors: Radiologic-pathologic correlation. *Radiographics.* 2013;33(3):803–831. doi:10.1148/rg.333135005

11. Grünewald TG, Cidre-Aranaz F, Surdez D, et al. Ewing sarcoma. *Nat Rev Dis Primers.* 2018;4(1):5. doi:10.1038/s41572-018-0003-x

12. Nesbit ME Jr, Gehan EA, Burgert EO Jr, et al. Multimodal therapy for the management of primary, nonmetastatic Ewing's sarcoma of bone: a long-term follow-up of the first intergroup study. *J Clin Oncol.* 1990;8(10):1664–1674. doi:10.1200/JCO.1990.8.10.1664

13. Womer RB, West DC, Krailo MD, et al. Randomized controlled trial of interval-compressed chemotherapy for the treatment of localized Ewing sarcoma: a report from the Children's Oncology Group. *J Clin Oncol.* 2012;30(33):4148–4154. doi:10.1200/JCO.2011.41.5703

14. Haeusler J, Ranft A, Boelling T, et al. The value of local treatment in patients with primary, disseminated, multifocal Ewing sarcoma (PDMES). *Cancer.* 2010;116(2):443–450. doi:10.1002/cncr.24740

15. Saylors RL 3rd, Stine KC, Sullivan J, et al. Cyclophosphamide plus topotecan in children with recurrent or refractory solid tumors: a Pediatric Oncology Group phase II study. *J Clin Oncol.* 2001;19(15):3463–3469. doi:10.1200/JCO.2001.19.15.3463

16. Casey DA, Wexler LH, Merchant MS, et al. Irinotecan and temozolomide for Ewing sarcoma: the Memorial Sloan Kettering experience. *Pediatr Blood Cancer.* 2009;53(6):1029–1034. doi:10.1002/pbc.22206

17. Van Winkle P, Angiolillo A, Krailo M, et al. Ifosfamide, carboplatin, and etoposide (ICE) reinduction chemotherapy in a large cohort of children and adolescents with recurrent/refractory sarcoma: the Children's Cancer Group (CCG) experience. *Pediatr Blood Cancer.* 2005;44(4):338–347. doi:10.1002/pbc.20227

18. Aran V, Devalle S, Meohas W, et al. Osteosarcoma, chondrosarcoma and Ewing sarcoma: clinical aspects, biomarker discovery and liquid biopsy. *Crit Rev Oncol Hematol.* 2021;162:103340. doi:10.1016/j.critrevonc.2021.103340

19. Enneking WF, Spanier SS, Goodman MA. A system for the surgical staging of musculoskeletal sarcoma. *Clin Orthop Relat Res.* 2003(415):4–18. doi:10.1097/01.blo.0000093891.12372.0f

20. Gelderblom H, Hogendoorn PC, Dijkstra SD, et al. The clinical approach towards chondrosarcoma. *Oncologist.* 2008;13(3):320–329. doi:10.1634/theoncologist.2007-0237

21. Chow W, Frankel P, Ruel C, et al. Results of a prospective phase 2 study of pazopanib in patients with surgically unresectable or metastatic chondrosarcoma. *Cancer.* 2020;126(1):105–111. doi:10.1002/cncr.32515

22. Schuetze SM, Bolejack V, Choy E, et al. Phase 2 study of dasatinib in patients with alveolar soft part sarcoma, chondrosarcoma, chordoma, epithelioid sarcoma, or solitary fibrous tumor. *Cancer.* 2017;123(1):90–97. doi:10.1002/cncr.30379

23. Tap WD, Villalobos VM, Cote GM, et al. Phase I study of the mutant *IDH1* inhibitor ivosidenib: safety and clinical activity in patients with advanced chondrosarcoma. *J Clin Oncol.* 2020;38(15):1693–1701. doi:10.1200/JCO.19.02492

24. D'Angelo SP, Mahoney MR, Van Tine BA, et al. Nivolumab with or without ipilimumab treatment for metastatic sarcoma (Alliance A091401): two open-label, non-comparative, randomised, phase 2 trials. *Lancet Oncol.* 2018;19(3):416–426. doi:10.1016/S1470-2045(18)30006-8

25. Tawbi HA, Burgess M, Bolejack V, et al. Pembrolizumab in advanced soft-tissue sarcoma and bone sarcoma (SARC028): a multicentre, two-cohort, single-arm, open-label, phase 2 trial. *Lancet Oncol.* 2017;18(11):1493–1501. doi:10.1016/S1470-2045(17)30624-1

26. Kostine M., Cleven AH, de Miranda NF, et al. Analysis of PD-L1, T-cell infiltrate and HLA expression in chondrosarcoma indicates potential for response to immunotherapy specifically in the dedifferentiated subtype. *Mod Pathol.* 2016;29(9):1028–1037. doi:10.1038/modpathol.2016.108

CHAPTER 23

Soft-Tissue Sarcoma

James Liu and Janai R. Carr-Ascher

INTRODUCTION

Soft-tissue sarcomas are a rare and heterogeneous group of tumors. There are more than 50 subtypes that vary in histology, patient demographics, and clinical behavior. These tumors can be further categorized into low grade and high grade based on pathological findings.[1] Among high-grade sarcomas, these can be further divided into translocation- and nontranslocation-driven subtypes. In adults, the most common translocation-driven sarcoma is synovial sarcoma, characterized by an *SSX-SYT* gene fusion. The nontranslocation subtypes are characterized by multiple chromosomal gains and losses (aneuploidy).[2] Common examples of nontranslocation-associated sarcomas are undifferentiated pleomorphic sarcoma, leiomyosarcoma, and dedifferentiated liposarcoma. Given the rare nature of soft-tissue sarcomas, patients should be referred to a specialty cancer center for treatment by a multidisciplinary team consisting of medical oncology, radiation oncology, orthopedic or surgical oncology, and a pathologist with expertise in sarcoma.

CASE SUMMARIES

Case 23.1: Localized Soft-Tissue Sarcoma

A 28-year-old female presents for 4 months of swelling and pain involving the right thigh. Initial workup with ultrasound (US) demonstrated a large soft-tissue mass in the posterior aspect of the right lower extremity. Subsequent MRI revealed a heterogeneous cystic and solid mass in the posterior medial thigh measuring 11 × 12.5 × 16 cm. Staging workup with chest, abdomen, and pelvis CT scans did not show any evidence of metastatic disease. She underwent biopsy of the lesion and pathology was consistent with synovial sarcoma including translocation t(X;18).

How Is a Diagnosis Established?

- A biopsy is required for the diagnosis of soft-tissue sarcoma. Given there are more than 50 distinct subtypes, immunohistochemistry (IHC) as well as fluorescent in situ hybridization (FISH) are needed to determine a specific sarcoma subtype.

Patient Diagnosis
- *Synovial sarcoma with translocation t(X;18)*

How Are Soft-Tissue Sarcomas Staged?

- Soft-tissue sarcoma typically presents as an enlarging mass in the extremities, thorax, retroperitoneum, or head and neck region. Retroperitoneal soft-tissue sarcomas are typically liposarcomas and leiomyosarcomas.[3] Certain histological subtypes of soft-tissue sarcoma are commonly associated with cytogenetic translocations which can be used to assist with diagnosis.[4] For example, t(X;18)(p11;q11) is commonly observed in synovial sarcomas leading to a fusion protein, SS18-SSX. Staging for soft-tissue sarcoma typically follows tumor, node, metastasis (TNM) staging established by the American Joint Committee on Cancer (AJCC). Of note, the most recent (eighth edition) AJCC staging includes separate staging for soft-tissue sarcoma of the extremities and retroperitoneum.

What Is the Approach to Treatment?

- For all soft-tissue sarcomas, regardless of location, surgical resection with clear margins is the cornerstone of therapy and the primary predictor of prognosis. Radiation is considered for all tumors greater than 5 cm and has equal benefits in regard to local control in the neoadjuvant or adjuvant setting. Of note, the addition of radiation to surgery does not lead to an improvement in overall survival (OS).[5] Neoadjuvant radiation has several advantages. The total radiation dose is lower, the response to therapy can be evaluated, and tumor size can be reduced to facilitate surgical resection. Yet, there is an increased rate of wound complications related to neoadjuvant radiation that is not seen with adjuvant radiation. Adjuvant radiation has the added benefit of evaluating tumor histology at resection.[6]
- The use of chemotherapy in localized soft-tissue sarcomas has been controversial as conflicting data exists and improvements in OS across trials have been inconsistent.[7,8] This is likely related to the rarity of the disease. In clinical trials, due to limited numbers of patients, all soft-tissue sarcomas are grouped together which limits clinical applicability. In general, chemotherapy with doxorubicin and ifosfamide (AIM) should be considered for healthy and fit patients who would benefit from downstaging the disease to ensure an R0 resection.[9–11] For those with high-grade sarcomas greater than 10 cm in size or with histologies that are traditionally more sensitive to chemotherapy such as synovial sarcoma, chemotherapy can be discussed. Chemotherapy can be given in the neoadjuvant or adjuvant setting with equal efficacy.[12]

Patient's Stage and Treatment Course
- *The patient was treated with 6 cycles of AIM chemotherapy with an interim MRI showing partial response. After completion of neoadjuvant chemotherapy, she underwent neoadjuvant radiation followed by surgical resection with negative margins (stage pT3N0M0).*

What Are the Toxicities of Treatment?

- Patients receiving AIM chemotherapy should have limited comorbidities. This intensive regimen has a high rate of neutropenic fever and requires growth factor support. Side effects include cardiac toxicity, secondary malignancy, and infertility associated with doxorubicin. Ifosfamide can lead to neurotoxicity and hemorrhagic cystitis. Mesna should be given with this regimen.

What Is the Recommended Surveillance for Soft-Tissue Sarcoma?

- In patients without radiographic evidence of disease after treatment, the National Comprehensive Cancer Network (NCCN) recommends close interval follow-up with imaging of the primary site, chest, and other potential sites of metastatic disease depending on histology. Imaging every 3 to 6 months for the first 2 to 3 years, then every 6 months for 2 additional years, and annual imaging thereafter, is recommended. Of note, data for intensive imaging follow-up is limited and clinical trials are ongoing to determine the optimal time interval and mode of imaging.[13]

Case 23.2: Metastatic Soft-Tissue Sarcoma

A 68-year-old female presented for evaluation of an enlarging right thigh mass. Initial workup including an MRI of the right thigh revealed a 11.9-cm elliptical mass in the vastus lateralis muscle. Further CT staging did not identify any sites of distant metastasis. A biopsy of the thigh mass showed high-grade, undifferentiated pleomorphic sarcoma. She underwent neoadjuvant radiation therapy (RT) followed by surgical resection with pathology revealing a 14.2-cm undifferentiated pleomorphic sarcoma. The surgical margins were negative. A follow-up CT scan of her chest a month after surgical resection unfortunately identified multiple new pulmonary nodules, the largest being one 3 cm in size located in the left lower lobe. A biopsy showed metastatic undifferentiated pleomorphic sarcoma. She received two cycles of doxorubicin; however, due to poor tolerance, she was transitioned to gemcitabine and docetaxel, which resulted in stable disease.

How Is a Diagnosis Established?

- The lungs are the most common site of metastasis for sarcomas. For a patient with sarcoma and new lung nodules, a biopsy can be considered to provide a definitive diagnosis, although in the correct clinical context it is not required. For lesions outside of the lungs, given the rarity, biopsy is required to confirm the diagnosis of metastatic sarcoma.

Patient's Diagnosis

- *Metastatic, high-grade, undifferentiated pleomorphic sarcoma*

What Is the Typical Pattern of Metastasis for Soft-Tissue Sarcomas?

- While sarcomas vary significantly in histological appearance, location, and patient characteristics, nearly all tumors metastasize to the lung. A small number of sarcomas such as angiosarcoma will metastasize to local lymph nodes, but this is uncommon.[14] Metastasis to other sites such as bone is seen, but the lung remains the most common site of metastasis. Metastasis to other organs (outside of the lung) as well as the central nervous system (CNS) are exceedingly rare but have been reported.[15]

How Are Metastatic Soft-Tissue Sarcomas Treated?

- Nearly all subtypes of sarcoma, once metastatic, are treated with systemic therapy. Surgical resection or radiation can be considered for oligometastatic disease although data to support this approach is limited. There is a growing list of targeted therapy options in specific subtypes of sarcoma, such as the recent approval of tazemetostat for INI-1 deficient epithelioid sarcoma.[16] Despite this, the majority of soft-tissue sarcomas are treated similarly once metastatic. Chemotherapy is first-line therapy, generally with an anthracycline such as doxorubicin. Regimens such as gemcitabine and docetaxel in leiomyosarcoma and eribulin in liposarcoma have increased subtype-specific efficacy, but these agents can be used across soft-tissue sarcoma subtypes.[17,18] Other chemotherapy options include trabectedin and liposomal doxorubicin.[19,20] Tyrosine kinase inhibitors (TKIs), in particular pazopanib, have also demonstrated a response across sarcoma subtypes.[21]

- There is increasing interest in the use of immunotherapy in sarcomas. Two trials, SARC028 and Alliance A091401, showed limited responses in sarcomas. A small number of patients responded who had undifferentiated pleomorphic sarcoma, liposarcoma, and angiosarcoma, which has prompted further trials focused on these subtypes that are ongoing.[22, 23]

Case 23.3: Rhabdomyosarcoma

A 78-year-old male presented for evaluation for right orbital swelling and was found to have alveolar rhabdomyosarcoma (ARMS). Initial workup including CT scan of the orbit demonstrated a 2.8 × 2.8 × 1.3 cm mass impinging upon the right medial rectus muscle. A follow-up MRI re-demonstrated the orbital mass and an additional left maxillary ostium mass. Subsequent PET scan was notable for focal uptake at the site of the orbital mass and additional focal uptake at the left iliac bone. Pelvic MRI identified a 2.5-cm posterior iliac crest lesion suggestive of metastatic spread. A biopsy of the left orbital mass revealed ARMS, and a follow-up biopsy of the left iliac lesion confirmed rhabdomyosarcoma (RMS). He then underwent surgical resection of the orbital mass with final pathology consistent with a 4.5-cm ARMS with extensive involvement of the connective tissue and submucosal glands; all five parotid lymph nodes and margins were also noted to be positive. PAX3-FOXO1 fusion was identified through FISH testing. He then underwent RT to the tumor bed and was unable to complete the full course of radiation due to mucositis. A follow-up MRI of the head, spine, and pelvis showed granulation tissue at the site of prior orbital exenteration, innumerable pelvic lesions, and diffuse metastatic disease of the axial skeleton including the T12 vertebral body. Given the rapid progression of his disease, he initiated treatment with vincristine, doxorubicin, and cyclophosphamide. However, during his treatment course he developed acute renal failure and was transitioned to hospice.

How Are Head and Neck Sarcomas Staged?

- RMS can arise from any part of the body. The most common sites of primary disease include the head and neck, genitourinary tract, and the extremities.[22] RMSs typically do not follow AJCC staging systems for soft-tissue sarcoma. The Intergroup Rhabdomyosarcoma Study Group (IRSG) combines information from TNM staging along with surgical-pathological clinical groups to divide patients into four risk categories (low-risk subset A, low-risk subset B, intermediate risk, and high risk).[23]

Patient's Clinical Stage
- *Stage IV metastatic RMS*

What Are the Types of Rhabdomyosarcoma?

- The two most common subtypes of RMS consist of ARMS and embryonal rhabdomyosarcoma (ERMS); these have been traditionally differentiated based on light microscopic features. Additionally, ARMS is typically associated with balanced chromosomal translocations, either t(2;13)(q35;q14) or a variant t(1;13)(p36;q14). This juxtaposition results in the formation of fusion genes *PAX3–FOXO1* by t(2;13) and *PAX7–FOXO1* by t(1;13) detectable by FISH. The World Health Organization (WHO) also recognizes two rare subtypes of RMS: pleomorphic RMS (typically seen in older adults and treated as general soft-tissue sarcomas) and a spindle cell/sclerosing RMS.[22]

Patient's Rhabdomyosarcoma Subtype
- *Based on the* PAX3-FOXO1 *fusion gene, he has an ARMS.*

How Is Localized and Metastatic Disease Treated?

- Data for treatment of adults with RMS is limited, which supports the referral of patients to a center with sarcoma expertise. In general, treatment follows that of the pediatric population and is determined by the risk of disease recurrence. Systemic treatment is guided by IRSG risk groups utilizing vincristine, doxorubicin, and cyclophosphamide (VAC) or vincristine and doxorubicin (VA). For low-risk patients, a doublet of VA or a modified VAC with reduced cyclophosphamide are acceptable treatment options. For those with intermediate- and high-risk disease VAC is the recommended therapy. Treatment with surgical excision remains the standard of care when feasible. Adjuvant radiation for low-risk patients remains controversial while radiation is indicated for intermediate- and high-risk groups. Those with embryonal/fusion-negative subtypes do not benefit from radiation; therefore, this should not be offered.[22,24]

What Are the Treatment Toxicities?

- Both VAC and VA chemotherapy are associated with fatigue, nausea, cytopenias, and alopecia. Vincristine can lead to neuropathy, which should be closely monitored. Doxorubicin as well as other anthracyclines can cause cardiac toxicity and secondary malignancy. Cyclophosphamide is associated with hemorrhagic cystitis; therefore, mesna should be administered with this regimen.

Case 23.4: Gastrointestinal Stromal Tumor

A 74-year-old female presented for evaluation at the ED for flank pain. She underwent CT scan of her abdomen and was found to have a 5.5-cm gastric mass. She underwent surgical excision of the mass with pathology consistent with gastrointestinal stromal tumor (GIST), spindled type. Pathological assessment was notable for a high mitotic activity of 10 mitosis/50 high power field (HPF). IHC was positive for CD117 and DOG1 and mutational studies were notable for a PDGFRA Exon 18 mutation not associated with D842V.

How Is a Diagnosis Established?

- Pathology showing a mesenchymal tumor with IHC positive for *c-KIT* (CD-117) and *DOG1* are diagnostic for GIST.

Patient's Diagnosis
- *PDGFR-mutated GIST*

How Is a Gastrointestinal Stromal Tumor Staged?

- GIST is a soft-tissue sarcoma that is commonly associated with aberrations in genes encoding *KIT* and *PDGFRA*. Although staging for GIST tumors follows conventions set by the AJCC TNM staging system, additional histological features (mitotic rate in addition to size) are typically utilized to provide prognostic information and to guide adjuvant therapy.[25]

Patient's Clinical Stage
  • *Stage IIIA (T3N0M0, high mitotic rate)*

Which Patients Should Receive Adjuvant Therapy?

  • Patients who undergo surgical resection for GIST are classified as low, intermediate, or high risk based on a combination of tumor size and mitotic rate. In general, tumors that are 5 cm or less and with 5 mitosis/50 HPF or less are associated with low potential for metastasis. These patients can be managed with observation alone after definitive surgical resection. However, those with intermediate- or high-risk disease require adjuvant therapy given the high risk for metastasis.[25] Imatinib is the adjuvant treatment of choice in patients with intermediate- and high-risk disease.[26] The optimal duration of adjuvant therapy is controversial, though patients are treated a minimum of 3 years. Ongoing trials are evaluating the efficacy of prolonged adjuvant therapy for up to 6 years of therapy.[26,27]

Patient's Treatment
  • *The patient started adjuvant imatinib 400 mg daily and completed 3 years of therapy without disease recurrence.*

What Are the Treatment Options for Metastatic Disease?

  • Mutational assessment for *KIT* and *PDGFRA* is important to guide therapeutic options for unresectabele or metastatic GIST. Imatinib 400 mg daily is considered the treatment of choice for the majority of patients with unresectable or metastatic disease. Those harboring a *PDGFRA* exon 18 D842V mutation are typically insensitive to imatinib, and avapritinib is the agent of choice.[28,29] The presence of *KIT* exon 9 mutation is also attributed to resistance to imatinib at the 400-mg dose; however, treatment at a higher dose of 800 mg daily can ameliorate this resistance.[30] Sunitinib is typically considered in the second-line setting after progression on imatinib.[31] Alternatively, for those with *PDGFRA* mutations insensitive to imatinib (including D842V), dasatinib can be used.[32]

What Are the Treatment Toxicities?

  • Side effects of imatinib and other TKIs include edema, rash, nausea, diarrhea, cytopenias, and athralgias. In addition to these side effects, avapritinib has been associated with cognitive dysfunction and intracranial hemorrhage.

REVIEW QUESTIONS

1. Which of the following characteristics is associated with the lowest risk for metastatic potential for gastrointestinal stromal tumor (GIST)?
   A. Mitotic rate greater than 5, tumor size 2.5 cm
   B. Mitotic rate of 5 or lower, tumor size 5.5 cm
   C. Mitotic rate greater than 5, tumor size 5.5 cm
   D. Mitotic rate of 5 or lower, tumor size 12 cm

2. A 24-year-old female presents to the hospital with worsening left leg pain and was found to have a 6-cm soft-tissue mass in the left thigh. A biopsy of the lesion reveals rhabdomyosarcoma (RMS), alveolar subtype. Which of the following translocations are typically associated with alveolar rhabdomyosarcoma (ARMS)?
   A. t(2;13)(q35;q14)
   B. t(X;18)(p11;q11)
   C. Inversion 12q13
   D. t(1;3)(p36;q25)

3. A 55-year-old male who presented to the hospital with abdominal pain was found to have metastatic gastrointestinal stromal tumor (GIST) with extensive pulmonary involvement. Further molecular testing identified a *PDGFRA D842V* mutation. What is the best initial treatment for this patient?
   A. Imatinib 400 mg daily
   B. Imatinib 400 mg twice daily
   C. Avapritinib 300 mg daily
   D. Dasatinib 70 mg twice daily

4. A previously healthy 27-year-old woman presented with an enlarging mass in the upper thigh. A biopsy demonstrates synovial sarcoma and imaging does not show other sites of disease. The mass is 12.2 cm and abutting the neurovascular bundle, making a complete resection unlikely. What would you recommend?
   A. Neoadjuvant chemotherapy and radiation followed by resection
   B. Neoadjuvant radiation followed by resection
   C. Amputation
   D. Surgical resection followed by adjuvant chemotherapy

5. A 62-year-old man was found to have a 9.3-cm soft-tissue mass invading the rectus femoris. Imaging did not show other sites of disease. Biopsy demonstrated undifferentiated pleomorphic sarcoma. He is evaluated by orthopedic oncology who states the mass is amendable to a wide local excision (WLE). What are the next steps in treatment?
   A. Neoadjuvant radiation followed by resection
   B. Neoadjuvant chemotherapy followed by resection and adjuvant chemotherapy
   C. Neoadjuvant chemoradiation
   D. Surgical resection

6. A 45-year-old woman presents with shortness of breath. She is found to have numerous lung nodules on CT scans. A CT of the abdomen and pelvis demonstrates a pelvic mass.

Biopsy of the lung nodules shows metastatic dedifferentiated liposarcoma that is *MDM2-*positive. What therapy would you recommend?

A. Pazopanib

B. Dacarbazine

C. Pembrolizumab

D. Doxorubicin

7. Neoadjuvant radiation of extremity soft-tissue sarcomas is associated with which of the following as compared to adjuvant radiation?

A. Higher risk of local recurrence

B. Higher total dose of radiation

C. Increased risk of wound complications

D. Larger field of radiation

ANSWERS AND RATIONALES

1. **B. Mitotic rate of 5 or lower, tumor size 5.5 cm.** Typically GIST that are 5 cm or lower in size and have a mitotic rate of 5 / 50 high power field (HPF) or less are associated with low risk for metastatic potential. For patient with tumors 5 to 10 cm in size with low mitotic rate of 5 or lower, their risk of metastasis is also considered low (3.6%). However, a mitotic rate of 5 or greater and tumor size of 2 to 5 cm are considered moderate risk for metastasis (16%); adjuvant therapy should be considered in these patients.[25]

2. **A. t(2;13)(q35;q14).** ARMS is typically associated with t(2;13)(q35;q14) with a resulting formation of a *PAX3-FOXO1A* fusion gene. A less common fusion gene, t(1;13)(p36;q14), can also be seen in patients with *PAX7-FOXO1A* fusion. *FOXO1A* gene is also known as *FKHR* gene. Synovial sarcoma is typically associated with t(X;18)(p11;q11). Inversion 12q13 is typically seen in patients with solitary fibrous tumor. In patients with epithelioid hemangioendothelioma, t(1;3)(p36;q25) can also be identified.

3. **C. Avapritinib 300 mg daily.** This is the treatment of choice for patients with metastatic GIST with *PDGFRA D842V* mutation, given this mutation is associated with known resistance to imatinib therapy. Dasatinib is considered second-line therapy for those patients who had progressed on avapritinib.

4. **A. Neoadjuvant chemotherapy and radiation followed by resection.** This patient has a large tumor that is not amendable to complete resection. In soft-tissue sarcomas, resection with clear margins is the greatest predictor of survival. Therefore, this patient would benefit from downstaging the tumor with chemotherapy using AIM (doxorubicin and ifosfamide). The tumor is greater than 5 cm, so radiation should be given. Amputation has not been associated with improved survival as compared to limb-sparing resections.

5. **A. Neoadjuvant radiation followed by resection.** This patient should be evaluated for neoadjuvant radiation. For soft-tissue sarcomas over 5 cm, radiation should be considered. Perioperative chemotherapy is not the standard of care in soft-tissue sarcomas as listed in B. Chemotherapy could be considered given the size and histology, but chemoradiation alone would not be appropriate if the mass is resectable.

6. **D. Doxorubicin.** First-line therapy for metastatic soft-tissue sarcoma is doxorubicin. Pazopanib is approved for metastatic sarcoma, but the patients in the PALETTE trial leading to approval had all received an anthracycline. Response rates to doxorubicin are significantly higher as compared to pazopanib. Dacarbazine can be used in the metastatic setting but is inferior to doxorubicin. Responses to immunotherapy in trials have been limited in sarcomas; therefore, pembrolizumab would not be appropriate.

7. **C. Increased risk of wound complications.** Neoadjuvant radiation has an increased risk of wound complications as compared to adjuvant radiation. Advantages of neoadjuvant radiation are that the total dose of radiation is lower (50 Gy vs. 66 Gy) and the field of radiation is smaller. There is not a difference in the rates of local recurrence between neoadjuvant and adjuvant chemotherapy.

REFERENCES

1. Fletcher CDM, Bridge JA, Hogendoorn PC, Mertens F, World Health Organization, and International Agency for Research on Cancer. *WHO Classification of Tumours of Soft Tissue and Bone.* 4th ed. IARC Press; 2013:468.

2. Helman LJ, Meltzer P. Mechanisms of sarcoma development. *Nat Rev Cancer.* 2003;3(9):685–694. doi:10.1038/nrc1168

3. Lawrence W Jr, Donegan WL, Natarajan N, et al. Adult soft tissue sarcomas. A pattern of care survey of the American College of Surgeons. *Ann Surg.* 1987;205(4):349–359. doi:10.1097/00000658-198704000-00003

4. Italiano A, Di Mauro I, Rapp J, et al. Clinical effect of molecular methods in sarcoma diagnosis (GENSARC): a prospective, multicentre, observational study. *Lancet Oncol.* 2016;17(4):532–538. doi:10.1016/S1470-2045(15)00583-5

5. Yang JC, Chang AE, Baker AR, et al. Randomized prospective study of the benefit of adjuvant radiation therapy in the treatment of soft tissue sarcomas of the extremity. *J Clin Oncol.* 1998;16(1):197–203. doi:10.1200/JCO.1998.16.1.197

6. O'Sullivan B, Davis AM, Turcotte R, et al. Preoperative versus postoperative radiotherapy in soft-tissue sarcoma of the limbs: a randomised trial. *Lancet.* 2002;359(9325):2235–2241. doi:10.1016/S0140-6736(02)09292-9

7. Saponara M, Stacchiotti S, Casali PG, Gronchi A. (Neo)adjuvant treatment in localised soft tissue sarcoma: the unsolved affair. *Eur J Cancer.* 2017;70:1–11. doi:10.1016/j.ejca.2016.09.030

8. Pasquali S, Gronchi A. Neoadjuvant chemotherapy in soft tissue sarcomas: latest evidence and clinical implications. *Ther Adv Med Oncol.* 2017;9(6):415–429. doi:10.1177/1758834017705588

9. Judson I, Verweij J, Gelderblom H, et al. Doxorubicin alone versus intensified doxorubicin plus ifosfamide for first-line treatment of advanced or metastatic soft-tissue sarcoma: a randomised controlled phase 3 trial. *Lancet Oncol.* 2014;15(4):415–423. doi:10.1016/S1470-2045(14)70063-4

10. Pervaiz N, Colterjohn N, Farrokhyar F, et al. A systematic meta-analysis of randomized controlled trials of adjuvant chemotherapy for localized resectable soft-tissue sarcoma. *Cancer.* 2008;113(3):573–581. doi:10.1002/cncr.23592

11. Network NCC. *Soft Tissue Sarcoma (Version 3.2021).* March 2, 2022. https://www.nccn.org/professionals/physician_gls/pdf/sarcoma.pdf

12. Almond LM, Gronchi A, Strauss D, et al. Neoadjuvant and adjuvant strategies in retroperitoneal sarcoma. *Eur J Surg Oncol.* 2018;44(5):571–579. doi:10.1016/j.ejso.2018.02.001

13. Glasbey JC, Bundred J, Tyler R, et al. The impact of postoperative radiological surveillance intensity on disease free and overall survival from primary retroperitoneal, abdominal and pelvic soft-tissue sarcoma. *Eur J Surg Oncol.* 2021;47(7):1771–1777. doi:10.1016/j.ejso.2021.01.021

14. Fong Y, Coit DG, Woodruff JM, Brennan MF. Lymph node metastasis from soft tissue sarcoma in adults. Analysis of data from a prospective database of 1772 sarcoma patients. *Ann Surg.* 1993;217(1):72–77. doi:10.1097/00000658-199301000-00012

15. Chaigneau L, Patrikidou A, Ray-Coquard I, et al. Brain metastases from adult sarcoma: prognostic factors and impact of treatment. A retrospective analysis from the French Sarcoma Group (GSF/GETO). *Oncologist.* 2018;23(8):948–955. doi:10.1634/theoncologist.2017-0136

16. Gounder M, Schöffski P, Jones RL, et al. Tazemetostat in advanced epithelioid sarcoma with loss of INI1/SMARCB1: an international, open-label, phase 2 basket study. *Lancet Oncol.* 2020;21(11):1423–1432. doi:10.1016/S1470-2045(20)30451-4

17. Schöffski P, Chawla S, Maki RG, et al. Eribulin versus dacarbazine in previously treated patients with advanced liposarcoma or leiomyosarcoma: a randomised, open-label, multicentre, phase 3 trial. *Lancet.* 2016;387(10028):1629–1637. doi:10.1016/S0140-6736(15)01283-0

18. Hensley ML, Maki R, Venkatraman E, et al. Gemcitabine and docetaxel in patients with unresectable leiomyosarcoma: results of a phase II trial. *J Clin Oncol.* 2002;20(12):2824–2831. doi:10.1200/JCO.2002.11.050

19. Demetri GD, von Mehren M, Jones RL, et al. Efficacy and safety of trabectedin or dacarbazine for metastatic liposarcoma or leiomyosarcoma after failure of conventional chemotherapy: results of a phase III randomized multicenter clinical trial. *J Clin Oncol.* 2016;34(8):786–793. doi:10.1200/JCO.2015.62.4734

20. Judson I, Radford JA, Harris M, et al. Randomised phase II trial of pegylated liposomal doxorubicin (DOXIL/CAELYX) versus doxorubicin in the treatment of advanced or metastatic soft tissue sarcoma: a study by the EORTC Soft Tissue and Bone Sarcoma Group. *Eur J Cancer.* 2001;37(7):870–877. doi:10.1016/s0959-8049(01)00050-8

21. van der Graaf WT, Blay J-Y, Chawla SP, et al. Pazopanib for metastatic soft-tissue sarcoma (PALETTE): a randomised, double-blind, placebo-controlled phase 3 trial. *Lancet.* 2012;379(9829):1879–1886. doi:10.1016/S0140-6736(12)60651-5

22. D'Angelo SP, Mahoney MR, Van Tine BA, et al. Nivolumab with or without ipilimumab treatment for metastatic sarcoma (Alliance A091401): two open-label, non-comparative, randomised, phase 2 trials. *Lancet Oncol.* 2018;19(3):416-426. doi:10.1016/S1470-2045(18)30006-8

23. Tawbi HA, Burgess M, Bolejack V, et al. Pembrolizumab in advanced soft-tissue sarcoma and bone sarcoma (SARC028): a multicentre, two-cohort, single-arm, open-label, phase 2 trial. *Lancet Oncol.* 2017;18(11):1493-1501. doi:10.1016/S1470-2045(17)30624-1

24. Skapek SX, Ferrari A, Gupta AA, et al. Rhabdomyosarcoma. *Nat Rev Dis Primers.* 2019;5(1):1. doi:10.1038/s41572-018-0051-2

25. Hettmer S, Li Z, Billin AN, et al. Rhabdomyosarcoma: current challenges and their implications for developing therapies. *Cold Spring Harb Perspect Med.* 2014;4(11):a025650. doi:10.1101/cshperspect.a025650

26. Crist WM, Anderson JR, Meza JL, et al. Intergroup rhabdomyosarcoma study-IV: results for patients with non-metastatic disease. *J Clin Oncol.* 2001;19(12):3091–3102. doi:10.1200/JCO.2001.19.12.3091

27. Miettinen M, Lasota J. Gastrointestinal stromal tumors: pathology and prognosis at different sites. *Semin Diagn Pathol.* 2006;23(2):70–83. doi:10.1053/j.semdp.2006.09.001

28. Whooley P, Correa E, von Mehren M. Deciding on the duration of adjuvant therapy in gastrointestinal stromal tumor. *Expert Rev Anticancer Ther.* 2021;21(5):547–556. doi:10.1080/14737140.2021.1863149

29. Eriksson M, Joensuu H. Adjuvant imatinib for GIST: duration likely matters. *Ann Oncol.* 2021;32(4):434–436. doi:10.1016/j.annonc.2021.01.073

30. Heinrich MC, Jones RL, von Mehren M, et al. Avapritinib in advanced *PDGFRA D842V*-mutant gastrointestinal stromal tumour (NAVIGATOR): a multicentre, open-label, phase 1 trial. *Lancet Oncol.* 2020;21(7):935–946. doi:10.1016/S1470-2045(20)30269-2

31. Kang Y-K, George S, Jones RL, et al. Avapritinib versus regorafenib in locally advanced unresectable or metastatic GI stromal tumor: a randomized, open-label phase III study. *J Clin Oncol.* 2021;39(28):3128–3139. doi:10.1200/JCO.21.00217

32. Casali PG, Zalcberg J, Le Cesne A, et al. Ten-year progression-free and overall survival in patients with unresectable or metastatic GI stromal tumors: long-term analysis of the European Organisation for Research and Treatment of Cancer, Italian Sarcoma Group, and Australasian Gastrointestinal Trials group intergroup phase III randomized trial on imatinib at two dose levels. *J Clin Oncol.* 2017;35(15):1713–1720. doi:10.1200/JCO.2016.71.0228

33. Demetri GD, van Oosterom AT, Garrett CR, et al. Efficacy and safety of sunitinib in patients with advanced gastrointestinal stromal tumour after failure of imatinib: a randomised controlled trial. *Lancet.* 2006;368(9544):1329–1338. doi:10.1016/S0140-6736(06)69446-4

34. Montemurro M, Cioffi A, Dômont J, et al. Long-term outcome of dasatinib first-line treatment in gastrointestinal stromal tumor: a multicenter, 2-stage phase 2 trial (Swiss Group for Clinical Cancer Research 56/07). *Cancer.* 2018;124(7):1449–1454. doi:10.1002/cncr.31234

CHAPTER 24

Primary Brain Tumors

Akaolisa S. Eziokwu and Jacob Mandel

INTRODUCTION

Central nervous system (CNS) cancers account for about 1.3% of all new cancer diagnoses and 3.1% of all cancer deaths in the United States, with estimated new cases of 24,500 and 18,600 deaths in 2021. The 5-year relative survival remains poor at about 32.6% (National Cancer Institute [NCI]: Surveillance, Epidemiology, and End Results [SEER]). CNS tumors can present with different symptoms ranging from headaches, seizures, focal neurological deficits affecting speech or mobility, and/or neurocognitive dysfunction depending on tumor size and location.

Treatment of primary CNS cancers often involves some combination of surgical resection, radiation therapy (RT), and chemotherapy; a multidisciplinary team that includes neurosurgeons, medical oncologists, neuroradiologists, neurologists, radiation oncologists, and physical and occupational therapists is important to appropriately manage these patients.

This chapter employs a case-based approach to discuss the clinical, histopathological, and molecular diagnosis; World Health Organization (WHO) staging; evidence-based management; and post-treatment follow-up of primary CNS cancers, focusing on *adult-type diffuse gliomas* (glioblastoma, isocitrate dehydrogenase [*IDH*] wildtype; oligodendroglioma, *IDH* mutant 1p/19q co-deleted; and astrocytoma, *IDH* mutant).

CASE SUMMARIES

Case 24.1: Glioblastoma, *IDH* Wildtype

A 73-year-old male with a past medical history (PMH) of hypertension, hyperlipidemia, and type 2 diabetes presents to the ED due to a fall secondary to left-sided weakness. His family reports he had been having difficulty with his memory for the past few weeks. Additionally, he has been having morning headaches for the past week or two. His wife also has noted that he has been staying up later, is more quiet and reserved, and has had spells of tangential conversations over the past several weeks. The patient reports that he is not aware of these symptoms and "feels fine." The patient is a former smoker, but denies alcohol or drug use. His exam reveals hyperreflexia in his left lower extremity and 4+/5 weakness on his left side. On presentation to the ED, a CT of the head was performed which showed a mass in the right frontal lobe with midline shift to the left measuring approximately 9 mm. Subsequent MRI of the brain revealed a heterogeneously enhancing mass expanding the cortex of the right frontal lobe anteriorly, inferiorly, and in the paramedian location. Extensive vasogenic edema in the right frontal lobe is identified, which extends posteriorly to

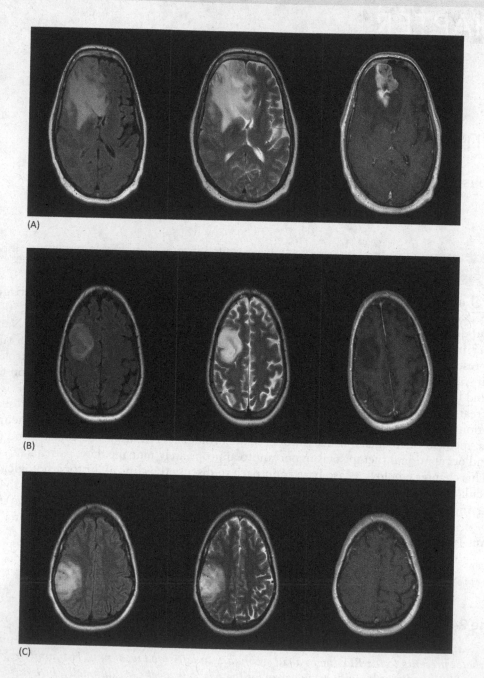

Figure 24.1 MR imaging of adult newly diagnosed adult-type diffuse gliomas. (A) Glioblastoma, *IDH* wildtype: MRI of the brain axial FLAIR, axial T2, and axial T1 post contrast (left to right) demonstrating a *heterogeneously enhancing mass* expanding the cortex of the right frontal lobe anteriorly, inferiorly, and in the paramedian location. *Extensive vasogenic edema* in the right frontal lobe is identified which extends posteriorly to involve the external capsule, insula, genu of the corpus callosum, and hypothalamus, and superiorly to involve the superior right frontal gyrus. (B) Astrocytoma, *IDH* mutant, grade 2: MRI of the brain axial FLAIR, axial T2, and axial T1 post contrast (left to right) demonstrating a *nonenhancing 4.6cm mass* in the right middle frontal gyrus with mass effect on the adjacent cortical sulci and gyri without evidence for vasogenic edema in the adjacent parenchyma. T2-FLAIR mismatch sign (presence of complete/near-complete hyperintense signals on a T2-weighted image and a relatively hypointense signal on FLAIR except for a hyperintense peripheral rim) is present. (C) Oligodendroglioma, *IDH* mutant, 1p/19q co-deleted, grade 3: MRI brain axial FLAIR, axial T2, and axial T1 post contrast (left to right) demonstrating a *T1 isointense, T2 hyperintense nonenhancing expansile lesion* involving the right posterior frontal and anterior parietal cortex and subcortical white matter with "bubbly" appearance of the cortex at the caudal margin of the lesion and mass effect.

involve the external capsule, insula, genu of the corpus callosum, and hypothalamus, and superiorly to involve the superior right frontal gyrus (Figure 24.1A).

How Is a Diagnosis Established?

- Maximal safe resection is the preferred approach if possible. Biopsy can be used in situations of poor performance status (PS) or when the mass is in a location not amenable to surgery.

Patient's Diagnosis

- *The patient underwent a right frontal craniotomy for mass resection.*
- *Pathology: specimen contains a highly cellular tumor which has moderate to severe atypia, multifocal necrosis with some pseudopalisading of tumor cells, vascular proliferation, and frequent mitotic activity. Immunoperoxidase stains for GFAP are strongly positive in nearly all tumor cells. IDH–1 immunoperoxidase stains are negative in tumor.*

What Further Molecular or Genomic Testing Is Required?

- All newly diagnosed glioblastoma should undergo testing for *IDH* mutation status. Immunohistochemistry (IHC) for the most common *IDH* mutation in gliomas, *IDH1* R132H, captures approximately 90% of *IDH* mutations in gliomas. If R132H mutant *IDH1* IHC is negative, sequencing of *IDH1* and *IDH2* should be performed in younger patients (younger than 55 years), as *IDH*-mutation status is integral to an accurate diagnosis.[1]
- While not required for diagnosis, O6-methylguanine-DNA methyltransferase (*MGMT*) promotor methylation status should be tested. *MGMT* is an enzyme that is integral for DNA repair after alkylating-agent chemotherapy. The *MGMT* gene can be silenced by methylation of its promoter during tumor development, thus inhibiting repair of DNA damage and enhancing the possible effectiveness of alkylating agent chemotherapy. Methylated tumors have a better prognosis and are predictive of response to alkylating-agent chemotherapy.[2]
- Due to the limited effectiveness of treatment options at disease recurrence, more extensive molecular sequencing is encouraged to evaluate for potential clinical trials and/or possible targetable mutations (*BRAF* mutation, *NTRK* fusion, and so on), although this is also not required for diagnostic purposes.

Patient's Molecular and Genomic Testing

- *Testing involves IDH wildtype (based on IHC and subsequent molecular testing). Molecular testing revealed PTEN and TERT promoter mutations, CDKN2A and CDKN2B loss, and EGFR copy number gain.*
- *MGMT promotor was methylated.*

How Is This Tumor Staged?

- The 2021 *WHO Classification of Tumors of the Central Nervous System* is used to stage cancers of the CNS.
- Glioblastoma, *IDH* wildtype is an integrated diagnosis based upon histopathological and molecular parameters with a WHO grade 4.
- Glioblastoma, *IDH* wildtype is an astrocytic tumor that is histopathologically defined by microvascular proliferation and/or necrosis and molecularly defined by a lack of an *IDH* mutation.

- Additionally, recent updates allow a glioblastoma, *IDH* wildtype CNS WHO grade 4 designation even in cases that otherwise appear histologically lower grade if *TERT* promoter mutation, *EGFR* amplification, and +7/–10 copy number changes are seen in an *IDH* wildtype diffuse astrocytoma.[1]

Patient's Clinical Stage
- Glioblastoma, IDH *wildtype WHO grade 4*

What Are Appropriate Treatment Options?

- The standard of care for newly diagnosed glioblastoma is maximal safe resection followed by 6 weeks of focal intensity modulated RT (60 Gy in 30 fractions) plus concomitant oral temozolomide 75 mg/m² body surface area (BSA), followed by 6 cycles of adjuvant temozolomide (150 to 200 mg/m² for 5 days during each 28-day cycle). This was shown in a randomized clinical trial to prolong median survival by an additional 2.5 months compared to radiation alone (14.6 months vs. 12.1 months) as well as increase long-term 5-year overall survival (OS; 9.8% vs. 1.9%)[3,4] (Table 24.1).
- Many neuro-oncologists will give up to 12 cycles of adjuvant temozolomide if there is no disease progression, although the benefit of more than 6 cycles remains uncertain.[5]
- Alternating electric fields (tumor treating fields [TTFields]) delivered by a portable medical device put onto the scalp was examined in an open-label randomized trial along with monthly temozolomide in patients with newly diagnosed glioblastoma in the post-radiation setting with stable disease. The TTFields device had improved progression-free survival (PFS) compared with those assigned to temozolomide alone (6.7 vs. 4.0 months). OS from the time of randomization was also improved (20.9 vs. 16.0 months).[6]
- The TTFields trial lacked a sham device in the control arm, raising concern that differences in supportive care may have impacted survival in the device arm. Additionally, patients must shave their heads and the device needs to be worn at least 18 hours per day, which may be burdensome and may limit the interest for many patients.
- For patients with *MGMT* promotor methylation, the addition of lomustine to standard of care was examined comparing standard temozolomide chemoradiotherapy (75 mg/m² per day concomitant to radiotherapy [59 to 60 Gy] followed by six courses of temozolomide 150 to 200 mg/m² per day on the first 5 days of the 4-week course) or to up to six courses of lomustine (100 mg/m² on day 1) plus temozolomide (100 to 200 mg/m² per day on days 2 to 6 of the 6-week course) in addition to radiotherapy (59 to 60 Gy). Median OS (mOS) was improved from 31.4 months with temozolomide to 48.1 months (32.6 months-not assessable) with lomustine-temozolomide. However, the findings should be interpreted with caution, owing to the small size of the trial (*n* = 129), lack of difference in PFS between the groups (16.7 months in both), and increase in toxicity seen in the combination arm.[7]
- Patients with very low PS (non-ambulatory and fully dependent on others for activities of daily living [ADLs]) are best treated with maximal supportive care alone due to very poor prognosis.

Recommended Treatment Plan for This Patient
- *Treatment involves 6 weeks of concurrent chemoradiation (60 Gy in 30 fractions plus concomitant oral temozolomide 75 mg/m² BSA), followed by up to 12 cycles of adjuvant temozolomide (150 to 200 mg/m² for 5 days during each 28-day cycle).*

What Are the Toxicities Associated With Standard of Care Treatment?

- Radiation can acutely cause hair loss, lack of energy, decreased appetite/weight loss, headaches, nausea/vomiting and radiation dermatitis.
- Patients receiving concurrent chemoradiation with temozolomide chemotherapy require weekly complete blood counts (CBCs) and comprehensive metabolic panels (CMPs) to examine for hematologic effects or hepatotoxicity. The most common hematologic adverse effect is thrombocytopenia. Patients may also develop lymphopenia, and *Pneumocystis jirovecii* pneumonia (PJP) prophylaxis should be given to all patients with significant lymphopenia and/or those on high-dose steroids.
- A CBC should be obtained prior to each adjuvant temozolomide cycle to monitor for hematologic toxicity.
- Temozolomide-linked aplastic anemia, myelodysplasia, plasmablastic lymphoma, and treatment-related acute myeloid leukemia (t-AML) has been rarely reported.
- Common nonhematologic side effects of temozolomide include constipation, nausea/vomiting, decreased appetite, weight loss, rash and fatigue. Hepatotoxicity can occur and a CMP should also be obtained prior to each adjuvant temozolomide cycle.
- In both pregnant patients and pregnant partners of male patients, fetal harm and adverse developmental outcomes associated with temozolomide exposure have been reported. Patients should be on effective contraception if they have reproductive potential.
- The most common side effects when using TTFields include scalp irritation (redness and itchiness), headaches, malaise, muscle twitching, falls, and skin ulcers/infections.

What Are Other Treatment Considerations?

Pseudoprogression

- This refers to the phenomenon of increased contrast enhancement and surrounding T2/FLAIR hyperintensity within the radiation treatment field that may be noticed on post-chemoradiation scan obtained 4 weeks after concurrent chemoradiation, compared to prechemoradiation scan (or may even occur several months after chemoradiation). This is considered the "treatment effect," hence the term "tumor pseudoprogression." This is different from new contrast enhancement *outside of the radiation treatment field* which should be considered tumor progression and treated accordingly.
- Patients with suspected pseudoprogression should continue with adjuvant temozolomide cycles as planned. If symptomatic a short course of steroids or bevacizumab can be used to decrease edema and mass effect.
- Glioblastoma patients with *MGMT* promoter methylation have been found to have a higher incidence of tumor pseudoprogression compared to unmethylated *MGMT* promoter patients.[8]

Treatment De-Escalation

- For patients with a poor performance score or older patients (70 or older), a de-escalation of treatment may be appropriate.
- A shorter course (40 Gy in 15 fractions) of chemoradiation with concurrent temozolomide followed by adjuvant temozolomide was found to prolong survival in patients 65 years or older compared to a shorter course of radiation alone (9.3 months vs. 7.6 months).[9]
- Radiotherapy alone resulted in a modest improvement in survival compared to supportive care only (29.1 weeks, as compared with 16.9 weeks). Radiotherapy alone is preferable to temozolomide alone in patients with *MGMT* unmethylated tumors.[10,11]
- For older adult patients with *MGMT* methylated tumors in need of de-escalation of treatment, temozolomide alone is a reasonable option.[11,12]

What Is Required for This Patient's Follow-Up and Survivorship?

- MRI of the brain with and without contrast postoperatively to determine the extent of surgical resection, repeated 3 to 4 weeks after the completion of chemoradiation and then after every 2 to 3 adjuvant cycles for the first 2 years, is required. Subsequently, scans can be performed less frequently thereafter as long as the tumor continues to remain without evidence of disease progression.
- Physical therapy (PT)/occupational therapy (OT)/speech therapy evaluations should be performed following surgery to identify patients who may benefit from rehab or outpatient therapies.
- Patients who have had seizures should remain on antiepileptic prophylaxis, while those who have not had seizures can be tapered off if started prior to surgery.
- Patients should be clinically monitored for deep-vein thrombosis (DVT) and pulmonary emblism (PE) as venous thromboembolism (VTE) can occur in 20% to 30% of glioblastoma patients.[13]
- Patients should be evaluated for fatigue, changes in mental status, and mood, including depression and anxiety.
- Many patients will require short-term or permanent disability secondary to neurological deficits and/or change in their cognition, potentially preventing them from being able to return to their prior occupation.

Case 24.2: Astrocytoma, *IDH* Mutant

A 33-year-old female with no PMH reportedly lost consciousness and had a seizure in which coworkers witnessed her body shaking. She was taken to the ED, where she had a second seizure. Her husband witnessed this and stated that she was talking, then suddenly turned her head to the left and both arms were shaking rhythmically. CT of the head was performed, showing a right frontal mass. Subsequent MRI of the brain with and without contrast revealed a nonenhancing 4.6-cm mass in the right middle frontal gyrus with mass effect on the adjacent cortical sulci and gyri without evidence for vasogenic edema in the adjacent parenchyma (Figure 24.1B). She reports having rare brief self-limited staring episodes for a few weeks prior to the seizure. She was started on levetiracetam and dexamethasone. Her neurological exam was unremarkable. She was felt to be appropriate for awake craniotomy, and was discharged home with planned readmission for surgery following neuropsychology testing.

How Is a Diagnosis Established?

- Maximal safe resection is the preferred approach if possible. Biopsy can be used in situations of poor PS or when the mass is in a location not amenable to surgery.
- T2-FLAIR mismatch sign is a highly specific imaging marker of *IDH*-mutant astrocytomas. It is defined as the presence of complete/near-complete hyperintense signals on a T2-weighted image and a relatively hypointense signal on FLAIR except for a hyperintense peripheral rim. While helpful in presurgical counseling, even in patients with a T2-FLAIR mismatch sign, maximal safe resection is indicated for confirmation and reduction of tumor disease burden.[14,15]

Patient's Diagnosis

- The patient underwent a right frontal craniotomy for mass resection.
- Pathology: The tumor is moderately to highly cellular and contains scattered multinucleate and atypical tumor cells. No vascular proliferation or necrosis is identified. Infiltration of the cortex by secondary structures of Scherer is noted. No mitoses are identified in any portion of the tumor. Both specimens are examined in their entirety. Immunoperoxidase stains

for GFAP stain the majority of tumor cells. P53 immunoperoxidase stains scattered and atypical tumor nuclei. IDH1 is strongly positive in the majority of tumor cells. The MIB1 labeling index is mostly less than 1% in the majority of the tumor; however, a small focus of tumor has a labeling index of 7.1%.

What Further Molecular or Genomic Testing Is Required?

- All newly diagnosed astrocytoma should undergo testing for *IDH* mutation status. IHC for the most common *IDH* mutation in gliomas, *IDH1* R132H, captures approximately 90% of *IDH* mutations in gliomas. If R132H-mutant *IDH1* IHC is negative, sequencing of *IDH1* and *IDH2* should be performed in younger patients (younger than 55 years), as *IDH*-mutation status is integral to an accurate diagnosis.[1]
- Testing for whole-arm deletion of 1p and 19q due to an unbalanced translocation between chromosomes 1 and 19 is an essential feature of oligodendroglial tumors and should be performed unless examining an astrocytic *IDH*-mutant tumor with unequivocal evidence of *TP53* or *ATRX* mutations.[16]
- Alpha-thalassemia/intellectual disability syndrome X-linked (*ATRX*) mutations are regularly found in diffuse astrocytic gliomas. *ATRX* mutations are closely correlated with *IDH1/2* and *TP53* mutations and are mutually exclusive with 1p/19q co-deletion. IHC staining for *ATRX* expression has diagnostic value for establishing diffuse astrocytic tumors, where lack of nuclear staining for *ATRX* signifies the presence of an *ATRX* mutation.
- Most *IDH*-mutant astrocytomas have missense somatic mutations in the *TP53* gene. Robust nuclear staining for mutant *p53* is often seen with these tumors.
- More extensive molecular sequencing is encouraged to evaluate for *CDKN2A/B* homozygous deletion, which can effect tumor grading, and to look for potentially targetable mutations (*BRAF* mutation, *NTRK* fusion, and so on).

Patient's Molecular and Genomic Testing

- IDH-*mutated (based on IHC and subsequent molecular testing—IDH1 p.R132H)*
- *The 1p/19q status was negative for co-deletion.*
- *Molecular testing revealed ATRX and p53 mutations.*

How Is This Tumor Staged?

- The 2021 *WHO Classification of Tumors of the Central Nervous System* is used to stage cancers of the CNS.
- In the most recent classification, all *IDH*-mutant diffuse astrocytic tumors are deemed a single type (*Astrocytoma*, IDH-*mutant*) and then graded as CNS WHO grade 2, 3, or 4.[1]
- *IDH*-mutant diffuse astrocytic tumor grading is based upon histopathological features in conjunction with molecular testing results.
- Astrocytomas, *IDH*-mutant, grade 2 tumors are diffusely infiltrative astrocytic gliomas with increased cellularity and atypia, but lack mitoses, endothelial proliferation, or necrosis.
- Astrocytomas, *IDH*-mutant, grade 3 tumors are diffusely infiltrative astrocytic gliomas that display greater cellularity, more prominent nuclear atypia and hyperchromasia, and mitoses, but lack endothelial proliferation or necrosis.
- Astrocytomas, *IDH*-mutant, grade 4 tumors are heavily cellular, pleomorphic astrocytic gliomas with mitotic activity as well as microvascular proliferation and/or necrosis.

- Additionally, grading is no longer exclusively histological, since the occurrence of CDKN2A/B homozygous deletion results in a CNS WHO grade of 4, even in the absence of microvascular proliferation or necrosis.[1]

Patient's Clinical Stage
- Astrocytoma, IDH-mutant, grade 2

What Are Appropriate Treatment Options?

Astrocytoma, IDH-Mutant, grade 2
- A study looking at low-grade astrocytoma and oligodendroglioma in adults (EORTC 22845) examined early radiotherapy of 54 Gy in fractions of 1.8 Gy or deferred radiotherapy until the time of progression. Median PFS (mPFS) was 5.3 years in the early radiotherapy group and 3.4 years in the control group. However, OS was similar between groups: median survival in the radiotherapy group was 7.4 years compared with 7.2 years in the control group. This suggested that radiotherapy could be deferred for patients with low-grade glioma who are carefully monitored.[17]
- A subsequent study (RTOG9802) examined "high risk" grade 2 astrocytoma, oligoastrocytoma, or oligodendroglioma in those who were younger than 40 years of age and had undergone subtotal resection or biopsy or who were 40 years of age or older, and compared RT alone or to RT followed by 6 cycles of procarbazine, lomustine (also called CCNU), and vincristine (PCV). The PCV regimen consisted of 42-day cycles of lomustine 110 mg/m² orally, day 1 (max 200 mg), procarbazine 60 mg/m² orally, days 8 to 21, and vincristine 1.4 mg/m² intravenously (max 2 mg per dose), days 8 and 29. Patients who received RT plus chemotherapy had longer mOS than did those who received RT alone (13.3 vs. 7.8 years).[18]
- A post hoc analysis of RTOG 9802 also found that patients with IDH-mutant high-risk low-grade glioma irrespective of co-deletion status derive benefit from the addition of PCV.[19]
- Low-risk (less than 40 years old with a gross total resection) astrocytoma, IDH-mutant, grade 2 patients can be monitored with surveillance alone with periodic MRI of the brain scans deferring immediate postsurgery radiation and/or chemotherapy (Table 24.1).
- High-risk (less than 40 years old with a biopsy or subtotal resection or older than 40) astrocytoma, IDH-mutant, grade 2 patients should receive postoperative RT (54 Gy in 30 fractions) followed by adjuvant chemotherapy (6 cycles of adjuvant PCV chemotherapy or 12 cycles of adjuvant temozolomide; Table 24.1).

Astrocytoma, IDH-Mutant, Grade 3
- The CATNON (EORTC study 26053-22054) trial investigated the addition of concurrent, adjuvant, and both concurrent and adjuvant temozolomide to radiotherapy in adults with newly diagnosed 1p/19q non-co-deleted anaplastic gliomas. This study found that adjuvant temozolomide chemotherapy, but not concurrent temozolomide chemotherapy, was associated with a survival benefit in patients with 1p/19q non-co-deleted anaplastic glioma.[20]
- Regardless of age or resection status, astrocytoma, IDH-mutant, grade 3 patients should receive postoperative RT (59.4 to 60 Gy in 1.8 to 2 Gy fractions) followed by adjuvant chemotherapy (12 cycles of adjuvant temozolomide; Table 24.1).

Table 24.1 Treatment Recommendations Following Maximal Safe Surgical Resection in Newly Diagnosed Adult-Type Diffuse Gliomas

WHO Diagnosis	Recommended Treatments	Clinical Trial(s) Supporting Recommendation
Glioblastoma, IDH *wildtype, grade 4*	6 weeks of concurrent chemoradiation (60 Gy) with daily temozolomide followed by 6–12 cycles of adjuvant temozolomide	EORTC 26981-22981
Astrocytoma, IDH-*mutant, grade 2*	Radiation (54 Gy) alone followed by 6 cycles of adjuvant PCV or 12 cycles of adjuvant temozolomide if "high risk"	RTOG 9802
	or	or
	Observation alone	EORTC 22845
Astrocytoma, IDH-*mutant, grade 3*	6 weeks of radiation alone (60 Gy) followed by 12 cycles of adjuvant temozolomide	CATNON
Astrocytoma, IDH-*mutant, grade 4*	6 weeks of concurrent chemoradiation (60 Gy) with daily temozolomide followed by 6–12 cycles of adjuvant temozolomide	EORTC 26981-22981
Oligodendroglioma, IDH-*mutant 1p/19q co-deleted, grade 2*	Radiation (54 Gy) alone followed by 6 cycles of adjuvant PCV or 12 cycles of adjuvant temozolomide if "high risk"	RTOG 9802
	or	or
	Observation alone	EORTC 22845
Oligodendroglioma, IDH-*mutant 1p/19q co-deleted, grade 3*	PCV up to 4 cycles followed by immediate involved-field radiation (59.4 Gy)	RTOG 9402
	or	or
	59.4 Gy of RT followed by 6 cycles of adjuvant PCV or 12 cycles of adjuvant temozolomide	EORTC 26951

IDH, isocitrate dehydrogenase; PCV, procarbazine, lomustine, and vincristine; RT, radiation therapy, WHO, World Health Organization.

Astrocytoma, *IDH*-Mutant, Grade 4

- Historically, these tumors have been included in trials for glioblastoma. Treatment is similar to glioblastoma *IDH* wildtype with maximal safe resection followed by 6 weeks of focal intensity modulated RT (60 Gy in 30 fractions) plus concomitant oral temozolomide 75 mg/m² BSA, followed by 6 cycles of adjuvant temozolomide (150 to 200 mg/m² for 5 days during each 28-day cycle)[3] (Table 24.1).

Recommended Treatment Plan for This Patient
- *Surveillance imaging alone (patient was a "low risk" astrocytoma, IDH-mutant, grade 2 patient who was 33 years old with a gross total resection)*

What Are the Toxicities Associated With Standard of Care Treatments?

Radiation
- Radiation can acutely cause hair loss, lack of energy, decreased appetite/weight loss, headaches, nausea/vomiting, and radiation dermatitis.
- Potential long-term effects of radiation include progressive delayed neurocognitive impairment and a low risk of secondary tumor formation (meningioma).

Concurrent Chemoradiation With Daily Temozolomide
- Patients receiving concurrent chemoradiation with temozolomide chemotherapy require weekly CBCs and CMPs to examine for hematologic effects or hepatotoxicity. The most common hematologic adverse effect is thrombocytopenia. Patients may also develop lymphopenia, and PJP prophylaxis should be given to all patients with significant lymphopenia and/or those on high-dose steroids.

Adjuvant Temozolomide
- A CBC should be obtained prior to each adjuvant temozolomide cycle to monitor for hematologic toxicity.
- Temozolomide-linked aplastic anemia, myelodysplasia, plasmablastic lymphoma, and t-AML have been rarely reported.
- Common nonhematologic side effects of temozolomide include constipation, nausea/vomiting, decreased appetite, weight loss, rash, and fatigue. Hepatotoxicity can occur and a CMP should also be obtained prior to each adjuvant temozolomide cycle.
- In both pregnant patients and pregnant partners of male patients, fetal harm and adverse developmental outcomes associated with temozolomide exposure have been reported. Patients should be on effective contraception if they have reproductive potential.

Procarbazine, Lomustine, and Vincristine
- PCV can also cause hematologic effects or hepatotoxicity. Before day 1 of each cycle, a CBC and CMP should be completed. Weekly CBCs are often done starting at week 4.
- Dose adjustments of lomustine and procarbazine are typically performed for hematologic toxicity depending on the extent of nadir and length of recovery.
- Dose adjustments may be necessary for all three drugs based on the timing and severity of hepatotoxicity.
- Lomustine and procarbazine can cause nausea/vomiting, and patients should receive premedication with antiemetics before each dose.
- Lomustine can very rarely lead to serious pulmonary toxicity (infiltrates, fibrosis).
- Procarbazine has possible drug–drug and drug–food interactions based on weak inhibition of monoamine oxidase (MAO) in the gastrointestinal system. Tyramine-rich foods (for example, aged cheese, smoked meats) should not be eaten, and concomitant use of an MAO inhibitor is contraindicated due to the risk of hypertensive crisis. Alcohol use is also not allowed due to the risk of a disulfiram-like reaction. Additionally, procarbazine hypersensitivity can lead to cutaneous maculopapular rash and should be discontinued if a rash develops.
- Vincristine can commonly cause constipation secondary to autonomic neuropathy and/or length-dependent sensory peripheral neuropathy.

What Are Other Treatment Considerations?

Procarbazine, Lomustine, and Vincristine Versus Temozolomide

- PCV and temozolomide are both rational options for adjunctive therapy in astrocytoma, *IDH*-mutant, grade 2 tumors. Use of PCV is supported by results of the RTOG 9802, whereas temozolomide was used in CATNON. Temozolomide is easier to administer as it does not require an IV infusion and has better patient tolerance due to typically fewer side effects.[18,20]

Necessity of Vincristine in Procarbazine, Lomustine, and Vincristine Regimen

- Vincristine has been demonstrated to not cross an intact blood-brain barrier, so its usefulness in this combination regimen is uncertain. However, studies comparing PCV with a two-drug regimen (lomustine and procarbazine) are limited, but due to the unclear benefit of vincristine it is frequently stopped quickly if neurotoxicity is seen.[21]

What Is Required for This Patient's Follow-Up and Survivorship?

- *The requirement is MRI of the brain with and without contrast postoperatively to determine the extent of surgical resection, then every 3 months for the first 2 years, then every 4 months for 2 years, then every 6 months for several years, then yearly as long as there is no evidence of recurrent tumor.*
- *PT/OT/Speech therapy evaluations should be performed following surgery to identify patients who may benefit from rehab or outpatient therapies.*
- *Patients who have had seizures should remain on antiepileptic prophylaxis, while those who have not had seizures can be tapered off if started prior to surgery. Radiation and chemotherapy are also correlated with better seizure control in patients.[22]*
- *Patients with reproductive potential in whom chemotherapy is planned should be informed of the potential for infertility. Men can be referred for sperm banking, and women can be referred to reproductive specialists for discussion of fertility preservation possibilities such as embryo and oocyte cryopreservation if interested in future paternity. This is ideally to be done prior to the patient starting chemotherapy.*
- *Patients should be routinely evaluated for fatigue, changes in mental status, and mood, including depression and anxiety.*
- *Glioma patients are at high risk for neurocognitive deficits. Baseline neurocognitive testing can be helpful for comparison if neurocognitive changes are reported during or after treatments. Cognitive rehabilitation can be beneficial in certain patients with deficits.*
- *Many patients will require short or permanent disability secondary to neurological deficits, seizures, and/or change in their cognition, potentially preventing them from being able to return to their prior occupation.*

Case 24.3: Oligodendroglioma, *IDH* Mutant, 1p/19q Co-Deleted

A 39-year-old female with no PMH reports that she was typing notes and noticed that she could not control her hand to write the word she wanted. She described a loss of coordination and fine motor movement of the left hand. She also felt a sensation of coldness moving from her head down her body. Her symptoms persisted for about 15 minutes, then resolved. She states about 2 weeks ago she had a similar episode. She was typing notes at work and felt like she could not type the word she wanted as her hands were fumbling on the keyboard. This episode lasted only minutes and so she did not have it further investigated. CT of the head was performed that revealed mass effect, vasogenic edema and some loss of the overlying gray-white junction within the posterior frontal and anterior parietal parenchyma. Subsequent MRI of the brain showed a T1 isointense, T2 hyperintense nonenhancing expansile lesion involving the right posterior frontal and anterior parietal cortex and subcortical white matter with "bubbly" appearance of the cortex at the caudal margin of the lesion and mass effect (Figure 24.1C). The patient had an EEG performed demonstrating focal slowing over the right hemisphere, most prominently in the right central-parietal and right temporal-parietal regions as well as occasional lateralized periodic discharges (LPD) in the right temporal more than the frontal region. She was started on levetiracetam and dexamethasone. Her neurological exam was unremarkable.

How Is a Diagnosis Established?

- Maximal safe resection is the preferred approach if possible. Biopsy can be used in situations of poor PS or when the mass is in a location not amenable to surgery.

Patient's Diagnosis

- The patient underwent a right awake frontotemporal craniotomy for mass resection.
- Pathology: The tumor has moderately high cellularity focally with rare mitoses, but no vascular proliferation or necrosis. It exhibits a typical oligodendroglial phenotype. Immunperoxidase stains for GFAP are positive in surrounding neuropil and membranously. S100 is positve in tumor cell nuclei. Immunoperoxidase stains for p53 stain a rare tumor cell nucleus. IDH1 is strongly and diffusely positive in tumor nuclei and cytoplasm. Focally, the MIB1 labeling index is as high as 15.6%.

What Further Molecular or Genomic Testing Is Required?

- All newly diagnosed oligodendroglioma should undergo testing for IDH mutation status. IHC for the most common IDH mutation in gliomas, IDH1 R132H, captures approximately 90% of IDH mutations in gliomas. If R132H-mutant IDH1 IHC is negative, sequencing of IDH1 and IDH2 should be performed in younger patients (younger than 55 years), as IDH-mutation status is integral to an accurate diagnosis.[1]
- Testing for whole-arm deletion of 1p and 19q due to an unbalanced translocation between chromosomes 1 and 19 is an essential feature of oligodendroglial tumors and should be performed as well. Oligodendroglioma are molecularly classified, diffusely infiltrating gliomas that must contain both an IDH1 or IDH2 mutation and co-deletion of chromosome arms 1p and 19q.

Patient's Molecular and Genomic Testing

- IDH-mutated (based on IHC and subsequent molecular testing—IDH1 p.R132H)
- 1p/19q status revealed a co-deletion. Both 1p36 and 19q13 deletions were detected, as determined with FISH analysis.
- Molecular testing also demonstrated TERT (telomerase reverse transcriptase), CIC (capicua transcriptional repressor), and NOTCH1 mutations.

How Is This Tumor Staged?

- The 2021 WHO Classification of Tumors of the Central Nervous System is used to stage cancers of the CNS.
- In the most recent classification, all IDH-mutant, 1p/19q co-deleted, diffuse oligodendroglial tumors are deemed a single type (oligodendroglioma, IDH-mutant, 1p/19q co-deleted) and then graded as CNS WHO grade 2 or 3.[1]
- IDH-mutant, 1p/19q co-deleted, diffuse oligodendroglial tumor grading is based upon histopathological features.

- Oligodendrogliomas are histologically well-differentiated, diffusely infiltrating tumors arranged primarily of cells similar to oligodendrocytes. The usual appearance is that of sheets of isomorphic round nuclei surrounded by clear cytoplasm ("fried egg" look). Delicate, branching capillaries and microcalcifications are characteristic.
- Oligodendroglioma, *IDH*-mutant, 1p/19q co-deleted, grade 3 tumors are characterized by the presence of high cell density, mitosis, nuclear atypia, microvascular proliferation, and necrosis.

Patient's Clinical Stage
- *Oligodendroglioma, IDH-mutant, 1p/19q co-deleted, grade 3*

What Are Appropriate Treatment Options?

Oligodendroglioma, *IDH*-Mutant, 1p/19q Co-Deleted, Grade 2
- A study looking at low-grade astrocytoma and oligodendroglioma in adults (EORTC 22845) examined early radiotherapy of 54 Gy in fractions of 1.8 Gy or deferred radiotherapy until the time of progression. mPFS was 5.3 years in the early radiotherapy group and 3.4 years in the control group. However, OS was similar between groups: median survival in the radiotherapy group was 7.4 years compared with 7.2 years in the control group. This suggested that radiotherapy could be deferred for patients with low-grade glioma who are carefully monitored.[17]
- A subsequent study (RTOG9802) examined "high risk" grade 2 astrocytoma, oligoastrocytoma, or oligodendroglioma in those who were younger than 40 years of age and had undergone subtotal resection or biopsy or who were 40 years of age or older, and compared RT alone or to RT followed by 6 cycles of PCV. The PCV regimen consisted of 42-day cycles of lomustine 110 mg/m^2 orally, day 1 (max 200 mg), procarbazine 60 mg/m^2 orally, days 8 to 21, and vincristine 1.4 mg/m^2 intravenously (max 2 mg per dose), days 8 and 29. Patients who received RT plus chemotherapy had longer mOS than did those who received RT alone (13.3 vs. 7.8 years).[18]
- A post hoc analysis of RTOG 9802 also found that patients with *IDH*-mutant high-risk low-grade glioma irrespective of co-deletion status derive benefit from the addition of PCV.[19]
- *Low-risk (less than 40 years old with a gross total resection) oligodendroglioma, IDH-mutant, 1p/19q co-deleted, grade 2 patients can be monitored with surveillance alone with periodic MRI of the brain scans deferring immediate postsurgery radiation and/or chemotherapy (Table 24.1).*
- *High-risk (less than 40 years old with a biopsy or subtotal resection or older than 40) oligodendroglioma, IDH-mutant, 1p/19q co-deleted, grade 2 patients should receive postoperative RT (54 Gy in 30 fractions) followed by adjuvant chemotherapy (6 cycles of adjuvant PCV chemotherapy or 12 cycles of adjuvant temozolomide; Table 24.1).*

Oligodendroglioma, *IDH*-Mutant, 1p/19q Co-Deleted, Grade 3
- The RTOG 9402 trial included anaplastic oligodendrogliomas or anaplastic oligoastrocytomas and inspected 4 cycles of intensified PCV followed by RT or immediate RT without chemotherapy. OS was found to be increased in patients receiving PCV followed by RT compared with only RT initially (median 14.7 vs. 7.3 years).[23]
- The EORTC study 26951 also examined newly diagnosed anaplastic oligodendroglial tumors, which were randomly assigned to either 59.4 Gy of RT or the same RT followed by 6 cycles of adjuvant. PFS was significantly increased when patients were treated with RT plus PCV compared with RT alone (median 157 vs. 50 months), and there was

a trend toward increase in OS (median not reached vs. 112 months) for patients with 1p/19q co-deletions.[24]

- *Regardless of age or resection status, oligodendroglioma, IDH-mutant, 1p/19q co-deleted, grade 3 patients should receive postoperative RT (59.4 to 60 Gy in 1.8 to 2 Gy fractions) followed by adjuvant chemotherapy (6 cycles of adjuvant PCV chemotherapy or 12 cycles of adjuvant temozolomide; Table 24.1).*

Recommended Treatment Plan for This Patient
- *Postoperative RT (59.4 to 60 Gy in 1.8 to 2 Gy fractions) followed by adjuvant chemotherapy (12 cycles of adjuvant temozolomide)*

What Are the Toxicities Associated With Standard of Care Treatments?

Radiation
- Radiation can acutely cause hair loss, lack of energy, decreased appetite/weight loss, headaches, nausea/vomiting, and radiation dermatitis.
- Potential long-term effects of radiation include progressive delayed neurocognitive impairment and a low risk of secondary tumor formation (meningioma).

Adjuvant Temozolomide
- A CBC should be obtained prior to each adjuvant temozolomide cycle to monitor for hematologic toxicity.
- Temozolomide-linked aplastic anemia, myelodysplasia, plasmablastic lymphoma, and t-AML have been rarely reported.
- Common nonhematologic side effects of temozolomide include constipation, nausea/vomiting, decreased appetite, weight loss, rash, and fatigue. Hepatotoxicity can occur and a CMP should also be obtained prior to each adjuvant temozolomide cycle.
- In both pregnant patients and pregnant partners of male patients, fetal harm and adverse developmental outcomes associated with temozolomide exposure have been reported. Patients should be on effective contraception if they have reproductive potential.

Procarbazine, Lomustine, and Vincristine
- PCV can also cause hematologic effects or hepatotoxicity. Before day 1 of each cycle, a CBC and CMP should be completed. Weekly CBCs are often done starting at week 4.
- Dose adjustments of lomustine and procarbazine are typically performed for hematologic toxicity depending on the extent of the nadir and length of recovery.
- Dose adjustments may be necessary for all three drugs based on the timing and severity of hepatotoxicity.
- Lomustine and procarbazine can cause nausea/vomiting, and patients should receive premedication with antiemetics before each dose.
- Lomustine can very rarely lead to serious pulmonary toxicity (infiltrates, fibrosis).
- Procarbazine has possible drug–drug and drug–food interactions based on weak inhibition of MAO in the gastrointestinal system. Tyramine-rich foods (for example, aged cheese, smoked meats) should not be eaten, and concomitant use of an MAO inhibitor is contraindicated due to the risk of hypertensive crisis. Alcohol use is also not allowed due to the risk of a disulfiram-like reaction. Additionally, procarbazine hypersensitivity can lead to cutaneous maculopapular rash and should be discontinued if a rash develops.
- Vincristine can commonly cause constipation secondary to autonomic neuropathy and/or length-dependent sensory peripheral neuropathy.

What Are Other Treatment Considerations?

Procarbazine, Lomustine, and Vincristine Versus Temozolomide for Adjunctive Therapy in High-Risk Astrocytoma, *IDH*-Mutant, Grade 2 Tumors

- PCV and temozolomide are both rational options for adjunctive therapy in astrocytoma, *IDH*-mutant, Grade 2 tumors. Use of PCV is supported by results of the RTOG 9802, whereas temozolomide was used in CATNON. Temozolomide is easier to administer as it does not require an IV infusion and has better patient tolerance due to typically fewer side effects.[18,20]

Necessity of Vincristine in Procarbazine, Lomustine, and Vincristine Regimen

- Vincristine has been demonstrated to not cross an intact blood-brain barrier, so its usefulness in this combination regimen is uncertain. However, studies comparing PCV with a two-drug regimen (lomustine and procarbazine) are limited, but due to the unclear benefit of vincristine it is frequently stopped quickly if neurotoxicity is seen.[21]

What Is Required for This Patient's Follow-Up and Survivorship?

- *Requirements are MRI of the brain with and without contrast postoperatively to determine the extent of surgical resection, then every 3 months for the first 2 years, then every 4 four months for 2 years, then every 6 months for several years, then yearly as long as there is no evidence of recurrent tumor.*
- *PT/OT/Speech therapy evaluations should be performed following surgery to identify patients who may benefit from rehab or outpatient therapies.*
- *Patients who have had seizures should remain on antiepileptic prophylaxis, while those who have not had seizures can be tapered off if started prior to surgery. Radiation and chemotherapy are also correlated with better seizure control in patients.[22]*
- *Patients with reproductive potential in whom chemotherapy is planned should be informed of the potential for infertility. Men can be referred for sperm banking, and women can be referred to reproductive specialists for discussion of fertility preservation possibilities such as embryo and oocyte cryopreservation if interested in future paternity. This is ideally to be done prior to the patient starting chemotherapy.*
- *Patients should be routinely evaluated for fatigue, changes in mental status, and mood, including depression and anxiety.*
- *Glioma patients are at high risk for neurocognitive deficits. Baseline neurocognitive testing can be helpful for comparison if neurocognitive changes are reported during or after treatments. Cognitive rehabilitation can be beneficial in certain patients with deficits.*
- *Many patients will require short-term or permanent disability secondary to neurological deficits, seizures, and/or change in their cognition, potentially preventing them from being able to return to their prior occupation.*

REVIEW QUESTIONS

1. A 65-year-old man with no major past medical history (PMH) except for hyperlipidemia is seen in the ED for right-sided weakness and falls for a few weeks. CT of the head without contrast reveals a left frontal lobe mass with vasogenic edema. This is confirmed with MRI of the brain with and without contrast. He has excellent performance status (PS) and the neurosurgery team thinks he is a good surgical candidate. What is the most appropriate next step?
   A. Radiation oncology consult for stereotactic brain radiation
   B. Neoadjuvant chemoradiotherapy with oral temozolomide
   C. Craniotomy and maximal safe resection
   D. Lumbar puncture

2. The patient in question 1 undergoes resection of the mass, and histopathological features are suggestive of glioblastoma. Which of these molecular testing methods is also necessary to diagnose his disease?
   A. *MGMT* promoter methylation status
   B. *BRAF* mutation status
   C. *NTRK* fusion status
   D. *IDH* mutation status

3. A 72-year-old woman with a history of hypertension, type 2 diabetes mellitus, and fibromyalgia is found to have a mass in the left parietal lobe during evaluation of new-onset seizure. Her Eastern Cooperative Oncology Group (ECOG) is 0. She undergoes craniotomy and surgical resection. Her diagnosis is glioblastoma *IDH* wildtype. What is the most appropriate next step in her treatment?
   A. 6 weeks of concomitant chemoradiotherapy with oral temozolomide followed by 6 cycles of adjuvant temozolomide
   B. Sequential induction with 6 cycles of oral temozolomide followed by 6 weeks of focal radiation treatment
   C. 12 cycles of oral temozolomide
   D. Observation

4. The woman in question 3 is scheduled to start chemoradiotherapy with oral temozolomide soon. Presence of which of these molecular features in her tumor predicts greater response to oral temozolomide?
   A. *IDH* wildtype status
   B. Methylated *MGMT* promoter
   C. *P53* mutation
   D. *BRAF* mutation

5. The same patient as in questions 3 and 4 presents for follow-up in a medical oncology clinic 4 weeks after completing chemoradiotherapy. She is now on adjuvant oral temozolomide. She reports intermittent 4/10 generalized headache for the past 2 weeks that improves with over-the-counter (OTC) oral acetaminophen. She has no new focal deficit. Urgent MRI of the brain with and without contrast reveals increased contrast enhancement and T2 hyperintensity within the treatment field compared to prechemoradiation scan. Which of these interventions is least reasonable at this time?

   A. Short course oral dexamethasone
   B. Repeat MRI of the brain in 4 weeks

C. Continue adjuvant oral temozolomide

D. Discontinue oral temozolomide and start procarbazine, lomustine, and vincristine (PCV)

6. A 37-year-old man with past medical history (PMH) of obesity and type 2 diabetes mellitus on oral medications is found to have a mass in the right frontal cortex during a workup of left-sided arm weakness and persistent headache. He underwent a craniotomy, and postoperative imaging revealed a gross total surgical resection. Histopathology is consistent with infiltrating glioma, grade 2. Further molecular testing of tumor cells is positive for *IDH1* mutation as well as co-deletion of 1p and 19q. What is the most likely diagnosis?

A. Astrocytoma

B. Meningioma

C. Oligodendroglioma

D. Glioblastoma

7. What is the next best step in the treatment of the patient in question 6?

A. Surveillance with periodic MRI brain

B. 6 weeks of concomitant chemoradiotherapy with oral temozolomide followed by 6 cycles of adjuvant temozolomide

C. Post-op radiation only

D. Post-op radiation followed by adjuvant chemotherapy

8. A 55-year-old woman is diagnosed with astrocytoma, *IDH*-mutant, grade 3 after she had maximal resection of a left parietal lobe mass. Her Eastern Cooperative Oncology Group (ECOG) is 0. What is the most appropriate next step in her treatment?

A. Surveillance with periodic MRI of the brain

B. 6 weeks of concomitant chemoradiotherapy with oral temozolomide followed by 6 cycles of adjuvant temozolomide

C. Post-op radiation only

D. Post-op radiation followed by adjuvant temozolomide chemotherapy

9. A 66-year-old man is diagnosed with astrocytoma *IDH*-mutant, grade 4 after a maximal resection of a right temporal lobe mass. His Eastern Cooperative Oncology Group (ECOG) is 1. What is the most appropriate next step in his treatment?

A. Surveillance with periodic MRI brain

B. 6 weeks of concomitant chemoradiotherapy with oral temozolomide followed by 6 cycles of adjuvant temozolomide

C. Post-op radiation only

D. Post-op radiation followed by adjuvant procarbazine, lomustine, and vincristine (PCV) chemotherapy

10. Which of these molecular findings would not be expected for diffuse astrocytic gliomas?

A. *ATRX* mutation

B. *IDH1/2* mutation

C. 1p/19q co-deletion

D. *P53* mutation

ANSWERS AND RATIONALES

1. **C. Craniotomy and maximal safe resection.** Maximal safe resection is the preferred approach if possible. Biopsy can be used in situations of poor PS or when the mass is in a location not amenable to surgery. Lumbar puncture could precipitate herniation and should be avoided.

2. **D. *IDH* mutation status.** All newly diagnosed glioblastoma should undergo testing for *IDH* mutation status. Immunohistochemistry (IHC) for the most common *IDH* mutation in gliomas, *IDH1* R132H, captures approximately 90% of *IDH* mutations in gliomas. If R132H-mutant *IDH1* IHC is negative, sequencing of *IDH1* and *IDH2* should be performed in younger patients (younger than 55 years), as *IDH*-mutation status is integral to an accurate diagnosis. A glioblastoma must be *IDH wildtype*. The other molecular tests are not necessary to diagnose glioblastoma.

3. **A. 6 weeks of concomitant chemoradiotherapy with oral temozolomide followed by 6 cycles of adjuvant temozolomide.** The standard of care for newly diagnosed glioblastoma is maximal safe resection followed by 6 weeks of focal intensity modulated radiation therapy (60 Gy in 30 fractions) plus concomitant oral temozolomide 75 mg/m^2 body surface area (BSA), followed by 6 cycles of adjuvant temozolomide (150 to 200 mg/m^2 for 5 days during each 28-day cycle). This was shown in a randomized clinical trial to prolong median survival by an additional 2.5 months compared to radiation alone (14.6 months vs. 12.1 months) as well as increase long-term 5-year overall survival (9.8% vs. 1.9%).[3,4]

4. **B. Methylated *MGMT* promoter.** *MGMT* is an enzyme that is integral for DNA repair after alkylating-agent chemotherapy. The *MGMT* gene can be silenced by methylation of its promoter during tumor development, thus inhibiting repair of DNA damage and enhancing the possible effectiveness of alkylating agent chemotherapy. Methylated tumors have a better prognosis and are predictive of response to alkylating-agent chemotherapy.[2]

5. **D. Discontinue oral temozolomide and start procarbazine, lomustine, and vincristine (PCV).** This patient has pseudoprogression. This refers to the phenomenon of increased contrast enhancement and surrounding T2/FLAIR hyperintensity within the radiation treatment field that may be noticed on postchemoradiation scan obtained 4 weeks after concurrent chemoradiation, compared to prechemoradiation scan (or may even occur several months after chemoradiation). This is considered the "treatment effect," hence the term "tumor pseudoprogression." This is different from new contrast enhancement outside of the radiation treatment field, which should be considered tumor progression and treated accordingly.

   Patients with suspected pseudoprogression should continue with adjuvant temozolomide cycles as planned. If symptomatic, a short course of steroids or bevacizumab can be used to decrease edema and mass effect.

6. **C. Oligodendroglioma.** Oligodendroglioma are molecularly classified, diffusely infiltrating gliomas that must contain both an *IDH1* or *IDH2* mutation and co-deletion of chromosome arms 1p and 19q.

7. **A. Surveillance with periodic MRI of the brain.** Low-risk (less than 40 years old with a gross total resection) oligodendroglioma, *IDH*-mutant, 1p/19q co-deleted, grade 2 patients can be monitored with surveillance alone with periodic MRI of the brain scans, deferring immediate post-surgery radiation and/or chemotherapy.

8. **D. Post-op radiation followed by adjuvant temozolomide chemotherapy.** Regardless of age or resection status, astrocytoma, *IDH*-mutant, grade 3 patients should receive postoperative radiation therapy (RT; 59.4 to 60 Gy in 1.8 to 2 Gy fractions) followed by adjuvant chemotherapy of 12 cycles of adjuvant temozolomide based on The CATNON (EORTC study 26053-22054) trial, which found that adjuvant temozolomide chemotherapy, but not concurrent temozolomide chemotherapy, was associated with a survival benefit in patients with 1p/19q non-co-deleted anaplastic glioma.

9. **B. 6 weeks of concomitant chemoradiotherapy with oral temozolomide followed by 6 cycles of adjuvant temozolomide.** Historically, astrocytoma *IDH*-mutant, grade 4 tumors have been included in trials for glioblastoma. Treatment is similar to glioblastoma *IDH* wildtype, with maximal safe resection followed by 6 weeks of focal intensity modulated radiation therapy (RT; 60 Gy in 30 fractions) plus concomitant oral temozolomide 75 mg/m^2 body surface area (BSA), followed by 6 cycles of adjuvant temozolomide (150 to 200 mg/m^2 for 5 days during each 28-day cycle).

10. **C. 1p/19q co-deletion.** Alpha-thalassemia/mental retardation syndrome X-linked (*ATRX*) mutations are regularly found in diffuse astrocytic gliomas. *ATRX* mutations are closely correlated with *IDH1/2* and *TP53* mutations and are mutually exclusive with 1p/19q co-deletion.

REFERENCES

1. Louis DN, Perry A, Wesseling P, et al. The 2021 WHO classification of tumors of the central nervous system: a summary. *Neuro-Oncology.* 2021;23(8):1231–1251. doi:10.1093/neuonc/noab106
2. Hegi ME, Diserens AC, Gorlia T, et al. *MGMT* gene silencing and benefit from temozolomide in glioblastoma. *N Engl J Med.* 10 2005;352(10):997–1003. doi:10.1056/NEJMoa043331
3. Stupp R, Mason WP, van den Bent MJ, et al. Radiotherapy plus concomitant and adjuvant temozolomide for glioblastoma. *N Engl J Med.* 2005;352(10):987–996. doi:10.1056/NEJMoa043330
4. Stupp R, Hegi ME, Mason WP, et al. Effects of radiotherapy with concomitant and adjuvant temozolomide versus radiotherapy alone on survival in glioblastoma in a randomised phase III study: 5-year analysis of the EORTC-NCIC trial. *The Lancet Oncology.* 2009;10(5):459–466. doi:10.1016/s1470-2045(09)70025-7
5. Balana C, Vaz MA, Manuel Sepúlveda J, et al. A phase II randomized, multicenter, open-label trial of continuing adjuvant temozolomide beyond 6 cycles in patients with glioblastoma (GEINO 14-01). *Neuro-oncology.* 2020;22(12):1851–1861. doi:10.1093/neuonc/noaa107
6. Stupp R, Taillibert S, Kanner A, et al. Effect of tumor-treating fields plus maintenance temozolomide vs maintenance temozolomide alone on survival in patients with glioblastoma: a randomized clinical trial. *Jama.* 2017;318(23):2306–2316. doi:10.1001/jama.2017.18718
7. Herrlinger U, Tzaridis T, Mack F, et al. Lomustine-temozolomide combination therapy versus standard temozolomide therapy in patients with newly diagnosed glioblastoma with methylated *MGMT* promoter (CeTeG/NOA-09): a randomised, open-label, phase 3 trial. *Lancet (London, England).* 2019;393(10172):678–688. doi:10.1016/s0140-6736(18)31791-4
8. Brandes AA, Franceschi E, Tosoni A, et al. *MGMT* promoter methylation status can predict the incidence and outcome of pseudoprogression after concomitant radiochemotherapy in newly diagnosed glioblastoma patients. *Am J Clin Oncol.* 2008;26(13):2192–2197. doi:10.1200/jco.2007.14.8163
9. Perry JR, Laperriere N, O'Callaghan CJ, et al. Short-course radiation plus temozolomide in elderly patients with glioblastoma. *N Engl J Med.* 2017;376(11):1027–1037. doi:10.1056/NEJMoa1611977
10. Keime-Guibert F, Chinot O, Taillandier L, et al. Radiotherapy for glioblastoma in the elderly. *N Engl J Med.* 2007;356(15):1527–1535. doi:10.1056/NEJMoa065901
11. Wick W, Platten M, Meisner C, et al. Temozolomide chemotherapy alone versus radiotherapy alone for malignant astrocytoma in the elderly: the NOA-08 randomised, phase 3 trial. *Lancet Oncol.* 2012;13(7):707–715. doi:10.1016/s1470-2045(12)70164-x
12. Malmström A, Grønberg BH, Marosi C, et al. Temozolomide versus standard 6-week radiotherapy versus hypofractionated radiotherapy in patients older than 60 years with glioblastoma: the Nordic randomised, phase 3 trial. *The Lancet Oncology.* 2012;13(9):916–926. doi:10.1016/s1470-2045(12)70265-6

13. Yust-Katz S, Mandel JJ, Wu J, et al. Venous thromboembolism (VTE) and glioblastoma. *J Neurooncol.* 2015;124(1):87–94. doi:10.1007/s11060-015-1805-2

14. Broen MPG, Smits M, Wijnenga MMJ, et al. The T2-FLAIR mismatch sign as an imaging marker for non-enhancing *IDH*-mutant, 1p/19q-intact lower-grade glioma: a validation study. *Neuro-Oncol.* 2018;20(10):1393–1399. doi:10.1093/neuonc/noy048

15. Deguchi S, Oishi T, Mitsuya K, et al. Clinicopathological analysis of T2-FLAIR mismatch sign in lower-grade gliomas. *Scientific Reports.* 2020;10(1):10113. doi:10.1038/s41598-020-67244-7

16. Louis DN, Giannini C, Capper D, et al. cIMPACT-NOW update 2: diagnostic clarifications for diffuse midline glioma, H3 K27M-mutant and diffuse astrocytoma/anaplastic astrocytoma, *IDH*-mutant. *Acta Neuropathol.* 2018;135(4):639–642. doi:10.1007/s00401-018-1826-y

17. van den Bent MJ, Afra D, de Witte O, et al. Long-term efficacy of early versus delayed radiotherapy for low-grade astrocytoma and oligodendroglioma in adults: the EORTC 22845 randomised trial. *Lancet (London, England).* 2005;366(9490):985–990. doi:10.1016/s0140-6736(05)67070-5

18. Buckner JC, Shaw EG, Pugh SL, et al. Radiation plus procarbazine, CCNU, and vincristine in low-grade glioma. *N Engl J Med.* 2016;374(14):1344–1355. doi:10.1056/NEJMoa1500925

19. Bell EH, Zhang P, Shaw EG, et al. Comprehensive genomic analysis in NRG oncology/RTOG 9802: a phase III trial of radiation versus radiation plus procarbazine, lomustine (CCNU), and vincristine in high-risk low-grade glioma. *Am J Clin Oncol.* 2020;38(29):3407–3417. doi:10.1200/jco.19.02983

20. van den Bent MJ, Tesileanu CMS, Wick W, et al. Adjuvant and concurrent temozolomide for 1p/19q non-co-deleted anaplastic glioma (CATNON; EORTC study 26053-22054): second interim analysis of a randomised, open-label, phase 3 study. *The Lancet Oncol.* 2021;22(6):813–823. doi:10.1016/s1470-2045(21)00090-5

21. Webre C, Shonka N, Smith L, et al. PC or PCV, that is the question: primary anaplastic oligodendroglial tumors treated with procarbazine and CCNU with and without vincristine. *Anticancer Res.* 2015;35(10):5467–5472. https://ar.iiarjournals.org/content/35/10/5467

22. Koekkoek JA, Kerkhof M, Dirven L, et al. Seizure outcome after radiotherapy and chemotherapy in low-grade glioma patients: a systematic review. *Neuro-Oncology.* 2015;17(7):924–934. doi:10.1093/neuonc/nov032

23. Cairncross G, Wang M, Shaw E, et al. Phase III trial of chemoradiotherapy for anaplastic oligodendroglioma: long-term results of RTOG 9402. *J Clin Oncol.* 2013;31(3):337–343. doi:10.1200/jco.2012.43.2674

24. van den Bent MJ, Brandes AA, Taphoorn MJ, et al. Adjuvant procarbazine, lomustine, and vincristine chemotherapy in newly diagnosed anaplastic oligodendroglioma: long-term follow-up of EORTC Brain Tumor Group study 26951. *J Clin Oncol.* 2013;31(3):344–350. doi:10.1200/jco.2012.43.2229

CHAPTER 25

Cancer of Unknown Primary

Marcus Geer, Jennifer Girard, and Francis P. Worden

INTRODUCTION

Cancers of unknown primary (CUPs) are metastatic tumors with an unidentified primary site that are heterogenous in their histological subtype with variable clinical presentation and overall poor prognosis. CUPs account for 2% to 9% of all tumors with approximately 32,000 new cases each year.[1,2] The average age at diagnosis is 60 to 75 years. Histological subtypes include well, moderate, and poorly differentiated adenocarcinoma (most common is about 50% to 70% of cases); squamous cell carcinoma (SCC); poorly differentiated carcinomas; carcinomas with neuroendocrine differentiation; and undifferentiated. For about 80% of patients diagnosed with CUP, prognosis is poor with a median overall survival (mOS) of 3 to 10 months.[1] There is a subset of CUPs with favorable prognosis (about 20%) with mOS of 12 to 36 months that includes those with a resectable tumor, isolated inguinal adenopathy involving SCC, women with adenocarcinoma only involving axillary lymph nodes (LNs), women with papillary adenocarcinoma of the peritoneum, and poorly differentiated neuroendocrine tumor.[1,3]

Clinical Presentation: Patients with CUP present with variable symptoms usually related to sites of disease. Fifty precent of patients present with multiple sites of involvement, with the most common sites including the liver, lungs, bone, and LNs.[3] A prognostic model to predict overall survival (OS) in patients demonstrated a high neutrophil-to-lymphocyte ratio as the strongest predictor of poor OS; other predictors of poor OS in the model included male gender at birth, poor Eastern Cooperative Oncology Group (ECOG) progression-free survival (PFS; 2 or greater), and adenocarcinoma histology, In other studies, additional indicators of poor prognosis include the presence of liver metastases and elevated lactate dehydrogenase (LDH).[4]

Staging: CUPs are metastatic by definition. Diagnosis and staging start with a thorough history, with a physical exam that includes rectal, pelvic, and breast examination. Laboratory studies should include serum complete blood count (CBC), chemistry panel, and LDH as well as serum assessment of alpha-fetoprotein (AFP), beta-human chorionic gonadotropin (beta-hCG), chromogranin A, and prostate-specific antigen (PSA). One can consider sending urinalysis and urine cytology, carbohydrate antigen (CA)-19-9, carcinoembryonic antigen (CEA), CA-15-3, and CA-27.29 in clinical context. Diagnostic imaging should include a minimum of CT of the chest, abdomen, and pelvis. The role of a whole body 2-deoxy-2-[18F]fluoro-D-glucose PET (FDG PET) is to establish a diagnosis of CUP. This is under investigation. A comprehensive review of 10 published studies concluded PET is a useful diagnostic tool in those with cervical nodal metastatic sites and those with a single site of disease with treatment aimed at cure.[5] Endoscopy should be guided based on clinical symptoms and laboratory results.

Patients with suspected CUP should complete a core needle biopsy with sufficient tissue to send for multiple immunohistochemistry (IHC) markers as well as for microsatellite instability (MSI)/mismatch repair (MMR) status and tumor molecular profiling. IHC is critical and identifies a primary origin of chemosensitive or curable tumors 30% of the time. Large panels of markers should be avoided. Typically, cytokeratins CK7/CK20, PSA (men), estrogen receptor (ER)/progesterone receptor (PR) status (women), thyroid transcription factor 1 (TTF-1), NapsinA, thyroglobulin, calcitonin, chromogranin, synaptophysin, AFP, OCT4, hcg, S1000, and vimentin/desmin should be considered within clinical context to attempt to identify a primary tumor site[1,3] (Table 25.1).

Certain patterns of cytokeratin markers lend clues to primary sites that should prompt addition IHC stains to attempt to identify a primary tumor (Table 25.2).

There exists a subset of patients, about 20% of those diagnosed with CUP, that present with a defined, favorable risk disease (Table 25.3) and should be treated accordingly.

Additionally, molecular gene expression profiling to predict tissue of origin is important as it can identify origin and allow for site-specific therapy. A prospective trial completed at the Sarah Cannon Research Institute in 2013 used a 92-gene reverse transcription polymerase chain reaction (RT-PCR) cancer classification assay on 252 patients with CUP and predicted a tumor of origin in 98% of patients. The most common tumor origins predicted were biliary (18%), urothelium (11%), colorectal (10%), and non-small cell lung cancer (NSCLC; 7%). In the study, 232 patients were treated and 194 received assay-directed therapy with median survival of 12.5 months, with statistically significant improvement in OS for those patients with chemo-responsive tumor origins versus those with poorly responsive tumor origins (13.4 vs. 7.6 months; $p = 0.04$). It remains unclear if site-directed therapy improves OS in patients with CUP from this one study; however, it does suggest that identifying a subset of patients that will respond favorably to treatment can improve survival over the historical mOS of 10 months.[6-9]

Table 25.1 Probable Primaries Based on Immunohistochemistry Staining

Cancer Type	Cytokeratin Status	IHC Staining Pattern
Undifferentiated carcinoma	Positive	± ER/PR ± Vimentin/desmin
Prostate cancer		+ PSA
Breast cancer		± ER/PR ± Vimentin/desmin
Colorectal cancer		CK20+ CK7- CDX2+
Lung adenocarcinoma		TTF1, NapsinA
Thyroid cancer		+ Thyroglobulin, calcitonin ± Chromogranin, synaptophysin ± TTF1
Neuroendocrine		+ Chromogranin, synaptophysin ± Thyroglobulin, calcitonin ± TTF1/NapsinA
Germ cell		+ OCT4, AFP, hCG, PLAP ± Vimentin/desmin
Melanoma	Negative	+ S100/HMB45 ± Vimentin/desmin
Sarcoma		+ Vimentin/desmin ± S100/HMB45

AFP, alpha-fetoprotein; CK, cytokeratin; ER, estrogen receptor; hCG, human chorionic gonadotropin; IHC, immunohistochemistry; LCA, leukocyte common antigen; NSE, neuron-specific enolase; PR, progesterone receptor; PLAP, placental alkaline phosphatase; PSA, prostate-specific antigen; TTF1, thyroid transcription factor 1.

Table 25.2 Immunohistochemistry Markers for Cancer of Unknown Primary

Stain	Possible Primary Site	Additional IHC Stains
CK7- CK20+	Colorectal Merkel cell	CEA, CDX2
CK7+ CK20-	Lung Breast Pancreatic/cholangiocarcinoma Thyroid Cervical/Endometrial	TTF1 ER/PR GCDFP-15 CK19
CK7+ CK20+	Urothelial Ovarian Pancreatic/Cholangiocarcinoma	Urothelin, GATA3 WT-1
CK7- CK20-	Hepatocellular Renal cell Prostate Squamous cell	PSA Hep Par 1
AE1/AE3	Carcinoma	
CK5/6, p63/p40	Squamous cell	
Calretinin	Mesothelial tumor	

Table 25.3 Favorable Risk Cancers of Unknown Primary

CUP Subtype	Tumor Equivalent	Treatment
Poorly differentiated neuroendocrine tumor of unknown primary	Poorly differentiated neuroendocrine tumors	Platinum (carboplatin, cisplatin) Etoposide
Well-differentiated neuroendocrine tumor of unknown primary	Well-differentiated neuroendocrine tumor	Somatostatin analogues Streptozocin+ 5-FU Sunitinib Everolimus
Peritoneal serous papillary adenocarcinoma	Ovarian	Surgical debulking Carboplatin and taxol
SCC of non-supraclavicular cervical LNs	Head and neck SCC	Neck dissection +/- radiation Chemoradiation with platinum
Colorectal IHC (CK20+ CDX2+ CK7-)	Metastatic colon cancer	Oxaliplatin-containing regimen: FOLFOX, FOLFIRI +/- bevacizumab
Single metastatic site		Resection Radiation therapy Consider systemic therapy
Men with blastic bone lesions and elevated PSA	Prostate cancer	Androgen deprivation therapy +/- Radiation therapy

CK, cytokeratin; 5-FU, 5-fluorouracil; FOLFIRI, 5-FU and irinotecan; FOLFOX, 5-FU and oxaliplatin; IHC, immunohistochemistry; LN, lymph node; PSA, prostate- specific antigen; SCC, squamous cell carcinoma.

CASE SUMMARIES

Case 25.1: Squamous Cell Carcinoma of the Head and Neck

A 56-year-old male with a 45 pack-year smoking history notices a neck mass just under his jaw that is causing a nagging pain when he chews. He feels the mass increased in size over the last several months. He has no medical comorbidities and no personal or family history of diabetes. Performance status is 0—he works full time and is active outdoors on the weekend. He has lost 10 pounds over the last month as he is having difficulty swallowing. He undergoes direct laryngoscopy under anesthesia with otolaryngology with no identifiable mass in the nasopharynx, hypopharynx, or larynx. CT of the neck identifies 4 × 3 cm level II right-sided cervical LN with two to three additional borderline enlarged LNs.

How Is a Cancer of Unknown Primary of the Head and Neck Diagnosed?

- Obtain fine needle aspiration (FNA) of the cervical LN or core needle biopsy to make a tissue diagnosis.
- Direct visualization with fiberoptic examination under anesthetic and biopsies should be completed to attempt to identify a primary tumor.
- Complete staging to attempt to identify a primary source with CT of the neck, chest, abdomen, and pelvis or PET/CT.
- Common histologies of a neck mass with unknown primary include SCC, adenocarcinoma, anaplastic/undifferentiated epithelial tumors, lymphoma, thyroid cancer, and melanoma.
- Core needle biopsy or FNA should undergo testing for Epstein-Barr virus-encoded RNA in situ hybridization (EBER-ISH) and p16 for SCC, thyroglobulin, calcitonin, PAX8, and TFF if anaplastic histology to identify a thyroid primary.
- **Note: For unknown primary tumors that stain positive for EBER, the T stage becomes T0, and they are treated as Epstein-Barr virus (EBV)+ nasopharyngeal carcinomas. For unknown primary tumors that stain positive for p16, the T stage becomes T0, and they are treated as human papillomavirus (HPV)+ oropharyngeal carcinomas.**
- For level I, II, III, and upper V cervical LN masses positive for malignancy, consider tonsillectomy in addition to the previously noted recommendations.
- For level IV and lower V cervical LNs positive for malignancy, consider esophagogastroduodenoscopy (EGD) and bronchoscopy in addition to the previously noted recommendations (Figure 25.1).

Case Update

- *The patient undergoes core needle biopsy of the enlarged right-sided LN which demonstrates a poorly differentiated SCC; p63-positive, p16-negative, negative for EBV. PET/CT demonstrates fluorodeoxyglucose (FDG)-avid level II right cervical LNs, with the largest measuring 4 cm with two borderline enlarged 1 cm LNs; it is otherwise normal. He undergoes tonsillectomy including lingual tonsillectomy, which is negative for malignancy.*

How Do You Establish Regional Lymph Node Involvement?

- Involvement is based on the American Joint Committee on Cancer (AJCC) eighth edition tumor, lymph node, metastasis (TNM) staging system for cervical LNs and unknown primary tumors of the head and neck (Table 25.4).

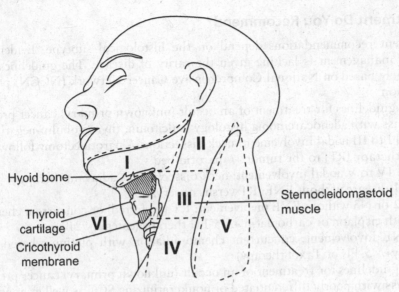

Figure 25.1 Labeled diagram of neck

Case Update

- *Based on staging, our patient has an SCC of unknown primary involving three right-sided level II cervical LNs, with the largest 4 cm in size with no evidence for extranodal extension (ENE) on imaging, therefore N2 disease.*

Table 25.4 N Staging for p16-, p16+, and EBV+ Squamous Cell Cancers of the Head and Neck

N staging for p16 [HPV]-negative cancer of unknown primary of the head and neck

N1	Metastasis in single ipsilateral LN, ≤3 cm without ENE
N2	a: Metastasis in single ipsilateral LN >3 cm but ≤6 cm without ENE b: Metastases in multiple ipsilateral nodes ≤6 cm without ENE c: Metastases in bilateral or contralateral LNs ≤6 cm without ENE
N3	a: Metastasis in single LN >6 cm without ENE b: Metastasis in any nodes ENE+

N staging for p16 [HPV]-positive cancer of unknown primary of the head and neck

N1	One or more ipsilateral LNs, none larger than 6 cm
N2	Contralateral or bilateral LNs, none larger than 6 cm
N3	LN(s) larger than 6 cm

N staging for EBER-ISH [EBV]-positive cancer of unknown primary of the head and neck

N1	Unilateral metastasis in LN(s), 6 cm or less in greatest dimension, above the supraclavicular fossa.
N2	Bilateral metastasis in LN(s) 6 cm or less in greatest dimension, above the supraclavicular fossa
N3	Metastasis in a LN(s) a: Greater than 6 cm in dimension b: Extension to the supraclavicular fossa

EBER-ISH, Epstein-Barr virus-encoded RNA in situ hybridization; EBV, Epstein-Barr virus; ENE, extranodal extension; HPV, human papillomavirus.

What Treatment Do You Recommend?

- Treatment recommendations depend on the histological subtype. Evidence to guide clinical management is lacking given the rarity of disease. The guidelines that follow are largely based on National Comprehensive Cancer Network (NCCN) panel member discussion.
- NCCN guidelines for treatment of an occult (unknown primary) cancer presenting as a neck mass with adenocarcinoma histology (calcitonin, thyroglobulin-negative):
  - Level I to III nodal involvement: neck dissection +/- parotidectomy followed by radiation therapy (RT) to the tumor +/- parotid bed.
  - Level IV to V nodal involvement: neck dissection +/- adjuvant therapy
    - N1 disease without ENE: RT versus observation
    - N2 or N3 without ENE involvement: RT (preferred) or concurrent chemoradiation with cisplatin or carboplatin +/- 5-FU therapy (category 2B)
    - ENE involvement: concurrent chemoradiation with platinum-based chemotherapy +/- 5-FU or Taxol therapy)
- NCCN guidelines for treatment of an occult (unknown primary) cancer presenting as a neck mass with poorly differentiated or nonkeratinizing SCC as well as anaplastic carcinoma that is not of thyroid origin:
  - Definitive therapy for N1 disease:
    - Neck dissection (preferred) with postoperative RT or observation.
    - RT (cat 2B); based on retrospective single institution study from M. D. Anderson involving 52 patients, with 13 patients receiving radiation (intensity modulated radiation therapy [IMRT]) followed by neck dissection and 13 receiving neck dissection prior to radiation, 14 patients with N1 disease who had excisional biopsy, and 14 who received chemotherapy with the study demonstrating 8% disease-free survival and 89% OS.[10]
  - Definitive therapy for N2 or N3 disease:
    - Neck dissection (preferred); postoperative management in those patients without ENE with RT is preferred and concurrent chemoradiation is a category 2B recommendation. When ENE is present, treat with concurrent chemoradiation. (category 1).
    - Concurrent chemoradiation (category 2B).
    - Induction chemotherapy followed by concurrent chemoradiation is useful in certain circumstances but is a category 3 recommendation.
- Principles of surgery, radiation, and systemic therapy:
  - Ipsilateral neck dissection should include level I to IV LNs sampling 18 LNs.
  - Postoperative chemoradiation 60 Gy in 2.2 Gy/fraction over 6 to 7 weeks with either weekly cisplatin 40 mg/m^2 or every 3 weeks 100 mg/m^2.
  - Definitive chemoradiation with 70 Gy IMRT in 2 Gy fractions and 100 mg/m^2 cisplatin every 3 weeks or carboplatin 70 mg/m^2 days 1 to 4 and 600 mg/m^2/day infusional 5-FU for 96 hours every 3 weeks.

Case Update

- *Based on staging, our patient has an SCC of unknown primary involving three right-sided level II cervical LNs, the largest being 4 cm in size with no evidence for ENE on imaging, therefore suggesting N2 disease. He underwent right neck dissection of level I to IV LNs and 19 nodes were removed; three of the LNs were positive for SCC with extranodal extension from the largest 4 cm LN. Therefore, he underwent adjuvant therapy with concurrent chemoradiation therapy with 40 mg/m^2 cisplatin weekly while receiving 66 Gy radiation Monday through Friday in 2.2 Gy fractions.*

Treatment of Recurrent or Persistent Disease

- *Case Update: Our patient was doing well for 5 years. He then noted abdominal back pain and bloating and lost about 20 to 30 lbs. His energy has been much lower than normal for the past 2 or 3 months. He reports to the ED. CT of the abdomen and pelvis is performed and demonstrates multiple 1- to 2-cm masses in the liver concerning for metastatic disease with note of incompletely characterized lung nodules. CT of the chest shows multiple bilateral 1- to 3-cm lung nodules. The patient undergoes a core needle biopsy of a liver mass and it is positive for a poorly differentiated SCC: p63-positive, nonkeratinizing, p16-negative.*
- Patients with distant metastatic disease with recurrent SCC of unknown primary of the head and neck should be treated as very advanced head and neck cancers (see Chapter 1, "Head and Neck Cancer").

Case 25.2: Poorly Differentiated Carcinoma of Unknown Primary

A 67-year-old female presents to the ED with failure to thrive. She notes about 1 year ago she was in her usual state of health, working and running her household. About 6 months ago she noted fatigue and started to lose weight, and about 4 months ago she noted abdominal pain, bloating, and back pain at the level of her bra strap. Over the past 2 weeks she noted yellowing in her eyes, vomiting, and confusion. Labs in the ED are notable for a white count of 15,000, neutrophil count of 13,000, hemoglobin of 10.3 milligrams/deciliter, platelet count of 120,000, creatinine of 1.3 with elevated aspartate aminotransferase (AST) 100, alanine aminotransferase (ALT) 98, Tbili 4.9, Alk Phos 480, and LDH 490. CT with contrast of the chest, abdomen, and pelvis reveals a T7 compression fracture without cord impingement, blastic appearing lesions in the spine and iliac bone with innumerable liver mets ranging in size from 0.5 to 2 cm with intrahepatic ductal dilatation and enlarged mesenteric, and retroperitoneal and perigastric LNs measuring from 2 to 3 cm in size.

What Additional Workup Is Required?

- Initial workup should focus on finding a primary site for the tumor. Additional workup should be based on the patient's history, symptoms, and clinical signs.
- *Case Update: The patient reports that she has noticed intermittent dark stools. She also notes occasional vaginal spotting without bleeding. Her last mammogram was 4 months ago and was BI-RADS 2. Her last colonoscopy was 7 years ago at the age of 60. She has never had an EGD. Her mother had breast cancer in her 70s. She has two sisters—no cancer history. No family history of colon, prostate, or pancreatic cancer.*
- The next step would be to obtain a tissue diagnosis. She has masses suspicious for cancer in the bone, lung, and liver. The decision on where to biopsy is an important consideration. Bone biopsies should be avoided when possible due to limited tissue and the inability to complete molecular testing and next-generation sequencing (NGS). When requesting biopsy for CUP, request multiple core biopsies as extended IHC testing, NGS, and MMR/MSI status should be considered to fully characterize the sample. In our patient's case, the best site for a biopsy would be the liver.
- Molecular gene expression profiling to predict tumor of origin is important as it can identify the origin and allow for site-specific therapy based on a prospective trial completed at the Sarah Cannon Research Institute, as previously discussed. Biliary tract was most commonly predicted (18%), followed by urothelium (11%), colorectal (10%), and NSCLC (7%). In the study, 232 patients were treated and 194 received

assay-directed therapy with median survival of 12.5 months. There was statistically significant improved OS for chemoresponsive directed therapy of 13.4 versus 7.6 months ($p = 0.04$).[6]

- The role of FDG PET/CT in CUP may be helpful in cervical nodal disease or single-site disease, but is not likely to add much to our patient's case.
- Given abdominal disease, the clinician would also consider a transvaginal ultrasound (US) to visualize the ovaries.
- The role of EGD and colonoscopy should be symptom driven. Given our patient's presentation and history, she should complete these studies.
- The role of tumor markers is suggestive but not conclusive of a primary site. Given female sex and the location of the metastatic disease focused in the abdomen, it would be reasonable to send testing for CA-19-9 (elevations suggestive for pancreatic cancer), CEA (suggestive of colorectal or ovarian cancer), CA-125 (suggestive of ovarian cancer), and CA-15-3 and CA-27-29 (suggestive of breast cancer), as well as AFP (suggestive of hepatocellular carcinoma).
- The role of CNS imaging should be based on symptoms. MRI of the brain is recommended, CT of the head with contrast is acceptable.
- Additionally in this patient's case, magnetic resonance cholangiopancreatography (MRCP) and possibly endoscopic retrograde cholangio-pancreatography (ERCP) could be helpful given obstructive liver disease.

Case Update

- *The patient undergoes successful biopsy of the liver with three core samples. IHC staining demonstrates CK7+ CK20+ AE1/AE3 + poorly differentiated carcinoma; additional stains are negative for p63, s100, HMB45, ER/PR, PAX8, TTF1, chromogranin, vimentin, and synaptophysin. In addition, 6/6 MMR are present on IHC staining. The NGS panel is pending. EGD demonstrates chronic gastritis; biopsies are taken and are negative for neoplasm. Colonoscopy is completed; there are two sessile polyps removed that are noncancerous, and random biopsies of the sigmoid, ascending, and terminal ileum are negative for neoplasm. Tumor markers demonstrate a normal AFP, CA-15-3, and CA-27-29; CEA is 13 (normal range 0–2.5 ug/L), CA-19-9 200 (normal range 0–37 U/mL), and CA-125 85 (normal range 0–35 U/mL). MRCP is completed that demonstrates liver metastases causing intrahepatic ductal dilatation not amenable to stenting. Transvaginal US shows a normal endometrial stripe and normal appearing ovaries.*

What Is the Role of Molecular Gene Expression Profiling in Poorly Differentiated Carcinoma of Unknown Primary?

- Two prospective double-blinded studies of patients with poorly differentiated neoplasms of unknown primary demonstrated statistically significant improvement in identifying a site of origin using tissue of origin molecular profiling rather than IHC (91% vs. 71%; $p = 0.02$).[11]

Case Update

- *Gene expression profiling is unable to identify a tissue of origin, but suggests hepatobiliary or lung origin. You share the results of the biopsy with the patient and the patient's husband. She is tearful and does not understand how a site of cancer cannot be identified from all the testing. Her husband appears distressed and states the house just does not run without her. She remains hospitalized and can get up to go to the bathroom with one person assisting.*

She is only eating about 400 or 500 calories per day, mostly from nutrition supplements. Ursodiol and intravenous (IV) hydration are initiated. Bilirubin and alkaline phosphatase remain elevated. Care management is involved in her discharge planning.

What Is Our Patient's Prognosis?

- Her prognosis is poor as she falls into the high-risk group (elevated LDH, leukocytosis greater than 10 with high neutrophil/lymphocyte ratio, PS 2, visceral involvement with liver mets). Her OS is on the order of 5 to 8 months.

What Treatment Do You Recommend for This Patient?

- Psychosocial distress often accompanies a diagnosis of CUP for the patient and the family. A study completed by Hyphantis et al. noted rates of anxiety and depression in patients with CUP were higher than for all other cancer types.
- End of life and early involvement of palliative care is important given the short OS, especially in patients with poor prognosis where systemic therapies will often not improve OS and therefore may not be offered.

If She Was a Treatment Candidate, What Treatment Could Be Offered?

- Poorly differentiated carcinoma of unknown primary is treated similarly to adenocarcinoma of unknown primary. Systemic therapy in CUP has been determined through Phase II clinical trials in an attempt to improve OS; however despite this, the regimen response rates (RRs) are around 20% with mOS of around 6 months with no clear standard of care between regimens. It is expert consensus to treat with site-specific therapy if the gene expression profile predicts an origin. Treatment should be carefully considered given questionable benefit and considerable toxicity.
  - *Carboplatin and paclitaxel:* Phase II Hellenic Cooperative demonstrated an objective response rate (ORR) of 39%. The German CUP Group compared carboplatin and paclitaxel versus gemcitabine and vinorelbine. The mOS was 11 months, 1 year OS 38%, and ORR 24% for carbo/Taxol versus 7 months, 29% and 20% for gem/vinorelbine. This regimen may be appropriate for our patient's histology.[12]
  - *Cisplatin or carboplatin and docetaxel:* A Phase II Hellenic group trial included 29 patients, of which 28% had an undifferentiated carcinoma. The mOS was 16 months. This regimen may be appropriate for our patient's histology.[13]
  - *Cisplatin and gemcitabine (or docetaxel):* A randomized Phase II trial of gemcitabine and cisplatin (GEFCAPI 01) included mostly well-differentiated adenocarcinoma and would be less appropriate for our patient. This trial demonstrated median ORR of 55% with mOS of 8 months.[14]
  - *Capecitabine and oxaliplatin:* Phase II data in the front-line setting suggest a 12% RR and mOS of 8 months. Use in the second line from a Phase II trial suggests a 19% ORR and mOS of 9.7 months. These trials mainly included patients with adenocarcinoma and would not be appropriate for our patient.[15,16]
- There are a few poorly differentiated carcinomas with good clinical outcomes as they are responsive to chemotherapy:
  - Poorly differentiated carcinoma of midline distribution (extranodal germ cell) should be treated as poor prognosis germ cell tumors (see Chapter 15, "Testicular Cancer").[3]

- ○ Poorly differentiated neuroendocrine carcinomas (NECs) are treated with platinum plus etoposide +/- atezolizumab, much like a small cell carcinoma.[3]
- *NUT* midline carcinoma is identified by the rearrangement of the *NUT* gene with translocation of *BRD3* or *BRD4*. Median age is 24 years with overall poor prognosis, with mOS of 6.5 months regardless of therapy.[17]

The Patient Presents to Your Clinic Outpatient; What Do You Recommend for Treatment?

- *Case Update: The patient is discharged home from the hospital on day 5. She returns to your outpatient clinical 2 weeks later to discuss therapy. Her husband pushes her in a wheelchair to the room. At home she can walk around but feels too tired to go out to eat or go to the store. She is eating some solid foods but still relying on nutritional supplements for most of her calories. She spends most waking hours on the couch and must rest after walking from the couch to the kitchen. Labs at today's visit demonstrate white count of 17,000, neutrophil count of 15,000, hemoglobin of 9.3, platelets of 110, creatinine of 1.4, total bilirubin of 5.4, alk phos of 480, and LDH of 600.*
- Systemic chemotherapy is usually reserved for patients with good function status PS 0 to 2. Her PS currently is 3. Additionally, she has impaired renal function, with elevated bilirubin increasing the risk of toxicity from platinum-based regimen, docetaxel, or paclitaxel, which are the regimens with the highest RRs for patients with poorly differentiated carcinoma. Therefore, discussion of hospice and palliative care is most appropriate.

Case 25.3: Neuroendocrine Cancer of Unknown Primary

A 63-year-old man presents to his primary care provider (PCP) for evaluation of progressive abdominal bloating and epigastric pain. He is generally healthy with well-controlled hypertension. He has a 10 pack-year tobacco history and quit smoking 20 years prior. His pain has progressed over the last 3 weeks and has been accompanied by fatigue and unintentional weight loss of 8 lbs. He has not had any change in stool caliber or bleeding. He has not had any hematuria or lower urinary tract symptoms. On physical exam, he is found to have palpable hepatomegaly without any other stigmata of long-standing liver disease. Lab testing reveals normal blood counts and normal renal function. Liver function testing shows an elevated AST: 89, ALT: 55, and alkaline phosphatase: 234 with normal total bilirubin. Calcium is mildly elevated at 10.5 with a normal albumin of 4.1. CT imaging reveals innumerable hepatic lesions of mostly less than 1 cm, mediastinal and hilar lymphadenopathy without a corresponding pulmonary mass, and diffuse osseous disease. Biopsy of a liver lesion is described as poorly differentiated carcinoma with neuroendocrine features.

How Is the Diagnosis of Neuroendocrine Cancer of Unknown Primary Confirmed?

- Neuroendocrine cancer of unknown primary is rare, representing less than 5% of all CUP.[18]
  - ○ Detection of chromogranin, synaptophysin, and the cytoplasmic protein PGP9.5 by IHC are specific markers of neuroendocrine differentiation. CD56 is a more sensitive marker but less specific.[19]

- o Other markers may provide insight into the possible tissue of origin. For example, TTF1 is expressed in poorly differentiated tumors and well-differentiated tumors of the lung. CDX2 is expressed in tumors of intestinal origin.[19,20]
- o Abnormal P53, P16, or RB expression portends a poorly differentiated NECs.[21,22]

Case Update

- *Pathology: IHC staining demonstrates tumor cells that are positive for chromogranin, cytokeratin, and synaptophysin while negative for CD45, desmin, and Sox 10.*

How Are Neuroendocrine Cancers of Unknown Primary Classified?

- Histological differentiation and tumor grade are the major determinants of clinical course. Accurate pathological evaluation is critical to treatment planning and prognosis.
- Well-differentiated neuroendocrine tumors with G1 and G2 grades have typically more indolent courses.
- Poorly differentiated tumors are classified as NECs, are all G3, and herald aggressive clinical behavior.
- Rarely, well-differentiated NEC will have a higher mitotic rate with a G3 grade.

Case Update

- *Diagnosis. Based on the lack of clear primary lesion, the patient is diagnosed with NEC of unknown primary.*

What Other Imaging Should Be Included in the Evaluation of Neuroendocrine Cancers of Unknown Primary?

- CT imaging of the chest and CT or MRI imaging of the abdomen and pelvis should be obtained for initial staging.
- For patients with well-differentiated tumors or clinical symptoms consistent with functionally active tumors, imaging with somatostatin receptor integrated PET/CT scan (gallium Ga-68 DOTATATE or copper Cu-64 DOTATATE) should be considered.
- FDG-PET/CT and dedicated brain imaging are only recommended for poorly differentiated neuroendocrine carcinoma.
- Endoscopic studies including EGD and colonoscopy should be considered based on symptoms, pattern of spread, and overall clinical suspicion.

Case Update: Imaging

- *MRI of the brain did not reveal intracranial metastases.*
- *FDG-PET/CT showed metabolically avid mediastinal, supraclavicular, and cervical LNs with extensive involvement of the liver.*
- *DOTATATE PET was deferred given the high-grade nature of the disease.*

What Additional Laboratory Testing Should Be Considered?

- Elevation in chromogranin A is associated with nonfunctioning tumors. It may be used to compliment medical decision-making but does not guide therapy.
- Measuring specific hormone levels is important to identify functioning tumors and for potential monitoring of therapy response.

- Biochemical testing should be dictated by patient symptoms and disease biology. For symptomatic patients, serotonin secretion can be measured via 24-hour urine or spot serum measurements of 5-hydroxyindoleacaetic acid (5-HIAA). More extensive hormonal studies including glucagon, gastrin, insulin, vasoactive intestinal peptide (VIP), metanephrines, adrenocorticotropic hormone (ACTH), and others could be considered in the appropriate context.
- Molecular testing for tumor mutational burden (TMB), MSI, and MMR deficiency does not affect front-line treatment recommendations. However, given the high rate of relapse and progressive disease, testing should be completed to assess eligibility for immune checkpoint inhibitor therapy in the second line.

Case Update: Lab Testing

- *Chromogranin A level was elevated to 1494 ng/mL (normal: less than 93). 5-HIAA was not detected in the plasma or urine. Further hormonal testing was deferred given the lack of symptoms associated with functioning tumors.*
- *NGS testing did not reveal an actionable mutation but reported a TMB of 23.*

What Is the Management of Localized Neuroendocrine Cancer of Unknown Primary?

- For localized, well-differentiated neuroendocrine tumors, surgical resection should be considered if feasible.
- Other modalities for locoregional management, such as transarterial embolization for liver predominant disease, could be considered in settings where surgery is contraindicated.
- There is no role for adjuvant systemic therapy for well-differentiated neuroendocrine tumors.[21]
- For localized poorly differentiated neuroendocrine carcinoma, management is dependent on individual patient presentation. Resection should be consolidated with neoadjuvant or adjuvant chemotherapy and potentially adjuvant radiation. Radiation and systemic chemotherapy alone or in combination are also viable therapeutic approaches.[22]

What Is the Management of Metastatic Well-Differentiated Tumors?

- Initial management options are similar regardless of the suspected primary site. Tumors that are asymptomatic or carry a low burden of disease may be appropriate for observation alone.[22]
- Tumors that demonstrate activity on somatostatin receptor integrated PET can be initially managed with somatostatin analogs: octreotide or lanreotide.
- For those with progressive or symptomatic disease that warrants therapy, several validated treatment options could be considered. For those with somatostatin receptor positivity, peptide receptor radionucleotide therapy (PRRT) should be considered in appropriate candidates.[23] Patients must have adequate blood counts and intact renal and liver function to be eligible for PRRT.
- For G1 or G2 tumors, everolimus is a therapeutic option per the RADIANT-4 trial and has well-demonstrated utility in those with a likely bronchopulmonary neuroendrocrine tumor (NET).[24]
- Cytotoxic chemotherapy options include the combination of capecitabine and temozolomide or platinum-based regimens, particularly in tumors with G3 grades.[25]

What Is the Management of Poorly Differentiated Neuroendocrine Carcinoma?

- Given the overall poor outcomes associated with this disease, appropriate assessment of functional status and discussions regarding intentions of therapy are critical.
- Platinum-based chemotherapy (carboplatin and cisplatin) regimens in combination with etoposide remain the standard front-line therapy for poorly differentiated disease. The choice of doublet is largely dependent on the individual patient and disease characteristics.[26]
- Oxaliplatin-fluoropyrimidine-based therapy has also been validated in high-grade NECs of the pancreas.[27]
- Spigel et al. reported an RR in neuroendocrine carcinoma of unknown primary to cytotoxic therapy of 70%, with 20% achieving a complete response (CR). The median survival was noted to be 15 months.[28]
- Immunotherapy, such as the combination of ipilimumab and nivolumab, is an option for those with progressive disease following initial chemotherapy.[29] Specifically, pembrolizumab is an option for those with MSI, MMR deficiency, or a high TMB that do not have other therapeutic options.[30,31]

Case Update: Treatment

- *Given his good functional status of ECOG:0, treatment was initiated with carboplatin and etoposide in 3-week cycles.*
- *After 2 cycles, he had improvement in his abdominal symptoms with substantial response of interim imaging. He required evaluation in the ED for refractory nausea following cycle 3 but otherwise tolerated 4 cycles well with a complete response of end-of-therapy CT imaging.*

What Surveillance Is Necessary?

- Monitoring during and after therapy is highly dependent on individual tumor and patient characteristics.
- For monitoring of asymptomatic disease, evaluation for clinical symptoms and repeat imaging should be completed on 3- to 6-month intervals depending on tumor characteristics.[22]
- Following resection or definitive therapy for localized disease with favorable biology, surveillance with clinical evaluation and repeat CT imaging of the involved regions every 3 to 6 months for up to 10 years is suggested. More frequent imaging should be obtained in the first year for poorly differentiated NEC and for 2 years in well-differentiated, G3 neuroendocrine tumors.
- The frequency of imaging and lab testing for those on active therapy must be tailored to the individual disease and adjusted as needed as symptoms indicate.
- Follow-up imaging following therapy consists largely of CT-based imaging of involved regions from 3 to 6 months. Specialized imaging with somatostatin receptor (SSR)-integrated or FDG PET should be obtained as clinically necessary.
- Biochemical markers should be obtained primarily based on clinical symptoms.
- Follow-up imaging and evaluation should continue for 10 years due to high rates of disease recurrence.
- Although data on long-term survival is limited, monitoring for sequelae of chemotherapy including development of secondary hematologic malignancy is important.

Case Update: Follow-Up
- *Approximately 6 months after completion of therapy, his chromogranin A started to trend up with appearance of recurrent adenopathy. Given his TMB of greater than 10, he was a candidate for the programmed death-ligand 1 (PD-L1) immune checkpoint inhibitor pembrolizumab. He remains on pembrolizumab every 3 weeks until progression.*

Case 25.4: Adenocarcinoma of Unknown Primary

A 73-year-old woman is seen in the ED after a motor vehicle accident. She is generally healthy with well-controlled hypertension and diabetes that is managed with metformin. She has no significant exposure to tobacco, alcohol, or other drugs. She has had age-appropriate cancer screen to date with no abnormal or concerning findings on prior mammograms, Pap smears, or colonoscopies. CT imaging of the abdomen and pelvis in the ED did not reveal any evidence of traumatic injury but discovered multiple peritoneal and soft-tissue implants concerning for peritoneal carcinomatosis. There were no masses identified in the liver, pancreas, or gastrointestinal (GI) tract and no evidence of biliary or pancreatic ductal dilatation. There was nonspecific thickening of the uterus involving the left adnexa noted without a definitive mass. Initial lab testing demonstrated normal blood counts and differential as well as normal kidney and liver function. She underwent a CT guided core needle biopsy of a 3.2 × 4.4 × 2.6 cm soft-tissue implant in the abdominal wall. The initial pathology interpretation revealed a moderately differentiated adenocarcinoma.

How Is Adenocarcinoma of Unknown Primary Diagnosed?

- Obtaining an adequate tissue sample for evaluation is critical. Decisions regarding the mode of biopsy (FNA vs. core needle, vs. surgical) should be determined by the safety of the procedure, anticipated need for multiple samples for expanded testing, and the type of testing required.
- Adenocarcinoma is the most common histological subtype of cancer of unknown primary, making up approximately 60% of cases.[18]
- Glandular formations recognized under light microscopy are the unifying structures that define adenocarcinoma.
- IHC is useful to confirm the classification of a tumor. Initial IHC staining for CK7 and CK20 may lend suspicion for primary tissue type; however, other stains are more specific for individual primary sites (Table 25.2). However, extensive testing is unlikely to add additional benefit as staining patterns are variable and less often diagnostic of a specific tissue of origin.[1] Communication with the performing pathologist is critical to thorough yet efficient testing.[18]

Case Update: IHC Staining
- *IHC staining of the tumor was positive for CK7 and negative for CK20. There was moderate positivity for CDX2. It was negative for WT 1, PAX8, p53, and TTF-1. This is a nonspecific pattern and could be compatible with pancreas or upper GI primary.*

What Further Molecular or Genomic Testing Is Required?

- Recent advances in genomic profiling serve two purposes: compare a tumor genomic expression to historical controls to determine the tissue of origin and determine the presence of actionable mutations for which specific therapies are available.
- Testing for DNA MMR proficiency and MSI should be completed. Similarly, assessment of the TMB by NGS or another validated assay should be completed. There is tissue agnostic approval for the use of immunotherapies in those with tumors that are MMR deficient/MSI-high or have a TMB of 10 or greater.

- The rate of detection of therapeutically actionable mutations by NGS varies widely in the literature. Ross et al. and Vargese et al. reported a genomic abnormality with a corresponding therapy backed by high-level clinical evidence in about one out of three patients.[32,33] Studies comparing the use of targeted therapies identified by NGS with empiric platinum-based regimens are ongoing (NCT03498521).
- As previously described, molecular identified assays can be used to assign a probable tissue of origin to tailor therapies, but the overall benefit to this approach over empiric therapy remains to be determined. Routine use is not currently recommended by the NCCN.[1]

Case Update: Additional Molecular Testing
- *Additional testing showed MMR proficiency and MSI-low.*
- *Molecular identifier assay assigned a 69% probability to pancreaticobiliary tissue of origin.*
- *NGS showed a TMB of 0 and no actionable mutations.*

What Further Workup Is Necessary for Adenocarcinoma of Unknown Primary?

- Appropriate testing largely depends on which anatomical regions are involved and clinical presentation.
- Complete staging imaging with CT scans of the neck, chest, abdomen, and pelvis should be completed to determine the extent of disease.
- FDG PET should be considered in localized disease where curative therapies could be considered.
- For males over the age of 40, a PSA level should be measured.
- Females should have a mammogram followed by breast MRI or US if further investigation is warranted.
- For males with retroperitoneal disease, and both males and females with mediastinal disease, workup should include markers for germ cell tumors: AFP and beta-hCG.
- Urine cytology should also be obtained in the presence of retroperitoneal disease to assess for genitourinary malignancy.
- CA-125 should be measured in women with disease in a distribution compatible with ovarian malignancy, including the chest, abdomen, pelvis, retroperitoneal space, or inguinal nodes.
- Endoscopic evaluation should be considered in those with disease localized to the liver, supraclavicular, or inguinal nodes. Otherwise, it should be reserved for those with symptoms or an IHC pattern concerning for GI disease.
- Particular awareness should be given to the psychosocial stress associated with the workup and diagnosis of cancer of unknown primary.

Case Update: Additional Workup
- *PET imaging revealed hypermetabolic peri-gastric and peri-caval LNs in addition to the known peritoneal and soft-tissue masses. There was no other evidence of focal uptake.*
- *Expanded lab testing showed mild and nonspecific elevation in CA-125 and CEA.*
- *The patient was referred to gynecologic oncology for further evaluation. On bimanual exam she had no evidence of palpable masses. Uterine tissue biopsy was negative for cytological abnormality.*
- *Based on the available data, including imaging characteristics, IHC staining pattern, and genomic expression profile, concern was greatest for a metastatic adenocarcinoma of pancreatic origin.*
- *During her initial consultation, she repeatedly expressed shock at the diagnosis given she was generally feeling well without obvious symptoms related to the disease. On follow-up visits, her goals of care were discussed, including her desire to continue traveling for as long as possible.*

What Is Appropriate Management for Localized Disease?

- Appropriate treatment of localized disease is largely tailored to the individual region that is involved and the clinical factors discovered during workup.
- If the primary is discovered or determined during workup, it should be approached per appropriate guidelines.
- Those with isolated head, neck, and supraclavicular adenocarcinoma should be managed following the head and neck occult primary algorithm.
- Females with isolated axillary nodal disease can be approached similarly to breast cancer with locoregional involvement. Axillary node dissection with consideration of radiation or systemic therapy is appropriate for men presenting with isolated axillary disease.
- Localized mediastinal disease should be approached as a poor risk testicular germ cell tumor for male patients or ovarian germ cell in female patients under the age of 40. For those over the age of 40, treatment with an NSCLC paradigm could be considered; for those over 50, it is recommended.
- Surgical resection +/- radiation or systemic therapy should be considered for appropriate candidates with a single site of metastasis or resectable isolated retroperitoneal, inguinal, liver, and boney disease.
- Disease limited to pleural or peritoneal fluids should have appropriate symptom management with priority given to systemic therapy.

What Treatment Could Be Considered for Widely Disseminated or Unresectable Disease?

- Consideration must be given to patient PS and intent of treatment prior to embarking on therapy.
- Clinical trial enrollment remains a preferred option as treatment outcomes have been historically poor for this cancer and there is no established standard of care for the chemotherapeutic regimen.
- There are ongoing studies regarding the benefit of treatment directed by tissue of origin testing compared to empiric chemotherapy. It is expert consensus to treat with site specific therapy if a tissue of origin is identified.
- Multiple chemotherapy regimens have been studied in Phase II and Phase III clinical trials and are appropriate front-line therapy. For patients eligible for systemic therapy, the combinations of carboplatin and paclitaxel, cisplatin and gemcitabine, and docetaxel and gemcitabine are preferred.[34,35] For those with suspected GI or pancreaticobiliary origins, the use of fluoropyrimidine-based therapies could also be considered with platinum agents or irinotecan if not platinum eligible (CapeOx, mFOLFOX, FOLFIRI). The evidence for these regimens is summarized in the section on poorly differentiated carcinoma as these tumors demonstrate a higher degree of response to chemotherapy.
- More intensive three-drug regimens including paclitaxel, carboplatin, etoposide, and FOLFIRINOX should be reserved for fit patients with ECOG 0-1 due to additional toxicity.[36]
- Given their utility as single agents in GI malignancies with generally favorable toxicity profiles, the fluoropyrimidines capecitabine and 5-fluorourocil could be considered in CUPs.
- Immunotherapy with the immune check point inhibitor pembrolizumab is an option for tumors with MMR deficiency, MSI-high, and TMB of 10 or greater. Approval for this indication was based on the KEYNOTE-158 trial. This Phase II study of pembrolizumab after failure of front-line therapy in patients with MSI-H/MMR-deficient tumors of 27 different lineages demonstrated an ORR of 34.3%, median PFS of 4 months, and OS

of 24 months.[30] Retrospective analysis of the same cohort demonstrated that in patients with TMB of 10 or greater, there was an ORR of 29% with 4% of these being CR. For patients who had a response, 50% had a response lasting for at least 24 months.[31,37-39]

Case Update: Treatment Options

- *Given extensive peritoneal disease and intra-abdominal nodal disease with IHC and molecular profiles suggestive of a pancreaticobiliary origin, surgical debulking was deferred.*
- *Discussions regarding possible cytotoxic chemotherapy options included a platinum agent in combination with either gemcitabine, fluorouracil (and additional leucovorin), or paclitaxel. Single-agent gemcitabine was also considered. She was not a candidate for immunotherapy based on her MMR, MSI, and TMB testing. She was not interested in referral to another center for clinical trial consideration.*
- *She declined chemotherapy and wished to pursue supportive care measures alone. Referral was placed for enrollment in hospice services.*

REVIEW QUESTIONS

1. What subtype of cancer of unknown primary (CUP) is considered favorable risk?
   A. Poorly differentiated adenocarcinoma
   B. Poorly differentiated carcinoma
   C. Well-differentiated adenocarcinoma with metastatic disease to bone, liver, and lung
   D. Poorly differentiated neuroendocrine tumor
   E. *NUT* carcinoma

2. What clinical feature is not considered a poor prognostic indicator?
   A. Female gender at birth
   B. Performance status (PS) 3
   C. Leukocyte count of 15,000 with neutrophil count of 14,000
   D. Metastatic disease to the liver
   E. Adenocarcinoma histology

3. Which subtype of cancer of unknown primary (CUP) is not correctly associated with its recommended therapy?
   A. Poorly differentiated neuroendocrine tumor; carboplatin and etoposide +/- atezolizumab
   B. Squamous cell carcinoma (SCC) of the head and neck with unknown primary; neck dissection followed by chemoradiation
   C. Poorly differentiated carcinoma; carboplatin and docetaxel
   D. CUP with colorectal immunohistochemistry (IHC; CK7+CK20-CDX2+); carboplatin and Taxol
   E. Well-differentiated neuroendocrine tumor of unknown primary; somatostatin analogues

4. Which immunohistochemistry (IHC) is correctly paired with its tumor of origin?
   A. CK7+CK-CDX2+; pancreatic
   B. AE1/AE3+, cytokeratin +; sarcoma
   C. OCT4, alpha-fetoprotein (AFP), placental alkaline phosphatase (PLAP); germ cell tumor
   D. HMB45, s100; poorly differentiated carcinoma
   E. Cytokeratin -, vimentin +; adenocarcinoma

5. A 68-year-old female with past medical history (PMH) of hypertension, diabetes, and a 30 pack-year smoking history has had a slow clinical decline over the past 2 years. She sought care from her primary care provider (PCP) and urgent care for abdominal pain and back pain. The PCP recommended treatment for dyspepsia and physical therapy; within the last 6 months she has lost 30 lbs. She had to retire due to fatigue and she presents to the ED after 5 days of nausea, vomiting, and being unable to keep down food or water. CT of the chest, abdomen, and pelvis demonstrated metastatic disease to bone, liver, and lung. Her creatinine is 1.9 and bilirubin is 2.0. Core needle biopsy demonstrates a poorly differentiated adenocarcinoma mismatch repair (MMR)/microsatellite instability (MSI) stable; molecular profiling does not predict a tumor of origin. Which do you recommend as next steps?
   A. Recommend palliative care, assess performance status (PS) in an outpatient setting, and, if improved, discuss systemic chemotherapy with carboplatin and Taxol
   B. Start inpatient chemotherapy as it is her only hope to improve her symptoms and PS
   C. Initiate end-of-life discussion and plan for discharge home on hospice

D. Recommend outpatient therapy with cisplatin and gemcitabine

E. Send for programmed death-ligand 1 (PD-L1) status and treat with pembrolizumab if positive

6. A 57-year-old male 50 pack-year smoker presents with a new lump in the groin. Ultrasound (US) identifies a 3-cm right inguinal lymph node (LN). Core needle biopsy is attained and histology demonstrates a moderately differentiated squamous cell carcinoma (SCC) with tumor mutational burden (TMB) of 8. Immunohistochemistry (IHC) stains demonstrate CK5/6, p63/p40; negative for S100, synaptophysin, and desmin. Fluorodeoxyglucose (FDG)-PET/CT is obtained and demonstrates the right inguinal LNs with standardized uptake value (SUV) of 13 with no other sites of disease. How would you treat this patient?

A. Surgical resection

B. Radiation therapy (RT)

C. Systemic chemotherapy with carboplatin and gemcitabine

D. Immunotherapy with pembtolizumab

E. Observation

7. A 68-year-old female presents with abdominal pain, bloating, and weight loss of about 15 pounds in the last 2 months. She presents to the ED with abdominal pain. CT of the abdomen and pelvis demonstrates studding of the peritoneum. Transvaginal ultrasound of the abdomen is negative for ovarian masses and demonstrates endometrial stripes of appropriate thickness for a postmenopausal woman. CT of the chest is normal. Biopsy of one of the peritoneal nodules demonstrates serous papillary carcinoma. CA-125 is 980. Which is the best next step in management?

A. Discuss hospice as there are no treatment options for this type of cancer of unknown primary (CUP)

B. Radiation therapy (RT) to the peritoneum

C. Hold off on therapy until next-generation sequencing (NGS) is complete

D. Systemic therapy only with carboplatin and paclitaxel; there is no role for surgery

E. Consider surgical debulking and systemic therapy with carboplatin and paclitaxel

8. A 48-year-old female presents with abdominal pain. Ultrasound (US) of the liver demonstrates multiple masses in the liver up to 5 cm in size. Biopsy of the liver demonstrates a tumor that is well differentiated, positive for synaptophysin and chromogranin, grade 1 with Ki-57 of 3%. How would you classify this tumor and what would you recommend for the next step in staging?

A. Small cell carcinoma; obtain a fluorodeoxyglucose (FDG) PET/CT

B. Merkel cell carcinoma (MCC); obtain a CT of the chest, abdomen, and pelvis

C. Well-differentiated neuroendocrine tumor; obtain a PET DOTATATE scan

D. Poorly differentiated neuroendocrine tumor; obtain a FDG PET/CT

9. A 73-year-old female presents with abdominal pain, flushing, and diarrhea. She presented to the ED with these symptoms. In the ED, CT of the chest, abdomen, and pelvis demonstrate multiple lesions in the liver and bilateral lungs, with the largest in size being 3 cm. Chromogranin is 11,000. Biopsy of the lesion is positive for a well-differentiated grade 1 neuroendocrine tumor. PET DOTATATE scan demonstrates somatostatin uptake in the lesions in the liver and lung. What do you recommend for treatment?

A. Lanreotide; consider referral for peptide receptor radionucleotide therapy (PRRT)

B. Observation

C. Carboplatin and etoposide

D. Radiation therapy (RT) to the lesions in the liver as they are causing symptoms

10. A 52-year-old male 50 pack-year smoker presents with back pain that has not responded to 5 months of physical therapy, as well as complaints of abdominal pain. His primary care physician (PCP) obtains an MRI of the spine that notes many lesions suspicious for neoplasm and a compression fracture at L1. The radiologist also notes masses in the liver. The patient is referred to oncology, which obtains a fluorodeoxyglucose (FDG) PET/CT that demonstrates FDG-avid lesions in the lungs and liver as well as the thoracic spine and lumbar spine. No primary tumor is identified. Biopsy of the lung nodule is positive for an epithelioid-type tumor that is synaptophysin-positive with Ki-67 of 82%. Microsatellite instability (MSI) stable, tumor mutational burden (TMB) of 5. Up until this appointment he was working full time, and up until about 1 month ago he was walking. Renal and liver function are normal. What do you recommend for treatment?

A. Systemic therapy with carboplatin and paclitaxel

B. Referral to radiation oncology for palliative radiation to the spine and systemic therapy with carboplatin and etoposide.

C. Immunotherapy with pembrolizumab

D. Radiation therapy (RT) only to the spine; observation otherwise.

ANSWERS AND RATIONALES

1. **D. Poorly differentiated neuroendocrine tumor.** This is considered favorable risk given the responsiveness to treatment with platinum and etoposide regimens. Adenocarcinoma subtype predicts poor prognosis. *NUT* carcinoma is a rare subtype of unknown primary with no effective treatment and poor prognosis.

2. **A. Female gender at birth.** Male gender predicts poor prognosis in cancer of unknown primary (CUP).

3. **D. CUP with colorectal immunohistochemistry (IHC; CK7+CK20-CDX2+); carboplatin and Taxol.** This is a favorable subtype of CUP and should be treated with a metastatic colorectal regimen such as 5-FU and oxaliplatin (FOLFOX).

4. **C. OCT4, alpha-fetoprotein (AFP), placental alkaline phosphatase (PLAP); germ cell tumor.** The others are incorrectly paired. CK7+CK-CDX2+ is colorectal; AE1/AE3+, cytokeratin + is carcinoma; HMB45, s100 is melanoma; cytokeratin -, vimentin + is sarcoma.

5. **A. Recommend palliative care, assess performance status (PS) in an outpatient setting, and, if improved, discuss systemic chemotherapy with carboplatin and Taxol .** There is not an indication to treat inpatient for cancer of unknown primary (CUP) and she is not yet hospice appropriate. It is best to have the patient recover from her hospitalization and, if her PS improves, consider chemotherapy.

6. **A. Surgical resection.** For cancer of unknown primary (CUP) with good prognosis and single metastatic site, recommend surgical resection of the inguinal LN. One could consider adjuvant radiation after excision.

7. **E. Consider surgical debulking and systemic therapy with carboplatin and paclitaxel.** With CUP, ovarian type, guidelines are to treat similar to ovarian primary and consider surgical debulking as well as systemic therapy (carboplatin and paclitaxel) to improve overall survival.

8. **C. Well-differentiated neuroendocrine tumor; obtain a PET DOTATATE scan.** Low-grade well-differentiated neuroendocrine tumor given Ki-67 is less than 15% and that it is grade 1. This is not a poorly differentiated neuroendocrine tumor or small cell given the low grade and low Ki-67. Immunohistochemistry (IHC) staining does not support a diagnosis of MCC.

9. **A. Lanreotide, consider referral for peptide receptor radionucleotide therapy (PRRT).** The patient is symptomatic with a well-differentiated neuroendocrine tumor that demonstrates somatostatin uptake. The clinician would recommend treatment with a somatostatin analogue that is long acting such as lanreotide.

10. **B. Referral to radiation oncology for palliative radiation to the spine and systemic therapy with carboplatin and etoposide.** Presentation represents a poorly differentiated neuroendocrine tumor or a small cell, with unknown primary; however, given the smoking history, it is likely lung primary. Poorly differentiated neuroendocrine tumors are chemo responsive and are treated similarly to small cell carcinoma with carboplatin and etoposide. Given that he is experiencing pain from a compression fracture from metastatic issues, one could consider palliative radiation to relieve pain.

REFERENCES

1. National Comprehensive Cancer Network. Occult Primary (Version 1.2022). https://www.nccn.org/guidelines/guidelines-detail?category=1&id=1451
2. Massard C, Loriot Y, Fizazi K. Carcinomas of an unknown primary origin—diagnosis and treatment. *Nat Rev Clin Oncol.* 2011;8(12):701–710. doi:10.1038/nrclinonc.2011.158
3. Varghese AM, Arora A, Capanu M, et al. Clinical and molecular characterization of patients with cancer of unknown primary in the modern era. *Ann Oncol Off J Eur Soc Med Oncol.* 2017;28(12):3015–3021. doi:10.1093/annonc/mdx545
4. Raghav K, Hwang H, Jácome AA, et al. Development and validation of a novel nomogram for individualized prediction of survival in cancer of unknown primary. *Clin Cancer Res.* 2021;27(12):3414–3421. doi:10.1158/1078-0432.CCR-20-4117
5. Zhu L, Wang N. ^{18}F-fluorodeoxyglucose positron emission tomography-computed tomography as a diagnostic tool in patients with cervical nodal metastases of unknown primary site: a meta-analysis. *Surg Oncol.* 2013;22(3):190–194. doi:10.1016/j.suronc.2013.06.002
6. Hainsworth JD, Rubin MS, Spigel DR, et al. Molecular gene expression profiling to predict the tissue of origin and direct site-specific therapy in patients with carcinoma of unknown primary site: a prospective trial of the Sarah Cannon Research Institute. *J Clin Oncol.* 2013;31(2):217–223. doi:10.1200/JCO.2012.43.3755
7. Greco FA, Lennington WJ, Spigel DR, Hainsworth JD. Poorly differentiated neoplasms of unknown primary site: diagnostic usefulness of a molecular cancer classifier assay. *Mol Diagn Ther.* 2015;19(2):91–97. doi:10.1007/s40291-015-0133-8
8. Moran S, Martínez-Cardús A, Sayols S, et al. Epigenetic profiling to classify cancer of unknown primary: a multicentre, retrospective analysis. *Lancet Oncol.* 2016;17(10):1386–1395. doi:10.1016/S1470-2045(16)30297-2
9. Yoon HH, Foster NR, Meyers JP, et al. Gene expression profiling identifies responsive patients with cancer of unknown primary treated with carboplatin, paclitaxel, and everolimus: NCCTG N0871 (Alliance). *Ann Oncol.* 2016;27(2):339–344. doi:10.1093/annonc/mdv543
10. Frank SJ, Rosenthal DI, Petsuksiri J, et al. Intensity-modulated radiotherapy for cervical node squamous cell carcinoma metastases from unknown head-and-neck primary site: M. D. Anderson cancer center outcomes and patterns of failure. *Int J Radiat Oncol Biol Phys.* 2010;78(4):1005–1010. doi:10.1016/j.ijrobp.2009.09.006
11. Varadhachary GR, Raber MN. Cancer of unknown primary site. *N Engl J Med.* 2014;371(8):757–765. doi:10.1056/NEJMra1303917
12. Briasoulis E, Kalofonos H, Bafaloukos D, et al. Carboplatin plus paclitaxel in unknown primary carcinoma: a phase II Hellenic Cooperative Oncology Group study. *J Clin Oncol.* 2000;18(17):3101–3107. doi:10.1200/JCO.2000.18.17.3101
13. del Muro XG, Marcuello E, Gumá J, et al. Phase II multicentre study of docetaxel plus cisplatin in patients with advanced urothelial cancer. *Br J Cancer.* 2002;86(3):326–330. doi:10.1038/sj.bjc.6600121
14. Culine S, Lortholary A, Voigt J-J, et al. Cisplatin in combination with either gemcitabine or irinotecan in carcinomas of unknown primary site: results of a randomized phase II study--trial for the French Study Group on Carcinomas of Unknown Primary (GEFCAPI 01). *J Clin Oncol.* 2003;21(18):3479–3482. doi:10.1200/JCO.2003.12.104
15. Hainsworth JD, Spigel DR, Burris HA 3rd, et al. Oxaliplatin and capecitabine in the treatment of patients with recurrent or refractory carcinoma of unknown primary site: a phase 2 trial of the Sarah Cannon Oncology Research Consortium. *Cancer.* 2010;116(10):2448–2454. doi:10.1002/cncr.25029
16. Schuette K, Folprecht G, Kretzschmar A, et al. Phase II trial of capecitabine and oxaliplatin in patients with adeno- and undifferentiated carcinoma of unknown primary. *Onkologie.* 2009;32(4):162–166. doi:10.1159/000201125
17. Chau NG, Ma C, Danga K, et al. An anatomical site and genetic-based prognostic model for patients with nuclear protein in testis (NUT) midline carcinoma: analysis of 124 patients. *JNCI Cancer Spectr.* 2020;4(2):pkz094. doi:10.1093/jncics/pkz094
18. Greco FA, Hainsworth JD. Cancer of unknown primary site. In: DeVita VT Jr, Lawrence TS, Rosenberg SA, eds. *DeVita, Hellman, and Rosenberg's Cancer: Principles and Practice of Oncology.* 10th ed. Wolters Kluwer; 2015:1720–1737.
19. Oien KA. Pathologic evaluation of unknown primary cancer. *Semin Oncol.* 2009;36(1):8–37. doi:10.1053/j.seminoncol.2008.10.009
20. La Rosa S, Chiaravalli AM, Placidi C, Papanikolaou N, Cerati M, Capella C. TTF1 expression in normal lung neuroendocrine cells and related tumors: immunohistochemical study comparing two different monoclonal antibodies. *Virchows Arch.* 2010;457(4):497–507. doi:10.1007/s00428-010-0954-05
21. Tang LH, Untch BR, Reidy DL, et al. Well-differentiated neuroendocrine tumors with a morphologically apparent high-grade component: a pathway distinct from poorly differentiated neuroendocrine carcinomas. *Clin Cancer Res an Off J Am Assoc Cancer Res.* 2016;22(4):1011–1017. doi:10.1158/1078-0432.CCR-15-0548
22. Shah MH, Goldner WS, Halfdanarson TR, et al. NCCN guidelines insight: neuroendocrine and adrenal tumors, version 2.2018. *J Natl Compr Canc Netw.* 2020;16(6):693–702. doi:10.6004/jnccn.2018.0056

23. Baum RP, Kulkarni HR, Singh A, et al. Results and adverse events of personalized peptide receptor radionuclide therapy with ^{90}Yttrium and ^{177}Lutetium in 1048 patients with neuroendocrine neoplasms. *Oncotarget.* 2018;9(24):16932–16950. doi:10.18632/oncotarget.24524

24. Singh S, Carnaghi C, Buzzoni R, et al. Everolimus in neuroendocrine tumors of the gastrointestinal tract and unknown primary. *Neuroendocrinol.* 2018;106(3):211–220. doi:10.1159/000477585

25. Fine RL, Gulati AP, Krantz BA, et al. Capecitabine and temozolomide (CAPTEM) for metastatic, well-differentiated neuroendocrine cancers: the Pancreas Center at Columbia University experience. *Cancer Chemother Pharmacol.* 2013;71(3):663–670. doi:10.1007/s00280-012-2055-z

26. Frizziero M, Spada F, Lamarca A, et al. Carboplatin in combination with oral or intravenous etoposide for extra-pulmonary, poorly-differentiated neuroendocrine carcinomas. *Neuroendocrinology.* 2019;109(2):100–112. doi:10.1159/000497336

27. Spada F, Antonuzzo L, Marconcini R, et al. Oxaliplatin-based chemotherapy in advanced neuroendocrine tumors: clinical outcomes and preliminary correlation with biological factors. *Neuroendocrinology.* 2016;103(6):806–814. doi:10.1159/000444087

28. Spigel DR, Hainsworth JD, Greco FA. Neuroendocrine carcinoma of unknown primary site. *Semin Oncol.* 2009;36(1):52–59. doi:10.1053/j.seminoncol.2008.10.003

29. Klein O, Kee D, Markman B, et al. Immunotherapy of ipilimumab and nivolumab in patients with advanced neuroendocrine tumors: a subgroup analysis of the CA209-538 clinical trial for rare cancers. *Clin Cancer Res.* 2020;26(17):4454–4459. doi:10.1158/1078-0432.CCR-20-0621

30. Marabelle A, Le DT, Ascierto PA, et al. Efficacy of pembrolizumab in patients with noncolorectal high microsatellite instability/mismatch repair-deficient cancer: results from the phase II KEYNOTE-158 study. *J Clin Oncol Off J Am Soc Clin Oncol.* 2020;38(1):1–10. doi:10.1200/JCO.19.02105

31. Marabelle A, Fakih M, Lopez J, et al. Association of tumour mutational burden with outcomes in patients with advanced solid tumours treated with pembrolizumab: prospective biomarker analysis of the multicohort, open-label, phase 2 KEYNOTE-158 study. *Lancet Oncol.* 2020;21(10):1353–1365. doi:10.1016/S1470-2045(20)30445-9

32. Ross JS, Sokol ES, Moch H, et al. Comprehensive genomic profiling of carcinoma of unknown primary origin: retrospective molecular classification considering the CUPISCO study design. *Oncologist.* 2021;26(3):e394-e402. doi:10.1002/onco.13597

33. Cancers of unknown primary site: ESMO Clinical Practice Guidelines for diagnosis, treatment and follow-up. *Annals of Oncology.* 2015;26:v133-v138

34. Greco FA, Gray J, Burris HA 3rd, et al. Taxane-based chemotherapy for patients with carcinoma of unknown primary site. *Cancer J.* 2001;7(3):203–212.

35. Huebner G, Link H, Kohne CH, et al. Paclitaxel and carboplatin vs gemcitabine and vinorelbine in patients with adeno- or undifferentiated carcinoma of unknown primary: a randomised prospective phase II trial. *Br J Cancer.* 2009;100(1):44–49. doi:10.1038/sj.bjc.6604818

36. Hainsworth JD, Spigel DR, Clark BL, et al. Paclitaxel/carboplatin/etoposide versus gemcitabine/irinotecan in the first-line treatment of patients with carcinoma of unknown primary site: a randomized, phase III Sarah Cannon oncology research consortium trial. *Cancer J.* 2010;16(1):70–75. doi:10.1097/PPO.0b013e3181c6aa89

37. National Comprehensive Cancer Network. Head and Neck Occult Primary (Version 3.2021). Accessed November 29, 2021.

38. Hainsworth JD, Fizazi K. Treatment for patients with unknown primary cancer and favorable prognostic factors. *Semin Oncol.* 2009;36(1):44–51. doi:10.1053/j.seminoncol.2008.10.006

39. Sève P, Billotey C, Broussolle C, et al. The role of 2-deoxy-2-[F-18]fluoro-D-glucose positron emission tomography in disseminated carcinoma of unknown primary site. *Cancer.* 2007;109(2):292–299. doi:10.1002/cncr.22410

CHAPTER 26

Hodgkin Lymphoma

Radhika Takiar, Lisa P. Chu, and Tycel J. Phillips

INTRODUCTION

Hodgkin lymphoma (HL) is a lymphoid malignancy that accounts for 10% of all lymphoma cases.[1] Although the exact etiology of pathogenesis is unknown, Epstein-Barr virus (EBV) infection, autoimmune diseases, HIV, and immunosuppression have been shown to increase the risk of developing HL. Additionally, there is a familial predisposition as risk is higher among identical twins or same-sex siblings. HL presents in a bimodal distribution affecting patients who are 15 to 30 years old or older than 55 to 60 years old and tends to have a slight male predominance (male:female incidence ratio of 1.3).[1,2]

HL is derived from B cells and can be subdivided into classical HL (cHL), which accounts for the majority of cases (95%), and nodular lymphocyte-predominant HL (NLPHL), which is the remaining minority. The four histological subtypes within cHL are nodular sclerosis (NS), mixed cellularity (MC), lymphocyte rich (LR), and lymphocyte depleted. Treatment for cHL is the same across all subtypes except for NLPHL; treatment for NLPHL is unique as it is immunophenotypically distinct from cHL, lacks CD15 and CD30 positivity, and clinically behaves similar to a low grade non-Hodgkin lymphoma.[2]

The majority of patients can be cured with systemic chemotherapy alone with or without radiation. Since this disease presents in young adults, there is an ongoing effort to limit late, treatment-related toxicities. Several novel agents, such as brentuximab vedotin and immunotherapy, are being incorporated into not only relapsed/refractory disease, but also actively investigated as frontline agents.

CASE SUMMARIES

Case 26.1: Early-Stage, Favorable Risk Hodgkin Lymphoma

A 25-year-old female developed acute onset of chest pain and dyspnea while exercising. Her symptoms resolved with rest. A few days later, she began to notice a dry cough without obvious triggers. She is otherwise healthy, a lifelong nonsmoker, and very active. For the chest pain, she was told to try nonsteroidal anti-inflammatory drugs (NSAIDs) in case the pain was musculoskeletal in etiology. Due to persistent cough, a chest x-ray was performed which showed an enlarged cardiac silhouette but no obvious consolidation or effusions. Despite a trial of proton pump inhibitors (PPIs), her cough persisted and she developed generalized itching and drenching night sweats along with right neck swelling. Physical exam was notable for a 2-cm right cervical chain lymph node (LN).

How Is a Diagnosis Established?

- A diagnosis is preferably established through excisional or image-guided core biopsy. Fine needle aspiration (FNA) does not provide sufficient material for adequate architecture or histology evaluation.
- PET is also necessary to evaluate for distant disease.

Patient's Diagnosis

- PET scan shows fluorodeoxyglucose (FDG)-avid right level III cervical lymphadenopathy along with right hilar lymphadenopathy.
- Excisional biopsy of the cervical LN: Sections show cores of LN effaced by atypical lymphoid infiltrate with evidence of Reed-Sternberg cells. Large, atypical cells are positive for CD30, CD15, and PAX5 (weak), but negative for CD20 and CD3. Diagnosis: cHL, NS subtype.

What Are the Different Subtypes of Hodgkin Lymphoma?

- Considering all HL cases, cHL accounts for 95%. Among cHL, there are several subtypes: NS (accounts for 70% of cases), MC (20% to 25%), LR (5%), and lymphocyte depleted (1%).[1]
- NLPHL accounts for 5% of cases.[1] NLPHL is immunophenotypically and morphologically different from cHL as it has a predominance of "lymphocyte-predominant" cells known.as "popcorn cells" that have lobulated, vesicular nuclei with several nucleoli at the periphery. These "popcorn cells" in NLPHL are typically CD30 and CD15 negative, but positive for CD19, CD20, CD45, and CD79a. In contrast to cHL, NLPHL expresses markers seen with germinal-center B cells.[2]

Which Molecular Feature Is Important in Distinguishing Between Classical Hodgkin Lymphoma and Anaplastic Large-Cell Lymphoma?

- Both cHL and anaplastic large-cell lymphoma are CD30 positive with large, atypical cells; however, HL also expresses PAX-5, which is not seen with anaplastic large-cell lymphoma.[3]

Which Age Groups Are Most Likely to Develop Hodgkin Lymphoma?

- Typically presentation with HL occurs in a bimodal fashion, affecting those who are 15 to 30 years old and those who are older than 55 to 60 years.

How Is This Tumor Staged?

- PET/CT is the preferred modality for staging.
- The Ann Arbor staging system is used to stage HL (Table 26.1).[4]
- Early or limited-stage disease includes stages I to II, whereas advanced-stage disease includes stages III to IV. Stage II-bulky disease is classified as advanced-stage disease.[4]

Patient's Clinical Stage

- The patient's stage is early-stage cHL (stage II-B) due to the presence of two LN regions on the same side of the diaphragm.

Table 26.1 Ann Arbor Staging System

Stage	Involvement
I	Single lymph node region or localized involvement of a single extralymphatic organ/site (IE)
II	≥2 nodal regions on the same side of the diaphragm or localized involvement of a single associated extralymphatic organ/site and its regional lymph node(s) with or without involvement of other lymph node regions on the same side of the diaphragm (IIE)
III	Lymph nodes on both sides of the diaphragm
IV	Diffuse or disseminated involvement of ≥1 extranodal organs with or without associated lymph node involvement

A - No systemic symptoms
B - Presence of B symptoms such as unexplained fever greater than 38°C, drenching night sweats, or weight loss greater than 10% of body weight in the previous 6 months
X - Bulky disease—defined as a mediastinal mass with a maximum width of one-third or more of the diameter of the thorax or a nodal mass of 10 cm or more in maximum dimension
E - Involvement of a single extranodal site contiguous or proximal to the known nodal site

Source: Cheson BD, Fisher RI, Barrington SF, et al. Recommendations for initial evaluation, staging, and response assessment of Hodgkin and non-Hodgkin lymphoma: the Lugano classification. *J Clin Oncol.* 2014;32(27):3059–3068. doi:10.1200/JCO.2013.54.8800

What Determines Favorable Versus Unfavorable Risk?

- A few risk factors that determine risk for early-stage HL are age, erythrocyte sedimentation rate (ESR), B symptoms, and LN involvement.
- The European Organization for the Research and Treatment of Cancer (EORTC) defines "unfavorable risk" as patients with 1 or more of the following features: age older than 50 at diagnosis, bulky mediastinal adenopathy, involvement of four or more LN regions, and B symptoms with ESR greater than 30 mm/hr or ESR greater than 50 mm/hr without B symptoms.[5]
- The German Hodgkin's Study Group (GHSG) utilizes similar variables to the EORTC group but does not incorporate age and defines "unfavorable risk" as three or more LN regions involved.[6]

Patient's Risk

- *ESR 25 and no B symptoms.*
- *The patient has early-stage favorable risk disease as she is young, has only two LN regions involved, lacks bulky mediastinal lymphadenopathy, and has a low ESR without B symptoms.*

What Are the Possible Treatment Options for Early-Stage Favorable Risk Classical Hodgkin Lymphoma?

- Combined modality therapy is the standard of care and typically consists of adriamycin, bleomycin, vinblastine, and dacarbazine (ABVD) with involved-field radiation therapy (IFRT).[2]
- The HD-10 trial randomized previously untreated cHL with early-stage, favorable risk (based on GHSG criteria) into four groups: ABVD for 2 cycles with 30 Gray (Gy) IFRT, ABVD for 2 cycles with 20 Gy IFRT, ABVD for 4 cycles with 30 Gy IFRT, and ABVD for

4 cycles with 20 Gy IFRT. At 5 years, there was no significant difference in freedom from treatment failure (FFTF) between 2 or 4 cycles of ABVD (91% vs. 93%, respectively, P = 0.39) or overall survival (OS), P = 0.61. There was also no difference in FFTF (P = 1) or OS between 20 Gy and 30 Gy (P = 0.61). This established the regimen of ABVD for 2 cycles with 20 Gy IFRT as the standard of care.[7]

- PET-adapted approaches to therapy were explored in the RAPID trial. Patients with stage IA or IIA cHL without bulky disease received 3 cycles of ABVD followed by interim PET. Those who were PET negative (defined as Deauville score of 1 to 2) were randomized to 30 Gy IFRT or no further therapy. Those with PET-positive disease were treated with 1 additional cycle of ABVD and IFRT. The primary endpoint of non-inferiority with no further treatment was not met; however, outcomes were excellent with both IFRT and no further therapy (97% vs. 99%, 95% confidence interval [CI]: 97.6 to 100, respectively). Based on these results, treatment with 3 cycles of ABVD may be sufficient if patients have an interim PET scan that is negative.[8]

- A similar PET-adapted approach for early-stage favorable risk cHL was evaluated by CALGB 50604, though it included patients with B symptoms or extranodal disease. All patients received ABVD for 2 cycles followed by interim PET. Those who were PET negative (Deauville score of 1 to 3) were treated with an additional 2 cycles of ABVD. PET-positive patients received intensified chemotherapy with dose-intense bleomycin, etoposide, doxorubicin, cyclophosphamide, vincristine, procarbazine, and prednisone (escalated BEACOPP) with IFRT. Outcomes were excellent among those who were PET negative with 3-year progression-free survival (PFS) at 91% as compared to PET positive 66% (P = 0.01). Among patients with stage I to II cHL with B symptoms or extranodal disease, treatment with ABVD for 4 cycles is also an option if interim PET after 2 cycles is negative.[9]

Patient's Treatment Plan

- *As she had B symptoms, that would favor the treatment approach per CALGB 50604, which is ABVD for 2 cycles followed by interim PET. If PET negative, she will get 2 additional cycles of ABVD.*
- *Often in younger patients in their early 20s, radiation is omitted due to potential long-term toxicities such as cardiovascular toxicity and risk of secondary malignancies.[10]*

What Are the Toxicities Associated With Chemoradiotherapy?

- Radiation increases the risk of cardiovascular toxicity (such as coronary heart disease [CHD]) and secondary malignancies.
- Toxicities specific to ABVD are the following: neutropenia, alopecia, nausea/vomiting, heart failure/valvular disease (related to doxorubicin), pneumonitis (related to bleomycin), infertility, and secondary malignancies (both solid tumors and leukemia).

Case 26.2: Early-Stage, Unfavorable Risk Hodgkin Lymphoma

A 60-year-old female developed fullness near her right supraclavicular region and attributed it to a viral illness. About 3 months later, the swelling became more pronounced and she presented to her primary care doctor. On physical exam, she had a 1.5-cm palpable right supraclavicular node. PET revealed FDG-avid right supraclavicular LN along with left cervical, bilateral axillary and mediastinal lymphadenopathy. Excisional biopsy of the right supraclavicular LN confirmed lymphocyte-rich cHL. Labs were normal besides ESR, which was 60 mm/hr.

Patient's Stage and Risk
- *Stage II, early-stage unfavorable risk (as she had an elevated ESR and 4 LN regions involved)*

Treatment Options for Early-Stage Unfavorable Risk

- The GHSG HD-11 trial randomized early-stage unfavorable risk patients in four arms: ABVD for 4 cycles with 20 Gy IFRT, ABVD for 4 cycles with 30 Gy IFRT, BEACOPP for 4 cycles with 20 Gy IFRT, or BEACOPP for 4 cycles with 30 Gy IFRT. The 5-year FFTF was similar between ABVD and BEACOPP when 30 Gy IFRT was incorporated ($P = 0.65$). Of the four arms, the combination of 4 cycles of ABVD with 20 Gy IFRT was inferior to the other groups; thus, if ABVD is utilized, it should incorporate 30 Gy IFRT. Since there is not a difference between the chemotherapy arms, the recommendation based on this trial is ABVD for 4 cycles with 30 Gy IFRT.
- To determine whether dose-intensification for early-stage unfavorable risk improved FFTF, the GHSG HD-14 trial was performed. Patients were randomized to ABVD for 4 cycles or escalated BEACOPP for 2 cycles followed by ABVD for 2 cycles (2+2) and all patients were then treated with 30 Gy IFRT. Although the 2+2 arm demonstrated improved 5-year FFTF (95% vs. 88%, P less than 0.001), the OS was similar across both groups (~97%). Additionally, a dose-intensified regimen with BEACOPP led to more grade 3 to 4 toxicities (87.1% vs. 50.7%) compared to ABVD alone.[11]
- The EORTC H-10 trial evaluated both favorable (F) and unfavorable (U) early-stage HL patients with PET-based versus non–PET-based treatment approaches. Both groups received ABVD for 2 cycles followed by PET; the control arm proceeded to 2 additional cycles of ABVD with involved node radiation therapy (INRT); however, the experimental arm stratified treatment based on PET results. Patients with PET-negative disease (Deauville score of 1 to 3) were treated with 4 cycles of ABVD, but those with PET-positive disease were given 2 cycles of escalated BEACOPP with INRT. Among the U group, 5-year PFS was 92.1% versus 89.6% (hazard ratio [HR] 1.45, 95% CI 0.8 to 2.5) in the 2 ABVD + IFRT versus ABVD alone, respectively. Additionally, among PET-positive patients (19%), intensification to escalated BEACOPP + INRT improved 5-year PFS from 77.4% to 90.6% as compared to ABVD + INRT ($P = 0.002$). Based on these results, another therapy option for early-stage unfavorable risk is ABVD for 6 cycles without radiation.[12]

Patient's Treatment Plan
- *Options for treatment would be ABVD for 4 cycles with 30 Gy INRT or ABVD for 6 cycles without radiation (if interim PET is negative).*
- *Patient is treated with ABVD for 4 cycles followed by 30 Gy INRT. Follow-up PET shows complete response (Deauville score 1).*

What Is Required for This Patient's Follow-Up?

- This may vary between institutions, but typically is guided by the National Comprehensive Cancer Network (NCCN)[13] and Childhood Oncology Group (COG).
- According to the NCCN guidelines, the recommendation is for follow-up visits with history and physical examination every 3 to 6 months for 1 to 2 years, then 6 to 12 months for year 3 and annually thereafter.[13]

- Patients who are PET negative upon completion of therapy do not require surveillance imaging. Imaging should only be performed if there is clinical or physical exam evidence concerning for relapse.
- Patients should get annual labs to monitor for secondary hematologic malignancies: complete blood count (CBC) with differential, comprehensive metabolic panel (CMP), lactate dehydrogenase (LDH)/ESR, and thyroid-stimulating hormone (TSH; if history of neck irradiation).

What Is Required for This Patient's Survivorship?

- For cardiac surveillance, patients should get an echocardiogram within 1 year post-treatment and repeated as clinically indicated.
- Patients with neck irradiation should also get surveillance for radiation-induced carotid artery stenosis with carotid ultrasound (US) at 10 years post-treatment and every 10 years thereafter, or sooner if indicated.[14]
- All patients should have routine cancer surveillance for colorectal, lung, and breast cancers. Among females who receive chest irradiation (at younger than 30 years old), breast cancer screening should begin 8 years after radiation or at age 30, whichever occurs last.
- Patients should remain up-to-date on vaccines per the Centers for Disease Control and Prevention (CDC) guidelines.

Case 26.3: Advanced-Stage Hodgkin Lymphoma

A 62-year-old male is seeing his primary care physician (PCP) for the first time in 10 years. He has noticed frequent fevers, his pants are too loose, and he has been having to change his sheets most nights of the week due to drenching night sweats. His energy level has been low and he is no longer exercising. On physical exam, he has bilateral cervical lymphadenopathy. CBC is notable for a hemoglobin of 10 g/DL, and white blood cell count of 16,000/mm³. His PCP orders a PET/CT which shows FDG uptake in LNs above and below the diaphragm. Additionally, there are multiple foci of pathological skeletal FDG uptake. He undergoes an excisional biopsy of an enlarged cervical LN which shows lymphocyte-rich cHL.

Patient's Stage

- *Stage IV given LN involvement on both sides of the diaphragm and bone marrow involvement*

What Is the Patient's Risk?

- Risk is based on the International Prognostic Score (IPS), developed from a retrospective review of over 5000 patients with cHL.[15]
- One point is given for each of the following factors:
  - Serum albumin less than 4 g/dL
  - Hemoglobin less than 10.5 g/dL
  - Male gender
  - Age greater than 45 years
  - Stage IV disease
  - White blood cell count of 15,000/microL or more
  - Lymphopenia
- Based on the IPS, there are associated 5-year freedom from progression and 5-year OS estimates (Table 26.2).
- *Patient's risk: 5 (for anemia, lymphocytosis, age, male gender, and stage IV disease)*

Table 26.2 Prognostic Factors in Advanced-Stage Classical Hodgkin Lymphoma

Score	5-Year Freedom From Progression (%)	5-Year Overall Survival (%)
0	84	89
1	77	90
2	67	81
3	60	78
4	51	61
5–7	42	56

What Are Other Poor Prognostic Factors?

- Positive PET scan after 2 cycles of ABVD
- Increased density of lymphoma-associated macrophages (CD68-positive cells)

Treatment Options for Advanced-Stage Classical Hodgkin Lymphoma

- ABVD for 6 cycles. The RATHL trial studied the use of interim PET scan to de-escalate treatment; patients with newly diagnosed advanced cHL underwent a baseline PET scan, received 2 cycles of ABVD, and then underwent an interim PET scan. Based on the results of the PET scan, those with negative PET findings were randomly assigned to continued ABVD or assigned to AVD (bleomycin omitted) for the remaining 4 cycles. Of the patients who had a negative interim PET scan, there was no significant difference in OS (OS at 3 years—97.2% in the ABVD group versus 97.6% in the AVD group) and minimal risk of treatment failure with the AVD group.[16]
- The BV-AVD (brentuximab vedotin, doxorubicin, vinblastine, dacarbazine) regimen adds the anti-CD30 antibody brentuximab vedotin and omits bleomycin. In the ECHELON-1 trial, patients with untreated advanced-stage cHL were randomized to receive BV-AVD or ABVD. Based on the primary endpoint of modified PFS after a median follow-up of 60.9 months, BV-AVD had a higher PFS (84.9%) compared to ABVD (75.3%) with an HR of 0.68 ($P = 0.0017$); a more recent update has demonstrated that this regimen has an OS benefit compared to ABVD.[17,18] Of note, in this study, ABVD was not PET adaptive.
- The escalated BEACOPP (escBEACOPP) regimen was studied in the AHL2011 trial, where patients received either escBEACOPP for 6 cycles or 2 cycles. Those who received only 2 cycles had an interim PET and were either continued on escBEACOPP for 4 more cycles if interim PET was positive or switched to ABVD (for 4 cycles) if interim PET was negative. PET-driven treatment was found to have similar PFS (5-year PFS 86.2% standard 6-cycle escBEACOPP versus 85.7% in the PET-driven group, $P = 0.65$). However, more of the patients receiving standard treatment (escBEACOPP for 6 cycles) had infections and cytopenias.[19]
- Although Stanford V (adriamycin, vinblastine, mechlorethamine, vincristine, bleomycin, etoposide, prednisone) is listed in the NCCN guidelines, this is not given frequently in practice.

What Is Brentuximab Vedotin?

- It is an anti-CD30 monoclonal antibody conjugated to a mitotic spindle inhibitor. Its main toxicity is peripheral neuropathy.

Patient's Treatment Plan

- *The patient underwent 2 cycles of ABVD and his interim PET scan showed a Deauville score of 3. He was de-escalated to AVD for 4 more cycles, and his end-of-treatment PET was negative for disease.*

What Is the Role of Radiation?

- The patient may consider radiation therapy (RT) when there is residual PET-avid disease on the end of treatment scans.
- There is no benefit of radiation in PET-negative residual masses (those that are not metabolically active).

How Are Interim PET Scans Interpreted?

- They are interpreted based on the 5-point Deauville scoring system. Scores are assigned based on comparing the interim PET with the baseline PET.
  - 1: No residual uptake above background level
  - 2: Residual uptake less than or equal to mediastinal blood pool
  - 3: Residual uptake greater than mediastinal blood pool but not greater than liver
  - 4: Residual uptake moderately increased compared to liver
  - 5: Residual uptake markedly increased compared to liver OR with new sites of disease
- Typically, Deauville score of 1 to 3 is considered PET negative, whereas a score of 4 to 5 is considered PET positive. However, certain trials may define PET negativity differently, such as the RAPID trial.[8]

What Are Treatment Options for Relapsed/Refractory Hodgkin Lymphoma?

- The options are growing for relapsed/refractory disease with the advent of brentuximab vedotin (BV) and immunotherapy.
- One option is salvage chemotherapy with platinum (ifosfamide, carboplatin, and etoposide phosphate [ICE]) or gemcitabine-containing regimens with or without BV. If these patients achieve a remission and are candidates, they get consolidation with an autologous stem cell transplant.
- BV with bendamustine.
- Immune checkpoint inhibitors like pembrolizumab or nivolumab either as monotherapy or combinations (with BV or salvage chemotherapy).
- Chimeric antigen receptor T-cell therapy (CAR-T).

REVIEW QUESTIONS

1. A 28-year-old-male with no prior medical history presents with acute onset of dyspnea while playing soccer. He feels fullness in his neck along with drenching night sweats. CT scan is notable for non-bulky mediastinal disease along with right cervical chain lymphadenopathy. Lymph node (LN) biopsy shows abnormal cells which have expression of CD15+ and CD30+ and CD20-. Lab work shows an erythrocyte sedimentation rate (ESR) of 20 mm/hr. Which of the following is incorrect?
   A. Nodular sclerosis (NS) is the most common subtype of classical Hodgkin lymphoma (cHL)
   B. The cHL presents in a bimodal age distribution
   C. Nodular lymphocyte-predominant Hodgkin lymphoma (NLPHL) is treated the same as cHL
   D. There is a male predominance for cHL

2. What stage of disease does the patient from question 1 have and what would be the most appropriate treatment?
   A. Early-stage, favorable risk; adriamycin, bleomycin, vinblastine, and dacarbazine (ABVD) × 4 cycles + 30-Gy involved-field radiation therapy (IFRT)
   B. Early-stage, unfavorable risk; ABVD × 4 cycles + 30-Gy IFRT
   C. Early-stage, favorable risk; ABVD × 2 cycles + 20-Gy IFRT
   D. Early-stage, unfavorable risk; ABVD × 6 cycles without radiation

3. A 51-year-old female presents to discuss treatment options for stage I classical Hodgkin lymphoma (cHL). She developed an enlarging right groin lymph node (LN) that was biopsy-proven as cHL (lymphocyte-rich subtype). PET/CT confirms localized disease in the right groin. She lacks B symptoms. Labs were notable for erythrocyte sedimentation rate (ESR) of 90 mm/hr. What stage of disease does this patient have and what would be the recommended treatment?
   A. Early-stage, unfavorable risk; adriamycin, bleomycin, vinblastine, and dacarbazine (ABVD) × 4 cycles + 30-Gy involved-field radiation therapy (IFRT)
   B. Early-stage, unfavorable risk; ABVD × 6 cycles without radiation therapy (RT)
   C. Early-stage, favorable risk; ABVD × 2 cycles + 20-Gy IFRT
   D. Advanced-stage; Stanford V
   E. A or B

4. Which of the following is not a toxicity or side effect associated with adriamycin, bleomycin, vinblastine, and dacarbazine (ABVD)?
   A. Pulmonary fibrosis
   B. Cardiomyopathy
   C. Alopecia
   D. Hemorrhagic cystitis

5. A 30-year-old female who is 20 weeks' pregnant presents with chills and palpable bilateral axillary and posterior cervical chain lymph nodes (LNs). Imaging shows disease on both sides of the diaphragm. Biopsy is consistent with classical Hodgkin lymphoma (cHL). What is the most appropriate regimen for this patient?
   A. Adriamycin, bleomycin, vinblastine, and dacarbazine (ABVD) × 2 cycles + 20-Gy involved-field radiation therapy (IFRT)
   B. Escalated-dose bleomycin, etoposide, doxorubicin, cyclophosphamide, vincristine, procarbazine, and prednisone (BEACOPP) × 6 cycles + 30-Gy IFRT

C. ABVD × 6 to 8 cycles alone

D. Wait to start therapy until after delivery

6. An otherwise healthy 35-year-old male has completed 6 cycles of adriamycin, bleomycin, vinblastine, and dacarbazine (ABVD) for stage IV classical Hodgkin lymphoma (cHL). Nine months following completion of treatment, he noticed an enlarging cervical lymph node (LN), and a biopsy confirms relapse. PET scan shows diffuse disease. What is the next best step in management?

A. Start bleomycin, etoposide, doxorubicin, cyclophosphamide, vincristine, procarbazine, and prednisone (BEACOPP)

B. Start brentuximab vedotin

C. Start immunotherapy with pembrolizumab

D. Start salvage chemotherapy with ifosfamide, carboplatin, and etoposide phosphate (ICE) and plan for autologous stem cell transplant

E. Proceed to allogeneic stem cell transplant

7. Which of the following does not increase a patient's risk in advanced-stage classical Hodgkin lymphoma (cHL)?

A. Albumin 2.8 g/dL

B. Female gender

C. Age greater than 45 years

D. Hemoglobin 9.8 g/dL

8. A 55-year-old female was recently diagnosed with stage III classical Hodgkin lymphoma (cHL) involving mediastinal and inguinal lymph nodes (LNs) and has completed 2 cycles of adriamycin, bleomycin, vinblastine, and dacarbazine (ABVD). She undergoes PET scan which showed residual fluorodeoxyglucose (FDG) uptake in the inguinal nodes that is more than the uptake of the mediastinal blood pool but less than the uptake in the liver. What Deauville score does she have?

A. 1

B. 2

C. 3

D. 4

E. 5

9. For the patient in question 8, what does her Deauville score mean?

A. PET negative, she can continue on adriamycin, vinblastine, and dacarbazine (AVD)

B. PET negative, she should continue adriamycin, bleomycin, vinblastine, and dacarbazine (ABVD) to complete 4 cycles

C. PET positive, she should continue on ABVD to complete 4 cycles

10. A 35-year-old male with stage IIIA cHL completed 2 cycles of escalated bleomycin, etoposide, doxorubicin, cyclophosphamide, vincristine, procarbazine, and prednisone (BEACOPP) followed by interim PET showing Deauville score (DS) 4. He then went on to receive 4 additional cycles of escalated BEACOPP. End of treatment PET scan showed complete response in all regions besides left axilla, which remained mildly fluorodeoxyglucose (FDG)-avid. What would be the next best step?

A. Active surveillance

B. Consolidative radiation to left axilla

C. Salvage chemotherapy with ifosfamide, carboplatin, and etoposide phosphate (ICE)

D. Autologous stem cell transplant

ANSWERS AND RATIONALES

1. **C. Nodular lymphocyte-predominant Hodgkin lymphoma (NLPHL) is treated the same as cHL.** NLPHL is treated differently than cHL as it is immunophenotypically and morphologically distinct from cHL.

2. **C. Early-stage, favorable risk; ABVD × 2 cycles + 20-Gy IFRT.** He has stage II, favorable risk disease. Based on the HD-10 trial, there is no difference in freedom from treatment failure (FFTF) or overall survival (OS) when comparing ABVD × 2 cycles with 20-Gy IFRT versus 4 cycles or 30-Gy IFRT.

3. **E. A or B.** She has early-stage, unfavorable disease as ESR is greater than 50 without B symptoms. Either A or B is an appropriate treatment option.

4. **D. Hemorrhagic cystitis.** Bleomycin leads to pulmonary fibrosis, doxorubicin increases risk of cardiomyopathy, and ABVD can cause alopecia.

5. **C. ABVD × 6 to 8 cycles alone.** Chemotherapy is typically avoided in the first trimester due to the risk of teratogenic effects. Since this patient is in her second trimester, chemotherapy is feasible. However, radiation would be avoided due to the risk of radiation to the fetus.

6. **D. Start salvage chemotherapy with ifosfamide, carboplatin, and etoposide phosphate (ICE) and plan for autologous stem cell transplant.** Start salvage chemotherapy followed by autologous stem-cell transplantation (auto-SCT). Retreating with a combination chemotherapy regimen without auto-SCT would not be indicated in first relapse.

7. **B. Female gender.** Male gender is an unfavorable risk factor.

8. **C. 3.** Deauville score of 3 is when FDG uptake in the site of disease is greater than uptake in the mediastinal blood pool but equal to or less than uptake in the liver.

9. **A. PET negative, she can continue on adriamycin, vinblastine, and dacarbazine (AVD).** Given her interim PET was negative, the bleomycin can be dropped.

10. **B. Consolidative radiation to left axilla.** Consolidative radiation is an option for persistent FDG-avid disease on end of treatment scans.

REFERENCES

1. Kaseb H, Babiker HM. Hodgkin lymphoma. In: *StatPearls*. StatPearls Publishing; 2021. https://www.ncbi.nlm.nih.gov/books/NBK499969

2. Allen PM, Evens AM. Hodgkin lymphoma. In: Cuker A, Altman JK, Gerds AT, Wun T, eds. *American Society of Hematology Self-Assessment Program*. 7th ed. American Society of Hematology; 2019.

3. Döring C, Hansmann M-L, Agostinelli C, et al. A novel immunohistochemical classifier to distinguish Hodgkin lymphoma from ALK anaplastic large cell lymphoma. *Mod Pathol*. 2014;27(10):1345–1354.10.1038/modpathol.2014.44

4. Cheson BD, Fisher RI, Barrington SF, et al. Recommendations for initial evaluation, staging, and response assessment of Hodgkin and non-Hodgkin lymphoma: the Lugano classification. *J Clin Oncol*. 2014;32(27):3059–3068. doi:10.1200/JCO.2013.54.8800

5. Cosset JM, Henry-Amar M, Meerwaldt JH, et al. The EORTC trials for limited stage Hodgkin's disease. The EORTC Lymphoma Cooperative Group. *Eur J Cancer*. 1992;28A(11):1847–1850. doi:10.1016/0959-8049(92)90018-w

6. Eich HT, Diehl V, Görgen H, et al. Intensified chemotherapy and dose-reduced involved-field radiotherapy in patients with early unfavorable Hodgkin's lymphoma: final analysis of the German Hodgkin Study Group HD11 trial. *J Clin Oncol*. 2010;28:4199–4206. doi:10.1200/JCO.2010.29.8018

7. Engert A, Plütschow A, Eich HT, et al. Reduced treatment intensity in patients with early-stage Hodgkin's lymphoma. *N Engl J Med.* 2010;363(7):640–652. doi:10.1056/NEJMoa1000067

8. Radford J, Illidge T, Counsell N, et al. Results of a trial of PET-directed therapy for early-stage Hodgkin's lymphoma. *N Engl J Med.* 2015;372(17):1598–1607. doi:10.1056/NEJMoa1408648

9. Straus DJ, Jung S-H, Pitcher B, et al. CALGB 50604: risk-adapted treatment of nonbulky early-stage Hodgkin lymphoma based on interim PET. *Blood.* 2018;132(10):1013–1021. doi:10.1182/blood-2018-01-827246

10. van Leeuwen FE, Ng AK. Long-term risk of second malignancy and cardiovascular disease after Hodgkin lymphoma treatment. *Hematology Am Soc Hematol Educ Program.* 2016;(1):323–330. doi:10.1182/asheducation-2016.1.323

11. von Tresckow B, Plütschow A, Fuchs M, et al. Dose-intensification in early unfavorable Hodgkin's lymphoma: final analysis of the German Hodgkin Study Group HD14 trial. *J Clin Oncol.* 2012;20;30(9):907–913. doi:10.1200/JCO.2011.38.5807

12. André MPE, Girinsky T, Federico M, et al. Early positron emission tomography response-adapted treatment in stage I and II Hodgkin lymphoma: final results of the randomized EORTC/LYSA/FIL H10 trial. *J Clin Oncol.* 2017;35(16):1786–1794. doi:10.1200/JCO.2016.68.6394

13. National Comprehensive Cancer Network. Survivorship. Version 3.2021. https://www.nccn.org/professionals/physician_gls/pdf/survivorship.pdf

14. Ng AK. Current survivorship recommendations for patients with Hodgkin lymphoma: focus on late effects. *Blood.* 2014;124(23):3373–3379. doi:10.1182/blood-2014-05-579193

15. Hasenclever D, Diehl V, Armitage JO, et al. A prognostic score for advanced Hodgkin's disease. *N Engl J Med.* 1998;339:1506–1514. doi:10.1056/NEJM199811193392104

16. Johnson P, Federico M, Kirkwood A, et al. Adapted treatment guided by interim PET-CT scan in advanced Hodgkin's lymphoma. *N Engl J Med.* 2016;374:2419–2429. doi:10.1056/NEJMoa1510093

17. Connors JM, Jurczak W, Straus DJ, et al. Brentuximab vedotin with chemotherapy for stage III or IV Hodgkin's lymphoma. *N Engl J Med.* 2017;378:331–344. doi:10.1056/NEJMoa1708984

18. Straus DJ, Długosz-Danecka M, Connors JM, et al. Brentuximab vedotin with chemotherapy for stage III or IV classical Hodgkin lymphoma (ECHELON-1): 5-year update of an international, open-label, randomised, phase 3 trial. *Lancet Haematol.* 2021;8:e410–e421. doi:10.1016/S2352-3026(21)00102-2

19. Casasnovas R-O, Bouabdallah R, Brice P, et al. PET-adapted treatment for newly diagnosed advanced Hodgkin lymphoma (AHL2011): a randomised, multicentre, non-inferiority, phase 3 study. *Lancet Oncol.* 2019;20:202–215. doi:10.1016/S1470-2045(18)30784-8

CHAPTER 27

Non-Hodgkin Lymphoma

Alejandro Marinos, Colbert A. Parker, Akiva Diamond, and
Sravanti P. Teegavarapu

INTRODUCTION

Non-Hodgkin lymphomas (NHL) comprise a diverse group of hematologic malignancies derived from B-cells, T-cells, or natural killer (NK) cells. Clinical manifestations depend primarily on the cell of origin and the site of involvement. The disease can have a protracted course with few or no symptoms for several years or rapid progression with acute decompensation. Patients at diagnosis can present with enlarged lymph nodes (LNs), B symptoms (fevers, chills, night sweats, and weight loss), cytopenias, or organ-specific dysfunction due to lymphomatous involvement.

Risk factors for the development of NHL include chronic infections (HIV, hepatitis C virus [HCV], hepatitis B virus [HBV], Epstein-Barr virus [EBV], human T-lymphotropic virus type 1 [HTLV-1], human herpesvirus-8 [HHV8], *Helicobacter pylori*, *Chlamydia psittaci*, and *Campylobacter jejuni*) and a history of autoimmune or immune deficiency disorders. The pathogenesis of NHL is mainly related to errors in antigen receptor gene rearrangements (immunoglobulins or T-cell receptors), resulting in aberrant signaling of oncogenic pathways (Bruton's tyrosine kinase [*BTK*], phosphatidylinositol-4,5-bisphosphate 3-kinase catalytic subunit alpha [*PI3KCA*], Nuclear factor kappa B [*NF-KB*], mammalian target of rapamycin [*mTOR*], mitogen-activated protein kinases [*MAPK*], *myc*).

NHLs have an indolent course in 35% to 40% of cases; this group includes follicular lymphoma (FL), small lymphocytic lymphoma, some cases of mantle cell lymphoma (MCL), marginal zone lymphoma, lymphoplasmacytic lymphoma, and mycosis fungoides. About 50% of NHLs follow an aggressive course, which mainly consists of diffuse large B-cell lymphoma (DLBCL) and peripheral T-cell lymphomas. NHL with a very aggressive course accounts for about 5% of cases. Burkitt lymphoma (BL) and adult T-cell lymphoma/leukemia are representative of this last group (Table 27.1).

Common Issues to Non-Hodgkin Lymphomas

How Is a Diagnosis Established?

- An excisional LN biopsy is preferred, but multiple core needle biopsies are also acceptable. Submission of fresh tissue specimens with or without formalin-fixed tissue will allow performing necessary immunostaining and molecular studies.
- A PET/CT scan to determine the extent of disease is preferred; however, a contrasted CT chest abdomen and pelvis is often acceptable.
- Bone marrow biopsy is recommended for patients with cytopenias.
- Lumbar puncture is used for patients with neurological symptoms.

Table 27.1   2016 WHO Classification of Mature Lymphoid Neoplasms

2016 WHO Classification of Mature B-Cell Neoplasms

Chronic lymphocytic leukemia/small lymphocytic lymphoma

Monoclonal B-cell lymphocytosis*

B-cell prolymphocytic leukemia

Splenic marginal zone lymphoma

Hairy cell leukemia

Splenic B-cell lymphoma/leukemia, unclassifiable

   Splenic diffuse red pulp small B-cell lymphoma

   Hairy cell leukemia-variant

Lymphoplasmacytic lymphoma

   Waldenström macroglobulinemia

MGUS, IgM*

μ heavy-chain disease

γ heavy-chain disease

α heavy-chain disease

MGUS, IgG/A*

Plasma cell myeloma

Solitary plasmacytoma of bone

Extraosseous plasmacytoma

Monoclonal immunoglobulin deposition diseases*

Extranodal marginal zone lymphoma of MALT lymphoma

Nodal marginal zone lymphoma

  Pediatric nodal marginal zone lymphoma

Follicular lymphoma

  In situ follicular neoplasia*

  Duodenal-type follicular lymphoma*

Pediatric-type follicular lymphoma*

*Large B-cell lymphoma with IRF4 rearrangement**

Primary cutaneous follicle center lymphoma

MCL

  In situ mantle cell neoplasia*

DLBCL, NOS

  Germinal center B-cell type*

  Activated B-cell type*

T-cell/histiocyte-rich large B-cell lymphoma

Primary DLBCL of the CNS

Primary cutaneous DLBCL, leg type

EBV+ DLBCL, NOS*

*EBV+ mucocutaneous ulcer**

(continued)

Table 27.1 2016 WHO Classification of Mature Lymphoid Neoplasms (continued)

2016 WHO Classification of Mature B-Cell Neoplasms (cont.)

DLBCL associated with chronic inflammation

Lymphomatoid granulomatosis

Primary mediastinal (thymic) large B-cell lymphoma

Intravascular large B-cell lymphoma

ALK+ large B-cell lymphoma

Plasmablastic lymphoma

Primary effusion lymphoma

HHV8+ DLBCL, NOS*

BL

*Burkitt-like lymphoma with 11q aberration**

High-grade B-cell lymphoma, with *MYC* and *BCL2* and/or *BCL6* rearrangements*

High-grade B-cell lymphoma, NOS*

B-cell lymphoma, unclassifiable, with features intermediate between DLBCL and cHL

2016 WHO Classification of Mature T and NK Neoplasms

T-cell prolymphocytic leukemia

T-cell large granular lymphocytic leukemia

Chronic lymphoproliferative disorder of NK cells

Aggressive NK-cell leukemia

Systemic EBV+ T-cell lymphoma of childhood"

Hydroa vacciniforme-like lymphoproliferative disorder*

Adult T-cell leukemia/lymphoma

Extranodal NK-/T-cell lymphoma, nasal type

Enteropathy-associated T-cell lymphoma

Monomorphic epitheliotropic intestinal T-cell lymphoma*

*Indolent T-cell lymphoproliferative disorder of the GI tract**

Hepatosplenic T-cell lymphoma

Subcutaneous panniculitis-like T-cell lymphoma

Mycosis fungoides

Sézary syndrome

Primary cutaneous CD30+ T-cell lymphoproliferative disorders

    Lymphomatoid papulosis

    Primary cutaneous anaplastic large-cell lymphoma

Primary cutaneous γδ T-cell lymphoma

Primary cutaneous CD8+ aggressive epidermotropic cytotoxic T-cell lymphoma

Primary cutaneous acral CD8+ T-cell lymphoma*

Primary cutaneous CD4+ small/medium T-cell lymphoproliferative disorder*

Peripheral T-cell lymphoma, NOS

(continued)

Table 27.1   2016 WHO Classification of Mature Lymphoid Neoplasms (*continued*)

2016 WHO Classification of Mature T and NK Neoplasms (*cont.*)

AITL

Follicular T-cell lymphoma*

Nodal peripheral T-cell lymphoma with TFH phenotype*

Anaplastic large-cell lymphoma, ALK+

Anaplastic large-cell lymphoma, ALK-*

Breast implant–associated anaplastic large-cell lymphoma*

Provisional entities in the 2016 classification are listed in italics.
*Changes from the 2008 classification

AITL, angioimmunoblastic T-cell lymphoma; ALK, anaplastic lymphoma kinase; BL, Burkitt lymphoma; cHL, classical Hodgkin lymphoma; CNS, central nervous system; DLBCL, diffuse large B-cell lymphoma; EBV, Epstein-Barr virus; GI, gastrointestinal; HHV8, human herpesvirus-8; IRF4, interferon regulatory factor 4; MALT, mucosa-associated lymphoid tissue; MCL, mantle cell lymphoma; MGUS, monoclonal gammopathy of undetermined significance; NK, natural killer; NOS, not otherwise specified; TFH, t-follicular helper; WHO, World Health Organization.

Source: Data from Swerdlow SH, Campo E, Pileri SA. The 2016 revision of the World Health Organization classification of lymphoid neoplasms. *Blood*. 2016;127(20):2375–2390. doi:10.1182/blood-2016-01-643569

- Complete blood count (CBC), comprehensive metabolic panel (CMP), lactate dehydrogenase (LDH), HIV, hepatitis B, and uric acid are required.
- Echocardiogram is used if anthracyclines are being considered.

How Are Non-Hodgkin Lymphomas Staged?

- The Lugano classification is used to stage NHL.[1]
- Stage I: This stage has single LN region involvement or a single extra lymphatic site without nodal involvement.
- Stage II: This stage involves two or more involved LN regions on the same side of the diaphragm, or contiguous extra lymphatic extension from a nodal side with or without the involvement of other LN regions on the same side of the diaphragm.
- Stage III: In this stage, LN involvement occurs on both sides of the diaphragm.
- Stage IV: This stage involves diffuse or disseminated involvement of one or more different lymphatic organs, with or without associated LN involvement. Stage IV includes any involvement of the cerebrospinal fluid (CSF), bone marrow, liver, or multiple lung lesions. Spleen involvement is considered nodal involvement.
- Index E is used to define extranodal involvement for limited stage (I/II) disease.

Bulky disease: Bulky classification is limited to stage II disease. Definition of bulk depends on lymphoma histology.

CASE SUMMARIES

Case 27.1: Mantle Cell Lymphoma

A 63-year-old man presented to the clinic with a palpable right cervical LN enlarging over the last 4 months. A few weeks ago, he started experiencing fatigue and chills. He decided to seek medical care when his wife told him that his eyelids were looking droopy. He has a history of rheumatoid arthritis treated with adalimumab, but otherwise, he is active without physical limitations.

How Is a Diagnosis Established?

- Tissue biopsy, imaging with PET, and laboratory studies as recommended in general for NHLs

Patient's Diagnosis

- A cervical LN excisional biopsy revealed a monotypic B-cell population, CD20+, CD5+. Cyclin D1 immunostaining was positive. Fluorescent in situ hybridization (FISH) studies showed positivity for t(11:14). These features were compatible with MCL, which is usually positive for CD19, CD20, and CD5; in addition, nuclear staining for cyclin D1 is positive in 95% of the cases.[2] Although t(11:14) is not exclusive of MCL, it is present in 50% to 65% of cases.[3]
- The PET scan reported orbital, mandibular, right tonsillar, right neck mass, shoddy adenopathy throughout the abdomen and pelvis, and increased standardized uptake value (SUV) activity in the spleen.
- White blood cell (WBC) count was 17.2, platelets of 120, LDH 200 (upper normal limit [UNL] 120), and uric acid was within normal limits. HIV and HBV serologies were negative.
- A bone marrow biopsy was performed due to the thrombocytopenia and showed involvement by MCL.
- CSF was negative for lymphomatous involvement.

How Is Mantle Cell Lymphoma Staged and Risk-Stratified?

- Staging is performed using the Lugano staging system (see the previous text).
- Stage I or II require confirmation with endoscopy and colonoscopy.
- Risk stratification is based on the Mantle Cell Lymphoma International Prognostic Index (MIPI) score (age, LDH, WBC, Eastern Cooperative Oncology Group (ECOG), Ki-67).[4]
- Bulky disease is defined as longest diameter of 5 cm or more.[5]

Patient's Clinical Stage

- The patient has stage IV disease based on bone marrow infiltration.

What Are Appropriate Treatment Options?

- Most patients require initiation of treatment soon after diagnosis due to being symptomatic. Some patients with low risk, low stage disease may have an indolent course and can be observed.
- In advanced disease, surgery and radiation are reserved for symptom control (for example, gastrointestinal bleeding and pain control).
- Patients with stage I or contiguous non-bulky stage II disease can be treated with radiotherapy alone or an abbreviated course of chemotherapy and involved-site radiation therapy (ISRT). For noncontiguous, non-bulky stage II disease patients, less aggressive immunochemotherapy is preferred. Possible regimens include R-CHOP (rituximab, cyclophosphamide, doxorubicin, vincristine, and prednisone), CHOP (cyclophosphamide, doxorubicin, vincristine, and prednisone), bendamustine-rituximab (BR), and VR-CAP (rituximab, cyclophosphamide, doxorubicin, bortezomib, and prednisone).[6]
- Patients with aggressive stage II bulky and stage III or IV disease should be assessed for autologous stem-cell transplantation (auto-SCT) candidacy. Patients who are candidates should receive aggressive chemotherapy regimens (Nordic regimen, alternating R-CHOP/R-DHAP [rituximab, cyclophosphamide, doxorubicin, vincristine, prednisone, dexamethasone, cytarabine, and cisplatin], hyper-CVAD [cyclophosphamide, vincristine sulfate, doxorubicin hydrochloride (Adriamycin), and dexamethasone]) followed by high-dose

chemotherapy and autologous stem cell rescue. Following autologous transplant, maintenance with rituximab is indicated. For patients who are not appropriate for transplant, less aggressive immunotherapy is an option. For those who receive R-CHOP, maintenance with rituximab every 8 weeks until relapse or intolerance is indicated.[6] For patients who receive bendamustine rituximab, there is less clear benefit of maintenance.

Patient's Treatment

- The patient received 6 cycles of the Nordic regimen (dose-intensified rituximab, cyclophosphamide, vincristine, doxorubicin, prednisone alternating with rituximab, and high-dose cytarabine).
- He underwent an autologous transplant with BEAM (carmustine [bcnu], etoposide, cytarabine, melphalan) conditioning, followed by rituximab maintenance every 8 weeks for 3 years.

Follow-Up and Relapsed Disease

- Patients should undergo clinical surveillance with history and physical (H&P) every 3 to 6 months for 5 years with imaging as clinically indicated.[6]
- For patients with relapsed disease, treatment options include Bruton's tyrosine kinase (BTK) inhibitors and lenalidomide/rituximab. Allogeneic stem cell transplant can be considered for patients who have a second-line response as a consolidation strategy. Finally, brexucabtagene autoleucel is a new chimeric antigen receptor T (CAR-T) cell therapy that can be used in the third-line setting for patients who have received chemoimmunotherapy and a BTK inhibitor.[6,7]

Case 27.2: Follicular Lymphoma

A 66-year-old female presents to the ED for evaluation of fever, chills, and flank pain that started 3 days prior. She is otherwise healthy, but does report that her primary physician had diagnosed her with urinary tract infections (UTIs) twice within the past 2 months and she had completed a course of antibiotics 2 weeks ago with improvement in her symptoms. She also reports intermittent nausea and vomiting during this time period leading to decreased appetite and weight loss of approximately 10 pounds. On examination she is noted to be febrile and tachycardic with abdominal and costovertebral angle tenderness. The remainder of the physical exam was normal. She is admitted to the hospital for treatment of pyelonephritis with intravenous (IV) antibiotics. Over the next 48 hours her symptoms significantly improve; however, she continues to have fevers and chills. A CT scan of the abdomen is ordered to evaluate for a perinephric abscess; however, she is instead revealed to have diffuse retroperitoneal, mesenteric, and inguinal lymphadenopathy concerning for a lymphoproliferative disorder.

How Is a Diagnosis Established?

- Tissue diagnosis can be confirmed by core needle or excisional (preferred) LN biopsy.
- If a PET scan is available, the most PET avid node should be biopsied to help rule out an aggressive transformation.
- Pathological grading is critical in FL and is based on the proportion of centroblasts seen on histology. Grade 3b disease features diffuse sheets of centroblasts (greater than15/high power field [HPF]) and is typically managed as DLBCL.[8]
- Typical immunophenotype: CD10+, CD20+, BCL6+, CD5-, although expression is variable. BCL2 overxpression related to t(14;18) translocation is very common, but can also be seen in other lymphomas.[8]

Patient's Diagnosis

- Retroperitoneal LN biopsy shows nodular proliferation of atypical lymphoid cells in a follicular pattern. Immunohistochemistry (IHC) staining is positive for CD10, CD20, BCL2, and BCL6, and negative for CD3, CD5 and cyclin D1. Ki-67 shows an overall proliferative index of approximately 20%.
- Initial core biopsy does not feature enough tissue for an accurate FL grading. An excisional biopsy of an inguinal node is performed and found to feature similar findings and morphology consistent with grade 1 to 2 FL.

How Is This Tumor Staged?

- Imaging of the chest, abdomen, and pelvis should be performed, either with PET/CT or traditional CT with contrast.
- Bone marrow biopsy should be performed in the event of unexplained cytopenias or in patients with limited-stage contiguous disease when definitive radiation is being considered.

Patient's Clinical Stage

- PET/CT: Scattered sites of nodal hypermetabolism are present both above and below the diaphragm, with the largest being a 5.7-cm retroperitoneal node conglomerate. The spleen is moderately enlarged (14.7 cm) with associated diffuse splenic hypermetabolism, consistent with the patient's known FL.
- Patient's CBC revealed mild thrombocytopenia and normal hemoglobin.
- LDH was within normal limits.
- Bone marrow biopsy: No evidence of involvement by FL.
- Final diagnosis: Low-grade FL, Lugano stage III.

Is Prognostic Risk Stratification Available for Follicular Lymphoma?

- The Follicular Lymphoma International Prognostic Index (FLIPI-1) is available and incorporates the patient's age, Ann Arbor staging, hemoglobin level, serum LDH, and number of involved nodal areas.[9]
- It should be noted that the FLIPI-1 scoring system was developed prior to the advent of anti-CD20 monoclonal antibody (rituximab) treatment; however, studies have validated its use in the post-rituximab era.[10]

Patient's Prognostic Score

Patient's FLIPI = 3 (age older than 60, stage III to IV, greater than 4 nodal sites) = high-risk disease

What Treatment Strategies Are Appropriate for Follicular Lymphoma?

- Patients with early-stage (Lugano stage I or contiguous stage II) FL should be considered for upfront treatment with ISRT as this can be curative in a number of patients.[6]
- For patients with more advanced disease, some asymptomatic patients can safely be observed without compromising overall survival (OS). The Groupe d'Etude des Lymphomes Folliculaires (GELF) criteria represent a group of commonly accepted indications for treatment as follows:
- Development of B symptoms
- Splenomegaly

- Pleural effusions or peritoneal ascites
- Lymphoma-related cytopenias
- A single nodal mass greater than 7 cm
  - Three nodal masses each greater than 3 cm[11]
- Treatment regimens for advanced disease typically involve anti–CD20-based chemoimmunotherapy regimens such as BR, R-CHOP, or R-CVP (rituximab, cyclophosphamide, vincristine, prednisolone). Although obinutuzumab treatment was associated with an increased progression-free survival (PFS), there was no improvement in OS and an increase in toxicity.[12] For patients who have an initial response to R-CHOP or R-CVP, maintenance rituximab can be considered as it has been shown in some studies to improve complete response rates and PFS, although it has not been shown to improve OS.[6]
- Any patient with grade 3b disease should be considered for immediate treatment similarly to DLBCL regardless of stage.[6]

Recommended Treatment

- *Our patient has advanced disease, but is symptomatic and has developed splenomegaly. Our decision is to pursue treatment with bendamustine-rituximab after a discussion of treatment options. End of treatment PET/CT showed a complete response with no evidence of active lymphoma.*

Surveillance and Relapse

- Baseline imaging should be repeated at the completion of treatment to document the patient's response.
- Patients should be monitored with serial history, physical examination, and laboratory work every 3 to 6 months for up to 5 years, and then annually.[6]
- Imaging should be performed as clinically indicated and should not be performed more frequently than every 6 months.[6]

What Treatment Options Are Available for Relapsed Follicular Lymphoma?

- Patients with suspected relapse should be strongly considered for re-biopsy to evaluate for histological transformation to a higher grade lymphoma.
- Patients can often be safely observed if they remain asymptomatic and have no other indications for treatment.
- For patients who require treatment, options include chemoimmunotherapy with a regimen that was not selected in the first line or lenalidomide-rituximab. An alternative option in the second (or later) lines includes radioimmunotherapy with Ibritumomab tiuxetan.[6]
- For multiply-relapsed patients, additional strategies might involve phosphatidyl inositol 3-kinase (PI3K) inhibitors, enhancer of zeste homolog 2 (EZH2) inhibitors, or CAR-T cell therapy.[6]
- It should be noted that early treatment failure (within 24 months of chemoimmunotherapy or within 12 months of rituximab monotherapy) has historically been associated with poor responses to traditional treatment strategies. In such cases, patients should be considered for clinical trials or high-dose chemotherapy followed by auto-SCT.[13]

Case 27.3: Diffuse Large B-Cell Lymphoma

A 57-year-old male presents to the hospital complaining of abdominal pain. He reports that approximately 2 months ago he started experiencing intermittent, mild abdominal pain. Around 4 to 5 days ago he reports that he started experiencing bloating followed by nausea and vomiting. He reports decreased appetite due to the pain and weight loss of approximately 25 pounds during the past 6 months. He has not noticed any blood in his stools. On examination, he is afebrile, tachycardic, and hypotensive with blood pressure 80/50, which improves with IV fluids. He is noted to be in mild distress with abdominal tenderness and mild distention. A CT of the abdomen is ordered and reveals a large cecal mass with associated mesenteric lymphadenopathy concerning for malignant obstruction with possible pending perforation. The patient is taken urgently for exploratory laparotomy and undergoes resection of the cecum, ascending colon, and terminal ileum. He does well postoperatively; however, the pathology is ultimately reported as consistent with DLBCL and he is referred by the surgeon to Oncology for further evaluation.

How Is the Diagnosis of Diffuse Large B-Cell Lymphoma Established?

- Diagnosis is established by tissue examination; excisional LN biopsy is preferred but multiple cores may be adequate, especially if the enlarged LNs are not accessible.
- Typical morphological findings involve diffuse infiltrate by atypical, large lymphoid cells resembling centroblasts or immunoblasts.
- Typical immunophenotype is positive for B-cell antigens CD19, CD20, CD22, Pax-5, and CD79a.[8]
- CD10 expression may be present and must be differentiated from FL or Burkitt lymphoma.[8]
- CD5 expression may be present and must be differentiated from MCL.[8]

What Additional Genetic Testing Should Be Performed?

- Testing to identify the cell of origin should be attempted either by IHC algorithms or gene expression profiling. Germinal center B cell type (GCB) DLBCL typically features improved outcomes in response to traditional R-CHOP chemotherapy when compared to the activated B-cell type (ABC), although at this time there is no change in management based on the cell of origin.[14]
- A commonly utilized method of determining cell or origin by IHC, the Hans algorithm, involves testing for CD10, Bcl6, and multiple myeloma 1 (MUM-1) in a stepwise progression to determine the cell of origin as pictured in Figure 27.1.[8]
- Testing for *MYC*, *BCL2*, and *BCL6* gene translocations should be performed. B-cell lymphomas that contain *MYC* translocations in conjunction with *BCL2* and/or *BCL6* translocations have traditionally been referred to as "double hit" or "triple hit" lymphomas and feature a worse prognosis. They are now considered a separate entity known as "high grade B-cell lymphomas with translocations of *MYC* and *BCL2* and/or *BCL6*" and may benefit from more intensive chemotherapy regimens.[6]

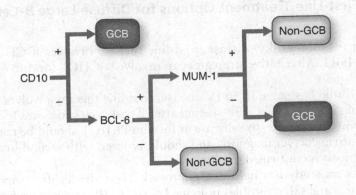

Figure 27.1   Hans algorithm for cell of origin by immunohistochemistry

- Further efforts to subclassify DLBCL subtypes based on genetic profiling are currently under investigation, and may provide new options for risk stratification and treatment strategies in the future.[15]

Patient's Diagnosis
- *Findings are consistent with DLBCL, activate B-cell subtype with re-arrangement of BCL6 but no MYC translocation, co-expression of MYC or BCL2 noted. Ki-67 greater than 50%, Epstein-Barr virus-encoded RNA (EBER) negative, positive for CD20, CD45, PAX-5, negative for CD3, CD5, and CD10.*

How Is Diffuse Large B-Cell Lymphoma Staged?

- Imaging of the chest, abdomen, and pelvis should be performed, either with PET/CT or traditional CT with contrast.
- Bone marrow biopsy should be performed in all patients except in cases where PET/CT confirms bone marrow involvement.

Staging Findings
- *PET/CT indicated a hypermetabolic cervical node (0.8 cm), left axillary node (1.0), celiac node (1.0 cm), and a retroperitoneal node (3.0 cm).*
- *Bone marrow biopsy did not show evidence of lymphoma.*
- *Serum LDH is normal; Hepatitis and HIV testing is negative.*

Does a Prognostic Stratification System Exist for Diffuse Large B-Cell Lymphoma?

- The International Prognostic Index (IPI) assigns a point for each of the following:
- Age older than 60 years
- Serum LDH greater than normal
- ECOG performance status 2 to 4
- Ann Arbor stage III or IV
  - Extranodal involvement greater than 1 site
- A score of 0 to 1 is considered low risk, 2 is low-intermediate risk, 3 is high-intermediate risk, and a score of 4 to 5 is considered high-risk disease.[16]

International Prognostic Index Score
- *1 (stage III or IV disease)—Low-risk disease*

What Are the First-Line Treatment Options for Diffuse Large B-Cell Lymphoma?

- For stage I to II (non-bulky) disease, first-line therapy involves R-CHOP for 3 cycles followed by ISRT. Alternative strategies can involve R-CHOP for 4 to 6 cycles without ISRT.
- For stage II (Bulky) or stage III to IV disease, first-line therapy involves R-CHOP for 6 cycles utilizing interim PET/CT re-staging after 2 to 4 cycles to assess response. Patients with no response or progressive disease at interim PET/CT should be considered for re-biopsy to confirm correct diagnosis and should proceed with second-line therapy if the original diagnosis is confirmed.
- Of note, a recent study has indicated improved 2-year disease-free survival rates with similar OS rates and safety profiles utilizing Pola-R-CHP, a regimen substituting polatuzumab vedotin for vincristine, when compared to R-CHOP.[17]

What Is the Role of Lumbar Puncture and Central Nervous System Prophylaxis?

- The Central Nervous System International Prognostic Index (CNS-IPI) model has been developed to assess risk for central nervous system (CNS) disease. A point is assigned for each of the following[18]:
  - Age older than 60 years
  - Serum LDH greater than normal
  - Performance status greater than 1
  - Ann Arbor stage III to IV disease
  - Involvement of greater than 1 extranodal site
- A CNS-IPI score of 4 or more, or the presence of kidney or adrenal gland involvement, is considered high risk for CNS disease and should be considered for lumbar puncture and CSF prophylaxis.[18]
- Additional indications for CNS prophylaxis include testicular lymphoma, "double/triple hit" lymphoma, HIV-associated lymphoma, primary cutaneous DLBCL of the leg, and stage IE DLBCL of the breast.[6]
- Commonly used regimens include intrathecal methotrexate and/or cytarabine (4 to 8 doses), or systemic high-dose methotrexate (2 to 4 cycles). High-dose methotrexate can be safely administered at the end of R-CHOP therapy without compromising R-CHOP delivery or increasing CNS events.[19]
- Although patients with a high CNS-IPI are at high risk of CNS relapse, it is unclear if CNS prophylaxis sufficiently mitigates that risk.[20]

First-Line Treatment
- *Our patient undergoes 3 cycles of R-CHOP with interim PET/CT showing excellent response to disease. He then completes 6 total cycles of R-CHOP.*
- *End of treatment PET/CT indicates complete response with no evidence of residual malignancy.*
- *Lumbar puncture and CNS prophylaxis are not indicated.*

Surveillance

- Baseline imaging should be repeated at completion of treatment to document remission.
- Patients should be monitored with serial history, physical examination, and laboratory work every 3 to 6 months for up to 5 years, and then annually.
- Imaging should not be performed more frequently than every 6 months during the first 2 years after completion of treatment, and then only as clinically indicated.
- If disease relapse is suspected based on clinical and imaging findings, repeat biopsy should be performed to confirm relapse.

Case Surveillance
- *Our patient does well post-treatment; however, at his 18-month follow-up he reports recent onset of night sweats and 15-pound weight loss.*
- *CT of the chest, abdomen, and pelvis is performed, and findings are concerning for new retroperitoneal and mesenteric lymphadenopathy.*
- *A biopsy is performed and confirms relapsed DLBCL.*

What Treatment Strategies Are Available on First Relapse?

- Second-line treatment strategies depend upon whether the patient is a candidate for eventual high-dose chemotherapy followed by auto-SCT.

- If a patient has primary refractory disease or relapses within the first 12 months, they should be referred for evaluation for CAR-T cell therapy.[21]
- In patients who are a candidate for transplant, second-line chemoimmunotherapy regimens include R-ICE (rituximab, ifosfamide, carboplatin, and etoposide) or R-GDP (rituximab, gemcitabine, dexamethasone, and cisplatin).[6]
- Patients who achieve a complete response with second-line treatment should proceed to transplant.[4,6] Patients who achieve only a partial response have traditionally had worse outcomes following autologous transplant, but it can still be considered.[22]
- For patients who are not candidates for transplant, second-line chemoimmunotherapy regimens include R-GemOx (rituximab, gemcitabine, oxaliplatin) or polatuzumab vedotin in combination with BR.[4] Patients who achieve a complete response can proceed with surveillance.

What Treatment Options Are Available for Multiply-Relapsed Disease?

- Third-line treatment can include anti-CD19 CAR-T cell therapy, regimens involving antibody–drug conjugates such as polatuzumab vedotin or loncastuximab tesirine, and tafasitamab in combination with lenalidomide, selinexor, or alternative chemoimmunotherapy regimens not utilized in the first or second line.[6]

Case 27.4: Peripheral T-Cell Lymphoma

A 62-year-old male presents to primary care due to fatigue. On exam he is found to have an irregular rhythm. Lab evaluation reveals hypercalcemia. The patient is treated medically for hypercalcemia with symptomatic relief. A CT scan at that time is unrevealing. Five months later he develops fevers, night sweats, and abdominal pain and is sent to the ED. He was found to be hypotensive, tachycardic, and febrile, and presumed to be septic. He was treated with broad spectrum IV antibiotics; his fevers persisted, and he was treated with IV steroids with significant improving. A CT scan was ordered to identify the source of infection and he was noted to have cervical, axillary, inguinal lymphadenopathy. An excisional biopsy is performed which revealed angioimmunoblastic T-cell lymphoma (AITL).

How Is the Diagnosis of T-Cell Lymphoma Established?

- Tissue diagnosis should be made by excisional or incisional biopsy. If unable to obtain surgical biopsy, then multiple cores may be adequate.
- Typical immunophenotype is positive for variable T-cell antigens and negative for B-cell antigens. Other than CD30+ in ALCL, T-cell antigens are variable. Rarely, aberrant CD20 may be expressed.
- The majority of cases are CD4+ and CD8-, but all combinations of CD4/CD8 are possible.

What Additional Genetic Testing Should Be Performed?

- In ALCL evaluate for ALK-1 status either by genetic analysis of t(2;5) or via IHC.
- EBER is identified in 40% of peripheral T-cell lymphomas and may be associated with a worse prognosis.
- Clonal T-cell receptor gene rearrangements are common, although it is not pathognomonic and false positives can be seen.

Patient's Diagnosis

- *Excisional biopsy with morphological review, IHC, and flow support diagnosis of peripheral T-cell lymphoma. Neoplastic cells are positive for CD3, TIA-1, CD2, CD5, and CD7 and negative for CD30, ALK1, BCL2, CD20, CD8, CD10, BCL6, Granzyme B, CD15, PAX5, and TdT. Ki-67 highlights a proliferative index of approximately 50% to 60% overall. Epstein-Barr virus-encoded RNA in situ hybridization (EBER ISH) is negative.*

How Is Peripheral T-Cell Lymphoma Worked Up and Staged?

- Staging is performed the same as in other aggressive lymphomas; physical exam, CBC, CMP, LDH, and staging scans with PET/CT or CT CAP with contrast (PET/CT is preferred). CT of the neck and/or MRI of the brain is used if there are concerning signs or symptoms for CNS involvement. There is increased importance of a skin exam as cutaneous manifestations are more common than in B-cell lymphomas.
- Bone marrow biopsy should be performed in all patients except in cases where PET/CT confirms bone marrow involvement.
- Echocardiogram should be obtained as anthracyclines remain a backbone of treatment.
- Consider HIV and HTLV-1 testing, as well as beta-2 microglobulin and C-reactive protein (CRP) for prognostic scoring.

Staging Findings

- *PET/CT indicated bilateral neck, axillary, and retroperitoneal adenopathy with hypermetabolic intramuscular activity concerning for extra nodal disease.*
- *Bone marrow biopsy showed an atypical lymphoid aggregate whose immunophenotype matched the LN biopsy, which is concerning for less than 5% involvement with peripheral T-cell lymphoma (PTCL).*
- *Serum LDH and beta-2 microglobulin were elevated at diagnosis. Hepatitis and HIV testing is negative.*

Does a Prognostic Stratification System Exist for Peripheral T-Cell Lymphoma?

- Although the IPI (see earlier in this chapter) was developed for B-cell lymphomas, it has shown to have prognostic significance in T-cell lymphomas as well;[23] however, this occurs with worse outcomes in IPI scores of 2 or greater. There are T-cell specific prognostic scores, but they have not been prospectively validated. The peripheral T-cell lymphoma unspecified (PTCLU) score assigns a point for each of the following:
  - Age older than 60 years
  - Serum LDH greater than normal
  - ECOG performance status 2 to 4
  - Bone marrow involvement
- Patients with zero points have a 5-year OS of 63%. One, two, and three to four of these adverse prognostic factors had 5-year OS of 53%, 33%, and 18%, respectively. A score of 0 to 1 is considered low risk, 2 is low-intermediate risk, 3 is high-intermediate risk, and a score of 4 to 5 is considered high-risk disease.

Peripheral T-Cell Lymphoma Unspecified Score

- *3—Poor risk disease*

What Are the First-Line Treatment Options for Peripheral T-Cell Lymphoma?

- Treatment of PTCL differs based on histology. ALCL-ALK–positive is the least aggressive PTCL; it has an available targeted therapy and is treated differently than all other histologies.

PTCL-NOS, ALCL-ALK–negative, and AITL are all treated with 6 cycles of CHOP, regardless of stage. Patients younger than 60 may benefit from the addition of etoposide. Brentuximab can be substituted for vincristine in patients with CD30-positive tumors, although the benefit of brentuximab was driven by the ALCL subgroup in the ECHELON-2 trial.[24]

- ALCL-ALK–positive is treated with brentuximab with CHP (cyclophosphamide, doxorubicin, prednisone); stage I to II is treated with 4 cycles + radiation or for 6 cycles +/- radiation, advanced stage is treated with 6 cycles +/- radiation.
- All patients should be re-staged after 3 to 4 cycles of chemotherapy, preferably with a PET scan; any progressive disease should be treated as relapse. Partial responses should be biopsied if possible.
- Consider consolidation with high-dose chemotherapy with autologous stem cell rescue for patients with ALCL, patients with ALK+ with a high IPI score, and for all patients with other histologies.

What Is the Role of Lumbar Puncture and Central Nervous System Prophylaxis?

- Consider lumbar puncture and MRI of the brain in patients with concerning signs or symptoms for CNS disease.
- Patients with PTCL are at low risk for CNS disease at presentation and at relapse.[25] There is a paucity of data regarding the necessity and efficacy of CNS prophylaxis in PTCL.[26]

First-Line Treatment

- *Our patient undergoes 4 cycles of CHOP with interim PET/CT showing excellent response. He completes an additional 2 cycles of CHOP.*
- *End of treatment PET/CT indicates complete response with no evidence of residual malignancy.*
- *He receives high-dose chemotherapy with autologous stem cell rescue as consolidation.*

Surveillance

- Surveillance recommendations are the same for PTCL as DLBCL (see Case 27.3 earlier in this chapter).

What Treatment Strategies Are Available on First Relapse?

- There is limited prospective data to guide second-line treatment of PTCL.
- For patients with ALCL, brentuximab is preferred. However, data supporting its use did not include patients treated with brentuximab in first line. Brentuximab may be considered if there was a long duration of remission after brentuximab in first-line treatment.
- Second-line treatment strategies depend upon whether the patient received high-dose chemotherapy and autologous stem cell rescue as part of first-line treatment and if the patient is a candidate for allogenic transplant.
- In patients who are a candidate for transplant, second-line options include combination chemotherapy (DHAP, ICE, and GDP are all acceptable) or single-agent chemotherapy. For non-transplant candidates, single-agent chemotherapy is recommended. Options include brentuximab if CD30-positive, belinostat, pralatrexate, and romidepsin. For ALK-positive ALCL, alectinib or crizotinib may be used. Bendamustine may be used in non-ALCL subtypes.
- Patients who achieve a complete response with second-line treatment should proceed to transplant. Patients who achieve only a partial response have traditionally had worse outcomes following autologous transplant, but it can still be considered.

What Treatment Options Are Available for Multiply-Relapsed Disease?

- Treatment recommendations remain the same for first and subsequent relapses.

Case 27.5: Burkitt Lymphoma

A 32-year-old male with a history of attention deficit hyperactivity disorder (ADHD) presented with progressively enlarging right neck mass for the last 2 months. He reported drenching night sweats, loss of appetite, difficulty swallowing, and hoarseness of voice. Physical exam confirmed a large right neck mass. Core biopsy of the right cervical LN showed high grade B-cell lymphoma with a Ki-67 greater than 99% and a "starry sky appearance." Immunophenotyping was positive for CD19, CD20, CD22, CD10, BCL6, and human leukocyte antigen (HLA)-DR, and negative for EBER, CD5, and BCL2. FISH studies were noted to be positive for MYC gene rearrangement/translocation t(8;14), and negative for BCL6 and BCL2 gene rearrangements, confirming BL.

How Is the Diagnosis of Burkitt Lymphoma Established?

- Tissue diagnosis is typically done by core or excisional biopsy.
- Morphology: Histologically, BL is characterized by complete effacement of LN architecture with sheets of lymphocytes, intermediate in size and nonpleomorphic, that contain basophilic cytoplasm, prominent vacuoles with round nuclei. Ki-67 typically approaches 100%. Classic "starry sky appearance" is caused by macrophages which have ingested the apoptotic tumor cells.
- IHC: The IHC is positive for CD20, CD10, BCL6, CD79a, HLADR, and CD45 and negative for CD5, BCL2, terminal deoxynucleotidyl transferase (TdT), and CD23. EBV positivity and CD21 expression is uniformly seen in endemic BL and 25% to 40% cases of sporadic BL.
- Genetics: A hallmark finding of BL is t(8;14), reciprocal translocation of the MYC gene, located on chromosome 8, to the immunoglobulin heavy chain (IGH) locus on chromosome 14. Rarely MYC translocations can involve chromosome 2 t(2;8) and chromosome 22 t(8;22). However, 5% of BL may lack MYC translocation and are now classified as Burkitt-like lymphoma with 11q aberration.
- Next-generation sequencing (NGS): Transcription factor *TCF3* or its negative regulator *ID3* was found to be mutated in 70% of sporadic and immunodeficiency associated BL and 40% of endemic cases.[27]

Patient's Diagnosis

- *Core biopsy of the right cervical LN showed high-grade B-cell lymphoma with Ki-67 greater than 99% and a "starry sky appearance." Immunophenotyping was positive for CD19, CD20, CD22, CD10, BCL6, and HLA-DR, and negative for EBER, CD5, and BCL2. FISH studies were noted to be positive for MYC gene rearrangement/translocation t(8;14), and negative for BCL6 and BCL2 gene rearrangements.*

Does Burkitt Lymphoma Have Subtypes?

- Sporadic BL is the most common subtype in the United States. It is common in males, more frequently involves extranodal sites (particularly the CNS), and is less commonly associated with EBV.
- Endemic BL is mostly seen in Africa, especially in areas where *Plasmodium falciparum* malaria is very prevalent. It is commonly associated with EBV, which plays a direct role in the pathogenesis of the lymphoma.

- Immunodeficient BL is primarily seen in HIV-positive patients and occurs in those with relatively high CD4 counts. Incidence of BL in HIV-positive patients has not changed despite the advent of highly active antiretroviral therapy (HAART).

Patient's Burkitt Lymphoma Subtype
- *Sporadic, negative for HIV and EBV*

How Is Burkitt Lymphoma Staged?

- The Ann Arbor and Murphy staging systems are commonly used for adults, whereas St. Jude's is used for pediatric patients.
- PET/CT or CT CAP is used for staging along with bone marrow biopsy.
- Given the high risk of CNS disease, lumbar puncture is routinely performed in all patients to look for CSF involvement.

Patient's Clinical Stage
- *PET/CT showed a biopsy-proven intensely hypermetabolic mass of 7.8 × 6.8 × 12.0 cm invading into the parapharyngeal soft tissues and extensive involvement along the cervical chains from the skull base to the base of neck. Additional sites of gastric, pancreatic, pleural/extrapleural, and intrathecal/perineural hypermetabolism were noted, representing additional sites of lymphoma. Bone marrow biopsy was positive for involvement by lymphoma. Lumbar puncture showed no evidence of malignant cells in the CSF. The previous findings were consistent with stage IV disease.*

Is There a Prognostic System for Burkitt Lymphoma?

- Age older than 40, impaired PS, elevated serum LDH, and CNS involvement were independently associated with adverse outcomes, forming the BL-IPI prognostic system.[28]
- BL-IPI consists of:
- Age 40 years or older
- ECOG PS (2 or greater)
- Serum LDH greater than 3X upper limit of normal (ULN)
  - CNS involvement
- Low risk (no risk factors; 18% of patients): 96% 3-year OS; 92% 3-year PFS.
- Intermediate risk (one risk factor; 36% of patients): 76% 3-year OS; 72% 3-year PFS.
- High risk (two or more risk factors; 46% of patients): 59% 3-year OS; 53% 3-year PFS.

Patient's Prognosis
- *BL-IPI Score -2, High Risk*

What Is the Front-Line Treatment for Burkitt Lymphoma?

- BL is very sensitive to chemotherapy and highly intensive combination chemotherapy regimens with CNS prophylaxis commonly used include:

  - Hyper-CVAD (which includes cyclophosphamide, vincristine, doxorubincin, dexamethasone, methotrexate, and cytarabine)
  - DA-EPOCH (dose adjusted, etoposide, vincristine, doxorubicin, cyclophosphamide, and prednisone)

- ○ CODOX-M (cyclophosphamide, vincristine, doxorubicin, and cytarabine)
- ○ CALGB 9251 (which includes cyclophosphamide, ifosfamide, methotrexate, vincristine, doxorubicin, cytarabine, and etoposide)
- Intensive multidrug chemotherapy results in remission rates of 65% to 100% and long-term survival of 40% to 80%.
- There have been no published randomized trials in BL comparing chemotherapy regimens.
- Recent retrospective study comparing CODOX-M/IVAC (ifosfamide, etoposide, cytarabine), hyper-CVAD, and R-EPOCH showed no difference in outcome.[29]
- The addition of rituximab to standard chemotherapy improved the event-free survival (EFS) and OS in a recent study.[30]
- Tumor lysis is an important complication in BL given the high rate of cell proliferation and turnover mandating the need for aggressive hydration and tumor lysis syndrome (TLS) prophylaxis with allopurinol.

What Is the Role of Lumbar Puncture and Central Nervous System Prophylaxis in Burkitt Lymphoma?

- CNS prophylaxis is a fundamental component of BL treatment given the 30% to 50% risk of CNS relapse without prophylaxis.[31]
- Intrathecal chemotherapy along with high-dose methotrexate and cytarabine are commonly employed for CNS prophylaxis along with use of more intense regimens for CNS involvement at baseline.

Patient's Treatment

- 'Given the high risk for TLS, the patient was started on aggressive hydration, allopurinol, and rasburicase. He received prephase treatment with steroids followed by DA-EPOCH-R (dose-adjusted etoposide, prednisone, vincristine, cyclophosphamide, doxorubicin, and rituximab) with intrathecal chemotherapy alternating with high-dose methotrexate/cytosine arabinoside (HD MTX/Ara-c). He completed 6 cycles and was noted to be in complete remission on the end of Rx PET. He is now on surveillance.

How Do You Treat Relapsed/Refractory Burkitt Lymphoma?

- The prognosis of relapsed/refractory BL is poor and patients should be encouraged to enroll in clinical trials.

Surveillance

- Follow-up visits include a history and physical examination, CBC, serum chemistries, and LDH every 3 to 4 months during the first year, every 6 months during the second year, and then annually.
- The role of follow-up imaging is not well defined but CT scans every 6 months for the first 2 years could be considered.

REVIEW QUESTIONS

1. A 57-year-old male with no prior medical history presents with fever, chills, night sweats, and an enlarging lymph node (LN) in the cervical area. He also thinks that he needs new glasses since his vision has recently worsened. On physical exam, he is thin, and a 4-cm mass is palpable in the anterior cervical LN chain. You also notice a right lateral rectus muscle palsy. He has an excisional biopsy that shows a CD20+, cyclin D1 is positive, and mantle cell lymphoma (MCL) is diagnosed. His PET scan shows only the LN biopsy area as avid. Which is the best next step?
   A. Start treatment with Nordic regimen
   B. Refer for bone marrow biopsy
   C. Start treatment with hyper-CVAD (cyclophosphamide, vincristine sulfate, doxorubicin hydrochloride [Adriamycin], dexamethasone)
   D. Refer for lumbar puncture
   E. Refer for endoscopy/colonoscopy

2. A 53-year-old female with a history of diabetes mellitus and end-stage renal disease (ESRD) on hemodialysis presents to your clinic. Her nephrologist has been administering intravenous (IV) iron for the last few months due to persistent iron deficiency anemia. About a month ago, she noticed an enlarging lump in the groin. She also reports that she has been very sweaty, especially at night, but she thinks it is her menopause. She goes to her primary care doctor, who decides to biopsy the lymph node (LN). The pathologist reports mantle cell lymphoma (MCL). Your physical exam is unremarkable, except for a 3.5-cm hard left inguinal mass. A PET scan only reports the inguinal mass as avid. Which is the best next step?
   A. Start treatment with Nordic regimen
   B. Refer for bone marrow biopsy
   C. Start treatment with hyper-CVAD (cyclophosphamide, vincristine sulfate, doxorubicin hydrochloride [Adriamycin], dexamethasone)
   D. Refer for lumbar puncture
   E. Refer for endoscopy

3. A 48-year-old female is referred to your clinic for recently diagnosed follicular lymphoma (FL). She had presented to the hospital with progressive low-grade fevers, night sweats, and weight loss over the past 3 months. She was noted to have mild anemia and thrombocytopenia. Imaging revealed diffuse lymphadenopathy above and below the diaphragm, and a cervical lymph node (LN) was biopsied and revealed low-grade FL (World Health Organization [WHO] grade 1). Serum lactate dehydrogenase (LDH), hepatitis, and HIV testing are negative. She undergoes cardiac testing and her ejection fraction is normal. A PET/CT was performed and revealed numerous LN groups above and below the diaphragm without evidence of bone marrow involvement. She was otherwise healthy prior to this diagnosis and is independent in her activities of daily living (ADLs) but is not currently working due to fatigue. Which of the following is the best next step in management?
   A. Bendamustine-rituximab (BR)
   B. R-CHOP (rituximab, cyclophosphamide, doxorubicin, vincristine, and prednisone)
   C. Bone marrow examination
   D. Diagnostic lumbar puncture
   E. R-CVP (rituximab, cyclophosphamide, vincristine, and prednisolone)

4. A 62-year-old male presents to establish care for recently diagnosed follicular lymphoma (FL). He had presented to the hospital with painless swelling in his neck and imaging

reveals significantly enlarged cervical lymph nodes (LNs), as well as further evidence of disease in the abdomen. He underwent a biopsy that revealed a nodular growth pattern consistent with FL, notable for solid sheets of centroblasts with greater than 15 centroblasts per high power field (HPF; grade 3b). He is otherwise healthy and has no comorbidities. Which of the following would be the best initial treatment option?

A. Bendamustine-rituximab (BR)
B. R-CVP (rituximab, cyclophosphamide, vincristine, and prednisolone)
C. R-CHOP (rituximab, cyclophosphamide, doxorubicin, vincristine, and prednisone)
D. Lenalidomide-rituximab
E. Rituximab monotherapy

5. A 52-year-old female presents for follow-up for diffuse large B-cell lymphoma (DLBCL). She had initially been diagnosed after presenting to the hospital with weight loss and abdominal pain. Imaging had revealed diffuse lymphadenopathy in the chest and abdomen and diagnosis was performed by an inguinal lymph node (LN) biopsy. She has completed 3 cycles of R-CHOP (rituximab, cyclophosphamide, doxorubicin, vincristine, and prednisone) therapy and has recently undergone a PET/CT that showed a complete response to therapy with no evidence of disease. What is the best next step in management?

A. Proceed with surveillance with imaging in 3 to 6 months
B. Proceed with surveillance with imaging in 12 months
C. Referral for involved-site radiation therapy (ISRT)
D. Continue R-CHOP

6. A 62-year-old female presents to the hospital with swelling in her neck accompanied by weight loss over the past 2 weeks. Imaging is performed and reveals a 3.3-cm cervical lymph node (LN) conglomerate as well as bilateral axillary lymphadenopathy. There is no lymphadenopathy noted in the abdomen or pelvis. Her complete blood count (CBC) reveals anemia and thrombocytopenia. Her serum lactate dehydrogenase (LDH) is 147 (upper limit of normal, 150). She reports that she has recently had to stop working due to fatigue but is otherwise independent at home. Which of the following is a risk factor for central nervous system (CNS) disease in this patient?

A. Age
B. Anemia/thrombocytopenia
C. Serum LDH
D. Performance status (PS)
E. Disease site(s)

7. A 66-year-old male is referred to your clinic for recently diagnosed anaplastic lymphoma kinase (ALK)-positive anaplastic large-cell lymphoma (ALCL), PET imaging reveals stage III disease. He has diabetes complicated by diabetic neuropathy, which causes some numbness and tingling in his toes, but balance remains intact. He has no neuropathy in his fingers. Which of the following is the best treatment option?

A. BV-CHP (brentuximab vedotin, cyclophosphamide, doxorubicin, and prednisone)
B. R-CHOP (rituximab, cyclophosphamide, doxorubicin, vincristine, and prednisone)
C. CHOP (cyclophosphamide, doxorubicin, vincristine, and prednisone)
D. CHEP (cyclophosphamide, Adriamycin, etoposide and prednisone)
E. CVP (cyclophosphamide, vincristine, and prednisolone)

8. A 35-year-old man, HIV-positive, presented to the ED with a 3-week history of fevers, night sweats, rapidly enlarging right jaw mass, and a painful left axillary mass. His CD4

count was 36 per cubic mm and HIV viral load 284,000/mm³. A biopsy of the left axillary mass revealed small to intermediate-sized cells with cleaved nuclei and a starry sky appearance under low power. Which cytogenetic abnormality is not associated with this description?

A. t(8;14)
B. t(2;8)
C. t(8;21)
D. t(8,22)

9. A 55-year-old man with no significant past medical history (PMH) presents with progressively worsening abdominal pain, fullness, and vomiting. CT of the abdomen and pelvis showed a 5 × 6 cm mesenteric mass along enlarged bilateral iliac lymph nodes (LNs) and moderate bilateral pleural effusions. Biopsy of the mesenteric mass showed a CD10+, kappa-restricted B-cell population with Ki-67 approaching 100%. Fluorescent in situ hybridization (FISH) was positive for MYC/immunoglobulin heavy chain (MYC/IGH). Which is the best treatment option for management of this patient?

A. R-CHOP (rituximab, cyclophosphamide, doxorubicin, vincristine, and prednisone)
B. DA-EPOCH-R (dose-adjusted etoposide, prednisone, vincristine, cyclophosphamide, doxorubicin, and rituximab) with central nervous system (CNS) therapy
C. R-CHOP with intrathecal chemotherapy (IT chemo)
D. Bendamustine-rituximab (BR)

ANSWERS AND RATIONALES

1. **D. Refer for lumbar puncture.** The patient should be referred for a lumbar puncture to rule out central nervous system (CNS) disease based on his symptoms and physical exam. The presence of CNS disease will change the stage of the disease from stage I, non-bulky, to stage IV.

2. **E. Refer for endoscopy.** The patient likely has stage I disease. However, this needs to be confirmed by performing an endoscopy and colonoscopy as lesions in the intestines can be missed by a PET scan. Furthermore, the persistent anemia in this patient could be related to an undiagnosed lesion in the bowel.

3. **C. Bone marrow examination.** This patient has otherwise unexplained cytopenias, and PET/CT did not indicate bone marrow involvement. She should undergo bone marrow biopsy to evaluate for lymphoma involvement prior to starting treatment.

4. **C. R-CHOP (rituximab, cyclophosphamide, doxorubicin, vincristine, and prednisone).** This patient has grade 3b FL which should be treated as diffuse large B-cell lymphoma (DLBCL). R-CHOP is the only answer choice that is considered a first-line treatment option in this case.

5. **D. Continue R-CHOP.** In patients with advanced DLBCL, interim PET/CT showing complete response should be followed by 3 more cycles of R-CHOP. However, 3 cycles of treatment would not be considered sufficient despite no evidence of disease on interim scans.

6. **A. Age.** Age older than 60 is considered a risk factor for CNS disease per Central Nervous System International Prognostic Index (CNS-IPI) guidelines. The patient does not meet any other CNS-IPI criteria and would be considered low risk for CNS involvement.

7. **A. BV-CHP (brentuximab vedotin, cyclophosphamide, doxorubicin, and prednisone).** Patients with ALK+ ALCL derived the most benefit in the ECHELON-2 trial, with a significant improvement in progression-free survival (PFS) and overall survival (OS). This patient's baseline peripheral neuropathy (PN) is grade 1 and was included in the trial. Although there was an increase in all-grade PN in the BV arm, there was not a significant increase in grade 3 or greater PN than was seen with vincristine treatment. If the patient develops grade 2 neuropathy, the brentuximab will need to be dose reduced. Although CHEP may be an attractive option for a patient with baseline grade 2 or higher PN, this has not been well studied in peripheral T-cell lymphoma (PTCL).

8. **C. t(8;21).** Burkitt lymphoma is commonly associated with reciprocal translocations of the *MYC* gene to IGH, t(8;14), κ t(2;8) and λ t(8;22). t(8;21) is a common chromosomal abnormality associated with acute myeloid leukemia (AML).

9. **B. DA-EPOCH-R (dose-adjusted etoposide, prednisone, vincristine, cyclophosphamide, doxorubicin, and rituximab) with central nervous system (CNS) therapy.** This patient has Burkitt lymphoma (BL). DA-EPOCH-R with CNS-directed therapy and prophylaxis has shown superior outcomes compared to the less intense regimens such as R-CHOP. CNS prophylaxis and therapy is a fundamental component of BL therapy given the high risk of CNS relapse.

REFERENCES

1. Cheson BD, Fisher RI, Barrington SF, et al. Recommendations for initial evaluation, staging, and response assessment of Hodgkin and non-Hodgkin lymphoma: the Lugano classification. *J Clin Oncol.* 2014;32(27):3059–3068. doi:10.1200/JCO.2013.54.8800

2. Zukerberg LR, Yang WI, Arnold A, Harris NL. Cyclin D1 expression in non-Hodgkin's lymphomas. Detection by immunohistochemistry. *Am J Clin Pathol.* 1995;103(6):756–760. doi:10.1093/ajcp/103.6.756

3. Bertoni F, Rinaldi A, Zucca E, Cavalli F. Update on the molecular biology of mantle cell lymphoma. *Hematol Oncol.* 2006;24(1):22–27. doi:10.1002/hon.767

4. Geisler CH, Kolstad A, Laurell A, et al. The Mantle Cell Lymphoma International Prognostic Index (MIPI) is superior to the International Prognostic Index (IPI) in predicting survival following intensive first-line immuno-chemotherapy and autologous stem cell transplantation (ASCT). *Blood.* 2010;115(8):1530–1533. doi:10.1182/blood-2009-08-236570

5. Rule S, Dreyling M, Goy A, et al. Outcomes in 370 patients with mantle cell lymphoma treated with ibrutinib: a pooled analysis from three open-label studies. *Br J Haematol.* 2017;179(3):430–438. doi:10.1111/bjh.14870

6. National Comprehensive Cancer Network. B-cell lymphomas (version 5.2021). https://www.nccn.org/professionals/physician_gls/pdf/b-cell.pdf

7. Wang M, Munoz J, Goy A, et al. KTE-X19 CAR T-cell therapy in relapsed or refractory mantle-cell lymphoma. *N Engl J Med.* 2020;382(14):1331–1342. doi:10.1056/NEJMoa1914347

8. Kaushansky K, Prchal JT, Bruns LJ, et al., eds. *Williams Hematology.* McGraw Hill; 2021.

9. Solal-Céligny P, Roy P, Colombat P, et al. Follicular lymphoma international prognostic index. *Blood.* 2004;104(5):1258–1265. doi:10.1182/blood-2003-12-4434

10. Nooka AK, Nabhan C, Zhou X, et al. Examination of the Follicular Lymphoma International Prognostic Index (FLIPI) in the national lymphocare study (NLCS): a prospective US patient cohort treated predominantly in community practices. *Ann Oncol.* 2013;24(2):441–448. doi:10.1093/annonc/mds429

11. Brice P, Bastion Y, Lepage E, et al. Comparison in low-tumor-burden follicular lymphomas between an initial no-treatment policy, prednimustine, or interferon alfa: a randomized study from the Groupe d'Etude des Lymphomes Folliculaires. Groupe d'Etude des Lymphomes de l'Adulte. *J Clin Oncol.* 1997;15(3):1110–1117. doi:10.1200/JCO.1997.15.3.1110

12. Marcus R, Davies A, Ando K, et al. Obinutuzumab for the first-line treatment of follicular lymphoma. *N Engl J Med.* 2017;377(14):1331–1344. doi:10.1056/NEJMoa1614598

13. Casulo C, Friedberg JW, Ahn KW, et al. Autologous transplantation in follicular lymphoma with early therapy failure: a national lymphocare study and center for international blood and marrow transplant research analysis. *Biol Blood Marrow Transplant.* 2018;24(6):1163–1171. doi:10.1016/j.bbmt.2017.12.771

14. Fu K, Weisenburger DD, Choi WWL, et al. Addition of rituximab to standard chemotherapy improves the survival of both the germinal center B-cell-like and non-germinal center B-cell-like subtypes of diffuse large B-cell lymphoma. *J Clin Oncol.* 2008;26(28):4587–4594. doi:10.1200/JCO.2007.15.9277

15. Chapuy B, Stewart C, Dunford AJ, et al. Molecular subtypes of diffuse large B cell lymphoma are associated with distinct pathogenic mechanisms and outcomes. *Nat Med.* 2018;24(5):679–690. doi:10.1038/s41591-018-0016-8

16. International Non-Hodgkin's Lymphoma Prognostic Factors Project. A predictive model for aggressive non-Hodgkin's lymphoma. *N Engl J Med.* 1993;329(14):987–994. doi:10.1056/NEJM199309303291402

17. Tilly H, Morschhauser F, Sehn LH, et al. Polatuzumab vedotin in previously untreated diffuse large B-cell lymphoma. *N Engl J Med.* 2022;386(4):351–363. doi:10.1056/NEJMoa2115304

18. Schmitz N, Zeynalova S, Nickelsen M, et al. CNS international prognostic index: a risk model for CNS relapse in patients with diffuse large B-cell lymphoma treated with R-CHOP. *J Clin Oncol.* 2016;34(26):3150–3156. doi:10.1200/JCO.2015.65.6520

19. Wilson MR, Eyre TA, Martinez-Calle N, et al. Timing of high-dose methotrexate CNS prophylaxis in DLBCL: an analysis of toxicity and impact on R-CHOP delivery. *Blood Adv.* 2020;4(15):3586–3593. doi:10.1182/bloodadvances.2020002421

20. Bobillo S, Joffe E, Sermer D, et al. Prophylaxis with intrathecal or high-dose methotrexate in diffuse large B-cell lymphoma and high risk of CNS relapse. *Blood Cancer J.* 2021;11(6):113. doi:10.1038/s41408-021-00506-3

21. Locke FL, Miklos DB, Jacobson CA, et al. Axicabtagene ciloleucel as second-line therapy for large B-cell lymphoma. *N Engl J Med.* 2022;386(7):640–654. doi:10.1056/NEJMoa2116133

22. Rodriguez J, Caballero MD, Gutierrez A, et al. Autologous stem-cell transplantation in diffuse large B-cell non-Hodgkin's lymphoma not achieving complete response after induction chemotherapy: The GEL/TAMO experience. *Ann Oncol.* 2004;15(10):1504–1509. doi:10.1093/annonc/mdh391

23. Schmitz N, Trümper L, Ziepert M, et al. Treatment and prognosis of mature T-cell and NK-cell lymphoma: an analysis of patients with T-cell lymphoma treated in studies of the German High-Grade Non-Hodgkin Lymphoma Study Group. *Blood.* 2010;116(18):3418–3425. doi:10.1182/blood-2010-02-270785

24. Horwitz S, O'Connor OA, Pro B, et al. Brentuximab vedotin with chemotherapy for CD30-positive peripheral T-cell lymphoma (ECHELON-2): a global, double-blind, randomised, phase 3 trial. *Lancet*. 2019;393(10168):229–240. doi:10.1016/S0140-6736(18)32984-2

25. Pro B, Perini G. Central nervous system prophylaxis in peripheral T-cell lymphoma. *Blood*. 2010;115(26):5427. doi:10.1182/blood-2010-02-266890

26. Zing N, Fischer T, Federico M, et al. Diagnosis, prevention and treatment of central nervous system involvement in peripheral T-cell lymphomas. *Crit Rev Oncol Hematol*. 2021;167:103496. doi:10.1016/j.critrevonc.2021.103496

27. Love C, Sun Z, Jima D, et al. The genetic landscape of mutations in Burkitt lymphoma. *Nat Genet*. 2012;44(12):1321–1325. doi:10.1038/ng.2468

28. Olszewski AJ, Jakobsen LH, Collins GP, et al. Burkitt lymphoma international prognostic index. *J Clin Oncol*. 2021;39(10):1129–1138. doi:10.1200/JCO.20.03288

29. Evens AM, Danilov A, Jagadeesh D, et al. Burkitt lymphoma in the modern era: real-world outcomes and prognostication across 30 US cancer centers. *Blood*. 2021;137(3):374–386. doi:10.1182/blood.2020006926

30. Ribrag V, Koscielny S, Bosq J, et al. Rituximab and dose-dense chemotherapy for adults with Burkitt's lymphoma: a randomised, controlled, open-label, phase 3 trial. *Lancet*. 2016;387(10036):2402–2411. doi:10.1016/S0140-6736(15)01317-3

31. Hill QA, Owen RG. CNS prophylaxis in lymphoma: who to target and what therapy to use. *Blood Reviews*. 2006;20(6):319–332. doi:10.1016/j.blre.2006.02.001

CHAPTER 28

Multiple Myeloma and Plasma Cell Neoplasms

Christopher T. Su, Jason C. Chen, and Matthew J. Pianko

INTRODUCTION

In 2021, there were an estimated 34,920 estimated new cases of multiple myeloma (MM), with a slight male predominance (55% vs. 45%). There were also an estimated 12,410 deaths, making MM the second most common hematologic malignancy following non-Hodgkin's lymphoma by both incidence and deaths in the United States.[1] Globally, the cumulative risk of being diagnosed with MM from birth to 74 years of age is 0.24% for men and 0.17% for women, making the diagnosis of MM 1.5 times more likely for men compared to women.[2] Encouragingly, 5-year survival has increased from 23.7% in 1976 to 53.9% in 2016, owing to rapid advances in MM therapy.[3]

Risk factors for MM include male sex, older age, African American race, and increased body mass index (BMI). As discussed previously, MM occurs more frequently in men. It is well known that MM is predominantly a disease of older adults, with over 60% of MM diagnosed over the age of 65 and less than 15% under the age of 55. The median age of death is 75 and 80% of deaths occur in those over the age of 65.[2] In terms of race, the incidence of MM is twice as common in African Americans when compared to whites, especially in patients younger than 50 years of age.[4] Finally, increased BMI has also been noted as a risk factor in developing MM.

MM is a disease caused by neoplastic plasma cells, characterized by the production of monoclonal immunoglobulin detected in the serum due to cellular expansion of the neoplastic cells in the bone marrow.[5] Typically, the secreted monoclonal proteins are IgG (most common) or IgA, and very rarely IgD or IgM.[6] MM is but one entity on the spectrum of plasma cell dyscrasias, which range from monoclonal gammopathy of undetermined significance (MGUS) to smoldering multiple myeloma (SMM), and finally active myeloma.

CASE SUMMARIES

Case 28.1: Precursor Disease (Monoclonal Gammopathy of Undetermined Significance, Smoldering Multiple Myeloma)

You are seeing a 72-year-old gentleman with a history of diabetes and hypertension and he was referred to you by his primary care physician (PCP) after an incidental finding of elevated total protein on routine labs. Serum protein electrophoresis (SPEP) and immunofixation (IFIX) showed a serum monoclonal IgG kappa protein level of 2.1 g/dL and an elevated serum free kappa/lambda light chain ratio of 14. Whole-body imaging with PET/CT did not show any concerning lytic lesions or plasmacytomas. MRI of the total spine and pelvis revealed no focal bone marrow lesions. Labs did not show any signs of renal failure, hypercalcemia, or anemia. A bone marrow biopsy showed involvement with atypical plasma cells, 20% to 25% of cellularity by CD138 immunohistochemistry (IHC), 23% clonal plasma cells by aspirate smear, and normal cytogenetics (46,XY[20]). Fluorescent in situ hybridization (FISH) testing showed no evidence of t(4;14), del17p, t(14;16), 1q abnormalities, or monosomy 13. The patient presents to your clinic for follow-up to review his diagnosis and management.

What Is the Diagnosis?

- The diagnostic criteria for MM, SMM, and MGUS as defined by the International Myeloma Working Group (IMWG)[7] are noted in the text that follows (Table 28.1).

Table 28.1 Diagnostic Criteria for MM, SMM, and MGUS as Defined by the International Myeloma Working Group

Diagnosis	Pathological Testing Results	Myeloma-Defining Events
MM	<ul><li>Clonal plasma cell ≥10% in the bone marrow OR</li><li>Biopsy-proven bone or extramedullary plasmacytoma</li></ul>	<ul><li>ANY one of:<ul><li>Hypercalcemia: serum calcium >1 mg/dL over the upper limit of normal, or >11 mg/dL</li><li>Renal insufficiency: creatinine clearance <40 mL/min, or serum creatinine >2 mg/dL, attributed to MM</li><li>Anemia: hemoglobin >2 g/dL below lower limit of normal, or <10 g/dL</li><li>Bone lesions: 1+ osteolytic lesions on x-ray, CT, or PET</li></ul></li><li>OR ANY one of:<ul><li>Clonal plasma cell ≥60% in the bone marrow</li><li>Involved: uninvolved serum free light chain ratio ≥100</li><li>>1 focal bone marrow lesion greater than 0.5 cm in size on MRI</li></ul></li></ul>Mnemonic: SLiM-CRAB (Sixty, Light, MRI, Calcium, Renal, Anemia, Bone)
SMM	<ul><li>Serum monoclonal protein (IgG or IgA) ≥3 g/dL OR</li><li>Urine monoclonal protein ≥500 mg per 24 hours AND/OR</li><li>Clonal plasma cells in bone marrow 10%–59%</li></ul>	No myeloma-defining events can be present.
MGUS	<ul><li>Serum monoclonal protein <3 g/dL AND</li><li>Clonal plasma cells in bone marrow <10%</li></ul>	No myeloma-defining events can be present.

Table 28.2 Mayo MGUS Model

Risk Group	Definition	Relative Risk	Absolute Risk of Progression at 20 Years
Low	• Serum monoclonal protein <1.5 g/dL AND • IgG subtype normal AND • FLC ratio 0.26–1.65	1	5%
Low-intermediate	1 factor abnormal	5.4	21%
High-intermediate	2 factors abnormal	10.1	37%
High	3 factors abnormal	20.8	58%

FLC, free light chain; MGUS, monoclonal gammopathy of undetermined significance.

Based on This Patient's Results, What Is the Diagnosis and What Are the Next Steps in the Evaluation?

• *This patient has a diagnosis of asymptomatic SMM, as his marrow showed greater than 10% plasma cells without evidence of end-organ damage or elevated biomarkers of malignancy that would meet the criteria for active MM. It is important to ensure that this patient does not have other findings of monoclonal protein-related disorders causing organ damage such as light chain deposition disease, or systemic amyloidosis, or other causes of monoclonal gammopathy of renal significance. Unexplained proteinuria should raise the question of whether a renal biopsy is needed or a fat pad biopsy could be considered. If suspected, additional biopsies and referrals to other specialists (for example, cardiology for endomyocardial biopsy) may be needed.*

How Is Monoclonal Gammopathy of Undetermined Significance Risk Stratified and Managed?

• MGUS can be risk-stratified based on the Mayo MGUS model (Table 28.2).[8]
• As MGUS is often incidentally diagnosed and most patients do not go on to develop MM (for low-risk disease risk of progression is approximately 1% every year), observation is generally recommended.[9]

Table 28.3 Mayo 2018 2/20/20 Criteria for SMM Risk Stratification

Risk Group	Definition	Estimated Rate of Progression in 2 Years	Estimated Rate of Progression in 5 Years	Estimated Rate of Progression in 10 Years
Low	None of the intermediate criteria	9.7%	22.5%	52.7%
Intermediate	• Serum monoclonal protein >2 g/dL OR • Clonal plasma cells in bone marrow >20% OR • Involved: uninvolved serum-free light chain ratio ≥20	26.3%	46.7%	65.3%
High	Two or more of the intermediate criteria	47.4%	81.5%	96.5%

Table 28.4   2020 IMWG SMM Risk Stratification Criteria

Risk Factor	Scoring
Involved:Uninvolved Serum-Free Light Chain Ratio	
>10–25	2
>25–40	3
>40	5
Serum Monoclonal Protein	
>1.5–3 g/dL	3
>3 g/dL	4
Clonal Plasma Cells in Bone Marrow	
>15–20%	2
>20–30%	3
>30–40%	5
>40%	6
Cytogenetic Abnormality on FISH Testing	
Any abnormality	2

FISH, fluorescent in situ hybridization; IMWG, International Myeloma Working Group; SMM, smoldering multiple melanoma.

How Is Smoldering Multiple Myeloma Risk Stratified and What Is This Patient's Risk?

- SMM can be risk stratified by using the Mayo 2018 2/20/20 criteria (Table 28.3).[10]
- The revised 2020 IMWG SMM risk stratification criteria include a scoring system that includes cytogenetic abnormalities (Table 28.4).[11]
- Out of a total possible 17 points in the previously described scoring schema, SMM patients can be categorized into four risk groups (Table 28.5).
- This patient has bone marrow plasma cells (BMPC) greater than 10% without signs of end-organ damage, so it meets the criteria for asymptomatic SMM. Based on the Mayo 2018 criteria, this patient has high-risk disease given BMPC greater than 20% and M-protein greater than 2 g/dL. Of note, he scores 8 points on the revised 2020 IMWG criteria (free light chain [FLC] ratio of 14—2 points; serum M-protein of 2.1 g/dL—3 points; 20% to 25% atypical plasma cells in bone marrow—3 points; no cytogenetic abnormality on FISH—0 points). This places him in the low-intermediate risk category with an estimated 26.2% rate of progression in 2 years.

Table 28.5   Risk Group Categorization for SMM Patients

Risk Group	Risk Scoring Range	Estimated Rate of Progression in 2 Years
Low	0–4	3.8%
Low-intermediate	5–8	26.2%
Intermediate	9–12	51.1%
High	>12	72.5%

SMM, smoldering multiple melanoma.

How Should Smoldering Multiple Myeloma Be Treated?

- Management of patients with newly diagnosed SMM depends on their risk stratification and comorbidities. Given the paucity of prospective data on SMM patients, enrollment in a clinical trial is recommended for all patients, if available. Otherwise, for patients with low- or intermediate-risk SMM, close observation is recommended. This includes labs every 3 to 6 months along with annual whole-body imaging, ideally using the same modality as during the initial evaluation for comparison. Patients with only one focal lesion detected on prior MRI scan should have imaging done every 6 months given the higher risk for symptomatic disease progression. For patients with rising markers, a repeat bone marrow biopsy may be needed as well.

- For patients with high-risk disease per Mayo 2018 2/20/20 criteria (two or more factors present), enrollment in a clinical trial, treatment with lenalidomide-based therapy, or observation can be considered. Two major randomized trials using either single-agent lenalidomide or combination therapy with lenalidomide and dexamethasone (RD) have established the role of treatment in asymptomatic high-risk SMM patients. The QuiRedex trial was an open-label Phase 3 trial conducted in Spain and Portugal which randomized high-risk SMM patients to lenalidomide plus dexamethasone versus observation.[12] High-risk SMM was defined as BMPC of 10% or greater, M-protein of greater than 3 g/dL (IgG) or greater than 2 g/dL (IgA), or Bence-Jones proteinuria greater than 1 g/24 hr, with immunoparesis (low level of 1 or more uninvolved immunoglobulins), and a flow cytometry-based assessment of the percentage of aberrant plasma cells in bone marrow aspirate (greater than 95%) instead of the Mayo 2018 criteria. In the long-term follow-up of the QuiRedex trial, with a median follow-up of 75 months, there was an improvement in progression-free survival (PFS) with lenalidomide and dexamethasone (hazard ratio [HR] 0.24, P less than 0.0001). While median overall survival (mOS) was not reached in either arm, there was an improvement in overall survival (OS) with lenalidomide and dexamethasone (HR 0.43, P = 0.024). Concerns regarding inadequate screening imaging and lack of widespread availability of tools used to define HR in the study were caveats that limited the uptake of RD as a standard of care for high-risk SMM. The Eastern Cooperative Oncology Group (ECOG) EAA173 Phase 3 trial conducted in the United States utilized single-agent lenalidomide versus observation for asymptomatic intermediate- and high-risk SMM patients.[13] Of note, this trial used the older Mayo 2008 risk stratification system, which considered M-protein greater than 3 g/dL, BMPC greater than 10%, and abnormal FLC ratio as high-risk features. After a median follow-up of 35 months, lenalidomide was associated with improved PFS (HR 0.28, P = 0.002) compared with observation, without a significant difference in OS. A post-hoc analysis demonstrated that the benefit of lenalidomide was only in the intermediate-risk group per Mayo 2008 criteria, and only in the high-risk group per Mayo 2018 criteria. Given the limitations of previously published trials and known long-term toxicities related to lenalidomide use (for example, secondary malignancies, cytopenia), patients should be counseled about the risks and benefits of active therapy. In addition, ongoing trials using novel agents and combinations such as the Phase 2 GEM-CESAR trial (carfilzomib-based combination therapy with autologous transplant) and the randomized Phase 3 ECOG EAA173/DETER-SMM trial (daratumumab, lenalidomide, and dexamethasone versus lenalidomide and dexamethasone) aim to demonstrate potential survival benefits with a more aggressive upfront approach for high-risk SMM patients.

Based on This Patient's Presentation, What Is the Recommended Treatment Plan?

- *Given that this patient has high-risk SMM by the Mayo 2018 risk stratification criteria, he should be considered for a clinical trial, observation, or lenalidomide-based therapy.*
- *Since no trials are available at your institution for SMM patients at this time, you discuss the role of lenalidomide versus observation for his high-risk SMM. The patient wishes to minimize*

any side effects at this time given his good quality of life, so he opts for close observation with clinic visits and labs every 3 months and annual MRI imaging according to IMWG imaging guidelines.[14]

Case 28.2: Newly Diagnosed, Transplant-Eligible Multiple Myeloma

You are seeing a 65-year-old gentleman who initially presented to his PCP with lower back pain. He was noted to have a serum IgG kappa monoclonal protein of 4.5 g/dL and evidence of lytic bone lesions on his MRI lumbar spine. His bone marrow biopsy shows approximately 60% to 65% involvement by aberrant kappa light chain plasma cells by CD138 IHC. Cytogenetics and FISH testing show trisomy 7 only and the absence of other high-risk features, and he was staged as having Revised International Staging System (R-ISS) stage II standard-risk MM. He has excellent health otherwise and walks 2 miles per day. He has normal renal function. His only medical comorbidity is hypertension, for which he takes hydrochlorothiazide. He presents to you to discuss treatment for MM.

What Is the Workup for Multiple Myeloma?

- Workup of MM generally consists of a comprehensive metabolic panel (CMP), complete blood count (CBC), serum β2 microglobulin, lactate dehydrogenase (LDH), SPEP, and urine protein electrophoresis (UPEP), followed by serum and urine IFIX. In addition, the serum FLC assay, which measures unbound kappa and lambda light chains in the serum, is

Table 28.6   Revised International Staging System Criteria for MM Staging

Prognostic Factor	Criteria
ISS Stage	
I	Serum β2 microglobulin <3.5 mg/L **AND** serum albumin ≥3.5 g/dL
II	Not ISS stage I or III
III	Serum β2 microglobulin ≥5.5 mg/L
Cytogenetics by FISH	
High-risk	Presence of del(17p) **AND/OR** t(4;14) **AND/OR** t(14;16)
Standard risk	No high-risk cytogenetics
Lactate Dehydrogenase	
Normal	Serum LDH <upper limit of normal
High	Serum LDH >upper limit of normal
R-ISS Staging	
I	ISS stage I **AND** standard-risk cytogenetics **AND** normal LDH
II	Not R-ISS stage I or III
III	ISS stage III **AND** either high-risk cytogenetics **OR** high LDH

FISH, fluorescent in situ hybridization; ISS, International Staging System; LDH, lactate dehydrogenase; MM, multiple melanoma; R-ISS, Revised International Staging System.

Source: Palumbo A, Avet-Loiseau H, Oliva S, et al. Revised international staging system for multiple myeloma: a report from International Myeloma Working Group. *J Clin Oncol.* 2015;33(26):2863–2869. doi:10.1200/JCO.2015.61.2267

important, as abnormal FLC ratios indicating the abnormal production of a characteristic light chain had been reported in 95% of MM patients.[15] The bone marrow biopsy is critical to the diagnosis of MM, which is used to determine the percentage of clonal plasma cells. The bone marrow biopsy sample should be sent for cytogenetics and FISH testing, which has prognostic significance. A complete evaluation of the skeletal system should be pursued, typically with CT, PET, or MRI to evaluate for any lytic bone lesions.

How Is Multiple Myeloma Staged?

- MM is staged using the R-ISS criteria (Table 28.6).[16]

How Is Multiple Myeloma Risk Stratified?

- The Mayo Clinic has proposed separate risk-stratification criteria for newly diagnosed MM, termed mSMART 3.0.[17] The Mayo model integrates additional genetic abnormalities compared to standard R-ISS staging (Table 28.7).

What Is the Diagnosis and Treatment?

- The patient is diagnosed with MM and urgent initiation of systemic therapy is indicated. The "standard" induction therapy is triplet therapy with lenalidomide, bortezomib, and dexamethasone (RVD), as established by the SWOG S0777 trial which demonstrated significant improvement in both PFS and OS with the addition of bortezomib to lenalidomide and dexamethasone over doublet therapy with lenalidomide and dexamethasone alone.[18] However, other regimens have been investigated, including carfilzomib, lenalidomide, and dexamethasone (KRD) in standard-risk MM in ENDURANCE,[19] and quadruplet therapy with the addition of daratumumab to RVD (D-RVD) in the phase 2 GRIFFIN trial.[20] The standard of care for a new diagnosis of high-risk multiple myeloma has not been defined; RVD, D-RVD, or KRD would be acceptable choices for this population. Research is ongoing to determine

Table 28.7 mSMART 3.0 Model

Risk Level	Definition

High risk	**ANY** of the following:
	• High-risk genetic abnormalities including **ANY** of the following:
	   ○ t(4;14)
	   ○ t(14;16)
	   ○ t(14;20)
	   ○ del(17p)
	   ○ *p53* mutation
	   ○ gain(1q)
	• R-ISS stage 3 disease
	• High plasma cell S phase
	• High-risk signature on gene expression profiling

Standard risk	None of the previously noted high-risk factors. Genetic abnormalities can include: • Trisomies • t(6;14) • t(11;14)

R-ISS, Revised International Staging System.

the optimal patient population that would benefit from KRD and D-RVD, although a standard induction chemotherapy regimen with RVD is appropriate in this case.

- Medically fit patients with minimal comorbidities should be considered for autologous hematopoietic cell transplantation (AHCT), as there is evidence of improved PFS over standard medical therapy, although OS improvements have yet to be observed.[21] The IFM2009 trial randomized newly diagnosed MM patients to induction chemotherapy with RVD followed by either consolidation chemotherapy with more RVD or high-dose chemotherapy followed by AHCT.[22] RVD with transplant had significantly prolonged PFS over RVD alone, although there were no significant OS differences. Two arms of the FORTE trial randomized MM patients to KRD followed by AHCT to KRD alone, and KRD followed by AHCT demonstrated improved responses compared to KRD alone.[23] Generally, allogeneic transplantation is not pursued for MM, and tandem autologous transplantation is seldom done except in very specific high-risk cases. Thus, we would generally recommend proceeding to a single AHCT following the completion of induction chemotherapy.

- Following AHCT, maintenance therapy should be considered. A meta-analysis comparing lenalidomide maintenance following AHCT against placebo or observation found improved PFS and OS with lenalidomide.[24] The BMT CTN 0702 trial compared maintenance therapies with a second tandem AHCT, additional cycles of RVD, or lenalidomide alone and found that the first two options did not improve PFS or OS, leaving a single AHCT followed by lenalidomide as the preferred consolidation and maintenance option.[25] Thus, we would generally also recommend lenalidomide maintenance following AHCT.

- Finally, this patient has lytic bone disease and thus is at risk for skeletal-related events (SREs), including pathological fracture, spinal cord compression, hypercalcemia, and need for radiation or surgery to bone. The use of osteoclast inhibitors (bisphosphonates such as pamidronate or zoledronic acid—or denosumab, a monoclonal antibody against receptor activator of nuclear factor kappa B ligand [RANKL]) has been shown to decrease SREs over placebo, with bisphosphonates and denosumab generally showing comparable efficacy. Considerations regarding the choice of therapy are generally dependent on renal function. Bisphosphonates are preferred over denosumab for patients with normal renal function, and the reverse for patients with impaired renal function (growth factor receptor [GFR] less than 30 mL/min).[26] Osteonecrosis of the jaw is an important toxicity to note for all osteoclast inhibitors, and flu-like symptoms are an adverse effect (AE) specific to bisphosphonates. Based on the patient's lytic bone lesions and normal renal function, we would recommend the addition of monthly bisphosphonate to his MM treatment for a total of 2 years of treatment according to current guidelines.[27]

Based on This Patient's Presentation, What Is the Recommended Treatment Plan?

- *Following discussion, you started the patient on RVD, zoledronic acid, and appropriate prophylactic medications including aspirin and acyclovir. Following 3 cycles of therapy, he achieved a partial response by IMWG MM criteria. At that time, you referred him to the bone marrow transplant (BMT) clinic for consideration of AHCT.*

Case 28.3: Newly Diagnosed, Transplant-Ineligible Multiple Myeloma

You are seeing an 83-year-old woman who presented to the hospital for overall weakness and fatigue. She was admitted and found to have elevated creatinine and bone lesions on CT imaging. She was subsequently found to have an IgG kappa serum monoclonal protein of 3.8 g/dL. Following a bone marrow biopsy, she was diagnosed with R-ISS stage II standard-risk MM. You speak to her daughter and she states that her mother is increasingly dependent on her care at home, including bathing. She is otherwise independent in her other activities of daily living

(ADLs). She requires assistance with all shopping trips, can prepare her meals if ingredients are provided to her, and can only travel with assistance in a car. She is also otherwise independent in her other instrumental ADLs. She is ambulatory and out of a chair for more than 50% of the day. She has diabetes on insulin with moderate peripheral neuropathy and mild chronic kidney disease (CKD), as well as chronic obstructive pulmonary disease (COPD) requiring two inhalers. Her daughter asks about treatment options for MM following discharge from the hospital.

What Is the Diagnosis and Treatment?

- The patient is diagnosed with MM and treatment should be considered. However, the treatment should be tailored to her overall medical and functional status. Treatment of MM in an older frail adult can be challenging, although there are several options. Initially, it is important to assess her performance status (PS) and degree of frailty. She appears to be ECOG grade 2 in functional status. In addition, the IMWG frailty scoring system is one of several tools that can be utilized to predict mortality and assess the risk of toxicity.[28,29] The scoring system considers the patient's age, Charlson comorbidity index, and degree of independence with ADLs and instrumental activities of daily living (iADLs) and categorizes patients into three categories of fit, intermediate fitness, and frail. Based on the scoring system, the patient is considered to be medically frail and not eligible for AHCT. In light of this, MM treatment should also be adjusted accordingly.
- The FIRST trial considered continuous treatment with RD in transplant-ineligible MM patients, and continuous RD until disease progression demonstrated significant response with no significant toxicities.[30] The MAIA trial considered the addition of daratumumab to RD (DaraRD), and the DaraRD group had further improvement of PFS and OS over RD, with no significant increase in toxicities.[31] Both of the previously described strategies avoid bortezomib due to the risk of increased toxicities, although a modified RVD strategy, termed RVD-lite with modified lenalidomide and bortezomib dosing, has been implemented with significant objective response rate (ORR) and PFS efficacy.[32] In this patient, we would generally avoid bortezomib given the peripheral neuropathy that is already present from diabetes. However, RD and DaraRD can both be considered as options at the hematology visit following discharge. A repeat functional assessment would be important at the outpatient appointment to determine whether there had been additional interval change since inpatient hospitalization.

Based on the Clinical Evaluation, What Is the Recommended Treatment Plan for This Patient?

- You discuss *with the daughter about starting the patient on RD in clinic for her newly diagnosed transplant-ineligible MM. The patient was stabilized and presents to your clinic 1 week following discharge from the hospital. Her functional status has improved from the hospitalization and reached her baseline again. You start her on daratumumab plus RD.*

Case 28.4: Relapsed/Refractory Multiple Myeloma

You continue to treat the 83-year-old woman in Case 28.3. She achieved a partial response based on IMWG response criteria.[33] After 22 cycles of treatment with good compliance overall, she was noted to have rising serum light chains and M-protein concerning for progressive disease. A repeat PET/CT was done due to worsening low back pain which showed new fluorodeoxyglucose (FDG)-avid bone lesions in her lumbar spine. A repeat bone marrow biopsy showed 25% plasma cells, and normal karyotype with a negative FISH testing panel. Her overall PS is relatively unchanged from her initial diagnosis, and she remains partially independent at home with some assistance from her daughter. She presents to your clinic after PET/CT and bone marrow biopsy are completed to discuss results and further management of her relapsed/refractory multiple myeloma (RRMM). The patient and her daughter are not interested in hospice at this time and are interested in pursuing further therapy if available.

What Is the Diagnosis and Treatment?

- At this time, this patient is considered lenalidomide-refractory and combinations utilizing other agents should be considered. Clinical trials should be considered at all stages of myeloma therapy, if available and the patient is interested. Outside of a clinical trial, there is no standardized sequence of agents to be used in relapsed disease, though recommendations based on prior studies, expert opinion, and institutional guidelines have been published. The mSMART guidelines for the treatment of myeloma, developed by the Mayo Clinic, are often used in practice.[17]

- For this frail, older patient, options recommended by mSMART include daratumumab-based regimens (DaraVD) or ixazomib-based regimens (ICD). Daratumumab (Dara) is a monoclonal antibody drug targeting CD38, a common marker on B-lymphocytes including myeloma tumor cells. Dara is administered subcutaneously or intravenously. The main side effects of this drug are infusion reactions, cytopenias, and increased risk of infections. Due to CD38 expression on red blood cells, Dara interferes with blood bank testing, so blood typing and screening should be done before starting Dara. The DaraVD regimen was evaluated in the CASTOR trial, a Phase 3 study in RRMM patients comparing the combinations of bortezomib and dexamethasone with or without daratumumab (DaraVD vs. VD).[34] After a median follow-up of 40 months, patients receiving DaraVD had an improvement in PFS (HR 0.39, P less than 0.001) with mOS not reached in either arm. Ixazomib is an oral proteasome inhibitor with a side effect profile similar to bortezomib, including the risk of neuropathy, GI toxicity, and cytopenia. The ICD regimen was evaluated in a Phase 2 single-arm study and demonstrated an ORR of 48% with a median PFS of 14.2 months.[35]

- As daratumumab is well-tolerated overall with minimal drug interactions, other combinations are also often used in practice for RRMM patients other than DaraVD. While this patient is lenalidomide-refractory, if she were thought to be sensitive to lenalidomide, one could consider the addition of daratumumab to her existing regimen (DaraRD) if other triplet options are not feasible. This combination was evaluated in the Phase 3 POLLUX trial comparing lenalidomide and dexamethasone with and without daratumumab (DaraRD vs. RD).[36] After long-term follow-up (median 3.5 years), there was an improvement in PFS (HR 0.44, P less than 0.0001) with mOS not reached in either arm. Another triplet combination is daratumumab plus carfilzomib (Kyprolis) and dexamethasone (DaraKD), which was recently evaluated in the Phase 3 CANDOR trial comparing KD +/- daratumumab which demonstrated improved PFS in the DaraKD arm (HR 0.63, P = 0.0027).[37] Yet another suitable option could be to use daratumumab plus pomalidomide and dexamethasone evaluated in the APOLLO trial.[38]

- For those patients with significant comorbidities or frailty, doublets can also be considered to reduce toxicity compared with standard triplet regimens. Options for this patient could include bortezomib with dexamethasone (VD), though at the risk of worsening her neuropathy, or pomalidomide with dexamethasone (PD), which is a newer immuno-modulatory agent with activity in lenalidomide-refractory disease.

- The variety of agents that have been shown to have efficacy in the RRMM space continues to grow and includes immunomodulators (lenalidomide, pomalidomide, thalidomide), proteasome inhibitors (bortezomib, ixazomib, carfilzomib), monoclonal antibodies (daratumumab, elotuzumab, isatuximab), alkylating chemotherapy (cyclophosphamide, melphalan, and bendamustine), nuclear export inhibitors (selinexor), antibody-drug conjugates (belantamab mafodotin), and cellular therapy such as chimeric antigen receptor T cells (CAR-T). However, many of these agents are not feasible in this case, given the patient's frailty and transplant-ineligible status.

Based on the Clinical Details of the Case, What Is the Recommended Treatment Plan?
After a discussion of treatment options with the patient and her family, the decision was made to start DaraKD regimen to reduce the risk of exacerbating her neuropathy, after an additional evaluation showed adequate cardiac function.

Case 28.5: Amyloid Light Chain Amyloidosis

A 56-year-old gentleman who is a former smoker with COPD was admitted to the hospital for shortness of breath, peripheral edema, ascites, and orthostatic hypotension. Chest imaging revealed pulmonary edema and cardiomegaly, so a transthoracic echocardiogram was done which showed biventricular wall thickening and abnormal longitudinal strain concerning for infiltrative disease such as cardiac amyloidosis. Cardiology was consulted and a Tc99m-PYP scan was done which was not suggestive of transthyretin amyloidosis (ATTR). Hematology was consulted and workup for amyloid light chain (AL) amyloidosis was done. Blood testing showed elevated serum lambda light chains with detectable IgG lambda M-protein. Bone marrow biopsy showed 12% lambda-restricted plasma cells and showed no material which stained positive with Congo Red. A fat pad biopsy was performed which also was negative for Congo Red staining. After further discussion with the primary team, an endomyocardial biopsy was done which was positive for amyloid deposition on Congo Red staining. You are consulted for further workup and management of presumed cardiac AL amyloidosis.

What Is the Diagnosis and Treatment?

- This patient has findings highly suggestive of AL amyloidosis given the negative PYP scan, bone marrow with significant plasma cells, elevated monoclonal light chains, and cardiac biopsy showing amyloid deposition. Criteria for diagnosis of systemic AL amyloidosis have also been defined by the IMWG.[7] However, confirmation of amyloid subtype should be done for all patients since treatment and prognosis for different amyloid etiologies varies significantly. Commonly used methods for amyloid subtype identification include immunofluorescence, immunoelectron microscopy, and mass spectrometry, with mass spectrometry as the preferred method if available. Ideally, tissue biopsy of the site of organ involvement is done to maximize diagnostic yield, though this may be associated with risk of harm depending on the location (heart, liver, kidney). Otherwise, obtaining a bone marrow biopsy, skin biopsy, or abdominal fat pad aspirate for analysis can be done, though with lower detection rates. High clinical suspicion of amyloidosis with negative initial biopsy results from bone marrow or fat pad biopsy should lead to further more invasive biopsies of involved organ tissue to obtain the diagnosis when safe to do so. This patient had amyloid typing via mass spectrometry done on his cardiac biopsy tissue, which was consistent with AL amyloidosis.
- Once the diagnosis is established, additional workup and specialist evaluations may need to be done to evaluate if other organs are involved, as AL amyloid can deposit in virtually any area outside the central nervous system (CNS). Common areas of involvement other than the bone marrow and heart include the liver, peripheral nerves, and kidneys. The recommended initial workup per National Comprehensive Cancer Network (NCCN) guidelines for all patients with suspected AL amyloidosis includes blood/urine testing for monoclonal protein and proteinuria, brain natriuretic peptide (BNP) and troponins to evaluate cardiac dysfunction, liver function testing to evaluate for liver damage, coagulation studies to evaluate for amyloid-associated coagulopathies, bone marrow biopsy to detect clonal plasma cell disorder, and any relevant tissue biopsies with amyloid typing to confirm the diagnosis. The Tc99m-PYP scan that this patient received uses a radiolabeled tracer that is specific for ATTR amyloid and can be helpful, though it is not

always available. Concurrent presence of monoclonal gammopathy with a positive PYP scan requires endomyocardial biopsy and amyloid peptide typing to obtain the correct diagnosis.

- The treatment of systemic AL amyloidosis has evolved significantly, now with the approval of daratumumab in combination with cyclophosphamide, bortezomib, and dexamethasone (DaraCyBorD) as the standard frontline treatment option. This was evaluated in the Phase 3 ANDROMEDA study which compared DaraCyBorD versus CyBorD, and demonstrated significantly improved hematologic and organ response rates (HR 0.58, $P = 0.02$).[39] In addition, patients should be started on doxycycline, which is thought to reduce amyloid formation, and in retrospective studies demonstrated high rates of hematologic response, though a recent Phase 3 trial using doxycycline in combination with CyBorD did not show an improvement in PFS compared with CyBorD alone.[40] Patients should also be evaluated for autologous stem cell transplant (auto-SCT) at the time of diagnosis with additional considerations when compared to MM patients without amyloidosis. In particular, patients need to have adequate renal function (creatinine clearance [CrCl] of 30 mL/min or more) and cardiac function (troponin T less than 0.06 ng/mL, systolic blood pressure of 90 mmHg or greater, New York Heart Association [NYHA] class I/II). Given the rarity of AL amyloidosis, clinical trials should be pursued if available. Treatment options for relapsed/refractory AL amyloidosis patients are similar to those for RRMM patients, albeit with less aggressive combinations to reduce exacerbating preexisting organ dysfunction. These include proteasome inhibitor-based regimens (VD, VMP, IxaDex, IRD), immunomodulator-based regimens (RD, CRD, PD), and melphalan-based regimens. For the rare subset of patients with t(11;14) mutation, venetoclax-based regimens have promising high efficacy and should be considered.

Based on the Clinical Findings, What is the Recommended Treatment Plan for This Patient?

- *Following further evaluation, the patient was found to have nephrotic range proteinuria and hepatomegaly consistent with kidney and liver involvement by amyloidosis. Thus, he was not deemed to be a transplant candidate despite his young biological age. You start the patient on DaraCyBorD therapy.*

REVIEW QUESTIONS

1. A 68-year-old woman is found to have hypercalcemia and anemia concerning for multiple myeloma (MM). She is started on aggressive intravenous (IV) fluid hydration and bisphosphonate therapy for symptomatic hypercalcemia. Further testing shows an elevated monoclonal protein, and bone marrow biopsy demonstrates 47% clonal plasma cells in her marrow. She has fluorescence in situ hybridization (FISH) testing done on her bone marrow sample. Which of the following abnormalities would not be considered a high-risk feature on FISH testing?
   A. Deletion (11q)
   B. Translocation (4;14)
   C. Translocation (14;16)
   D. Deletion (17p)
   E. Gain 1q

2. A 63-year-old gentleman presents to your office following a bone marrow biopsy and other testing that established a diagnosis of Revised International Staging System (R-ISS) stage II standard-risk multiple myeloma (MM). Serum calcium is 12 mg/dL, serum creatinine 1.1 mg/dL, hemoglobin 9.2 g/dL, and he has several lytic bone lesions noted on whole-body PET. He states he has significant lumbar pain due to bone lesions noted in that area. Following discussion, you decide to start him on lenalidomide, bortezomib, and dexamethasone (RVD) induction chemotherapy for his MM. You also decide to add a bone-strengthening agent. Which of the following is the best choice?
   A. Zoledronic acid
   B. Pamidronate
   C. Denosumab
   D. Clodronate

3. A 69-year-old woman with multiple myeloma (MM) presents to your clinic for further evaluation for a second opinion, after her first relapse with lenalidomide, bortezomib, and dexamethasone (RVD). After discussion, you recommend starting a regimen containing daratumumab for the treatment of relapsed disease. Before the first cycle, what testing is important to send for the patient?
   A. CD38 expression on serum
   B. CD38 expression on bone marrow
   C. Type and screen on serum
   D. B-cell quantification by flow cytometry on bone marrow
   E. Human leukocyte antigen (HLA) typing on serum

4. An 81-year-old gentleman presents with left hip pain for the past several months to his primary care provider (PCP). He is started on ibuprofen and physical therapy, then oxycodone as needed without relief. X-rays of the left hip show a large lytic lesion involving greater than 50% of the left femoral head, which is concerning for malignancy. Workup for suspected myeloma is ordered. Labs showed elevated light chain ratio, and bone marrow biopsy confirmed the diagnosis of multiple myeloma (MM). He is scheduled to meet with hematology to discuss systemic therapy options. However, he has ongoing worsening pain and weakness in his left leg and asks about potential management options. What is the next best approach for this patient?
   A. Wait to start systemic therapy for myeloma
   B. Recommend bed rest to reduce the impact on the left hip

C. Refer to physical medicine and rehabilitation (PM&R) for a steroid injection to the left hip for pain relief

D. Refer to Surgery for intervention

E. Refer to Radiation Oncology for definitive radiotherapy to the femoral lesion

5. A 67-year-old woman with previously diagnosed standard-risk multiple myeloma (MM) presents to your hematology clinic to establish care after moving from another state. She was initially treated with lenalidomide, bortezomib, and dexamethasone (RVD), followed by autologous stem cell transplant (auto-SCT), and achieved complete remission. After recovering from her transplant, she was started on lenalidomide maintenance and has been continued on this regimen for 4 years. About 8 months prior, she had Mohs surgery for a locally invasive melanoma lesion on her right shoulder, and several months afterward required resection of a squamous cell carcinoma (SCC) on her left ear. She is wondering about stopping therapy due to the costs and asks you about long-term side effects related to prolonged lenalidomide use. What is the most significant consideration for stopping maintenance therapy in this patient?

A. Cardiomyopathy

B. Neuropathy

C. Second primary malignancies

D. Autoimmune disease

E. Diarrhea

6. A fit 62-year-old man is diagnosed with standard-risk multiple myeloma (MM). At diagnosis, he presented with a serum IgG kappa M-protein of 4.2 g/dL, positive urine Bence-Jones protein, and 65% plasma cells on bone marrow biopsy. Despite his diagnosis, he remains extremely active and continues working at a local warehouse. You decide to start lenalidomide, bortezomib, and dexamethasone (RVD). He has now completed 3 cycles of therapy with a serum IgG kappa M-protein of 0.8 g/dL. You had discussed autologous hematopoietic cell transplantation (AHCT) with him previously and he would prefer to proceed to AHCT as soon as possible rather than at first relapse. What do you do?

A. Do not refer to bone marrow transplant (BMT) because the patient is not eligible

B. Continue therapy and refer once M-protein is undetectable

C. Continue therapy and refer to see BMT now

D. Change therapy due to suboptimal response

7. You are a hematology–oncology fellow and called to perform an inpatient bone marrow biopsy on a 72-year-old woman who presents with renal failure. It was a difficult tap, but you managed to acquire a decent sample for analysis. You receive the following results back on the pathology report: "4% clonal plasma cells on flow cytometry of aspirate and 8% aberrant lambda-restricted plasma cells via microscopy on May-Giemsa-stained biopsy and clot samples." Which is the most appropriate way to proceed?

A. No further testing is needed. She does not meet the diagnostic criteria for multiple myeloma (MM) because the higher percentage of clonal plasma cells should be chosen between the two quantification methods, and her clonal plasma cell percentage is less than 10%

B. Request CD138 immunohistochemistry (IHC) stains on biopsy and clot samples and re-evaluate

C. No further testing is needed. She does not meet the diagnostic criteria for MM because quantification of aberrant plasma cells via flow cytometry on aspirate is more accurate than microscopy on biopsy and clot samples

D. Request mass spectrometry on biopsy and clot samples and re-evaluate

8. A 78-year-old woman with multiple myeloma (MM) who completed 8 cycles of lenalido-mide, bortezomib, and dexamethasone (RVD) is transferring care to your practice from an external hematologist who has decided to retire. Today, she tells you that bortezomib has been discontinued 2 weeks ago due to worsening adverse effects (AEs), and she is cur-rently only on lenalidomide and dexamethasone. She is currently also taking acyclovir, fluconazole, and trimethoprim/sulfamethoxazole. Upon further questioning, she states that these medications were provided to her as prophylactic medications when she started RVD. She is not neutropenic today and does not have a history of significant bacterial or fungal infections in recent years. You want to streamline her medications. Which of the following choices is correct?
   A. Continue acyclovir, stop fluconazole, and stop trimethoprim/sulfamethoxazole
   B. Stop acyclovir, continue fluconazole, and stop trimethoprim/sulfamethoxazole
   C. Stop acyclovir, stop fluconazole, and continue trimethoprim/sulfamethoxazole
   D. Continue all three medications
   E. Stop all three medications

9. You have been referred from primary care a 52-year-old man who was found to have a serum IgG kappa monoclonal protein of 3.6 g/dL. His serum hemoglobin is 13.2 g/dL, creatinine 0.82 mg/dL, and calcium 9.2 mg/dL. His kappa/lambda free light chain (FLC) ratio is 62.5. You perform a bone marrow biopsy, and he has 13% clonal plasma cells seen on aspirate smears. To complete the workup, you order a skeletal survey which reveals no lytic lesions. After discussion with a colleague, you also order a PET/CT because of better specificity compared to the skeletal survey. It similarly shows no lytic lesions. What is the diagnosis?
   A. Smoldering multiple myeloma (SMM), given serum monoclonal protein greater than 3 g/dL, greater than 10% clonal plasma cells on bone marrow, and no myeloma-defining events
   B. Multiple myeloma (MM), given greater than 10% clonal plasma cells on the bone mar-row and kappa/lambda FLC ratio greater than 50, which is a myeloma-defining event
   C. Diagnosis is not yet established, as it requires further laboratory but not imaging tests
   D. Diagnosis is not yet established, as it requires further imaging but not laboratory tests

10. A 72-year-old woman presents to you with suspected newly diagnosed myeloma, based on elevated IgA kappa M-protein found during a workup of unexplained symptomatic anemia. Bone marrow biopsy demonstrates 39% clonal plasma cells. PET/CT shows fluo-rodeoxyglucose (FDG)-avid lesions in her thoracic spine and bilateral pelvis. She does not have any renal failure or hypercalcemia. She is started on induction therapy with lenalido-mide, bortezomib, and dexamethasone (RVD) and you discuss the role of adding bisphos-phonate therapy with zoledronic acid for bone health. What is the ideal dosing interval of zoledronic acid in this previously untreated, newly diagnosed myeloma patient?
    A. Every 1 month
    B. Every 4 months
    C. Every 6 months
    D. Every 12 months

ANSWERS AND RATIONALES

1. **A. Deletion (11q).** The Revised International Staging System (R-ISS) score includes t(4;14), t(14;16), and del(17p) as high-risk cytogenetics associated with a worse prognosis. Further cytogenetic abnormalities such as hypodiploidy and gain(1q) are also considered high-risk per the International Myeloma Working Group (IMWG), though not included in the R-ISS score. Del(11q) is not considered a high-risk feature.

2. **A. Zoledronic acid.** All of the options are osteoclast inhibitors that have been studied in the context of MM to reduce the risk of skeletal-related events (SREs; fractures, hypercalcemia, need for surgery, or radiation to stabilize bone). As the patient has hypercalcemia and bone pain due to his osteolytic disease, starting an osteoclast inhibitor is appropriate for treating his hypercalcemia, reducing bone pain, and reducing the risk of future fracture. Since he does not have renal insufficiency, there is no advantage to using denosumab over a bisphosphonate drug. Clodronate is a non–nitrogen-containing bisphosphonate (as opposed to zoledronic acid and pamidronate, which are nitrogen-containing) and is less potent (as demonstrated by the Myeloma IX trial[41]). Among the two remaining bisphosphonates, zoledronic acid is preferred over pamidronate, due to its greater efficacy in addressing the patient's hypercalcemia and also because of ease of administration (15 minutes vs. over 2 hours).

3. **C. Type and screen on serum.** Daratumumab is an anti-CD38 monoclonal antibody that binds to the surface of MM cells. However, red blood cells also express CD38, and treatment with daratumumab can cause pan-agglutination on the indirect Coombs test used in blood compatibility testing. Thus, patients starting daratumumab are advised to have a baseline type and screen performed in case future blood transfusions are needed (however, there are laboratory techniques to remove the CD38 interference, if needed, on a blood sample from a patient treated with daratumumab). The other choices do not have a role in the pretreatment planning of daratumumab.

4. **D. Refer to Surgery for intervention.** This patient has significant bony disease in his left femur with impending pathological fracture. Supportive measures such as bed rest and steroid injections alone are not sufficient in this case. This patient should consider prophylactic intramedullary nailing of the femur to prevent fracture after discussion with Surgery. Referral to Radiation Oncology also should be considered for palliative radiation therapy to his left hip bone lesion for pain relief, but for unstable lesions in the long bones, surgical fixation should be considered first.

5. **C. Second primary malignancies.** Previous trials utilizing lenalidomide in myeloma patients have shown an increase in second primary cancers, particularly cutaneous tumors, and leukemia. While lenalidomide is associated with increased thrombotic risk, it generally is not commonly associated with cardiac failure. Neuropathy is a common side effect of myeloma drugs such as bortezomib, though not with immunomodulators like lenalidomide. Autoimmune diseases are not associated with lenalidomide, though skin rashes can occur uncommonly. Diarrhea is a common problem with lenalidomide but can be managed with antidiarrheals and bile acid binders such as colesevelam or cholestyramine.

6. **C. Continue therapy and refer to see BMT now.** This patient is young and fit with great functional status. Thus, he should be considered for AHCT as consolidation therapy following induction chemotherapy. Disease reassessment after 3 cycles of RVD is appropriate. At this point, the patient has achieved partial response (PR) given

greater than 50% reduction in his serum M-protein and is eligible for AHCT. Current retrospective studies have not demonstrated a need for complete response (undetectable M-protein) prior to AHCT in terms of an advantage from a progression-free survival (PFS) or overall survival (OS) perspective. Thus, there is no clear benefit for additional cycles of RVD, especially as too many cycles of RVD (often greater than 6) can reduce yield during peripheral stem cell collection due to myelosuppression. There is no need to change therapy.

7. **B. Request CD138 immunohistochemistry (IHC) stains on biopsy and clot samples and re-evaluate.** Although the highest clonal plasma cell percentage should be chosen among reported quantification methods on the pathology report for diagnosis of MM, this pathology report is missing the percentage of clonal plasma cells via CD138 IHC staining, which is more accurate than the two methods presented. Aspirates are generally hemodilute and have lower plasma cell percentages compared to quantification on biopsy and clot samples. There is no role for mass spectrometry in quantifying the percentage of plasma cells, although it can be used to detect serum monoclonal proteins.

8. **A. Continue acyclovir, stop fluconazole, and stop trimethoprim/sulfamethoxazole.** Bortezomib is a proteasome inhibitor which is known to increase the risk of herpes zoster reactivation (shingles). Thus, prophylaxis with acyclovir during treatment is mandatory and is generally continued for a period of 3 to 12 months following discontinuation of proteasome inhibitor due to lingering drug effects. There is no routine role for antifungal and antibacterial prophylaxis in RVD therapy. Especially given the lack of neutropenia and history of significant infections, fluconazole and trimethoprim/sulfamethoxazole can be safely discontinued.

9. **D. Diagnosis is not yet established, as it requires further imaging but not laboratory tests.** The clinical vignette is of a patient who clearly has more than monoclonal gammopathy of undetermined significance (MGUS) given his serum monoclonal protein, and bone marrow biopsy findings. However, it is important to distinguish between SMM and MM. The key here is whether he has myeloma-defining events per the SLiM-CRAB criteria. He does not clearly meet any of the criteria (myeloma-defining light chain ratio is involved/uninvolved greater than 100 rather than greater than 50). Importantly, however, this patient only had a skeletal survey and PET/CT to evaluate for lytic bone lesions. Due to the low burden of disease in SMM, advisory groups such as the International Myeloma Working Group (IMWG) recommend whole-body MRI or at least a spine and pelvic MRI in these patients to rule out bone involvement. Thus, we would recommend MRI before arriving at a definitive diagnosis.

10. **A. Every 1 month.** This patient has untreated newly diagnosed myeloma with pathological bone lesions, so the recommendation for zoledronic acid dosing is every 1 month (3 to 4 weeks) for up to 2 years. Prior studies have demonstrated non-inferiority with every 3-month (12-week) dosing interval, and this can be considered in patients without myeloma-related bone disease or who are responding well on myeloma therapy. Renal function should be monitored closely when starting bisphosphonate therapy due to the potential need for dose adjustments.

REFERENCES

1. Siegel RL, Miller KD, Fuchs HE, Jemal A. Cancer statistics, 2021. *CA Cancer J Clin.* 2021;71(1):7–33. doi:10.3322/caac.21654
2. Padala SA, Barsouk A, Rawla P, et al. Epidemiology, staging, and management of multiple myeloma. *Med Sci (Basel).* 2021;9(1):3. doi:10.3390/medsci9010003
3. SEER. Data from: SEER*Stat Database: Incidence - SEER 9 Regs Research Data. November 2019 Sub (1975–2017). Deposited April 2020, based on the November 2019 submission. https://www.seer.cancer.gov
4. Waxman AJ, Mink PJ, Devesa SS, et al. Racial disparities in incidence and outcome in multiple myeloma: a population-based study. *Blood.* 2010;116(25):5501–5506. doi:10.1182/blood-2010-07-298760
5. Matsui W, Wang Q, Barber JP, et al. Clonogenic multiple myeloma progenitors, stem cell properties, and drug resistance. *Cancer Res.* 2008;68(1):190–197. doi:10.1158/0008-5472.CAN-07-3096
6. Bazarbachi AH, Avet-Loiseau H, Szalat R, et al. IgM-MM is predominantly a pre-germinal center disorder and has a distinct genomic and transcriptomic signature from WM. *Blood.* 2021;138(20):1980–1985. doi:10.1182/blood.2021011452
7. Rajkumar SV, Dimopoulos MA, Palumbo A, et al. International Myeloma Working Group updated criteria for the diagnosis of multiple myeloma. *Lancet Oncol.* 2014;15(12):e538–e548. doi:10.1016/S1470-2045(14)70442-5
8. Rajkumar SV, Kyle RA, Buadi FK. Advances in the diagnosis, classification, risk stratification, and management of monoclonal gammopathy of undetermined significance: implications for recategorizing disease entities in the presence of evolving scientific evidence. *Mayo Clin Proc.* 2010;85(10):945–948. doi:10.4065/mcp.2010.0520
9. Schmidt T, Callander N. Diagnosis and management of monoclonal gammopathy and smoldering multiple myeloma. *J Natl Compr Canc Netw.* 2020;18(12):1720–1729. doi:10.6004/jnccn.2020.7660
10. Lakshman A, Rajkumar SV, Buadi FK, et al. Risk stratification of smoldering multiple myeloma incorporating revised IMWG diagnostic criteria. *Blood Cancer J.* 2018;8(6):59. doi:10.1038/s41408-018-0077-4
11. Mateos MV, Kumar S, Dimopoulos MA, et al. International Myeloma Working Group risk stratification model for smoldering multiple myeloma (SMM). *Blood Cancer J.* 2020;10(10):102. doi:10.1038/s41408-020-00366-3
12. Mateos MV, Hernández MT, Giraldo P, et al. Lenalidomide plus dexamethasone versus observation in patients with high-risk smouldering multiple myeloma (QuiRedex): long-term follow-up of a randomised, controlled, phase 3 trial. *Lancet Oncol.* 2016;17(8):1127–1136. doi:10.1016/S1470-2045(16)30124-3
13. Lonial S, Jacobus S, Fonseca R, et al. Randomized trial of lenalidomide versus observation in smoldering multiple myeloma. *J Clin Oncol.* 2020;38(11):1126–1137. doi:10.1200/JCO.19.01740
14. Hillengass J, Usmani S, Rajkumar SV, et al. International Myeloma Working Group consensus recommendations on imaging in monoclonal plasma cell disorders. *Lancet Oncol.* 2019;20(6):e302-e312. doi:10.1016/S1470-2045(19)30309-2
15. Snozek CL, Katzmann JA, Kyle RA, et al. Prognostic value of the serum free light chain ratio in newly diagnosed myeloma: proposed incorporation into the international staging system. *Leukemia.* 2008;22(10):1933–1937. doi:10.1038/leu.2008.171
16. Palumbo A, Avet-Loiseau H, Oliva S, et al. Revised international staging system for multiple myeloma: a report from International Myeloma Working Group. *J Clin Oncol.* 2015;33(26):2863–2869. doi:10.1200/JCO.2015.61.2267
17. mSMART. Treatment guidelines: multiple myeloma. https://www.msmart.org/mm-treatment-guidelines
18. Durie BGM, Hoering A, Abidi MH, et al. Bortezomib with lenalidomide and dexamethasone versus lenalidomide and dexamethasone alone in patients with newly diagnosed myeloma without intent for immediate autologous stem-cell transplant (SWOG S0777): A randomised, open-label, phase 3 trial. *Lancet.* 2017;389(10068):519–527. doi:10.1016/S0140-6736(16)31594-X
19. Kumar SK, Jacobus SJ, Cohen AD, et al. Carfilzomib or bortezomib in combination with lenalidomide and dexamethasone for patients with newly diagnosed multiple myeloma without intention for immediate autologous stem-cell transplantation (ENDURANCE): a multicentre, open-label, phase 3, randomised, controlled trial. *Lancet Oncol.* 2020;21(10):1317–1330. doi:10.1016/S1470-2045(20)30452-6
20. Voorhees PM, Kaufman JL, Laubach J, et al. Daratumumab, lenalidomide, bortezomib, and dexamethasone for transplant-eligible newly diagnosed multiple myeloma: the GRIFFIN trial. *Blood.* 2020;136(8):936–945. doi:10.1182/blood.2020005288
21. Dhakal B, Szabo A, Chhabra S, et al. Autologous transplantation for newly diagnosed multiple myeloma in the era of novel agent induction: a systematic review and meta-analysis. *JAMA Oncol.* 2018;4(3):343–350. doi:10.1001/jamaoncol.2017.4600
22. Attal M, Lauwers-Cances V, Hulin C, et al. Lenalidomide, bortezomib, and dexamethasone with transplantation for myeloma. *N Engl J Med.* 2017;376(14):1311–1320. doi:10.1056/NEJMoa1611750
23. Gay F, Musto P, Rota-Scalabrini D, et al. Carfilzomib with cyclophosphamide and dexamethasone or lenalidomide and dexamethasone plus autologous transplantation or carfilzomib plus lenalidomide and dexamethasone, followed by maintenance with carfilzomib plus lenalidomide or lenalidomide alone for patients with newly diagnosed multiple myeloma (FORTE): a randomised, open-label, phase 2 trial. *Lancet Oncol.* 2021;22(12):1705–1720. doi:10.1016/S1470-2045(21)00535-0

24. McCarthy PL, Holstein SA, Petrucci MT, et al. Lenalidomide maintenance after autologous stem-cell transplantation in newly diagnosed multiple myeloma: a meta-analysis. *J Clin Oncol.* 2017;35(29):3279–3289. doi:10.1200/JCO.2017.72.6679

25. Stadtmauer EA, Pasquini MC, Blackwell B, et al. Autologous transplantation, consolidation, and maintenance therapy in multiple myeloma: results of the BMT CTN 0702 trial. *J Clin Oncol.* 2019;37(7):589–597. doi:10.1200/JCO.18.00685

26. Raje N, Terpos E, Willenbacher W, et al. Denosumab versus zoledronic acid in bone disease treatment of newly diagnosed multiple myeloma: an international, double-blind, double-dummy, randomised, controlled, phase 3 study. *Lancet Oncol.* 2018;19(3):370–381. doi:10.1016/S1470-2045(18)30072-X

27. Anderson K, Ismaila N, Flynn PJ, et al. Role of bone-modifying agents in multiple myeloma: American Society of Clinical Oncology clinical practice guideline update. *J Clin Oncol.* 2018;36(8):812–818. doi:10.1200/JCO.2017.76.6402

28. Palumbo A, Bringhen S, Mateos MV, et al. Geriatric assessment predicts survival and toxicities in elderly myeloma patients: an International Myeloma Working Group report. *Blood.* 2015;125(13):2068–2074. doi:10.1182/blood-2014-12-615187

29. Mian H, Brouwers M, Kouroukis CT, Wildes TM. Comparison of frailty scores in newly diagnosed patients with multiple myeloma: a review. *J Frailty Aging.* 2019;8(4):215–221. doi:10.14283/jfa.2019.25

30. Facon T, Dimopoulos MA, Dispenzieri A, et al. Final analysis of survival outcomes in the phase 3 FIRST trial of up-front treatment for multiple myeloma. *Blood.* 2018;131(3):301–310. doi:10.1182/blood-2017-07-795047

31. Facon T, Kumar SK, Plesner T, et al. Daratumumab, lenalidomide, and dexamethasone versus lenalidomide and dexamethasone alone in newly diagnosed multiple myeloma (MAIA): overall survival results from a randomised, open-label, phase 3 trial. *Lancet Oncol.* 2021;22(11):1582–1596. doi:10.1016/S1470-2045(21)00466-6

32. O'Donnell EK, Laubach JP, Yee AJ, et al. A phase 2 study of modified lenalidomide, bortezomib and dexamethasone in transplant-ineligible multiple myeloma. *Br J Haematol.* 2018;182(2):222–230. doi:10.1111/bjh.15261

33. Kumar S, Paiva B, Anderson KC, et al. International Myeloma Working Group consensus criteria for response and minimal residual disease assessment in multiple myeloma. *Lancet Oncol.* 2016;17(8):e328–e346. doi:10.1016/S1470-2045(16)30206-6

34. Palumbo A, Chanan-Khan A, Weisel K, et al. Daratumumab, bortezomib, and dexamethasone for multiple myeloma. *N Engl J Med.* 2016;375(8):754–766. doi:10.1056/NEJMoa1606038

35. Kumar SK, Grzasko N, Delimpasi S, et al. Phase 2 study of all-oral ixazomib, cyclophosphamide and low-dose dexamethasone for relapsed/refractory multiple myeloma. *Br J Haematol.* 2019;184(4):536–546. doi:10.1111/bjh.15679

36. Dimopoulos MA, Oriol A, Nahi H, et al. Daratumumab, lenalidomide, and dexamethasone for multiple myeloma. *N Engl J Med.* 2016;375(14):1319–1331. doi:10.1056/NEJMoa1607751

37. Dimopoulos M, Quach H, Mateos MV, et al. Carfilzomib, dexamethasone, and daratumumab versus carfilzomib and dexamethasone for patients with relapsed or refractory multiple myeloma (CANDOR): results from a randomised, multicentre, open-label, phase 3 study. *Lancet.* 2020;396(10245):186–197. doi:10.1016/S0140-6736(20)30734-0

38. Dimopoulos MA, Terpos E, Boccadoro M, et al. Daratumumab plus pomalidomide and dexamethasone versus pomalidomide and dexamethasone alone in previously treated multiple myeloma (APOLLO): an open-label, randomised, phase 3 trial. *Lancet Oncol.* 2021;22(6):801–812. doi:10.1016/S1470-2045(21)00128-5

39. Kastritis E, Palladini G, Minnema MC, et al. Daratumumab-based treatment for immunoglobulin light-chain amyloidosis. *N Engl J Med.* 2021;385(1):46–58. doi:10.1056/NEJMoa2028631

40. Shen KN, Fu WJ, Wu Y, et al. Doxycycline combined with bortezomib-cyclophosphamide-dexamethasone chemotherapy for newly diagnosed cardiac light-chain amyloidosis: a multicenter randomized controlled trial. *Circulation.* 2022;145(1):8–17. doi:10.1161/CIRCULATIONAHA.121.055953

41. Richardson PG, Laubach JP, Schlossman RL, et al. The medical research council myeloma IX trial: the impact on treatment paradigms. *Eur J Haematol.* 2012;88(1):1–7. doi:10.1111/j.1600-0609.2011.01721.x

CHAPTER 29

Acute Lymphoblastic Leukemia

Colbert A. Parker, Cyrus A. Iqbal, and Martha P. Mims

INTRODUCTION

Acute lymphoblastic leukemia (ALL) is a heterogeneous group of diseases caused by somatic mutations in lymphoid progenitor cells resulting in clonal proliferation of immature B- or T-lymphocytes. ALL accounts for ~15% of all leukemias diagnosed in the United States. The disease has a bimodal age distribution, with a peak between the ages of 1 and 4 (ALL is the most common malignancy diagnosed in patients younger than 15 years of age), and a second peak in patients older than 60 years of age.[1] ALL is more common in males than in females, and affects White and Hispanic patients more frequently than Black patients. There is no clear data supporting a link between ALL and environmental exposures to radiation, insecticides, and chemicals. However, Down syndrome and ataxia-telangiectasia are among the known genetic/heritable predisposing factors.[1,2]

The presentation of ALL varies, but common clinical features include lymphadenopathy, hepatomegaly, and splenomegaly, which are collectively present in approximately 50% of patients. Bone and joint pain are also frequently described. Laboratory findings include anemia and thrombocytopenia owing to infiltration of the bone marrow. Leukocytosis, as discussed in the cases to follow, can portend a poor prognosis. Central nervous system (CNS) involvement is present in 5% to 10% of cases, and predicts a worse prognosis.[3]

The classification of ALL includes stratification by modifiers such as age group, cell of origin (that is, B-cell or T-cell), and characteristic molecular signatures. For purposes of the case discussions to follow, the main age classifications are pediatric, adolescent-and-young-adult (AYA), and adult patients. B-cell ALL is much more common than T-cell ALL. The presence of the Philadelphia chromosome (derived from translocation 9;22) provides critical prognostic and therapeutic information in B-cell ALL. Other cytogenetic findings of prognostic relevance are discussed in the cases that follow.

Treatment of ALL depends on the cell of origin (T-cell or B-cell), the patient's age, the presence of specific cell surface markers, and the Philadelphia (Ph) chromosome. Ph+ ALL is treated with a tyrosine kinase inhibitor (TKI), and CD20+ cases permit the use of monoclonal antibodies targeting CD20 such as rituximab.[4]

Treatment can be summarized as follows:
- Induction therapy utilizing multi-agent combinations of drugs can be used, such as the hyper-CVAD regimen (comprised of hyperfractionated cyclophosphamide, vincristine, doxorubicin, and dexamethasone alternating with courses of methotrexate and cytarabine) or the CALGB 8811 regimen (featuring danorubicin, vincristine, prednisone, pegaspargase, and cyclophosphamide) with TKI and rituximab as appropriate. CNS prophylaxis as specified by the induction protocol is always used. CNS involvement at

Table 29.1   Complete Response Criteria in Acute Lymphoblastic Leukemia

No circulating lymphoblasts or extramedullary disease
Trilineage hematopoiesis and <5% blasts
ANC >1,000/microliter and platelets >100,000/microliter
No recurrence for 4 weeks

ANC, absolute neutrophil count.

Source: Berry DA, Zhou S, Higley H, et al. Association of minimal residual disease with clinical outcome in pediatric and adult lymphoblastic leukemia. *JAMA Oncol.* 2017;3:e170580. doi:10.1001/jamaoncol.2017.0580

diagnosis is relatively uncommon (5% to 10% of cases), but left untreated, 35% to 50% of cases will develop CNS disease.[5]

- Assessment of bone marrow response after induction to determine whether complete response (CR) has been achieved (Table 29.1).
- Ascertainment of minimal or measurable residual disease (MRD) status using reverse transcription polymerase chain reaction (RT-PCR), flow cytometry, or next-generation sequencing (NGS), as discussed in the cases that follow.
- Consolidation therapy in those achieving CR followed by allogeneic hematopoietic stem cell transplantation (allo-HSCT) or maintenance therapy, as guided by individualized evaluation of the risks and benefits of each option (that is, high-risk disease, MRD positivity, donor matching, ability to tolerate transplantation without prohibitive morbidity, and so on).
- In relapsed or refractory disease, the use of chimeric antigen receptor T-cell (CAR-T) therapy, bispecific T-cell engager (BiTE) treatment (such as blinatumomab), inotuzumab ozogamicin, or further multi-agent chemotherapy (Table 29.1).

CASE SUMMARIES

Case 29.1: Adolescent and Young Adult Acute Lymphoblastic Leukemia

A 26-year-old male presents to the ED with excessive bleeding from his gums following a dental cleaning and extraction 3 weeks earlier. He denies hemoptysis or melena. On questioning he reports low-grade fevers and fatigue that started approximately 2 months ago but had not bothered him enough to be evaluated. Vitals are normal, but he has gingival bleeding and conjunctival pallor. Initial laboratory evaluation demonstrates pancytopenia with white blood cell (WBC) 2,400/mL, hemoglobin (Hgb) 7.4 g/dL, and platelets 31,000/mL. A peripheral smear shows circulating blasts (approximately 40%).

How Is Acute Lymphoblastic Leukemia Diagnosed?

- A bone marrow aspirate and biopsy sample should be obtained to demonstrate at least 20% monoclonal lymphoblast involvement. Peripheral blood, while not ideal, can be used for diagnosis if there are sufficient circulating lymphoblasts and bone marrow examination is not clinically feasible.[6]
- Marrow samples should be examined for morphology and immunophenotyping, and sent for cytogenetic and molecular testing.

- Typically, B-cell ALL blasts are positive for CD19, CD22, CD79a, terminal deoxynucleotidyl transferase (TdT), or PAX5 in addition to variable expression of CD10 and CD20. Typical T-cell ALL blasts are positive for CD3 and CD7.[7]
- *BCR-ABL1* testing should be performed in all cases of B-cell ALL by fluorescence in situ hybridization or RT-PCR.[6]

Patient's Results
- *Peripheral blood flow cytometry is ordered and findings are consistent with a monoclonal B lymphoblast population (26% of events) that is CD10+, CD19+, CD22+, CD79a+, and/or TDT+. The population is CD3-, CD7-, CD13-, CD20-, CD33-, and/or MPO-. A bone marrow biopsy reveals a bone marrow that has been almost entirely replaced by leukemic blasts (98% blasts). Immunophenotype is similar to the peripheral blood flow. The final diagnosis is B-cell ALL. BCR-ABL testing is negative. Karyotyping is consistent with hyperdiploidy (55 chromosomes).*

What Further Workup Should Be Performed at Diagnosis?

- All patients should be evaluated for tumor lysis syndrome and disseminated intravascular coagulation (DIC).
- Hepatitis B and C, HIV testing, and transthoracic echocardiography (TTE) should be performed prior to chemotherapy.
- Testicular exam is performed for all males, as well as scrotal ultrasound (US) if clinically indicated.[6]
- Imaging of the brain and body is performed if indicated by clinical symptoms.[6]
- Fertility counseling should be performed in patients of child-bearing age, and fertility preservation should be offered; however, this is often not feasible due to the urgency of starting treatment. Studies of pediatric ALL survivors indicate that fertility is often preserved despite chemotherapy treatment; however, adolescents and young adults may be at higher risk due to higher cumulative doses.[8,9]

Patient's Results
- *The patient's labs are not concerning for tumor lysis or coagulopathy. Hepatitis and HIV testing are negative. TTE is normal with ejection fraction of 55% to 60%. He has no neurological findings at presentation to warrant brain imaging. Testicular exam is not concerning. CT scans of the chest, abdomen, and pelvis do not reveal any lymphadenopathy. After undergoing fertility counseling, the patient reports that he is interested in sperm banking, which is urgently arranged.*

What Is the Role of Lumbar Puncture and Intrathecal Chemotherapy?

- Lumbar puncture with intrathecal (IT) chemotherapy is recommended to evaluate for CNS involvement. Cerebrospinal fluid (CSF) should be sent for cytology and flow cytometry which is more sensitive.
- CNS-directed therapy is included in all current B-cell ALL regimens regardless of CNS status at diagnosis because a substantial portion of patients will develop CNS involvement if not treated with CNS-directed therapy.[10]
- CNS-directed therapy may involve IT chemotherapy (methotrexate or cytarabine), high-dose systemic chemotherapy (methotrexate or cytarabine), or cranial irradiation.
- In the absence of overt CNS involvement at diagnosis, current approaches typically feature both IT and high-dose systemic chemotherapy in the first line, reserving cranial irradiation for the relapsed/refractory setting.[11]

Patient's Initial Treatment
- *The patient is planned for induction chemotherapy and undergoes lumbar puncture on day 1 with administration of IT cytarabine. CSF is negative for lymphoblasts by cytology and flow cytometry.*

What Is the Initial Treatment for Acute Lymphoblastic Leukemia in the Adolescent and Young Adult Population?

- Induction regimens are comprised of combination chemotherapy including varying dosages of cyclophosphamide, vincristine, anthracyclines and glucocorticoids. Some regimens also involve alternating cycles of high-dose methotrexate and cytarabine.
- Supportive measures such as infection prophylaxis and tumor lysis monitoring should be a part of any treatment strategy.
- The addition of rituximab to treatment regimens for patients with CD20+ disease has shown a survival advantage in patients younger than 60.[12]
- Asparaginase, which has long been a key component in pediatric ALL regimens, has been shown to improve outcomes for adult ALL patients.[13] Widespread use of asparaginase in adults has been limited by significant toxicities; however, pediatric-inspired regimens have been shown to be safe and offer survival advantages in the adolescent and young adult population.[14]
- Toxicities associated with Asparaginase include serious infusion reactions/anaphylaxis, thrombosis, coagulopathy, hemorrhage, pancreatitis, hepatotoxicity, hyperglycemia, altered mental status, and nausea/vomiting. Pegylated formulations such as pegaspargase have significantly reduced (but not eliminated) the risk of hypersensitivity reactions; however, other toxicities remain a significant barrier to treatment in many adults.[15]

Patient's Initial Treatment
- *The patient undergoes induction treatment with cyclophosphamide, vincristine, daunorubicin, prednisone, and pegaspargase per the CALGB 10403 trial. Following count recovery after the first cycle, a bone marrow exam reveals a normocellular marrow with no lymphoblasts. Karyotyping and flow cytometry testing are normal, confirming remission with no MRD.*

What Is the Role of Post-Induction Therapy?

- Post-induction treatment in standard risk patients typically involves a consolidation phase consisting of multiple cycles of similar chemotherapy regimens to those used in induction. Patients with high-risk features can be considered for allo-HSCT.
- Following completion of induction and consolidation treatment, a 2- to 3-year period of maintenance chemotherapy is offered consisting of 6-mercaptopurine, methotrexate, vincristine, and glucocorticoids.
- 6-mercaptopurine toxicity can be significant in patients with mutations in the enzymes thiopurine methyltransferase (TPMT) or nucleoside diphosphate-linked moiety X motif 15 (NUDT15), causing prolonged, severe leukopenia requiring substantial dose reductions. TPMT mutations are more prevalent in patients of European or African ancestry, whereas NUDT15 mutations are more prevalent in patients of Asian or Hispanic ancestry. Pretreatment genetic testing should be considered, but is not considered mandatory given the relatively low prevalence of mutations in the general population.[16]

- CNS-directed therapy is continued during both the consolidation and maintenance phases, regardless of the initial CNS disease status.[6]

Patient's Further Treatment
- *The patient continues with consolidation chemotherapy using the same regimen utilized for induction for a total of 8 cycles. CNS prophylaxis is continued with methotrexate and cytarabine during each cycle. This was followed by 3 years of maintenance therapy with 6-mercaptopurine, methotrexate, vincristine, and glucocorticoids.*

What Further Surveillance Is Needed Posttreatment?

- Patients who complete induction, consolidation, and maintenance phases with no evidence of relapse can proceed with surveillance.
- Surveillance by routine history and physical examination with complete blood count (CBC) assessment is typical. Periodic monitoring for MRD with bone marrow aspiration and biopsy during the first 2 to 5 years can be considered given the availability of multiple salvage options in the MRD+ setting.[6]

Patient's Surveillance
- *The patient proceeds with bone marrow assessments every 6 months. At 12 months, CBC shows Hgb 8.7 g/dL and platelet count 72,000/mL. A bone marrow biopsy reveals recurrent disease with 35% lymphoblast involvement with similar cytogenetic profile to the initial biopsy.*

What Are Treatment Options in the Adolescent-and-Young-Adult Population in the Event of Relapse?

- Immunotherapeutic approaches such as blinatumomab or inotuzumab ozogamicin have shown improved outcomes over traditional chemotherapy although overall prognosis is much poorer for relapsed disease.[17,18]
  - Blinatumomab is a BiTE monoclonal antibody directed at CD19 on B-cell lymphoblasts and CD3 on cytotoxic T-cells.
  - Inotuzumab ozogamicin is a monoclonal anti-CD22 antibody conjugated to a cytotoxic agent. Inotuzumab is associated with veno-occlusive liver disease, and prophylactic ursodeoxycholic acid is recommended.
  - Head-to-head trials have not been performed for direct comparison.
- CD19-directed CAR-T therapy is also an option in the relapsed setting. Brexucabtagene autoleucel is available in first relapse at any age while tisagenlecleucel is approved for patients younger than 26 years of age in the refractory or multiple-relapsed setting.
- Patients who attain a CR following second-line induction therapy should be considered for consolidative allo-HSCT.[6]

Patient's Treatment at Relapse
- *The patient is treated with blinatumomab for relapsed disease. After 4 cycles of therapy, a bone marrow biopsy is performed and reveals CR with no lymphoblasts. Karyotyping and flow cytometry testing confirm that the patient has returned to MRD-negative status. The patient has four siblings; one is a human leukocyte antigen (HLA)-match, and the patient is planned for allo-HSCT as consolidation therapy.*

Case 29.2: Philadelphia Chromosome-Positive Acute Lymphoblastic Leukemia

A 40-year-old female presents to the ED with headaches, malaise, chills, and low-grade fevers over the preceding 8 weeks. She has a WBC count of 47,000/mL and a platelet count of 13,000/mL. Her peripheral smear demonstrates circulating blasts. She does not appear to be experiencing tumor lysis. She has no neurological findings on exam. A bone marrow biopsy is performed and aspirate flow cytometry demonstrates a monoclonal B lymphoblast population (30% of events); blasts are CD10+, CD19+, CD22+, CD79a+, and TDT+. The blast population is CD3-, CD7-, CD13-, CD20-, CD33-, and MPO-. Cytogenetic studies reveal t(9;22) in 10/20 metaphase cells and PCR demonstrates the p210 BCR-ABL transcript.

What Is the Significance of the Philadelphia Chromosome in Acute Lymphoblastic Leukemia?

- The Ph chromosome results from reciprocal translocation between chromosomes 9 and 22 and leads to the formation of an oncogenic *BCR-ABL1* fusion gene on chromosome 22. The *BCR-ABL1* is classically seen in chronic myelogenous leukemia (CML) but is also detected in approximately 25% of adult ALL cases with incidence increasing with age.
- The p190 variant, created by the fusion of the second exon of *ABL1* with the first exon of *BCR* (e1a2 transcript), is present in approximately two-thirds of Ph+ ALL patients. This variant is not commonly seen in CML.[19]
- The p210 variant, created by fusion of the second exon of *ABL1* with the 13th or 14th exons of *BCR* (e13a2 or e14a2 transcript), is present in the remaining third of ALL patients and is seen in most CML patients.[19]
- Historically, Ph+ ALL has been associated with poor outcomes; however, TKI therapy has improved outcomes considerably. TKI therapy should be included in induction, consolidation, and maintenance therapies.[6] Agent selection should take into account side effect profiles and patient comorbidities.

What Are Typical Induction Strategies for Philadelphia+ Acute Lymphoblastic Leukemia?

- The optimal induction strategy in Ph+ ALL has not been determined, but treatment is typically with TKI + multi-agent chemotherapy regimens similar to those used in Ph- disease.
- Approved TKIs include imatinib and dasatinib. Dasatinib offers higher CNS penetration and activity against many kinase domain mutations that cause imatinib resistance.[20] While not U.S. Food and Drug Administration (FDA) approved, nilotinib has been studied in ALL with reasonable response rates and may be an option for patients with contraindications to other available agents.[21]
- TKI use may allow for lower intensity induction strategies that omit anthracyclines and cyclophosphamide while maintaining reasonable remission rates.[22] Studies using TKIs with glucocorticoids alone have also reported excellent response rates.[23] These approaches have not been directly compared to higher intensity strategies, but may offer options for older or less fit patients.
- CNS prophylaxis, as in Ph- ALL, should be utilized routinely regardless of the presence of overt CNS disease.

Patient's Initial Treatment
- *The patient undergoes planned induction therapy with cyclophosphamide, vincristine, doxorubicin, dexamethasone, and dasatinib per the hyper-CVAD regimen. IT chemotherapy with methotrexate and cytarabine is administered, and CSF is negative for lymphoblasts by cytology and flow cytometry. Following count recovery after the first cycle, a bone marrow exam confirms complete hematologic and cytogenetic remission. PCR testing is negative for the BCR-ABL transcript and the patient is declared MRD negative.*

What Are Options for Post-Induction Therapy for Philadelphia+ Acute Lymphoblastic Leukemia?

- Allo-HSCT should be considered as consolidation if the patient is a candidate and a donor is available. Optimal timing is not clear and consolidation chemotherapy in combination with TKI can also be utilized.
- Nontransplant options include chemotherapy plus TKI, blinatumomab if MRD positive, or proceeding directly to maintenance therapy if MRD negative.
- Following consolidation, maintenance therapy with chemotherapy plus TKI or TKI alone is typically provided. MRD-negative patients may be able to safely proceed with active surveillance and resume TKI upon the development of MRD-positive disease.[24] The optimal strategy, including the duration of TKI therapy, is not well defined.
- CNS prophylaxis should be continued during consolidation and maintenance phases.[6]

Patient's Further Treatment

- *The patient is felt to be a transplant candidate. She has three siblings, and one is found to be an HLA match. She completes 8 total cycles of hyper-CVAD with dasatinib, followed by allogeneic transplant. She is then placed on maintenance treatment with dasatinib monotherapy.*

What Are the Principles of Surveillance in Philadelphia+ Acute Lymphoblastic Leukemia?

- Surveillance by routine history and physical examination with CBC assessment is typical.[6]
- Periodic monitoring of *BCR ABL* transcript by RT-PCR should be performed.[6]
- Periodic monitoring for MRD with bone marrow aspiration and biopsy during the first 5 years can also be considered.

What Treatment Options Are Available in the Relapse/Refractory Setting?

- Treatment options are similar to those utilized in Ph- disease but typically with the addition of TKI therapy. All patients should undergo mutational analysis of *BCR-ABL1* to detect potential kinase domain mutations that would guide TKI selection.
- Ponatinib is approved for use in patients who are resistant or intolerant to prior TKI therapy and is effective against the *T315I* mutation present in a significant number of ALL patients resistant to prior TKI therapy.[20] Asciminib is a TKI recently approved for CML that also has activity against the *T315I* mutation, but this drug has not been studied in ALL patients.

Case 29.3: Pre-B Cell Acute Lymphoblastic Leukemia

A 49-year-old man presented with 5 months of progressive bilateral knee and shin pain, which was worse at night. Laboratory evaluation revealed a WBC count of 120,000/µL, Hgb of 9.4 g/dL, and platelet count of 80,000/µL.

How Is Pre-B Cell Acute Lymphoblastic Leukemia Diagnosed?

- Clinical features of ALL include a subacute progression of aching bone pain, cytopenias, and leukocytosis (which, if markedly elevated, can predict a worse prognosis).
- Peripheral blood flow cytometry and bone marrow evaluation for morphology and cytogenetics should be performed.
- Detection of B-cell lineage markers, including CD19, CD22, CD10, and cytoplasmic CD79a, as well as general markers such as TdT, CD34, HLA-DR, and CD45, aid in the

Table 29.2. High-Risk Features in Pre–B-cell Acute Lymphoblastic Leukemia

Clinical	Age >35
Laboratory	WBC >30,000/μL
Cytogenetic	*BCR-ABL* translocation—t(9;22) *KMT2A* gene transcript—t(4;11)q(21;23) Hypodiploidy (<44 chromosomes) t(v;14q32)/IgH Complex karyotype (5 or more abnormalities) Intrachromosomal amplification of chromosome 21 (iAMP21) (17;19): TCF3-HLF fusion

WBC, white blood cell.

Source: Faderl S, O'Brien S, Pui CH, et al. Adult acute lymphoblastic leukemia: concepts and strategies. *Cancer*. 2010;116(5):1165–1176. doi:10.1002/cncr.24862; Hunger SP, Mullighan CG. Redefining ALL classification: toward detecting high-risk ALL and implementing precision medicine. *Blood*. 2015;125(26):3977–3987. doi:10.1182/blood-2015-02-580043

diagnosis of pre–B-cell ALL. The detection of CD20 enables the use of rituximab, and is present in approximately 65% of pre–B-cell ALL cases.[25]
- Cytogenetic features are important to define.

Diagnostic Workup Results
- *Flow cytometry demonstrated a large population of blasts that were CD19+, CD22+, CD20+, and CD10+. Bone marrow morphology showed 65% blasts, with immunophenotyping similar to that of peripheral blood. Cytogenetics revealed t(4;11)q(21;23) with KMT2A-AFF-1 fusion (formerly MLL-AF4). However, t(9;22) was not detected.*

What Are Important Prognostic and Risk Assessment Variables in Pre-B-Cell Acute Lymphoblastic Leukemia?

- Risk stratification and prognostic variables include patient, laboratory, and cytogenetic factors. Table 29.2 elaborates on these variables.

Patient's Risk Factors
- *In this patient, his age (older than 35 years), elevated WBC count (greater than 30,000/μL), and the presence of t(4;11), associated with the KMT2A (previously known as MLL) gene transcript, all predict a worse prognosis.*

What Is the Overall Approach to Treatment?

- Induction therapy is administered initially with regimens such as hyper-CVAD or CALGB 8811, followed by evaluation for CR (and MRD subsequently, if CR is achieved). More than 80% of patients achieve CR using such regimens.
- CNS-directed therapy (that is, CNS prophylaxis) is used routinely with IT chemotherapy using cytarabine and methotrexate.
- This patient's high-risk status suggests the need for stem cell transplantation early in his treatment course.[27]

Patient's Treatment
- *The patient received induction therapy with hyper-CVAD, with his first cycle complicated by gram-negative sepsis from which he recovered.*

How Is Response to Treatment Assessed?

- CR is determined by bone marrow exam at the completion of induction therapy. Any response other than CR is considered relapsed/refractory disease.
  - Failure to achieve CR is associated with a dismal prognosis, with 5-year survival rates below 10%.[26]
- Determination of MRD at the end of induction helps to allocate patients into prognostic and therapeutic subgroups.
  - MRD-positive patients are likely to benefit from treatment with blinatumomab prior to transplant. MRD-negative patients who undergo transplantation have a longer CR duration.[26]
- MRD can be determined by flow cytometric analyses, RT-PCR, and NGS-based assays detecting clonal rearrangements in *Ig/TCR* genes (immunoglobulin heavy chain and T-cell receptor).
- MRD-negativity is always defined relative to a preset threshold.

Final Clinical Course
- *The patient achieved CR by morphological criteria and MRD using RT-PCR. Given his high-risk features, he was referred for allo-HSCT.*

What Are Treatment Options in the Setting of Measurable Residual Disease-Positivity or Relapsed/Refractory Disease?

- In MRD-positive disease, blinatumomab, the BiTE, can be employed prior to allo-HSCT.
- For relapsed/refractory disease, next steps could include blinatumomab, inotuzumab ozogamicin, or CAR-T therapy.
- Allo-HSCT was considered early because of the patient's high-risk disease. If expected morbidity from transplantation is prohibitive, maintenance therapy would be preferable.

Case 29.4: T-Cell Acute Lymphoblastic Leukemia

A 29-year-old man presents for evaluation of fatigue, aching bone pain, petechiae, and unintended weight loss of 15 lb. His CBC demonstrates a WBC of 60,000/μL, Hgb of 7.4 g/dL, and platelet count of 70,000/μL.

How Is T-Cell Acute Lymphoblastic Leukemia Diagnosed?

- Peripheral blood flow cytometry and bone marrow biopsy and aspirate should be performed to evaluate morphology and to perform immunophenotyping and cytogenetic testing.
- Lymphoblasts in T-cell ALL are TdT-positive with variable expression of CD1a, CD2, CD3 (the only lineage-specific marker for lymphoblastic T-cell disease), CD4, CD5, CD7, and CD8. Cytoplasmic CD3 and CD7 are often positive.[28]
  - T-Lymphoblastic lymphoma is diagnosed in the same manner as T-cell ALL, except that bone marrow blasts are less than 20%.[29]
  - Expression of CD antigens defines pro–T-cell, pre–T-cell, cortical (thymic), and mature immunophenotypic groups.

Patient's Results
- *Peripheral blood flow cytometry revealed blasts that were CD1a+, CD3+, cD7+, and CD13-. Bone marrow biopsy reveals 40% blasts, with immunophenotyping similar to that of the peripheral blood. Cytogenetics reveals normal male karyotype. The final diagnosis is T-cell ALL.*

What Further Workup Should Be Performed?

- A CT of the chest, abdomen, and pelvis as well as TTE and hepatitis testing must be performed.
- As in B-cell ALL, lumbar puncture with IT chemotherapy should be performed. CSF flow cytometry is done to evaluate for CNS disease.
- Testicular involvement is even more common in T-cell ALL patients. If testicular abnormalities do not resolve by the end of induction therapy, consideration should be given to testicular irradiation.

Results of Diagnostic Workup

- CT CAP demonstrated mediastinal lymphadenopathy. Hepatitis serologies and TTE are unremarkable, and the CSF is negative for lymphoblasts by flow cytometry.

What Are Favorable Prognostic Features in This Case?

- The patient's age (younger than 35 years), WBC count below 100,000/μL, CD1a+, and normal karyotype are all favorable prognostic features. Note that elevated WBC count does not carry the same negative predictive value in T-cell ALL as it does on B-cell ALL.

Final Clinical Course

- The patient underwent induction with hyper-CVAD (including CNS prophylaxis), with day-28 bone marrow evaluation revealing CR. PCR testing confirms MRD negativity. He completed consolidation therapy and repeat marrow exam was negative; all lymphadenopathy had disappeared from the chest. He has remained in remission for 3 years.

What Treatment Options Are Available in the Relapsed/Refractory Setting?

- Nelarabine is the preferred agent, followed by evaluation for allo-HSCT, with 5-year survival data reported as 44% in one study.[30,31,32]

REVIEW QUESTIONS

1. A 30-year-old female presents to the hospital with abdominal pain and intermittent low-grade fevers that started 4 weeks prior. Physical examination is largely benign except for mild tenderness in the left upper quadrant and spleen palpable 8 cm below the left costal margin. A complete blood count (CBC) reveals a white blood cell (WBC) count of 65,000/mL, hemoglobin (Hgb) of 7.8 g/dL, and a platelet count of 12,000/mL. A peripheral smear is concerning for blasts. She undergoes bone marrow aspiration and biopsy which reveals a monoclonal lymphoblast population that is TdT+, CD3+, CD7+, CD19-, and/or CD20-. Which of the following is the most likely diagnosis?
   A. Pro–B-cell acute lymphoblastic leukemia (ALL)
   B. Mature–B-cell ALL
   C. T-cell ALL
   D. Pre–B-cell ALL

2. A 22-year-old male is admitted to the hospital to undergo his third cycle of consolidation chemotherapy for pre–B-cell acute lymphoblastic leukemia (ALL). He is receiving a multi-agent treatment regimen containing cyclophosphamide, glucocorticoids, doxorubicin, vincristine, and pegaspargase. He has tolerated treatment with the first 2 cycles without incident. He has a history of asthma and uses an albuterol inhaler once per week. Four hours after receiving an infusion of pegaspargase, he reports shortness of breath and pruritus. His temperature is 99.3°F (37.4°C), blood pressure 80/55, heart rate 118, and respiratory rate is 23. He feels like he is having an asthma attack, and requests an albuterol treatment. Which of the following is the most important next step in management?
   A. Albuterol nebulizer
   B. Intravenous (IV) diphenhydramine
   C. IV cetirizine
   D. Intramuscular (IM) epinephrine
   E. IV normal saline

3. A 65-year-old male presents to the hospital with low-grade fevers and a petechial rash that started 1 week prior. His complete blood count (CBC) demonstrates pancytopenia, and he is diagnosed with precursor B-cell acute lymphoblastic leukemia (ALL). Karyotyping performed on a bone marrow specimen reveals t(9;22). The patient is started on chemotherapy with dasatinib and initially attains complete response (CR). Several cycles later, BCR-ABL transcripts begin to rise and a T315I mutation is discovered. Which of the following tyrosine kinase inhibitors (TKIs) would be most likely to induce remission in this patient?
   A. Imatinib
   B. Dasatinib
   C. Nilotinib
   D. Asciminib
   E. Ponatinib

4. A 55-year-old female is diagnosed with pre–B-cell acute lymphoblastic leukemia (ALL) and the karyotype demonstrates t(9;22). She is planned for induction with multi-agent chemotherapy and dasatinib. Prior to treatment, a lumbar puncture is performed and does

not reveal any evidence of leukemic involvement of the CNS. Her neurological exam is within normal limits. Which of the following is true regarding central nervous system (CNS) management during induction?

A. CNS prophylaxis should be included in the induction regimen
B. Routine surveillance MRIs should be performed to monitor for CNS involvement
C. Lumbar puncture should be repeated after induction and treatment given if there is evidence of CNS involvement
D. No further CNS surveillance or treatment is warranted at this time

5. A 30-year-old male presents with 1 month of worsening fatigue and gum bleeding. A complete blood count (CBC) reveals a leukocyte count of 25,000/mL, hemoglobin of 6.2 g/dL, and platelets of 17,000/mL. The peripheral blood smear is concerning for numerous blasts, and bone marrow examination reveals a monoclonal population of CD19+, CD20+, CD22+, and/or CD10- cells. Which of the following findings would be considered a poor risk factor for this patient?

A. Hyperdiploidy
B. Hypodiploidy
C. Leukocyte count of 25,000/mL
D. Detection of ETV6-RUNX1 fusion transcripts
E. Age 30

6. A 50-year-old female is diagnosed with Philadelphia (Ph)- precursor B-cell acute lymphoblastic leukemia (ALL). She completes induction and consolidation treatment with appropriate multi-agent chemotherapy; however, at the completion of therapy a bone marrow examination reveals the presence of 12% lymphoblasts. She then undergoes 3 cycles of salvage therapy with inotuzumab ozogamicin and repeat bone marrow examination reveals she is in complete remission. She is otherwise in good health and has multiple healthy siblings. Which of the following is the most appropriate next step in management?

A. Continue inotuzumab ozogamicin
B. Start blinatumomab
C. Start monthly vincristine, prednisone, 6-mercaptopurine, and methotrexate
D. Referral for allogeneic hematopoietic stem cell transplant (allo-HSCT)
E. Referral for tisagenlecleucel

7. A 42-year-old male is diagnosed with precursor B-cell acute lymphoblastic leukemia (ALL) with cytogenetic testing revealing hyperdiploidy and no evidence of t(9;22) translocation. He undergoes multi-agent chemotherapy with appropriate central nervous system (CNS) prophylaxis. Following the completion of induction treatment, no minimal residual disease (MRD) is detected by multiparameter flow cytometry. He continues with further cycles and completes consolidation treatment without issue. He has multiple siblings and is otherwise healthy. Which of the following is the best next management strategy?

A. Referral for allogeneic hematopoietic stem cell transplantation (allo-HSCT)
B. Blinatumomab
C. Proceed with close routine surveillance
D. Start monthly vincristine, prednisone, 6-mercaptopurine, and methotrexate for 2 years
E. Referral for prophylactic cranial irradiation

8. A 40-year-old female of South Korean descent is diagnosed with Philadelphia (Ph-) precursor B-cell acute lymphoblastic leukemia (ALL). She is treated with multi-agent induction and consolidation chemotherapy, which is well tolerated. At the end of treatment she is confirmed to be in remission with no evidence of minimal residual disease (MRD). She is initiated on maintenance therapy with methotrexate, vincristine, 6-mercaptopurine (6-MP), and prednisone with periodic intrathecal (IT) chemotherapy. During the first cycle of maintenance therapy, she develops severe, prolonged neutropenia, ultimately requiring a 90% dose reduction of 6-MP. Which of the following enzyme deficiencies is most likely responsible for her intolerance of 6-MP?
   A. Thiopurine methyltransferase (TPMT)
   B. UDP Glucuronosyltransferase family 1 member A1 (UGT1A1)
   C. Nucleoside diphosphate-linked moiety X motif 15 (NUDT15)
   D. Glucose-6-phosphate dehydrogenase (G6PD)

9. Which of the following would be the best next step in management in a 30-year-old otherwise healthy patient with a history of T-cell acute lymphoblastic leukemia (ALL) who has just relapsed 1 year after second-line induction chemotherapy?
   A. Nelarabine
   B. Blinatumomab
   C. Inotuzumab ozogamicin
   D. Refer for allogeneic hematopoietic stem cell transplant (allo-HSCT)
   E. Polymerase chain reaction (PCR) testing for *BCR-ABL1*

10. A 42-year-old male is diagnosed with B-cell acute lymphoblastic leukemia (ALL). He undergoes multi-agent chemotherapy with appropriate central nervous system (CNS) prophylaxis. Following the completion of induction treatment, no minimal residual disease (MRD) is detected by multiparameter flow cytometry. He is started on maintenance therapy with prednisone, vincristine, 6-mercaptopurine, and methotrexate. Four months later, he presents to clinic reporting new onset numbness and tingling in his chin. Peripheral blood counts are slightly low but are consistent with his baseline counts since completing induction and consolidation. Which of the following is the most important next step in management?
    A. Start full dose acyclovir for suspected zoster infection
    B. Perform MRI of the brain followed by lumbar puncture with intrathecal (IT) chemotherapy and flow cytometry
    C. Reduce vincristine dosage for neuropathy
    D. Refer to dentist for thorough examination

ANSWERS AND RATIONALES

1. **C. T-cell ALL.** CD3 and CD7 are T-cell markers and are indicative of T-cell ALL in this patient.

2. **D. Intramuscular (IM) epinephrine.** While pegylated asparaginase products have significantly reduced the incidence of serious infusion reactions, they have not been completely eliminated and require early recognition and management. Other toxicities associated with asparaginase products include serious infusion reactions, thrombosis, coagulopathy, hemorrhage, hepatotoxicity, pancreatitis, hyperglycemia, altered mental status, and nausea/vomiting.

3. **E. Ponatinib.** All patients with relapsed or refractory Philadelphia (Ph)+ ALL should undergo kinase domain mutation testing to guide selection of TKI therapy. Ponatinib is the only TKI that has shown activity against *T315I* mutations in Ph+ ALL patients. While asciminib is another TKI approved for *T315I* patients in chronic myelogenous leukemia (CML), it has not yet been studied in ALL patients and ponatinib would be preferred in this patient.

4. **A. CNS prophylaxis should be included in the induction regimen.** While CNS involvement is uncommon at the time of diagnosis, patients who do not receive CNS-directed therapy as part of their treatment for ALL have much higher rates of later developing CNS disease. CNS-directed therapy is recommended as part of all phases of treatment in ALL regardless of initial CNS status. Patients who are initially CNS-negative are most often managed with intrathecal chemotherapy and high-dose systemic chemotherapy with CNS penetration.

5. **B. Hypodiploidy.** Hypodiploidy would be considered a poor risk factor in this patient with B-cell acute lymphoblastic leukemia (ALL). Additional poor cytogenetic risk factors would include *KMT2A* rearrangement, t(v;11q23.3), complex karyotype with five or more abnormalities, iAMP21, t(17;19), or possibly t(9;22). Additionally, patients with significant leukocytosis of greater than 30,000/mL in B-cell ALL or greater than 100,000/mL in T-cell ALL can be considered poor risk.

6. **D. Referral for allogeneic hematopoietic stem cell transplant (allo-HSCT).** Inotuzumab ozogamicin, a monoclonal anti-CD22 antibody conjugated to a cytotoxic agent, is an initial option for patients with refractory B-cell ALL that is CD22+ (greater than 90% of cases). It is associated with veno-occlusive liver disease and prophylactic ursodeoxycholic acid is recommended. While this treatment has shown improved outcomes compared to salvage chemotherapy, it is not considered curative and patients who obtain a complete response (CR) should be referred for allo-HSCT evaluation if they are considered a candidate. Blinatumomab, a bispecific T-cell engager (BiTE) monoclonal antibody, is an alternative option for refractory disease but would not be appropriate as consolidation after inotuzumab. Maintenance chemotherapy would similarly not be preferred for a patient with refractory disease after attaining second remission. Tisagenlecleucel is a chimeric antigen receptor T-cell (CAR-T) therapy that is an alternative option in refractory disease but is not approved in patients age 26 or older.

7. **D. Start monthly vincristine, prednisone, 6-mercaptopurine, and methotrexate for 2 years.** Induction and consolidation treatment should be followed by a maintenance phase regardless of MRD presence following induction. Maintenance chemotherapy regimens include

monthly vincristine/prednisone with or without 6-mercaptopurine and methotrexate for 2 to 3 years.

8. **C. Nucleoside diphosphate-linked moiety X motif 15 (NUDT15).** Both TPMT and NUDT15 mutations have been implicated in reduced metabolism of 6-MP causing severe, prolonged leukopenia necessitating dose reductions. TPMT is more prevalent in patients of European and African descent, whereas NUDT15 is more prevalent in patients of Asian or Hispanic descent. UGT1A1 has been implicated in severe neutropenia and diarrhea in patients receiving irinotecan. G6PD deficiency is associated with hemolytic anemia.

9. **A. Nelarabine.** This is a young patient with relapsed/refractory T-cell ALL. Nelarabine-based treatment would be the preferred option and is approved for T-cell ALL that has been relapsed/refractory after receiving two lines of chemotherapy. Blinatumomab and inotuzumab ozogamicin are treatment options for refractory B-cell ALL and are not used in T-cell ALL. Allogeneic transplant would be a potential option for consolidation if the patient is able to attain a second remission. *BCR-ABL1* testing would not be useful as *BCR-ABL1* has not been implicated in T-cell ALL.

10. **B. Perform MRI of the brain followed by lumbar puncture with intrathecal (IT) chemotherapy and flow cytometry.** Numb chin syndrome is an underrecognized complication of both solid and hematologic malignancies. It presents as a pure sensory neuropathy resulting from malignant infiltration of the mental nerve and should be evaluated by lumbar puncture with flow cytometry to assess for leptomeningeal involvement. MRI can also be considered; however, a standard MRI of the brain may not include full evaluation of the mental nerve. Traditional dental panoramic x-rays may be falsely normal.

REFERENCES

1. Bennett JM, Catovsky D, Daniel MT. Proposals for the classification of the acute leukemias. *Brit J Haem.* 1976;33:451–458. doi:10.1111/j.1365-2141.1976.tb03563.x
2. Paul S, Kantarjian H, Jabbour EJ. Adult acute lymphoblastic leukemia. *Mayo Clin Proc.* 2016;91:1645–1666. doi:10.1016/j.mayocp.2016.09.010
3. Jabbour E, O'Brien S, Konopleva M, Kantarjian H. New insights into the pathophysiology and therapy of adult acute lymphoblastic leukemia. *Cancer.* 2015;121:2517–2528. doi:10.1002/cncr.29383
4. Shah A, John BM, Sondhi V. Acute lymphoblastic leukemia with treatment—naive fanconi anemia. *Indian Pediatr.* 2013;50:508–510. https://www.indianpediatrics.net/may2013/508.pdf
5. Rowe JM, Buck G, Burnett AK, et al. Induction therapy for adults with acute lymphoblastic leukemia: results of more than 1500 patients from the international ALL trial: MRC UKALL XII/ECOG E2993. *Blood.* 2005;106:3760–3767. doi:10.1182/blood-2005-04-1623
6. National Comprehensive Cancer Network. Acute lymphoblastic leukemia (Version 4.2021). https://www.nccn.org/professionals/physician_gls/pdf/all.pdf
7. Larson RA. Acute lymphoblastic leukemia. In: Kaushansky K, Prchal JT, Burns LJ, Lichtman MA, Levi M, Linch DC, eds. *Williams Hematology.* 10e. McGraw Hill; 2021:1593–1616.
8. Byrne J, Fears TR, Mills JL, et al. Fertility of long-term male survivors of acute lymphoblastic leukemia diagnosed during childhood. *Pediatr Blood Cancer.* 2004;42(4):364–372. doi:10.1002/pbc.10449
9. Roshandel R, van Dijk M, Overbeek A, et al. Female reproductive function after treatment of childhood acute lymphoblastic leukemia. *Pediatr Blood Cancer.* 2021;68(4):e28894. doi:10.1002/pbc.28894
10. Surapaneni UR, Cortes JE, Thomas D, et al. Central nervous system relapse in adults with acute lymphoblastic leukemia. *Cancer.* 2002;94(3):773–779. doi:10.1002/cncr.10265
11. Larson RA. Managing CNS disease in adults with acute lymphoblastic leukemia. *Leuk Lymphoma.* 2018;59(1):3–13. doi:10.1080/10428194.2017.1326597
12. Thomas DA, O'Brien S, Faderl S, et al. Chemoimmunotherapy with a modified hyper-CVAD and rituximab regimen improves outcome in de novo Philadelphia chromosome-negative precursor B-lineage acute lymphoblastic leukemia. *J Clin Oncol.* 2010;28(24):3880–3889. doi:10.1200/JCO.2009.26.9456

13. Wetzler M, Sanford BL, Kurtzberg J, et al. Effective asparagine depletion with pegylated asparaginase results in improved outcomes in adult acute lymphoblastic leukemia: Cancer and Leukemia Group B study 9511. *Blood.* 2007;109(10):4164–4167. doi:10.1182/blood-2006-09-045351

14. Stock W, Luger SM, Advani AS, et al. A pediatric regimen for older adolescents and young adults with acute lymphoblastic leukemia: results of CALGB 10403 [published correction appears in *Blood.* 2019 September 26;134(13):1111]. *Blood.* 2019;133(14):1548–1559. doi:10.1182/blood-2018-10-881961

15. Chang A, Kim M, Seyer M, Patel S. Allergic reactions associated with pegaspargase in adults. *Leuk Lymphoma.* 2016;57(7):1665–1668. doi:10.3109/10428194.2015.1105369

16. Relling MV, Schwab M, Whirl-Carrillo M, et al. Clinical pharmacogenetics implementation consortium guideline for thiopurine dosing based on *TPMT* and *NUDT15* genotypes: 2018 update. *Clin Pharmacol Ther.* 2019;105(5):1095–1105. doi:10.1002/cpt.1304

17. Kantarjian H, Stein A, Gökbuget N, et al. Blinatumomab versus chemotherapy for advanced acute lymphoblastic leukemia. *N Engl J Med.* 2017;376(9):836–847. doi:10.1056/NEJMoa1609783

18. Kantarjian HM, DeAngelo DJ, Stelljes M, et al. Inotuzumab ozogamicin versus standard therapy for acute lymphoblastic leukemia. *N Engl J Med.* 2016;375(8):740–753. doi:10.1056/NEJMoa1509277

19. Melo JV. The diversity of *BCR-ABL* fusion proteins and their relationship to leukemia phenotype. *Blood.* 1996;88(7):2375–2384. doi:10.1182/blood.V88.7.2375.bloodjournal8872375

20. Pfeifer H, Wassmann B, Pavlova A, et al. Kinase domain mutations of *BCR-ABL* frequently precede imatinib-based therapy and give rise to relapse in patients with de novo Philadelphia-positive acute lymphoblastic leukemia (Ph+ ALL). *Blood.* 2007;110(2):727–734. doi:10.1182/blood-2006-11-052373

21. Kim D-Y, Joo Y-D, Lim S-N, et al. Nilotinib combined with multiagent chemotherapy for newly diagnosed Philadelphia-positive acute lymphoblastic leukemia. *Blood.* 2015;126(6):746–756. doi:10.1182/blood-2015-03-636548

22. Rousselot P, Coudé MM, Gokbuget N, et al. Dasatinib and low-intensity chemotherapy in elderly patients with Philadelphia chromosome-positive ALL. *Blood.* 2016;128(6):774–782. doi:10.1182/blood-2016-02-700153

23. Foà R, Vitale A, Vignetti M, et al. Dasatinib as first-line treatment for adult patients with Philadelphia chromosome-positive acute lymphoblastic leukemia. *Blood.* 2011;118(25):6521–6528. doi:10.1182/blood-2011-05-351403

24. Pfeifer H, Wassmann B, Bethge W, et al. Randomized comparison of prophylactic and minimal residual disease-triggered imatinib after allogeneic stem cell transplantation for *BCR-ABL1*-positive acute lymphoblastic leukemia. *Leukemia.* 2013;27(6):1254–1262. doi:10.1038/leu.2012.352

25. Chiaretti S, Zini G, Bassan R. Diagnosis and subclassification of acute lymphoblastic leukemia. *Mediterr J Hematol Infect Dis.* 2014;6(1):e2014073. doi:10.4084/MJHID.2014.073

26. Hunger SP, Mullighan CG. Redefining ALL classification: toward detecting high-risk ALL and implementing precision medicine. *Blood.* 2015;125(26):3977–3987. doi:10.1182/blood-2015-02-580043

27. Malard F, Mohty M. Acute lymphoblastic leukaemia. *Lancet.* 2020;395(10230):1146–1162. doi:10.1016/S0140-6736(19)33018-1

28. Borowitz MJ, Chan JKC. T-lymphoblastic leukaemia/lymphoma. In: Swerdlow SH, Campo E, Harris NL, et al., eds. *WHO Classification of Tumours of Haematopoietic and Lymphoid Tissues: World Health Organization Classification of Tumours.* 4th ed. International Agency for Research on Cancer (IARC); 2008:176–178.

29. Swerdlow SH, Campo E, Harris NL, et al., eds. *WHO Classification of Tumours of Haematopoietic and Lymphoid Tissues.* 4th ed. IARC Publications; 2008.

30. Marks DI, Paietta EM, Moorman AV, et al. T-cell acute lymphoblastic leukemia in adults: clinical features, immunophenotype, cytogenetics, and outcome from the large randomized prospective trial (UKALL XII/ECOG 2993). *Blood.* 2009;114(25):5136–5145. doi:10.1182/blood-2009-08-231217

31. DeAngelo DJ, Yu D, Johnson JL, et al. Nelarabine induces complete remissions in adults with relapsed or refractory T-lineage acute lymphoblastic leukemia or lymphoblastic lymphoma: cancer and leukemia group B study 19801. *Blood.* 2007;109:5136–5142. doi:10.1182/blood-2006-11-056754

32. Bakr M, Rasheed W, Mohamed SY, et al. Allogeneic hematopoietic stem cell transplantation in adolescent and adult patients with high-risk T-cell acute lymphoblastic leukemia. *Biol Blood Marrow Transplant.* 2012;18(12):1897–1904. doi: 10.1016/j.bbmt.2012.07.011

CHAPTER 30

Acute Myelogenous Leukemia

Elizabeth F. Eisenmenger, Maria Siddiqui, and Gustavo Rivero

INTRODUCTION

Acute myeloid leukemia (AML) accounts for about 90% of all acute leukemias. It is a hetero-geneous stem cell malignancy that results in the proliferation of immature hematopoietic cells leading to bone marrow and peripheral blood expansion. The median age at AML diagnosis is 68 years, with a male:female ratio of 1.5:1. The 5-year relative survival rate is 29.5% with an estimated 11,400 deaths per year.[1] Risk factors include genetic predisposition [that is, *RUNX1* thrombocytopenia familial disorder, *CEBPA*, and *DDX41* mutations, among others], aging, prior radiation and/or chemotherapy (particularly topoisomerase II inhibitors and alkylating agents), and antecedent hematologic disorders such as myelodysplastic syndrome or myelopro-liferative neoplasms.

Patients usually present with complications related to cytopenias; infection, fatigue, and shortness of breath. AML is diagnosed when the blast percentage is more than 20% in the peripheral blood or bone marrow; however, patients with certain karyotypic abnormalities, such as t(8;21), inv(16), t(16;16), and t(15;17), are diagnosed with AML regardless of blast count. Karyotyping, immunophenotyping, and molecular testing (ex. *NPM1, FLT3, TP53*) are important steps in diagnosis as results impact prognosis and treatment. The European LeukemiaNet (ELN) classification of AML incorporating cytogenetics and molecular mutations is presented in Table 30.1.[2] Standard induction chemotherapy for medically fit patients is "7 + 3," which is 7 days of infusional cytarabine and 3 days of anthracycline. A bone marrow biopsy is done after induction to check response to treatment. Consolidation chemotherapy is typically with high-dose cytarabine followed by allogeneic or autologous transplant for intermediate-risk and unfavorable risk patients. In recent years, new drugs and targeted therapies have been approved for induction and for relapsed AML. These new therapeutic opportunities have improved outcomes in older and high-risk AML patients. Recent drug approvals are outlined in Table 30.2.

CASE SUMMARIES

Case 30.1: Acute Promyelocytic Leukemia

A 28-year-old woman with no significant past medical history (PMH) was brought to the ED by her sister complaining of generalized weakness, excessive bruising, and continuous vaginal bleeding for 1 week. Her physical examination did not reveal lymphadenopathy or hepatospleno-megaly. She had ecchymoses on her thighs, arms, and upper torso that were not associated with

Table 30.1   2017 European LeukemiaNet Genetic Risk Stratification

Risk Category	Genetic Abnormality
Favorable	t(8;21)(q22;a22.1); *RUNX1-TUNX1T1*
	inv(16)(p13.1q22) or t(16;16)(p13.1;q22); *CBFB-MYH11*
	Mutated *NPM1* without *FLT3-ITD* or with *FLT3-ITD* low allelic expression
	Biallelic mutated *CEBPA*
Intermediate	Mutated *NPM1* and *FLT3-ITD* high allelic expression
	Wild-type *NPM1* without *FLT3-ITD* or with *FLT3-ITD* low allelic expression (without adverse-risk genetic lesions)
	t(9;11)(p21.3;q23.3); *MLLT3-KMT2A*
	Cytogenetic abnormalities not classified as favorable or adverse
Adverse	t(6;9)(p23;q34.1); *DEK-NUP214*
	t(v;11q23.3); *KMT2A* rearranged
	t(9;22)(q34.1;q11.2); *BCR-ABL1*
	inv(3)(q21.3q26.2) or t(3;3)(q21.3;q26.2); *GATA2, MECOM (EVI1)*
	-5 or del(5q); -7; -17/abn(17p)
	Complex karyotype, monosomal karyotype
	Wild-type *NPM1* and *FLT3-ITD* high allelic expression
	Mutated *RUNX1*
	Mutated *ASXL1*
	Mutated *TP53*

Source: Reproduced with permission from Döhner H, Estey E, Grimwade D, et al. Diagnosis and management of AML in adults: 2017 ELN recommendations from an international expert panel. *Blood*.2017;129(4):424–447. doi:10.1182/blood-2016-08-733196

trauma. There was oozing from IV line sites and some vaginal bleeding observed on a gyneco-logical examination. A complete blood count (CBC) showed a white blood cell (WBC) count of 1800/μL, hemoglobin (Hgb) level of 8.7 g/dL, and platelet count of 13,000/μL. The peripheral smear showed promyelocytes with large bilobed nuclei, prominent nucleoli, and several Auer rods. Coagulation parameters showed a prothrombin time (PT) of 18 s, partial thromboplastin time (PTT) of 38 s, and fibrinogen of 80 mg/dL.

What Is the Diagnosis?

- Morphological evidence of promyelocytes and coagulopathy suggest a diagnosis of acute promyelocytic leukemia (APL).
- APL represents 5% to 10% of all AML cases; the distinct cytogenetic signature is the presence of t(15;17) resulting in formation of the fusion gene transcript progressive mul-tifocal leukoencephalopathy/retinoic acid receptor alpha (*PML-RARα*).
- A presumptive diagnosis of APL is made with circulating promyelocytes containing abundant, often irregular nuclei. Primary azurophilic granules and Auer rods are a dis-tinctive feature of APL.

What Are the Types of Acute Promyelocytic Leukemia?

- There are two different forms of APL: the hypergranular and the microgranular variants.

Table 30.2 Drug Approvals in Acute Myeloid Leukemia Since 2017

Treatment	Type	FDA Approval	Indication
Midostaurin	FLT3 inhibitor	April 2017	Newly diagnosed *FLT3*-mutated AML
Gemtuzumab ozogamicin	Anti-CD33 antibody–drug conjugate	September 2017	Newly diagnosed CD33-positive AML Relapsed-refractory CD33-positive AML
CPX-351	Liposomal cytarabine and daunorubicin	August 2017	Newly diagnosed therapy-related AML Secondary AML AML with myelodysplasia-related changes
Glasdegib	Hedgehog pathway inhibitor	November 2018	Newly diagnosed AML aged ≥75 years or with comorbidities precluding intensive chemo-therapy (combined with low-dose cytarabine)
Venetoclax	BCL-2 inhibitor	November 2018	Newly diagnosed AML aged ≥60 years with comorbidities ineligible for intensive chemotherapy or eligible for BMT if unfavorable ELN2017. BCL2- inhibitor should be combined with hypomethylat-ing agents or low-dose cytarabine
Enasidenib	IDH2 inhibitor	August 2017	Relapsed-refractory IDH2-mutated AML and upfront therapy*
Ivosidenib	IDH1 inhibitor	July 2018	Relapsed or refractory IDH1-mutated AML Frontline for IDH1-mutated AML in patients ≥75 years or ineligible for intensive chemotherapy
Gilteritinib	FLT3 inhibitor	November 2018	Relapsed/Refractory *FLT3*-mutated AML
CC-486	Oral azacitidine	September 2020	AML in first CR or CRi after intensive induction chemotherapy and unable to complete intensive curative therapy
ASTX727	Oral decitabine-ceda-zuridine	July 2020	Pretreated/untreated MDS De novo/secondary MDS CMML

*Not U.S. Food and Drug Administration (FDA) approved, but suggested for de novo disease by National Comprehensive Cancer Network (NCCN).

AML, acute myeloid leukemia; BMT, bone marrow transplantation; CMML, chronic myelomonocytic leukemia; CR, complete remission; CRi, complete remission with incomplete blood count recovery; MDS, myelodysplastic syndrome.

- o In hypergranular APL, the promyelocytes have bilobed or kidney-shaped nuclei and the cytoplasm contains large basophilic granules.
- o In the microgranular variant, nuclei are bilobed and cytoplasm contains less con-spicuous granules. This type is associated with high leukocyte counts and rapid proliferation.

- APL is strongly myeloperoxidase (MPO) positive and cells express early myeloid markers: CD33 and C13. There is weak or absent expression of CD34, human leukocyte antigen (HLA)-DR, CD11b, or CD15.
- Clinically, APL is stratified into low and high risk based on initial WBC and platelet count.
  - The low-risk group includes patients with WBC of 10,000/µL or less and platelet count of 40,000/µL or more with relapse-free survival (RFS) of 98%.
  - The intermediate-risk group includes patients with WBC of 10,000/µL or less and platelets of 40,000/µL or less with RFS of about 90%.
  - The high-risk group includes patients with WBC greater than 10,000/µL and an RFS of 70%.

How Is Acute Promyelocytic Leukemia Diagnosed?

- If APL is suspected clinically, all-trans retinoic acid (ATRA) should be started promptly. The dosage is 45 mg/m^2/day in two divided doses.
- Following ATRA initiation, workup for APL including bone marrow exam, flow cytometry, cytogenetics, fluorescent in situ hybridization (FISH) for PML-RARα and reverse transcription polymerase chain reaction (RT-PCR) should be obtained.

How Is Acute Promyelocytic Leukemia Managed?

Treatment of APL is divided into:

- **Supportive Care**
  - This includes fresh frozen plasma (FFP), cryoprecipitate, and platelet transfusions to maintain fibrinogen concentration above 100 to 150 mg/ dL, platelet count greater than 30,000 to 50,000/µL, and international normalized ratio (INR) less than 1.5.
  - Leukapheresis, heparin, tranexamic acid, and other anticoagulant or antifibrinolytic therapy should not be used outside the context of a clinical trial.
  - Once treatment in begun, it is imperative to monitor closely for life threatening complications including:
    - **Differentiation syndrome (DS)** in patients on therapy is characterized by dyspnea, fever, weight gain, peripheral edema, pleural or pericardial effusion, unexplained hypotension, acute renal failure, and congestive heart failure (CHF).
      - Severe manifestations include respiratory failure or pleural/pericardial effusion.
      - Prophylactic corticosteroids should be considered (10 mg dexamethasone intravenously [IV] twice daily) in all APL cases, but should be started when WBC count is greater than 10,000/ µL or at the earliest symptoms or signs to prevent DS.
      - Discontinuation of ATRA or arsenic trioxide (ATO) is indicated in severe DS (acute renal failure or acute hypoxic respiratory failure necessitating intensive care).
    - **Coagulopathy:** Intracranial and pulmonary hemorrhages are life-threatening complications of APL coagulopathy.
      - Coagulation parameters are monitored frequently and transfusions given as indicated.
      - Strict fluid balance should be performed to avoid fluid overload.
- **Induction Therapy**
  - *Low- and Intermediate-Risk Acute Promyelocytic Leukemia*
    - Anthracyclines were the mainstay for APL before clinical trials showed superior disease-free survival (DFS) and overall survival (OS) with the addition of ATRA.[3,4]
    - Later, ATRA plus ATO showed synergism and promoted apoptosis and cellular differentiation.[5]

- The APL 0406 trial demonstrated that ATO + ATRA was noninferior to ATRA + chemotherapy with a 2-year event-free survival (EFS) of 97% versus 87.6%.[6] In a follow-up study, ATRA + ATO appeared more favorable than ATRA + chemotherapy.[7]
- ATO regimens require regular monitoring of electrolytes and QTc interval.
  - *High-Risk Acute Promyelocytic Leukemia*
    - Early institution of anthracyclines (idarubicin/daunorubicin with or without cytarabine [Ara-C]) with ATRA and ATO is the standard treatment approach based on the APML 4 study.[8]
    - Gemtuzumab ozogamicin is an alternative to anthracyclines in the management of high-risk APL.[9]

Clinical Course: Supportive Care and Induction Therapy

Based on risk stratification the patient was placed in the low-risk group. After a negative pregnancy test, she started on ATRA and was transfused with FFP, cryoprecipitate, and platelets. Soon after ATRA initiation, her WBC increased to 48,000/μL. Intravenous dexamethasone at 10 mg every 12 hours was administered, given the concern for DS. Hydroxyurea at 1000 mg orally every 12 hours was administered for cytoreduction. Two days later, her WBC was 16,000/μL. ATO at 0.15 mg/kg IV daily was added. She achieved complete hematologic and morphological remission based on a bone marrow examination performed 4 weeks after treatment with ATRA and ATO.

- **Consolidation Therapy in Acute Promyelocytic Leukemia**
  - Consolidation strategies depend on the risk classification and initial therapy.[10]
  - For low-risk disease in CR, 4 cycles of ATO at 0.15 mg/kg/day IV, 5 days per week, for 4 weeks every 8 weeks for 4 cycles, and ATRA 45 mg/m² for 2 weeks every 4 weeks for 7 cycles is recommended in first CR (CR1).
  - In high-risk APL, consolidation regimens incorporate ATRA plus ATO only, or in combination with chemotherapy.[11]

Clinical Course: Post Induction Therapy

The patient received consolidation therapy with the first cycle of ATRA and ATO. At the end of consolidation therapy, she attained a molecular remission.

- **Maintenance Therapy in Acute Promyelocytic Leukemia**
  - Studies by Gruppo Italiano Malattie EMatologiche dell'Adulto (GIMEMA) found no difference in relapse among maintenance arms in APL.[12]
  - Consideration for maintenance includes evaluation of initial disease risk (low vs. high risk), type, intensity, and duration of previous induction/consolidation and measurable residual disease (MRD) status by PML-RARα positivity.

Clinical Course (continued)

The patient continued PML-RARα PCR testing and has remained disease free for 3 years post-consolidation treatment.

What Is the Management of Relapsed Acute Promyelocyte Leukemia?

- APL relapse usually occurs within the first 3 years, and along with refractory disease comprises 5% to 10% of patients.
- For patients with confirmed molecular relapse (two successive PCR-positive assays with stable or rising PML-RARα transcript levels), preemptive therapy is started promptly to prevent frank relapse.
- ATO-based regimens are the first option for treatment of relapsed APL; ATRA plus chemotherapy can also be used as salvage therapy.[13]

- Autologous hematopoietic stem cell transplant (HSCT) should be considered for patients without detectable disease in the marrow (in second CR) and with an adequate PCR-negative harvest.
- Allogeneic HSCT (allo-HSCT) is recommended for patients failing to achieve a second molecular remission. For patients in whom HSCT is not feasible, available options include repeated cycles of ATO with or without ATRA /chemotherapy.

Is Central Nervous System Prophylaxis Routinely Used in Acute Promyelocytic Leukemia?

- Routine prophylaxis is not administered in low- or intermediate-risk disease as ATO crosses the blood–brain barrier and achieves therapeutic levels in cerebrospinal fluid (CSF).
- The CNS is the most common site of extramedullary disease in APL with 10% of relapsed disease cases accompanied by CNS involvement.
- Most CNS relapses occur in patients with hyperleukocytosis; hence, CNS prophylaxis is administered in high-risk patients after CR because lumbar puncture at presentation and during induction is dangerous.

Case 30.2: Acute Myeloid Leukemia With Favorable Risk in Younger Adults (18 to 60 Years Old)

A 48-year-old man with a history of hypertension presented to his primary physician with a 1-month history of generalized weakness, fatigue, easy bruising, and intermittent epistaxis. He also reported a 1-week history of exertional dyspnea and chest pain. Physical examination revealed pallor, although there was no hepatosplenomegaly or lymphadenopathy. There was no bruising, but some petechiae were visible on his lower extremities. WBC count was 46,000/μL with an Hgb of 6.8 g/dL and a platelet count of 18,000/μL. A peripheral blood smear showed a large number of monocytoid-appearing blasts and an increased number of eosinophils. A bone marrow aspirate and biopsy confirmed AML with cytogenetics showing inv(16). EKG and chest x-ray were normal. He was transfused for symptomatic anemia and aggressively hydrated in preparation for treatment. An echocardiogram demonstrated a normal ejection fraction (EF) with no wall motion abnormalities.

What Is the Management of Newly Diagnosed Favorable-Risk Acute Myeloid Leukemia?

There are four favorable-risk AML categories excluding APL (described in Table 30.1), and management is multifaceted.
- **Supportive Care**
  - Hyperleukocytosis (WBC count greater than 100,000/μL) leads to leukostasis and requires urgent treatment to prevent respiratory failure secondary to sludging of cells in the pulmonary circulation or spontaneous hemorrhages in the retina or CNS.
  - WBC count should be reduced rapidly to less than 50,000/μL with either leukapheresis or chemotherapy.
  - Excessive red blood cell (RBC) or platelet transfusions lead to increased blood viscosity in patients with high blast counts.
  - Renal function and uric acid should be evaluated, and allopurinol, rasburicase, and/or hemodialysis begun to prevent or treat tumor lysis syndrome.

Clinical Course: Supportive Care

The patient was started on allopurinol for tumor lysis prophylaxis and hydroxyurea to reduce his WBC count, while waiting to obtain bone marrow biopsy results, cardiac workup, and central line placement.

- **Induction Therapy**
  - Induction therapy is classically given with the "3 + 7" regimen, which includes 3 days of an anthracycline (for example, daunorubicin, at least 60 mg/m^2; idarubicin, 10 to 12 mg/m^2; or mitoxantrone, 10 to 12 mg/m^2) and 7 days of cytarabine (100 to 200 mg/m^2/day continuous IV infusion). CR is achieved in 70% to 80% of younger adults. The regimen is used across all subtypes of favorable-risk AML.
  - In younger adults with AML, induction therapy with daunorubicin at 90 mg/m^2 for 3 days versus 45 mg/m^2 improved CR and duration of remission.[14]
  - In de novo inv(16) and t(8;21), collectively called core binding factor AML (CBF AML), gemtuzumab ozogamicin can be added to standard induction based on superior EFS and OS, as demonstrated by the ALFA 0701 trial.[15]
  - An alternate regimen of fludarabine, high-dose cytarabine, idarubicin with granulocyte colony-stimulating factor (G-CSF), and a single dose of gemtuzumab ozogamicin can be considered.

Clinical Course: Induction Therapy

The patient achieved a CR with induction chemotherapy consisting of idarubicin, 12 mg/m^2, and 7 days of cytarabine (100 mg/m^2 continuous IV). He had prolonged cytopenias requiring frequent transfusion and developed transfusion-related acute lung injury (TRALI) and acute coronary syndrome that were medically managed.

- **Consolidation Therapy**
  - At day 14 to 21 bone marrow is done to assess response.
  - Patients with core binding factor (CBF) AMLs have good prognosis when consolidated with high-dose cytarabine without HSCT in first remission.
  - A landmark study showed that 4 cycles of high-dose cytarabine (3 g/m^2 per q12h on days 1, 3, and 5) are superior to 4 courses of 5 days of infusional cytarabine at either 100 mg/m^2 or 400 mg/m^2.[16]
  - High-dose Ara-C (HiDAC) is a reasonable choice for younger adults with mutated *NPM1* and wildtype *FLT3*/low *FLT3 ITD* and in patients with mutated biallelic *CEBPA*.
  - A meta-analysis showed significant OS benefit for allo-HSCT in intermediate- and high-risk AML as compared to consolidation chemotherapy.[17]

Clinical Course: Post Induction Therapy

Based on his favorable risk AML, induction was followed by 4 courses of consolidation with HiDAC. He has remained disease free for 3 years.

Case 30.3: Acute Myeloid Leukemia With Intermediate Risk/Unfavorable Risk in Younger Adults

A 57-year-old businessman with hypercholesterolemia and hypertension was brought to the hospital with an acute febrile illness and lethargy. On examination, he had mild hepatosplenomegaly with no lymphadenopathy. He had significant gingival hyperplasia and gum bleeding. Labs demonstrated a WBC of 60,000/μL with greater than 50% blasts, an Hgb of 9 g/dL, and a platelet count of 44,000/μL. Bone marrow biopsy confirmed AML and cytogenetic evaluation showed: 46XY, −7, +8, 21q-, and 11q- in all 20 of the analyzed cells. The patient was considered to have complex cytogenetics (greater than 3 cytogenetic abnormalities) and fell into the high-risk AML category with a poor prognosis.

What Is the Management of Intermediate and Unfavorable Risk Acute Myeloid Leukemia in Younger Adults (Younger Than 60 Years)?

- Induction Therapy
  - Induction strategy is based on comorbidities, performance status (PS), and the presence of an antecedent hematologic disorder.
  - The standard induction regimen is "3 + 7" as previously described. HiDAC induction and fludarabine + HiDAC with G-CSF are also options.
  - Patients in the ELN 2017 adverse risk category, especially those with *TP53* mutations, have poor outcomes with standard induction therapies; if available, a clinical trial is a better alternative.
  - Patients with *FLT3-ITD/TKD* mutations receive FLT3 inhibitors, midostaurin or sorafenib, on days 8 to 21 in addition to cytarabine and anthracyclines.
  - At the end of induction therapy, risk stratification is performed by obtaining a bone marrow exam.
    - If the bone marrow exam shows significant reduction in blasts, consolidation can be pursued immediately or delayed if marrow is hypoplastic.
    - If there is significant residual disease, reinduction is reasonable; however, treatment of refractory disease is challenging and allo-HSCT has a success rate of only about 10%.
  - In patients who achieve CR then relapse, subsequent response depends on the duration of CR.
    - If CR duration is greater than 12 months, 50% of patients achieve CR2 with cytarabine-containing regimens and should proceed to allo-HSCT.
    - Patients with shorter CR duration are best treated in clinical trials.

Clinical Course: Induction Therapy

The patient achieved complete remission after induction with 3 + 7. He received 2 cycles of HiDAC.

- Consolidation Therapy
  - For patients with intermediate- or poor-risk cytogenetics, allo-HSCT, preferably from a matched related donor, has shown benefit in CR1.[17]
  - Allo-HSCT outcomes from fully matched unrelated donors are similar to those from matched related donors.[18]
  - Long-term survival is about 30% for AML patients with adverse cytogenetics transplanted in CR1 from matched unrelated donors.[19]

Clinical Course: Post Induction Therapy

The patient had seven siblings and a younger brother was an HLA identical match. He proceeded to allo-SCT. Unfortunately, during a prolonged period of neutropenia he developed a perirectal abscess and succumbed to gram-negative sepsis despite antibiotic therapy.

- Maintenance Therapy
  - In patients older than 55 years who were unsuitable for bone marrow transplantation (BMT), attained CR after intense chemotherapy, and received partial or complete consolidation, oral azacitidine has demonstrated improved OS and RFS.[20]
  - In patients with *FLT3-ITD* mutation who are post-allogeneic transplantation and in remission, maintenance treatment with FLT3 inhibitor is recommended.[21]

Case 30.4: Acute Myeloid Leukemia in the Older Adult (Age Older Than 60 Years)

A 62-year-old man with poor PS presented to the ED with shortness of breath and fever. His physical exam revealed pallor and petechiae on his lower extremities. He had no hepatosplenomegaly, lymphadenopathy, or evidence of bleeding. WBC count was 500/mL, Hgb was 6 g/dL, and platelet count was 9,000/mL. Peripheral blood smear showed normal RBCs, few platelets, decreased WBCs, and few circulating blasts with high nuclear to cytoplasmic ratio and several nucleoli. No Auer rods were seen. Bone marrow exam showed 18% to 20% blasts and 60% cellularity. Flow cytometry showed a population of cells positive for CD34, CD117, CD13, and CD33 consistent with myeloid blasts.

How Is a Diagnosis Established?

- Peripheral blood smear or bone marrow has 20% blasts.

What Further Molecular or Genomic Testing Is Required?

- All AML patients should have cytogenetic and molecular testing on their bone marrow aspirate and biopsy to help with risk stratification (Table 30.1) and targeted therapies (Table 30.2).

Clinical Course
The patient's bone marrow exam revealed complex cytogenetics, and molecular studies were positive for a TP53 mutation.

What Are Appropriate Treatment Options?

- Older patients who are medically fit should receive more intensive induction chemotherapy.
- The "7+3" is appropriate for fit older patients. Liposomal cytarabine plus daunorubicin [CPX-351 formulation] is approved for therapy-related AML, myelodysplasia-related AML, or chronic myelomonocytic leukemia. CR rate is 29% to 32% in patients harboring *TP53* abnormalities.[5]

What Induction Options Are There for Older Patients Who Are Less Fit?

- Less-fit patients (multiple comorbidities, poor PS, adverse risk factor as in Table 30.1) may receive low-intensity treatment (low-dose cytarabine, azacitadine, and decitabine), clinical trials, or best supportive care.
- Older (greater than 75 years) or unfit patients may benefit from azacitidine plus venetoclax with superior OS (as compared to patients treated with single-agent hypomethylating agent [HMA]). OS was 14.7 months in the azacitidine-venetoclax group versus 9.6 months in the single-agent group.[22]
- Venetoclax plus low-dose cytarabine (LDAC) demonstrated superior CR in older patients with newly diagnosed AML ineligible for intensive chemotherapy. CR was 48% versus 13% in LDAC plus venetoclax versus the placebo arm.
  - Six-month follow-up demonstrated superior CR and OS for LDAC plus venetoclax in these patients.[23]

What Targeted Therapies Do We Have for Older, Less-Fit Patients?

- *IDH* mutations are present in 20% of AML cases. These mutations reduce alpha-ketoglutarate transformation into 2-hydroxyglutarate, an oncometabolite that inhibits *TET* proteins (which mediates DNA methylation).
- Ivosidenib (an *IDH1* inhibitor) is approved as monotherapy for newly diagnosed and relapsed/refractory AML (Table 30.2).[24]

- ○ Overall response rate (ORR) was 54.5% (CR = 30.3) in newly diagnosed AML patients. The median OS (mOS) was 12.6 months.[25]
- ○ In relapsed/refractory AML, the CR was 21.6%, and mOS was 8.8 months.[26]
- Enasidenib (an *IDH2* inhibitor) is approved for relapsed/refractory *IDH2*- mutated AML.
  - ○ CR+CRi was 27.9%, with an ORR of 39.6%.[27]
  - ○ mOS was 11.3 months for newly diagnosed disease and 8.8 months in the relapsed/ refractory setting.[27,28]
  - ○ OS was 22.9 months in those achieving CR and 10.6 months in those with CRi.[27]
  - ○ Enasidenib is not FDA approved for upfront therapy; however, the National Comprehensive Cancer Network (NCCN) recommends for de novo disease based on promising Phase 1/2 data.

Clinical Course: Induction Therapy

The patient received induction therapy with venetoclax and azacitidine because of his poor fitness.

What Monitoring Needs to Be Done for This Regimen?

- The patient should receive prophylaxis for tumor lysis syndrome.
- Kidney function, lactate dehydrogenase, uric acid, electrolytes, and CBC should be monitored.

What Is Required for Follow-Up?

- A bone marrow aspirate and biopsy should be done on day 21 to 28.
- Older, less-fit patients receiving HMA plus venetoclax should continue treatment until unacceptable toxicity or disease progression.
- In older, fit AML patients who received CPX351 and achieved CR, 1 to 2 additional cycles of CPX351 on days 1 and 3 could be administered as post-remission therapy.

REVIEW QUESTIONS

1. A 54-year-old female was admitted with left-sided hand and leg weakness. Her complete white count (WBC) showed a white count of 120,000/μL and platelets of 136 K/μL. Peripheral blood flow cytometry detected a CD34 negative and CD33, CD13, and CD117 positive monoblasts. What is the most likely etiology of her neurological defect?
   A. Hyperviscosity
   B. Leukostasis
   C. Intraparenchymal bleeding
   D. Toxoplasmosis

2. What is the most likely intervention that would produce faster resolution of symptoms in the patient described in question 1?
   A. Intravenous (IV) cytarabine
   B. Aspirin and IV heparin
   C. Leukapheresis
   D. High dose Bactrim

3. Your intervention for the patient in question 1 was successful, leading to improvement in muscle strength. Her bone marrow confirmed acute monocytic leukemia. Just 72 hours later, her *FLT3 ITD* was reported as positive with allele fraction (AF) of 0.35%. Cytarabine intravenously (IV) continuous infusion at 100 mg/m² for 7 days plus idarubicin at 12 mg/m² IV for 3 days were initiated. What is the most important next step in the patient therapy associated with improvement in overall survival (OS)?
   A. Increase cytarabine to 200 mg/m²
   B. Add cardioprotective agent
   C. Add midostaurin
   D. Wait for full next-generation sequencing (NGS) report

4. Her full next-generation sequencing (NGS) report arrived showing *DNTM3A* (allele fraction [AF] = 0.48) and *NPM1* mutations (AF = 0.55%). Her measurable residual disease (MRD) day 30 was 4.5%. What is the estimated overall survival (OS) at 5 years for this patient?
   A. 3%
   B. 11%
   C. 32%
   D. 18%

5. A 58-year-old male with previous history of testicular cancer was admitted with pancytopenia. He reports that he received chemotherapy about 2 years ago. His bone marrow was 20% cellular with blast aggregates that represent more than 80% of cellularity. His flow cytometry showed CD34, HLRDR, CD33, and CD117 positive myeloblasts. Karyotype was complex including monosomy 5, 7p deletion and trisomy 8. Next-generation sequencing (NGS) showed *P53* R248Q at allele fraction (AF) of 0.6%. What is the intervention that most likely would induce complete remission?
   A. Magrolimab
   B. Azacitidine
   C. Cytarabine plus idarubicin intravenously (IV)
   D. Liposomal cytarabine plus daunorubicin

6. For the patient in question 5, the intervention resulted in complete response (CR). The Phase III, open-label study demonstrated an overall remission rate and survival of:
   A. 28% and 5.95 months
   B. 15% and 3 months
   C. 47.7% and 8.2 months
   D. 47.7% and 9.56 months

7. A 61-year-old male presented with shortness of breath and white blood cell (WBC) count of 90,000/µL. His chest x-ray was normal. However, his hemoglobin (Hgb) was 6 g/dL and platelets 23,000/µL. His bone marrow biopsy showed 60% CD34 negative, but CD33 and CD13 positive myeloblasts. His karyotype was 47, XY +8 in 20 metaphases analyzed. Next-generation sequencing (NGS) showed *FLT3 ITD* and *IDH1* positive mutations with allele fraction (AF) of 0.95% and 0.12%, respectively. Cytarabine continuous infusion for 7 days plus idarubicin intravenously (IV) for 3 days were administered. Midostaurin 50 mg orally every 12 hours was added from day 8 to 21 of his cycle. A remission marrow evaluation showed 4% residual blasts. A bone marrow transplant search failed to identify a suitable donor. The patient received two additional cycles of high-dose cytarabine. His consolidation was held given two episodes of *Klebsiella* multiresistant bacteremia. What is the intervention most likely to improve the patient's overall survival (OS) and event-free survival (EFS)?
   A. IV maintenance decitabine
   B. Oral midostaurin
   C. Oral IDH inhibitor
   D. Oral azacitidine

8. The patient described in question 7 maintained complete remission for 6 months after induction/consolidation. However, he relapsed with normal karyotype acute myeloid leukemia (AML). A matched unrelated donor was subsequently identified. Next-generation sequencing (NGS) failed to demonstrate actionable mutations. Which of the following is he most likely to receive as part of his therapy for relapsed AML?
   A. Oral hypomethylating agents
   B. Intravenous (IV) hypomethylating agents plus IDH1 inhibitor
   C. Intermediate-dose cytarabine 1 to 1.5 g/m², 4 to 6 doses plus midostaurin
   D. Intermediate-dose cytarabine 1 to 2 g/m², 4 to 6 doses for 2 cycles

9. A 35-year-old female was admitted with diffuse bruising. Her complete blood count (CBC) showed a white blood cell (WBC) count of 6,000/µL. Hypogranular promyelocytic forms associated with Auer rods were observed in peripheral smear. Fluorescent in situ hybridization (FISH) progressive multifocal leukoencephalopathy/retinoic acid receptor alpha (*PML-RARα*) fusion was positive. All-trans retinoic acid (ATRA) plus arsenic trioxide (ATO) were administered. On day 3 of therapy, her WBC was 36,000/µL. Hydroxyurea at 1000 mg orally twice daily and intravenous (IV) dexamethasone were added. Nursing staff reports that her weight increased by 6 kg. Her next-generation sequencing (NGS) showed *FLT3 ITD* with allele frequency of 0.35%. What is the most likely next intervention?
   A. Continue ATRA plus ATO induction
   B. Continue ATRA + ATO + midostaurin
   C. Add anthracycline
   D. Add cytarabine plus anthracycline

10. In the acute promyelocytic leukemia (APL) patient from question 9, her bone marrow day 30 showed a blast count of 15%. Progressive multifocal leukoencephalopathy/retinoic acid receptor alpha (*PML-RARα*) reverse transcription polymerase chain reaction (RT-PCR) was 0.9%. What is the most likely intervention needed at this time?
    A. Proceed with low-risk APL maintenance
    B. Transition to high-risk APL maintenance
    C. Repeat 1 additional cycle of induction
    D. Add midostaurin to APL maintenance

ANSWERS AND RATIONALES

1. **B. Leukostasis.** Leukostasis is a life-threatening condition associated with intravascular blast aggregation resulting in organ failure. FAB M5 leukemias harboring *NPM1* and *FLT3 ITD* mutations commonly present with the complication. Acute myeloid leukemia (AML) patients who have developed severe thrombocytopenia and disseminated intravascular coagulation (DIC) are at risk for central nervous system (CNS) bleed. Hyperviscosity is frequently observed among multiple myeloma and Waldenstrom macroglobulinemia patients.

2. **A. Intravenous (IV) cytarabine.** A 100- to 200-mg continuous infusion is the preferred regimen for acute myeloid leukemia (AML) patients with leukostasis and hyperleukocytosis. Controlled studies have not demonstrated superior efficacy for leukapheresis over cytarabine. Leukapheresis should be avoided in acute promyelocytic leukemia (APL) patients given the high risk for hemorrhagic complications in the context of disseminated intravascular coagulation (DIC). High-dose Bactrim is administered in immunocompromised patients with evidence of central nervous system (CNS) toxoplasmosis.

3. **C. Add midostaurin.** Midostaurin is a first-generation tyrosine kinase inhibitor (TKI) that was approved by the U.S. Food and Drug Administration (FDA) in 2017 for the treatment of *FLT3*-mutated acute myeloid leukemia (AML). RATIFY trial demonstrated superior event-free survival (EFS) and overall survival (OS) in *FLT3*-mutated AML patients. In this patient, there is no need to wait for complete NGS report since the FLT3 inhibitor should be promptly administered in combination with intense induction. Cytarabine IV at 200 mg/m² is not superior to 100 mg/m² when administered for AML induction.

4. **D. 18%.** Triple positive acute myeloid leukemia (AML; *FLT3 ITD, NPM1,* and *DNMT3A*) is associated with an inferior outcome even after allogeneic stem cell transplantation (allo-SCT). In *NPM1/FLT3* high-risk patients, a lower complete response (CR) rate (59% vs. 78%, *P* = 0.01) was observed as compared with patients with wildtype *DNMT3A*.

5. **D. Liposomal cytarabine plus daunorubicin.** This is currently U.S. Food and Drug Administration (FDA) approved for myelodysplastic syndrome/chronic myelomonocytic leukemia (MDS/CMML)-derived and therapy-related acute myeloid leukemia (AML). Conventional 7+3 induction is not recommended for patients harboring *P53* mutations given the high induction failure risk. Magrolimab is an anti CD47 monoclonal antibody that enhances prophagocytic efficiency against malignant hemopoietic cells. Recent studies have demonstrated superior efficacy in *P53* MDS/AML; however, it is not currently approved by the FDA.

6. **D. 47.7% and 9.56 months.** Superior overall remission rate was demonstrated for liposomal cytarabine plus daunorubicin against "7+3" in acute myeloid leukemia (AML) patients. The study enrolled AML patients between the ages of 60 to 75 years with newly diagnosed therapy-related AML, AML arising from myelodysplastic syndrome (MDS) or chronic myelomonocytic leukemia (CMML), or de novo AML with MDS-related chromosomic abnormalities.

7. **D. Oral azacitidine.** This is an attractive option for patients older than 55 years in first remission who are not candidates for allogeneic stem cell transplantation (allo-SCT). The QUAZAR AML-001 trial demonstrated superior OS and relapse-free survival (RFS) for patients receiving the drug versus placebo. Oral *IDH1* inhibitor is currently approved for de novo and relapsed/refractory acute myeloid leukemia (AML) older than 60 years.

8. **D. Intermediate-dose cytarabine 1 to 2 g/m², 4 to 6 doses for 2 cycles.** High-dose Ara-C (HiDAC) is recommended for induction in AML patients with short complete response (CR) duration by the National Comprehensive Cancer Network (NCCN). HiDAC is as effective as HiDAC plus additional chemotherapy in this setting. FLT3 inhibitor is not needed since the FLT3 is wildtype. The patient should proceed with allogeneic transplantation after achieving measurable residual disease (MRD).

9. **A. Continue ATRA plus ATO induction.** Differentiation syndrome (DS) is a frequent complication observed in acute promyelocytic leukemia (APL) patients receiving differentiating therapy with ATRA and ATO. The condition is associated with a rapid increase in WBC. Respiratory and renal failure could develop if not quickly treated. Daily weight should be recorded since unexplained gain may signal DS. Treatment is directed to control WBC with hydroxyurea and initiation of prophylactic dexamethasone.

10. **A. Proceed with low-risk APL maintenance.** Low-risk APL patients who have completed all-trans retinoic acid (ATRA) plus arsenic trioxide (ATO) induction without evidence of complete response (CR) at day 30, should have bone marrow repeated 1 week after. The presence of cytogenetic or molecular markers would not influence the prognosis and therapeutic decisions. There is no need to repeat *PML-RARα* RT-PCR at the end of APL induction.

REFERENCES

1. National Cancer Institute. SEER cancer stat facts: leukemia—acute myeloid leukemia (AML). https://seer.cancer.gov/statfacts/html/amyl.html
2. Döhner H, Estey E, Grimwade D, et al. Diagnosis and management of AML in adults: 2017 ELN recommendations from an international expert panel. *Blood.* 2017;129(4):424–447. doi:10.1182/blood-2016-08-733196
3. Tallman MS, Andersen JW, Schiffer CA, et al. All-trans-retinoic acid in acute promyelocytic leukemia. *N Engl J Med.* 1997;337:1021–1028. doi:10.1056/NEJM199710093371501
4. Fenaux P, Chastang C, Chevret S, et al. A randomized comparison of all transretinoic acid (ATRA) followed by chemotherapy and ATRA plus chemotherapy and the role of maintenance therapy in newly diagnosed acute promyelocytic leukemia. *Blood.* 1999;94(4):1192–1200. doi:10.1182/blood.V94.4.1192
5. Gianni M, Koken MHM, Chelbi-Alix MK, et al. Combined arsenic and retinoic acid treatment enhances differentiation and apoptosis in arsenic-resistant NB4 cells. *Blood.* 1998;91(11):4300–4310. doi:10.1182/blood.V91.11.4300
6. Platzbecker U, Avvisati G, Cicconi L, et al. Improved outcomes with retinoic acid and arsenic trioxide compared with retinoic acid and chemotherapy in non-high-risk acute promyelocytic leukemia: final results of the randomized Italian-German APL0406 trial. *J Clin Oncol.* 2017;35(6):605–612. doi:10.1200/JCO.2016.67.1982
7. Cicconi L, Platzbecker U, Avvisati G, et al. Long-term results of all-trans retinoic acid and arsenic trioxide in non-high-risk acute promyelocytic leukemia: update of the APL0406 Italian-German randomized trial. *Leukemia.* 2020;34(3):914–918. doi:10.1038/s41375-019-0589-3
8. Iland HJ, Bradstock K, Supple SG, et al. All-trans-retinoic acid, idarubicin, and IV arsenic trioxide as initial therapy in acute promyelocytic leukemia (APML4). *Blood.* 2012;120(8):1570–1580. doi:10.1182/blood-2012-02-410746
9. Lancet JE, Moseley AB, Coutre SE, et al. A phase 2 study of ATRA, arsenic trioxide, and gemtuzumab ozogamicin in patients with high-risk APL (SWOG 0535). *Blood Adv.* 2020;4(8):1683–1689. doi:10.1182/bloodadvances.2019001278
10. Burnett AK, Russell NH, Hills RK, et al. Arsenic trioxide and all-trans retinoic acid treatment for acute promyelocytic leukaemia in all risk groups (AML17): results of a randomised, controlled, phase 3 trial. *Lancet Oncol.* 2015;16(13):1295–1305. doi:10.1016/S1470-2045(15)00193-X
11. Sanz MA, Montesinos P, Rayón C, et al. Risk-adapted treatment of acute promyelocytic leukemia based on all-trans retinoic acid and anthracycline with addition of cytarabine in consolidation therapy for high-risk patients: further improvements in treatment outcome. *Blood.* 2010;115(25):5137–5146. doi:10.1182/blood-2010-01-266007
12. Avvisati G, Lo-Coco F, Paoloni FP, et al. AIDA 0493 protocol for newly diagnosed acute promyelocytic leukemia: very long-term results and role of maintenance. *Blood.* 2011;117(18):4716–4725. doi:10.1182/blood-2010-08-302950

13. Raffoux E, Rousselot P, Poupon J, et al. Combined treatment with arsenic trioxide and all-trans-retinoic acid in patients with relapsed acute promyelocytic leukemia. *J Clin Oncol.* 2003;21(12):2326–2334. doi:10.1200/JCO.2003.01.149

14. Fernandez HF, Sun Z, Yao X, et al. Anthracycline dose intensification in acute myeloid leukemia. *N Engl J Med.* 2009;361(13):1249–1259. doi:10.1056/NEJMoa0904544

15. Lambert J, Pautas C, Terré C, et al. Gemtuzumab ozogamicin for *de novo* acute myeloid leukemia: final efficacy and safety updates from the open-label, phase III ALFA-0701 trial. *Haematologica.* 2019;104(1):113–119. doi:10.3324/haematol.2018.188888

16. Abdul Halim NA, Wong GC, Aloysius HY, Hwang WY, Linn YC, Lao Z. High dose cytarabine is superior to intermediate dose cytarabine as post-remission therapy for younger patients with favorable risk acute myeloid leukemia. *Blood.* 2016;128(22):4032. doi:10.1182/blood.V128.22.4032.4032

17. Koreth J, Schlenk R, Kopecky KJ, et al. Allogeneic stem cell transplantation for acute myeloid leukemia in first complete remission: systematic review and meta-analysis of prospective clinical trials. *JAMA.* 2009;301(22):2349–2361. doi:10.1001/jama.2009.813

18. Warlick ED, Peffault de Latour R, Shanley R, et al. Allogeneic hematopoietic cell transplantation outcomes in acute myeloid leukemia: similar outcomes regardless of donor type. *Biol Blood Marrow Transplant.* 2015;21(2):357–363. doi:10.1016/j.bbmt.2014.10.030

19. Slovak ML, Kopecky KJ, Cassileth PA, et al. Karyotypic analysis predicts outcome of preremission and post-remission therapy in adult acute myeloid leukemia: a Southwest Oncology Group/Eastern Cooperative Oncology Group study. *Blood.* 2000;96(13):4075–4083. doi:10.1182/blood.V96.13.4075

20. Wei AH, Döhner H, Pocock C, et al. Oral azacitidine maintenance therapy for acute myeloid leukemia in first remission. *N Engl J Med.* 2020;383(26):2526–2537. doi:10.1056/NEJMoa2004444

21. Burchert A, Bug G, Fritz LV., et al. Sorafenib maintenance after allogeneic hematopoietic stem cell transplantation for acute myeloid leukemia with FLT3-internal tandem duplication mutation (SORMAIN). *J Clin Oncol.* 2020;38(26):2993–3002. doi:10.1200/JCO.19.03345

22. DiNardo CD, Jonas BA, Pullarkat V, et al. Azacitidine and venetoclax in previously untreated acute myeloid leukemia. *New Eng J of Med.* 2020;383(7):617–629. doi:10.1056/NEJMoa2012971

23. Wei AH, Panayiotidis P, Montesinos P, et al. 6-month follow-up of VIALE-C demonstrates improved and durable efficacy in patients with untreated AML ineligible for intensive chemotherapy (141/150). *Blood Cancer J.* 2021;11(10):163. doi:10.1038/s41408-021-00555-8

24. Issa GC, DiNardo CD. Acute myeloid leukemia with IDH1 and IDH2 mutations: 2021 treatment algorithm. *Blood Cancer J.* 2021;11(6):107. doi:10.1038/s41408-021-00497-1

25. Roboz GJ, DiNardo CD, Stein EM, et al. Ivosidenib induces deep durable remissions in patients with newly diagnosed IDH1-mutant acute myeloid leukemia. *Blood.* 2020;135(7):463–471. doi:10.1182/blood.2019002140

26. DiNardo CD, Stein EM, de Botton S, et al. Durable remissions with ivosidenib in *IDH1*-mutated relapsed or refractory AML. *New Eng J of Med.* 2018;378(25):2386–2398. doi:10.1056/NEJMoa1716984

27. Stein EM, DiNardo CD, Fathi AT, et al. Molecular remission and response patterns in patients with mutant-IDH2 acute myeloid leukemia treated with enasidenib. *Blood.* 2019;133(7):676–687. doi:10.1182/blood-2018-08-869008

28. Pollyea DA, Tallman MS, de Botton S, et al. Enasidenib, an inhibitor of mutant IDH2 proteins, induces durable remissions in older patients with newly diagnosed acute myeloid leukemia. *Leukemia.* 2019;33(11):2575–2584. doi:10.1038/s41375-019-0472-2

CHAPTER 31

Chronic Myeloid Leukemia

Tamer Othman and Brian A. Jonas

INTRODUCTION

Chronic myeloid leukemia (CML) is a myeloproliferative neoplasm of hematopoietic stem cells that is marked in over 90% of cases by the presence of the Philadelphia (Ph) chromosome.[1] It encompasses 15% of adult leukemias and 0.5% of all cancers.[2] The incidence of CML is 1.9 per 100,000 people; it is estimated that 9110 new cases will be diagnosed in 2021, and that 1220 will die from the disease. CML is more commonly seen in older adults, with a median age of diagnosis of 65 years. It is diagnosed in the chronic phase (CP) in greater than 80% of cases and typically presents with fatigue, anorexia, and weight loss; however, about 40% are asymptomatic.[3]

The Ph chromosome, the hallmark of CML, results from a reciprocal translocation between the long arms of chromosomes 9 and 22, commonly referred to as t(9;22)(q34;q11), ultimately giving rise to the BCR-ABL1 oncoprotein.[1] The p210 isoform is typically encountered with CML, but less commonly the p190 or p230 isoforms are observed.[4] BCR-ABL1 serves as a constitutively active tyrosine kinase that drives leukemogenesis by promoting growth and replication via downstream signaling and disrupting the apoptotic pathway.[1] In the absence of treatment, CML will eventually progress to more aggressive variants, namely accelerated phase (AP) and blast phase (BP) CML, in ~3 to 5 years.[5]

Prior to the advent of BCR-ABL1 tyrosine kinase inhibitors (TKIs), which are now considered to be the cornerstone of CML management,[6] drug therapy was limited to hydroxyurea, busulfan, and interferon-alfa,[7] the latter of which carried with it an array of toxicities. Allogeneic hematopoietic stem cell transplantation (allo-HSCT), while curative, is only an option for young patients with an acceptable performance status (PS), organ function, and an appropriate donor given the morbidity and mortality associated with this procedure.[6] In the TKI era, however, management can be tailored to a patient's disease profile, comorbidities, treatment history, and goals of care to provide effective and tolerable therapy.[8] As a result, the life expectancy of a patient with chronic phase CML (CP-CML) harboring the Ph chromosome now approaches that of age-matched individuals in the Western population.[9]

CASE SUMMARIES

Case 31.1: Newly Diagnosed Chronic Myeloid Leukemia

A 38-year-old female with no past medical history (PMH) presents to her primary care provider (PCP) for left upper quadrant abdominal pain over the past 4 months. She endorses fatigue but denies fevers, night sweats, unintentional weight loss, nausea, vomiting, bruising, or bleeding. Physical exam was notable for left upper quadrant pain with palpation and a palpable spleen 12 cm below the costal margin. An ultrasound (US) performed in clinic showed marked splenomegaly with the spleen measuring 29.2 × 10.6 cm. Routine complete blood count (CBC) revealed a white blood cell (WBC) count of 363 × 10⁹, a hemoglobin (Hgb) of 8.5 g/dL, and a platelet count of 477 × 10⁹. Cell differential showed an elevation of absolute neutrophils, lymphocytes, eosinophils (6%), basophils (2%), metamyelocytes, myelocytes, and promyelocytes. The differential also detected 3% blasts. The patient was subsequently sent to the ED.

How Is a Diagnosis Established?

- Bone marrow aspirate and core biopsy are used to evaluate morphology and to calculate blast percentage to rule out occult accelerated phase CML (AP-CML) and blast phase CML (BP-CML; Table 31.1).
- Cytogenetics are used to confirm the presence of the Ph chromosome, which is defined by t(9;22)(q34;q11). This assay may also reveal additional chromosomal abnormalities (ACA). The diagnosis of typical CML requires documentation of the Ph chromosome by cytogenetics, or its associated oncoprotein, BCR-ABL1, by fluorescence in situ hybridization (FISH) or by polymerase chain reaction (PCR) in the presence of persistent and otherwise unexplained leukocytosis and/or thrombocytosis.[10]

Patient's Diagnosis

- Bone marrow biopsy morphology shows near 100% cellularity consisting primarily of myeloid precursors at various stages of maturation as well as increased basophils (10%) and eosinophils (15.5%), and dysplastic megakaryocytes suggestive of CML. Blast percentage is 0.5%.
- Cytogenetics show 46,XX,t(9;22)(q34.1;q11.2).

What Further Molecular or Genomic Testing Is Required?

- Quantitative reverse transcriptase polymerase chain reaction (qPCR) should be performed to confirm the presence of and quantify the BCR-ABL1 mRNA transcript.

Patient's Molecular and Genomic Testing

- qPCR quantifies the p210 isoform of BCR-ABL at 81.5693% on the international scale (IS).

How Is This Tumor Staged?

- CML is classified into three phases: CP, AP, and BP. While different models exist, AP-CML in clinical trials is most commonly defined by the Modified MD Anderson Cancer Center (MDACC) Criteria, while BP-CML is defined by the International Bone Marrow Transplant Registry (IBMTR; Table 31.1).[11,12]
- The Sokal and Hasford (Euro) scoring systems have been more commonly used in clinical trials for prognostication. The former stratifies patients into three risk groups based on age, spleen size, platelet count, and peripheral blood blast percentage while the latter incorporates these four factors in addition to the eosinophils and basophils in the peripheral blood.[13,14] The third scheme is the European Treatment and Outcome study long-term survival (ELTS) score, which uses the same variables as the Sokal score to predict CML-related death (Table 31.1).[15]

Table 31.1 Criteria for AP- and BP-CML

Modified MDACC Criteria for AP (Requires Only One of the Following)

Peripheral blood myeloblasts 15%–30%

Peripheral blood myeloblasts plus promyelocytes ≥20%

Peripheral blood basophils ≥20%

Platelets ≤100 × 10^9 not related to treatment

Clonal cytogenetic evolution[†]

IBMTR Criteria for BP (Requires Only One of the Following)

≥30% blasts in the blood, marrow, or both

Extramedullary involvement of blasts

[†]Refers to the development of both major route additional chromosomal abnormalities (ACAs; for example, a second Ph chromosome, trisomy 8, isochromosome 17q, +der[22]) and/or ACAs in Ph cells during treatment in the MDACC model.

AP-CML, accelerated phase-chronic myeloid leukemia; BP-CML, blast phase-chronic myeloid leukemia; IBMTR, International Bone Marrow Transplant Registry; MDACC, MD Anderson Cancer Center.

Patient's Chronic Myeloid Leukemia Phase and Risk-stratification
- *CP-CML, and low risk by all three scoring systems*

What Are Appropriate Treatment Options?

- TKIs are the standard of care for CP-CML. There are four approved TKIs in the first-line setting: the first-generation TKI, imatinib, and the second-generation TKIs, dasatinib, nilotinib, and bosutinib.
- Allo-HSCT is not recommended as frontline treatment for CP-CML.
- Long-term clinical trial data have demonstrated that all TKIs extend overall survival (OS) close to that of age-matched controls, and that second-generation TKIs typically lead to faster cytogenetic and molecular responses, as well as deeper molecular responses, with less progression to AP/BP compared to imatinib, but without a significant difference in long-term survival.[16–19]
- The selection of frontline TKI is based on the patient's age, comorbidities, ability to tolerate treatment, and risk-stratification, with second-generation TKIs being favored for intermediate/high-risk disease, drug interactions, and the patient's preference.

Recommended Treatment Plan for This Patient
- *Any of the four TKIs are appropriate in this patient given her lack of comorbidities, young age, and low-risk disease. She is started on dasatinib 100 mg daily.*

What Are the Toxicities Associated With Tyrosine Kinase Inhibitor Therapy?

- The TKIs are generally well-tolerated, and each has its own toxicity profile that should be considered when determining first-line TKI treatment.
- Imatinib can limit health-related quality of life, and can be associated with musculoskeletal pain and muscle cramps.[20]
- Dasatinib can cause pleural effusions and pulmonary hypertension, and thus, another TKI is preferred in patients with underlying lung disease or with preexisting conditions, making them susceptible to pleural effusion development.[21,22]

- Nilotinib can prolong the QT interval, is associated with increased peripheral arterial occlusive disease, and can induce diabetes through impaired glucose metabolism.[23-25] It may also lead to sudden cardiac death. Thus, nilotinib should be avoided in patients with a history of arrhythmias, coronary and arterial disease, and/or those on a QT prolonging medication.[26,27]
- Bosutinib can cause nausea, diarrhea, and transaminitis.[28]
- All TKIs can cause cytopenias requiring dose modifications, diarrhea, fluid retention, elevated liver enzymes, and rash.[29-31]

What Are Other Treatment Considerations?

Monitoring Response

- Response to TKI therapy is measured by hematologic, cytogenetic, and molecular response.
- Criteria for complete hematologic response (CHR)[32] is as follows:
  - WBC count within normal limits
  - Absolute neutrophil count at least $1 \times 10^9/L$
  - Platelet count 100 to $450 \times 10^9/L$
  - No immature granulocytes and basophils less than 2%
  - No extramedullary involvement (such as hepatomegaly or splenomegaly)
- CBC with cell differential should be obtained every 2 weeks until CHR is attained.
- Cytogenetic response is assessed via bone marrow cytogenetic analysis, and the percentage of Ph+ metaphases are documented. A complete cytogenetic response (CCyR) is defined as 0% Ph+ metaphases.
- Advances in monitoring techniques have allowed for less invasive monitoring of response to TKI, such that cytogenetic analyses on the bone marrow are rarely performed outside of a clinical trial, unless it becomes otherwise indicated (concern for treatment failure, progression to AP/BP, or a concurrent myelosuppressive process). In fact, a BCR-ABL1 level of 1% or less on the IS is equivalent to a CCyR.[33]
- qPCR on the peripheral blood to quantify BCR-ABL1 transcripts on the IS is a more convenient method to assess response and guide therapy, and should be obtained at least every 3 months.
- Early molecular response (EMR), defined as BCR-ABL1 of 10% or less at 3 and 6 months, has become a favorable prognosticator for long-term progression-free survival (PFS).[34,35]
- Major molecular response (MMR), defined as BCR-ABL1 of 0.1% or less, predicts a durable long-term cytogenetic response and decreases the risk of disease progression.[36-43]
- The criteria for a deep molecular response (DMR) varies based on the sensitivity of the qPCR assay: MR4.0 is defined as BCR-ABL1 of 0.01% or less while MR4.5 is BCR-ABL1 of 0.0032% or less on the IS.
- Table 31.2 summarizes treatment milestones and a response-adaptive approach to managing CML.

Patient's Response

- *The patient achieves CHR and EMR at 3 months, and MR4.5 at 1 year.*
- *She tolerates dasatinib well for 3.5 years without ever losing MR4.5.*

Long-Term Management and Monitoring

- Organizations such as the National Comprehensive Cancer Network (NCCN) and European LeukemiaNet (ELN) have provided guidelines on discontinuing TKI therapy after certain conditions have been met based on the Stop Imatinib (STIM) and EURO-SKI trials.[44,45]

Table 31.2 Treatment Milestones

Time After Starting Treatment	Response	Interpretation	Recommendations
3 months	– No CHR – Ph+ metaphases >95%	TKI-resistant	– Evaluate compliance and drug interactions – Switch TKI and evaluate for allo-HSCT – Consider bone marrow biopsy with cytogenetic response evaluation and ABL1 kinase domain mutational analysis
	– BCR-ABL1 >10% – Ph+ metaphases 36%–95%	Possibly TKI-resistant	– Evaluate compliance and drug interactions – Consider bone marrow biopsy with cytogenetic response evaluation and ABL1 kinase domain mutational analysis – Continue non-imatinib TKI, or increase dose if imatinib, or switch to alternate TKI – Consider evaluation for allo-HSCT
	– BCR-ABL1 <10% – Ph+ metaphases ≤35%	TKI-sensitive	– Continue TKI
6 months	– BCR-ABL1 >10%	TKI-resistant	– Evaluate compliance and drug interactions – Switch TKI and evaluate for allo-HSCT – Consider bone marrow biopsy with cytogenetic response evaluation and ABL1 kinase domain mutational analysis
	– BCR-ABL1 <10%	TKI-sensitive	– Continue TKI
12 months	– BCR-ABL1 >10%	TKI-resistant	– Evaluate compliance and drug interactions – Switch TKI and evaluate for allo-HSCT – Bone marrow biopsy with cytogenetic response evaluation and ABL1 kinase domain mutational analysis
	– BCR-ABL1 1%–10%	Possibly TKI-resistant	– Evaluate compliance and drug interactions – Consider bone marrow biopsy with cytogenetic response evaluation and ABL1 kinase domain mutational analysis – Continue non-imatinib TKI, or increase dose if imatinib, or switch to alternate TKI – Consider evaluation for allo-HSCT
	– BCR-ABL1 <1%	TKI-sensitive	– Continue TKI

allo-HSCT, allogeneic hematopoietic stem cell transplantation; CHR, complete hematologic response; Ph, Philadelphia; TKI, tyrosine kinase inhibitor.

Source: Data from Hochhaus A, Baccarani M, Silver RT, et al. European LeukemiaNet 2020 recommendations for treating chronic myeloid leukemia. *Leuk.* 2020;34(4):966–984. doi:10.1038/s41375-020-0776-2; National Comprehensive Cancer Network. Chronic myeloid leukemia (Version 3.2022). https://www.nccn.org/professionals/physician_gls/pdf/cml.pdf

- The NCCN criteria[46] are:
  - Age 18 years or older
  - CP-CML and no history of AP/BP
  - On an approved TKI therapy for a minimum of 3 years
  - Prior quantifiable BCR-ABL1 transcript
  - Stable molecular response (MR4 for 2 years and documented on four or more assays that were performed at least 3 months apart)
  - Access to a reliable qPCR assay with a minimum sensitivity to detect MR4.5 and a resulting turnaround time within 2 weeks
  - Monthly BCR-ABL1 monitoring for the first 6 months following discontinuation, then bimonthly during months 7 to 12, and every 3 months indefinitely thereafter for patients who remain in MMR
  - TKI resumption within 4 weeks of losing MMR with monthly BCR-ABL1 monitoring until re-establishing MMR, then every 3 months thereafter indefinitely for those restarting TKI therapy after losing MMR. For those unable to achieve MMR after 3 months of restarting a TKI, ABL1 kinase domain mutation testing should be performed, and monthly BCR-ABL1 monitoring should be continued for another 6 months
- The ELN 2020 criteria[9] are:
  - Mandatory:
    - CML in first CP only
    - Motivated patient with structured communication
    - Access to high-quality qPCR using the IS with rapid turn-around of PCR test results
    - Monthly BCR-ABL1 monitoring for the first 6 months, every 2 months for months 6 to 12, and every 3 months indefinitely thereafter
  - Minimal (stop allowed):
    - First-line therapy or second-line if intolerance was the only reason for changing TKI
    - Typical e13a2 or e14a2 BCR–ABL1 transcripts
    - TKI therapy duration greater than 5 years (greater than 4 years for a second-generation TKI)
    - MR4 or better duration greater than 2 years
    - No prior treatment failure
  - Optimal (stop recommended for consideration):
    - TKI therapy duration greater than 5 years
    - MR4 duration greater than 3 years or MR4.5 duration greater than 2 years
- Around 80% of CML recurrence takes place in the first 6 to 8 months after discontinuing TKI therapy.
- Some patients who discontinue their TKI may experience a polymyalgia-like syndrome that is generally self-limiting. However, some patients may require nonsteroidal anti-inflammatory drugs (NSAIDs) or corticosteroids.

The Patient's Outcome
- *She discontinues dasatinib and remains in MR4.5 2 years out.*

Case 31.2: Chronic Myeloid Leukemia With a *T315I* Mutation

A 57-year-old male with a PMH of hypertension presents to his family practitioner for 5 months of fatigue and night sweats. Physical exam is unremarkable. CBC reveals a WBC of 33.4 × 10⁹/L with an absolute neutrophilia of 23.9 × 10⁹/L, eosinophilia of 3.3 × 10⁹/L, and a basophilia of 1.3 × 10⁹/L on cell differential. No blasts are noted. Hgb is 13.4 g/dL and platelets are 1,135 10⁹/L. A bone marrow biopsy is performed which shows CP-CML. Cytogenetic analysis reveals 61%

Ph+ metaphases, and BCR-ABL1 by qPCR is 21.3515%. The patient is started on bosutinib 400 mg once daily. At 3 months, he achieves CHR and reports increased energy, but BCR-ABL1 level on peripheral blood is 11.0176%. He reports compliance with the TKI and is not on any other medications aside from amlodipine. At 6 months, BCR-ABL1 increases to 23.8667%.

What Further Genomic or Molecular Testing Is Required?

- At 3 months, the patient failed to meet the treatment milestone of a BCR-ABL1 less than 10% (see Table 31.2). At this juncture, options include continuing a second-generation TKI at the same dose as was done with this patient given the reduction in BCR-ABL1 from baseline and near EMR, or to switch to an alternate TKI.
- At 6 months, however, a change in TKI is necessary as he failed to reach the treatment milestone and his BCR-ABL1 level rose, consistent with TKI resistance.
- Referral to allo-HSCT and repeat bone marrow biopsy with aspirate for kinase domain mutational analysis is required at this point as well.

Patient's Diagnosis
- *Bone marrow biopsy shows 75% Ph+ metaphases and a T315I mutation.*
- *4% blasts are detected but is overall consistent with CP-CML.*

What Are Appropriate Treatment Options?

- Kinase domain mutations are a mechanism of TKI resistance and should be suspected when a patient fails to meet treatment milestones.
- Choice of second-line TKI depends on the mutation present, as only certain TKIs have activity against specific mutations (Table 31.3).[9,44]
- Ponatinib, a third-generation TKI, is the only TKI with activity against *T315I* mutations.[9]
- Very recently, the U.S. Food and Drug Administration (FDA) approved asciminib, the first-in-class STAMP (Specifically Targeting the ABL Myristoyl Pocket) inhibitor, for adults with CP-CML with a *T315I* mutation or CP-CML who have previously failed 2 or more TKIs (Table 31.3).[47]

Recommended Treatment Plan for This Patient
- *The patient is started on ponatinib 45 mg once daily and achieves an MMR at 3 months. Ponatinib is then reduced to 15 mg once daily.*

Table 31.3 Tyrosine Kinase Inhibitor Mechanisms of Resistance

TKI	Mutations Conferring Resistance to TKI
Bosutinib	*F317L, G250E, T315I, V299L*
Dasatinib	*F317L/V/I/C, T315I/A, V299L*
Nilotinib	*E255K/V, F359V/C/I, T315I, Y253H*
Ponatinib	None

TKI, tyrosine kinase inhibitor.

Source: Hochhaus A, Baccarani M, Silver RT, et al. European LeukemiaNet 2020 recommendations for treating chronic myeloid leukemia. *Leuk.* 2020;34(4):966–984. doi:10.1038/s41375-020-0776-2; National Comprehensive Cancer Network. Chronic myeloid leukemia (Version 3.2022). https://www.nccn.org/professionals/physician_gls/pdf/cml.pdf

What Are the Toxicities Associated With Ponatinib?

- As with other TKIs, ponatinib can induce cytopenias requiring dose modifications, rash, elevated liver enzymes, and fluid overload.[48]
- Arterial and venous thromboembolic events can occur with ponatinib, which can lead to serious vascular events like cerebral vascular accidents and myocardial infarctions.
- Pancreatitis has also been reported with ponatinib.

What Are Other Treatment Considerations?

- It is recommended that patients be screened for cardiovascular disease risk factors prior to starting ponatinib. A cardiology consult is preferrable if any risk factors are present prior to ponatinib initiation. Ocular toxicity, such as blindness or blurry vision, have been reported; thus, patients should undergo a comprehensive ophthalmologic exam at baseline and throughout treatment.[49]
- Given the toxicities associated with ponatinib, a dose reduction from 45 mg once daily to 15 mg once daily is recommended once a BCR-ABL1 of 1% or less has been reached, as was done with this patient.[44]
- Liver enzymes, CBC, and signs of heart failure and vaso-occlusion should be monitored while on therapy with ponatinib.
- Given his history of treatment failure, the patient would not be a candidate for discontinuing his TKI.

The Patient's Outcome

- *The patient achieves MR4.5 at 9 months and remains in MR4.5 while on ponatinib 15 mg once daily 2 years from his TKI switch.*

Case 31.3: Chronic Myeloid Leukemia With Lymphoid Blast Crisis

A 41-year-old male without any PMH was found to have a WBC of 227.4 × 10⁹/L with 29% myelocytes, 1% eosinophils, 0% basophils, and 2% blasts on the cell differential; an Hgb of 7.8 g/dL; and a platelet count of 234 × 10⁹/L after presenting with severe weakness and near syncope. A bone marrow biopsy and aspirate is performed, and is consistent with CP-CML. Cytogenetic analysis reveals 100% Ph+ metaphases and BCR-ABL quantification was 58.4913% by PCR. He was started on imatinib 400 mg once daily and achieved MMR by 3 months and MR4.5 by 12 months. At 15 months, BCR-ABL1 increased to 7.0421%. Kinase domain mutational analysis revealed an F317L mutation, and he was switched to nilotinib 300 mg twice daily. Subsequent BCR-ABL1 by PCR was 0.663% at 3 months, but increased to 18.0035% at 6 months. CBC shows a WBC of 79.0 × 10⁹/L with 24% blasts detected on the cell differential.

How Is a Diagnosis Established?

- With 24% blasts in the peripheral blood, the patient meets the criteria for AP, but a bone marrow biopsy with aspirate should be performed to distinguish between AP and BP as management differs between.

Patient's Diagnosis

- *The patient undergoes a bone marrow biopsy with aspirate which reveals a hypercellular marrow with 64% B-lymphoblasts, consistent with CML in lymphoid blast crisis (CML-LBC).*

- Cytogenetics reveal 65% Ph+ metaphases and +der(22), and qPCR quantifies BCR-ABL1 at 50.3150%.
- Kinase domain mutational analysis reveals a Y253H mutation.

What Are Appropriate Treatment Options?

- The preferred treatment for AP-CML is a second-generation TKI at an increased dose compared to CP-CML (for example, bosutinib 500 mg once daily, dasatinib 140 mg once daily, or nilotinib 400 mg twice daily) or a third-generation TKI. Imatinib at an increased dose of 600 mg once daily is acceptable, however.
- BP-CML is treated with induction chemotherapy for those fit for such treatment in combination with a TKI at the same increased dose as for AP-CML followed by consolidative allo-HSCT, whether a patient presents in BP or progresses to BP while on TKI therapy.
- The type of chemotherapy depends on the cell lineage of the proliferating blasts—acute myeloid leukemia (AML)-based chemotherapy is recommended for CML in myeloid blast crisis (CML-MBC) while acute lymphoblastic leukemia (ALL)-based chemotherapy is recommended for CML-LBC.
- Other instances where allo-HSCT is acceptable for managing CML include progression to AP while on TKI therapy, AP-CML failing to reach treatment milestones, and patients with CML who are resistant to or intolerant to multiple/all TKIs.
- Survival is superior for patients who proceed to allo-HSCT in second CP-CML versus AP/BP-CML.[50–52]
- In general, patients with CP-CML who progress to AP/BP while on TKI therapy have worse outcomes than those who present with de novo AP/BP-CML.
- Omacetaxine, an alkaloid that inhibits protein synthesis at the level of the ribosome, is also a treatment option for those who progress to AP-CML while on TKI therapy.[53]
- CML-LBC, like ALL, has been reported to involve the central nervous system (CNS); thus, cerebrospinal fluid (CSF) analysis and prophylactic intrathecal (IT) chemotherapy is recommended.[54–57]
- Dasatinib can cross the blood–brain barrier and can be considered for CNS leukemia.[58]

Recommended Treatment Plan for This Patient

- The patient undergoes 6 cycles of hyper-fractionated cyclophosphamide, vincristine, doxorubicin, and dexamethasone (hyper-CVAD) plus ponatinib and achieves CCyR after 1 cycle, and MR4.5 after 6 cycles.
- He undergoes allo-HSCT while in MR4.5 with thiotepa, busulfan, and fludarabine myeloablative conditioning.

What Are the Toxicities Associated With Hyper-CVAD and Allo-HSCT?

- Hyper-CVAD can induce cytopenias, which can lead to a period of blood product transfusion-dependence, as well as morbid or fatal bleeding and infections.[59]
- Other notable toxicities include hemorrhagic cystitis, peripheral neuropathy, anthracycline-induced cardiomyopathy, transaminitis, steroid-induced psychosis, mucositis, and secondary malignancies.
- Allo-HSCT can lead to myelosuppression and the potential consequences that come with pancytopenia, as well as many of the adverse events (AEs) previously mentioned that are seen with high-intensity chemotherapy. A unique toxicity with allo-HSCT is graft-versus-host-disease (GVHD), which can range from mild to life-threatening organ damage.[60,61]

What Are Other Treatment Considerations?

- For patients with advanced phase (i.e., AP/BP) CML, achieving CCyR post–allo-HSCT, TKI maintenance therapy for up to 1 year can be considered along with qPCR monitoring every 3 months for 2 years, then 3 to 6 months onward.[62-64]
- For those not achieving CCyR or relapse post–allo-HSCT, treatment options are limited but can include TKI with or without donor lymphocyte infusion, omacetaxine, or a clinical trial.[65-71]

The Patient's Outcome

- *The patient remains in CCyR and MR4.5 post–allo-HSCT, completes 1 year of post-HSCT ponatinib 15 mg once daily, and remains in molecular remission 3 years post–allo-HSCT.*

REVIEW QUESTIONS

1. A 51-year-old female presents to her primary care provider (PCP) for fatigue. Complete blood count (CBC) reveals a white blood cell (WBC) count of 34 × 10⁹/L and a platelet of 455 × 10⁹/L. Hemoglobin (Hgb) is within normal limits. Cell differential shows 68% neutrophils, 6% myelocytes, 3% metamyelocytes, 8% basophils, 11% lymphocytes, and 4% eosinophils. What studies must be obtained next to confirm a diagnosis?
   A. Flow cytometry on peripheral blood
   B. BCR-ABL1 kinase domain mutational analysis
   C. Bone marrow core biopsy and aspirate with cytogenetic analysis
   D. B and C
   E. All of the above

2. A 33-year-old male presents for a routine physical exam, and on complete blood count (CBC) is found to have a white blood cell (WBC) count of 88 × 10⁹/L, with 70% neutrophils, 5% myelocytes, 4% metamyelocytes, 7% basophils, 7% lymphocytes, and 7% eosinophils. Hemoglobin (Hgb) is 11.5 g/dL and platelet count is 556 × 10⁹/L. Bone marrow biopsy is consistent with chronic phase chronic myelogenous leukemia (CP-CML). BCR-ABL1 transcript level is 91.544% on the international scale (IS). He has no comorbidities or other remarkable past medical history (PMH). Which tyrosine kinase inhibitor (TKI) would not be appropriate for this patient?
   A. Imatinib
   B. Dasatinib
   C. Nilotinib
   D. Ponatinib
   E. Bosutinib

3. A 51-year-old male with a history of generalized anxiety disorder presents to the ED for increasing abdominal pain and distention. On physical exam, he is noted to have a spleen 11 cm below the costal margin. Complete blood count (CBC) with differential is notable for a white blood cell (WBC) count of 51 × 10⁹/L, 4% basophils, 6% eosinophils, and 2% blasts. Hemoglobin (Hgb) is 10.7 g/dL and platelet count is 421 × 10⁹/L. Bone marrow biopsy confirms chronic phase chronic myelogenous leukemia (CP-CML), and BCR-ABL by quantitative reverse transcriptase polymerase chain reaction (qPCR) is 66.820%. Which of the following would be the best treatment option for this patient?
   A. Dasatinib
   B. Imatinib
   C. Any tyrosine kinase inhibitor (TKI) as a bridge to allogeneic hematopoietic stem cell transplantation (allo-HSCT)
   D. Bosutinib
   E. A or D
   F. C and either A, B, or D

4. A 66-year-old female with a past medical history (PMH) notable for chronic phase chronic myelogenous leukemia (CP-CML) presents to the ED for shortness of breath. Vitals are notable for tachycardia to 107 bpm, and an O2 saturation of 90% requiring 2 L of nasal cannula (NC) to maintain greater than 95%. She has decreased breath sounds on the R base of her lung, but otherwise is clear to auscultation. A chest x-ray shows a right-sided pleural effusion. Hematology is consulted to determine if this finding is related to her

underlying disease. Which of the following is a plausible explanation for her pleural effusion that warrants evaluation from a hematology standpoint?

A. Progression to blast phase chronic myelogenous leukemia (BP-CML)

B. Dasatinib toxicity

C. Bosutinib toxicity

D. Mature granulocytic infiltration of the pleural space

E. None of the above

5. A 38-year-old male presents to the ED for debilitating fatigue and anorexia over the past 4 weeks. Exam yields no additional pertinent findings. Complete blood count (CBC) shows a white blood cell (WBC) count of 71×10^9/L and 11% myeloblasts. He is admitted and undergoes a bone marrow biopsy, which confirms chronic myelogenous leukemia (CML) with 17% myeloblasts. Which of the following is the most appropriate treatment option?

A. 7+3 induction plus tyrosine kinase inhibitor (TKI)

B. Dasatinib 100 mg daily

C. Bosutinib 500 mg daily

D. Imatinib 400 mg daily followed by allogeneic hematopoietic stem cell transplantation (allo-HSCT)

E. Immediate allo-HSCT

6. Which of the following regarding chronic myelogenous leukemia (CML) and its management is false?

A. Many patients with CML are asymptomatic at presentation

B. Second-generation tyrosine kinase inhibitors (TKIs) have led to superior overall and progression-free survival (PFS) compared to imatinib, and thus are preferred in intermediate- or high-risk CML

C. Blast phase CML (BL-CML) should be treated with multidrug combinational induction chemotherapy plus TKI followed by allogeneic hematopoietic stem cell transplantation (allo-HSCT) in first complete remission

D. Managing CML with TKIs requires a careful assessment of comorbidities as some of the non-overlapping toxicities with TKIs can help tailor treatment to each specific patient

7. A 49-year-old female is diagnosed with chronic phase chronic myelogenous leukemia (CP-CML) and is started on dasatinib 100 mg daily. Her baseline BCR-ABL1 by quantitative reverse transcriptase polymerase chain reaction (qPCR) is 77.201% on the international scale (IS). At 3 months, BCR-ABL1 level is 44.467% on the IS. The patient reports compliance with dasatinib, and review of medications shows no potential drug interactions. There are no signs of accellerated phase/blast phase (AP/BP) on the peripheral blood. Which of the following is the next appropriate step in management?

A. Bone marrow biopsy with cytogenetic response evaluation and ABL1 kinase domain mutational analysis

B. Increase dose of dasatinib to 100 mg twice daily and re-assess BCR-ABL1 level at 6 months

C. Repeat BCR-ABL1 level

D. A and/or B

8. A 65-year-old female with a past medical history (PMH) of coronary artery disease and a myocardial infarction 2 years ago was started on imatinib 400 mg daily after being diagnosed with chronic phase chronic myelogenous leukemia (CP-CML). Her baseline BCR-ABL1 level was 46.532%, and on 3-month assessment was 34.229%. Imatinib was increased to 600 mg daily, and at 6 months, her BCR-ABL level was 30.045%. A bone

marrow biopsy is performed that once again shows CP-CML. ABL kinase domain mutation reveals an *F317L* mutation and she is started on nilotinib. Which of the following should be performed prior to starting nilotinib?

A. Electrocardiogram
B. Echocardiogram
C. Pulmonary function tests
D. Ophthalmologic exam
E. Chest x-ray

9. A 47-year-old female is diagnosed with chronic phase chronic myelogenous leukemia (CP-CML) and is started on bosutinib 400 mg daily. At baseline, her BCR-ABL1 transcript level was 55.004% and at 3 months is 61.209%. A bone marrow biopsy is performed at this time, which reveals 17% myeloblasts. ABL domain mutational analysis shows a *T315I* mutation. Which of the following treatments would be most appropriate in addition to referral for allogeneic hematopoietic stem cell transplantation (allo-HSCT) evaluation?

A. Nilotinib
B. Ponatinib
C. Dasatinib
D. Asciminib
E. B or D

10. A 60-year-old male who was diagnosed with chronic phase chronic myelogenous leukemia (CP-CML) over 3 years ago had completed 3 years of dasatinib therapy and achieved a sustained MR4.5 for over 2 years. Dasatinib is discontinued; however, 1 month later BCR-ABL1 transcripts are detected. Which of the following is true?

A. Restarting the same tyrosine kinase inhibitor (TKI) at the same dose that was discontinued with quantitative reverse transcriptase polymerase chain reaction (qPCR) monitoring of BCR-ABL1 is reasonable
B. Patients with molecular relapse after TKI discontinuation must be referred for allogeneic hematopoietic stem cell transplantation (allo-HSCT) evaluation
C. Bone marrow core biopsy and aspirate, as well as ABL kinase domain mutational analysis, are mandatory at the time of molecular relapse upon discontinuation of a TKI
D. The same TKI that was discontinued can be restarted, but the dose should be increased from prior, and BCR-ABL1 levels should be closely followed
E. None of the above

ANSWERS AND RATIONALES

1. **C. Bone marrow core biopsy and aspirate with cytogenetic analysis.** Bone marrow core biopsy and aspirate must always be performed when chronic myeloid leukemia (CML) is suspected to evaluate morphology and to rule out the presence of occult accelerated phase/blast phase CML (AP/BP-CML). Cytogenetics should also be performed to confirm the presence of the Philadelphia (Ph) chromosome, t(9;22)(q34;q11), as well as additional chromosomal abnormalities (ACAs).

2. **D. Ponatinib.** The actual U.S. Food and Drug Administration (FDA) indications for ponatinib in CML are for those in any phase with no other TKIs indicated or who have a confirmed *T315I* mutation. As the patient has not failed a single TKI yet and has no contraindications to first- and second-generation TKIs, ponatinib would not be the first appropriate TKI.

3. **E. A or D.** The patient has intermediate-risk CP-CML based on the Sokal and Hasford scoring systems. Although imatinib is acceptable, it would not be the best treatment choice as the National Comprehensive Cancer Network (NCCN) guidelines recommend a second-generation TKI for first-line intermediate-risk CP-CML treatment. Allo-HSCT is no longer indicated for frontline treatment of CP-CML.

4. **B. Dasatinib toxicity.** Pleural effusions are well-recognized adverse events (AE) that occur more commonly with dasatinib than the other tyrosine kinase inhibitors (TKIs).[21] Pleural effusions as a result of an underlying disease-related process are very rare.[72]

5. **C. Bosutinib 500 mg daily.** Accelerated phase CML (AP-CML) is preferably treated with a second-generation TKI, but the doses would be higher for any TKI used for accelerated or blast phase CML (AP/BP-CML) compared to chronic phase CML (CP-CML). Although dasatinib would be acceptable, 140 mg daily as opposed to the 100 mg daily used for CP-CML would be the correct choice. Imatinib at an increased dose of 600 mg daily can also be used. Intensive acute leukemia-based regimens are generally reserved for BP-CML, followed by allo-HSCT in first complete remission. For AP-CML, allo-HSCT may be necessary, but only if the patient fails to reach treatment milestones on TKI therapy.

6. **B. Second-generation tyrosine kinase inhibitors (TKIs) have led to superior overall and progression-free survival (PFS) compared to imatinib, and thus are preferred in intermediate- or high-risk CML.** Long-term clinical trial data show that all TKIs extend overall survival (OS) close to that of age-matched controls, and that second-generation TKIs typically lead to faster cytogenetic and molecular responses, as well as deeper molecular responses, with less progression to accelerated phase or blast phase (AP/BP) compared to imatinib, but without a significant difference in long-term survival.

7. **A. Bone marrow biopsy with cytogenetic response evaluation and ABL1 kinase domain mutational analysis.** The patient has failed to achieve an early molecular response (EMR) at 3 months. At this juncture, it is necessary to evaluate compliance and drug interactions and to consider performing a bone marrow biopsy with cytogenetic response evaluation and ABL1 kinase domain mutational analysis. Non-imatinib tyrosine kinase inhibitors (TKIs) can be continued at their current dose (if there is no evidence of AP/BP), while the dose of imatinib, if started on it and continued at this time, should be increased. Switching to an alternate TKI is also reasonable, along with an allogeneic hematopoietic stem cell transplantation (allo-HSCT) evaluation. Dasatinib 100 mg twice daily is not a U.S. Food and Drug Administration (FDA)-approved dose for CML.

8. **A. Electrocardiogram.** Nilotinib can prolong the QT interval; thus, an EKG should be obtained to document baseline QT interval.

9. **E. B or D.** Ponatinib and asciminib have efficacy against *T315I* ABL domain mutations, while imatinib, dasatinib, bosutinib, and nilotinib do not. Other treatment options for patients with *T315I* mutations are omacetaxine and allo-HSCT.

10. **A. Restarting the same tyrosine kinase inhibitor (TKI) at the same dose that was discontinued with quantitative reverse transcriptase polymerase chain reaction (qPCR) monitoring of BCR-ABL1 is reasonable.** Upon molecular relapse, a TKI should be resumed within 4 weeks of losing major molecular response (MMR) with monthly BCR-ABL1 monitoring until re-establishing MMR, then every 3 months thereafter indefinitely for those restarting TKI therapy after losing MMR. For those unable to achieve MMR after 3 months of restarting a TKI, ABL1 kinase domain mutation testing should be performed, and monthly BCR-ABL1 monitoring should be continued for another 6 months. It is reasonable to restart the same TKI at the same dose that induced MR4.5 in this patient without a dose increase. Allo-HSCT referral is always reasonable, but is not absolutely mandatory until assessing how the patient will respond to restarting his TKI.

REFERENCES

1. Shet AS, Jahagirdar BN, Verfaillie CM. Chronic myelogenous leukemia: mechanisms underlying disease progression. *Leukemia*. 2002;16(8):1402–1411. doi:10.1038/sj.leu.2402577
2. Surveillance, Epidemiology, and End Results Program. Cancer stat facts: leukemia—chronic myeloid leukemia (CML). National Cancer Institute. https://seer.cancer.gov/statfacts/html/cmyl.html
3. Sawyers CL. Chronic myeloid leukemia. *N Engl J Med*. 1999;340(17):1330–1340. doi:10.1056/NEJM199904293401706
4. Melo JV. *BCR-ABL* gene variants. *Baillieres Clin Haematol*. 1997;10(2):203–222. doi:10.1016/s0950-3536(97)80003-0
5. Cortes J. Natural history and staging of chronic myelogenous leukemia. *Hematol Oncol Clin North Am*. 2004;18(3):569–584, viii. doi:10.1016/j.hoc.2004.03.011
6. Jabbour E, Kantarjian H. Chronic myeloid leukemia: 2020 update on diagnosis, therapy and monitoring. *Am J Hematol*. 2020;95(6):691–709. doi:10.1002/ajh.25792
7. Silver RT, Woolf SH, Hehlmann R, et al. An evidence-based analysis of the effect of busulfan, hydroxyurea, interferon, and allogeneic bone marrow transplantation in treating the chronic phase of chronic myeloid leukemia: developed for the American Society of Hematology. *Blood*. 1999;94(5):1517–1536. doi:10.1182/blood.V94.5.1517
8. Cortes J. How to manage CML patients with comorbidities. *Blood*. 2020;136(22):2507–2512. doi:10.1182/blood.2020006911
9. Hochhaus A, Baccarani M, Silver RT, et al. European LeukemiaNet 2020 recommendations for treating chronic myeloid leukemia. *Leuk*. 2020;34(4):966–984. doi:10.1038/s41375-020-0776-2
10. Jabbour E, Kantarjian H. Chronic myeloid leukemia: 2018 update on diagnosis, therapy and monitoring. *Am J Hematol*. 2018;93(3):442–459. doi:10.1002/ajh.25011
11. Kantarjian H, Deisseroth A, Kurzrock R, Estrov Z, Talpaz M. Chronic myelogenous leukemia: a concise update. *Blood*. 1993;82(3):691–703. doi:10.1182/blood.V82.3.691.691
12. Druker BJ, Marin D. Chronic myelogenous leukemia. In: DeVita VT Jr, Lawrence TS, Rosenberg SA, eds. *DeVita. Hellman, and Rosenberg's Cancer: Principles and Practice of Oncology*. 10th ed. Lippincott Williams & Wilkins; 2015:1644–1653.
13. Sokal JE, Cox EB, Baccarani M, et al. Prognostic discrimination in "good-risk" chronic granulocytic leukemia. *Blood*. 1984;63(4):789–799. doi:10.1182/blood.V63.4.789.789
14. Hasford J, Pfirrmann M, Hehlmann R, et al. A new prognostic score for survival of patients with chronic myeloid leukemia treated with interferon alfa. *J Natl Cancer Inst*. 1998;90(11):850–858. doi:10.1093/jnci/90.11.850
15. Pfirrmann M, Baccarani M, Saussele S, et al. Prognosis of long-term survival considering disease-specific death in patients with chronic myeloid leukemia. *Leukemia*. 2016;30(1):48–56. doi:10.1038/leu.2015.261
16. Hochhaus A, Larson RA, Guilhot F, et al. Long-term outcomes of imatinib treatment for chronic myeloid leukemia. *N Engl J Med*. 2017;376(10):917–927. doi:10.1056/NEJMoa1609324

17. Cortes JE, Saglio G, Kantarjian HM, et al. Final 5 year study results of DASISION: the dasatinib versus ima-tinib study in treatment-naïve chronic myeloid leukemia patients trial. *J Clin Oncol*. 2016;34(20):2333–2340. doi:10.1200/JCO.2015.64.8899

18. Hochhaus A, Saglio G, Hughes TP, et al. Long-term benefits and risks of frontline nilotinib vs imatinib for chronic myeloid leukemia in chronic phase: 5 year update of the randomized ENESTnd trial. *Leukemia*. 2016;30(5):1044–1054. doi:10.1038/leu.2016.5

19. Cortes JE, Gambacorti-Passerini C, Deininger MW, et al. Bosutinib versus imatinib for newly diagnosed chronic myeloid leukemia: results from the randomized BFORE trial. *J Clin Oncol*. 2018;36(3):231–237. doi:10.1200/JCO.2017.74.7162

20. Efficace F, Baccarani M, Breccia M, et al. Chronic fatigue is the most important factor limiting health-related quality of life of chronic myeloid leukemia patients treated with imatinib. *Leukemia*. 2013;27(7):1511–1519. doi:10.1038/leu.2013.51

21. Cortes JE, Jimenez CA, Mauro MJ, Geyer A, Pinilla-Ibarz J, Smith BD. Pleural effusion in dasatinib-treated patients with chronic myeloid leukemia in chronic phase: identification and management. *Clin Lymphoma Myeloma Leuk*. 2017;17(2):78–82. doi:10.1016/j.clml.2016.09.012

22. El-Dabh A, Acharya D. EXPRESS: pulmonary hypertension with dasatinib and other tyrosine kinase inhibitors. *Pulm Circ*. 2019;9(3):2045894019865704. doi:10.1177/2045894019865704

23. Sadiq S, Owen E, Foster T, et al. Nilotinib-induced metabolic dysfunction: insights from a translational study using in vitro adipocyte models and patient cohorts. *Leukemia*. 2019;33(7):1810–1814. doi:10.1038/s41375-018-0337-0

24. Racil Z, Razga F, Drapalova J, et al. Mechanism of impaired glucose metabolism during nilotinib therapy in patients with chronic myelogenous leukemia. *Haematologica*. 2013;98(10):e124–e126. doi:10.3324/haematol.2013.086355

25. Franklin M, Burns L, Perez S, Yerragolam D, Makenbaeva D. Incidence of type II diabetes mellitus among patients with chronic myelogenous leukemia (CML) receiving first or second line therapy with dasatinib or nilotinib. *J Clin Oncol*. 2016;34(15_suppl):e18126. doi:10.1200/JCO.2016.34.15_suppl.e18126

26. Cirmi S, El Abd A, Letinier L, Navarra M, Salvo F. Cardiovascular toxicity of tyrosine kinase inhibitors used in chronic myeloid leukemia: an analysis of the FDA Adverse Event Reporting System database (FAERS). *Cancers*. 2020;12(4):826. doi:10.3390/cancers12040826

27. Giles FJ, Mauro MJ, Hong F, et al. Rates of peripheral arterial occlusive disease in patients with chronic myeloid leukemia in the chronic phase treated with imatinib, nilotinib, or non-tyrosine kinase therapy: a retrospective cohort analysis. *Leukemia*. 2013;27(6):1310–1315. doi:10.1038/leu.2013.69

28. Pfizer. *Bosulif prescribing information*. December 2017. https://www.accessdata.fda.gov/drugsatfda_docs/label/2017/203341s009lbl.pdf

29. Mohanavelu P, Mutnick M, Mehra N, et al. Meta-analysis of gastrointestinal adverse events from tyrosine kinase inhibitors for chronic myeloid leukemia. *Cancers*. 2021;13(7):1643. doi:10.3390/cancers13071643

30. Masiello D, Gorospe G 3rd, Yang AS. The occurrence and management of fluid retention associated with TKI therapy in CML, with a focus on dasatinib. *J Hematol Oncol*. 2009;2:46. doi:10.1186/1756-8722-2-46

31. Jabbour E, Deininger M, Hochhaus A. Management of adverse events associated with tyrosine kinase inhibitors in the treatment of chronic myeloid leukemia. *Leukemia*. 2011;25(2):201–210. doi:10.1038/leu.2010.215

32. Fava C, Kantarjian HM, Jabbour E, et al. Failure to achieve a complete hematologic response at the time of a major cytogenetic response with second-generation tyrosine kinase inhibitors is associated with a poor prog-nosis among patients with chronic myeloid leukemia in accelerated or blast phase. *Blood*. 2009;113(21):5058–5063. doi:10.1182/blood-2008-10-184960

33. Cortes J, Quintás-Cardama A, Kantarjian HM. Monitoring molecular response in chronic myeloid leukemia. *Cancer*. 2011;117(6):1113–1122. doi:10.1002/cncr.25527

34. Hehlmann R, Lauseker M, Saußele S, et al. Assessment of imatinib as first-line treatment of chronic myeloid leukemia: 10 year survival results of the randomized CML study IV and impact of non-CML determinants. *Leukemia*. 2017;31(11):2398–2406. doi:10.1038/leu.2017.253

35. Hanfstein B, Müller MC, Hehlmann R, et al. Early molecular and cytogenetic response is predictive for long-term progression-free and overall survival in chronic myeloid leukemia (CML). *Leukemia*. 2012;26(9):2096–2102. doi:10.1038/leu.2012.85

36. Hughes TP, Hochhaus A, Branford S, et al. Long-term prognostic significance of early molecular response to imatinib in newly diagnosed chronic myeloid leukemia: an analysis from the international randomized study of interferon and STI571 (IRIS). *Blood*. 2010;116(19):3758–3765. doi:10.1182/blood-2010-03-273979

37. Druker BJ, Guilhot F, O'Brien SG, et al. Five year follow-up of patients receiving imatinib for chronic myeloid leukemia. *N Engl J Med*. 2006;355(23):2408–2417. doi:10.1056/NEJMoa062867

38. Press RD, Galderisi C, Yang R, et al. A half-log increase in BCR-ABL RNA predicts a higher risk of relapse in patients with chronic myeloid leukemia with an imatinib-induced complete cytogenetic response. *Clin Cancer Res*. 2007;13(20):6136–6143. doi:10.1158/1078-0432.CCR-07-1112

39. de Lavallade H, Apperley JF, Khorashad JS, et al. Imatinib for newly diagnosed patients with chronic myeloid leukemia: incidence of sustained responses in an intention-to-treat analysis. *J Clin Oncol*. 2008;26(20):3358–3363. doi:10.1200/JCO.2007.15.8154

40. Marin D, Milojkovic D, Olavarria E, et al. European LeukemiaNet criteria for failure or suboptimal response reliably identify patients with CML in early chronic phase treated with imatinib whose eventual outcome is poor. *Blood*. 2008;112(12):4437–4444. doi:10.1182/blood-2008-06-162388

41. Jabbour E, Kantarjian HM, O'Brien S, et al. Front-line therapy with second-generation tyrosine kinase inhibitors in patients with early chronic phase chronic myeloid leukemia: what is the optimal response? *J Clin Oncol*. 2011;29(32):4260–4265. doi:10.1200/JCO.2011.36.0693

42. Hehlmann R, Müller MC, Lauseker M, et al. Deep molecular response is reached by the majority of patients treated with imatinib, predicts survival, and is achieved more quickly by optimized high-dose imatinib: results from the randomized CML-study IV. *J Clin Oncol*. 2014;32(5):415–423. doi:10.1200/JCO.2013.49.9020

43. Saussele S, Hehlmann R, Fabarius A, et al. Defining therapy goals for major molecular remission in chronic myeloid leukemia: results of the randomized CML Study IV. *Leukemia*. 2018;32(5):1222–1228. doi:10.1038/s41375-018-0055-7

44. Mahon F-X, Réa D, Guilhot J, et al. Discontinuation of imatinib in patients with chronic myeloid leukaemia who have maintained complete molecular remission for at least 2 years: the prospective, multicentre Stop Imatinib (STIM) trial. *Lancet Oncol*. 2010;11(11):1029–1035. doi:10.1016/S1470-2045(10)70233-3

45. Saussele S, Richter J, Guilhot J, et al. Discontinuation of tyrosine kinase inhibitor therapy in chronic myeloid leukaemia (EURO-SKI): a prespecified interim analysis of a prospective, multicentre, non-randomised, trial. *Lancet Oncol*. 2018;19(6):747–757. doi:10.1016/S1470-2045(18)30192-X

46. National Comprehensive Cancer Network. Chronic myeloid leukemia (Version 3.2022). https://www.nccn.org/professionals/physician_gls/pdf/cml.pdf

47. Eşkazan AE. Asciminib in chronic myeloid leukemia: many questions still remain to be answered. *Blood Cancer J*. 2021;11(4):81. doi:10.1038/s41408-021-00475-7

48. Cortes JE, Kim D-W, Pinilla-Ibarz J, et al. A phase 2 trial of ponatinib in Philadelphia chromosome–positive leukemias. *N Engl J Med*. 2013;369(19):1783–1796. doi:10.1056/NEJMoa1306494

49. ARIAD Pharmaceuticals. ICLUSIG prescribing information. Revised November 2016. https://www.accessdata.fda.gov/drugsatfda_docs/label/2016/203469s022lbl.pdf

50. Saussele S, Lauseker M, Gratwohl A, et al. Allogeneic hematopoietic stem cell transplantation (allo SCT) for chronic myeloid leukemia in the imatinib era: evaluation of its impact within a subgroup of the randomized German CML study IV. *Blood*. 2010;115(10):1880–1885. doi:10.1182/blood-2009-08-237115

51. Boehm A, Walcherberger B, Sperr WR, et al. Improved outcome in patients with chronic myelogenous leukemia after allogeneic hematopoietic stem cell transplantation over the past 25 years: a single-center experience. *Biol Blood Marrow Transplant*. 2011;17(1):133–140. doi:10.1016/j.bbmt.2010.06.019

52. Khoury HJ, Kukreja M, Goldman JM, et al. Prognostic factors for outcomes in allogeneic transplantation for CML in the imatinib era: a CIBMTR analysis. *Bone Marrow Transplant*. 2012;47(6):810–816. doi:10.1038/bmt.2011.194

53. Gandhi V, Plunkett W, Cortes JE. Omacetaxine: a protein translation inhibitor for treatment of chronic myelogenous leukemia. *Clin Cancer Res*. 2014;20(7):1735–1740. doi:10.1158/1078-0432.CCR-13-1283

54. Rajappa S, Uppin SG, Raghunadharao D, Rao IS, Surath A. Isolated central nervous system blast crisis in chronic myeloid leukemia. *Hematol Oncol*. 2004;22(4):179–181. doi:10.1002/hon.737

55. Kim HJ, Jung CW, Kim K, et al. Isolated blast crisis in CNS in a patient with chronic myelogenous leukemia maintaining major cytogenetic response after imatinib. *J Clin Oncol*. 2006;24(24):4028–4029. doi:10.1200/JCO.2006.05.5608

56. Altintas A, Cil T, Kilinc I, Kaplan MA, Ayyildiz O. Central nervous system blastic crisis in chronic myeloid leukemia on imatinib mesylate therapy: a case report. *J Neurooncol*. 2007;84(1):103–105. doi:10.1007/s11060-007-9352-0

57. Aftimos P, Nasr F. Isolated CNS lymphoid blast crisis in a patient with imatinib-resistant chronic myelogenous leukemia: case report and review of the literature. *Leuk Res*. 2009;33(11):e178–e180. doi:10.1016/j.leukres.2009.04.023

58. Porkka K, Koskenvesa P, Lundán T, et al. Dasatinib crosses the blood-brain barrier and is an efficient therapy for central nervous system Philadelphia chromosome-positive leukemia. *Blood*. 2008;112(4):1005–1012. doi:10.1182/blood-2008-02-140665

59. Kantarjian H, Thomas D, O'Brien S, et al. Long-term follow-up results of hyperfractionated cyclophosphamide, vincristine, doxorubicin, and dexamethasone (Hhyper-CVAD), a dose-intensive regimen, in adult acute lymphocytic leukemia. *Cancer*. 2004;101(12):2788–2801. doi:10.1002/cncr.20668

60. Jacobsohn DA, Vogelsang GB. Acute graft versus host disease. *Orphanet J of Rare Dis*. 2007;2(1):35. doi:10.1186/1750-1172-2-35

61. Pérez-Simón JA, Sánchez-Abarca I, Díez-Campelo M, Caballero D, San Miguel J. Chronic graft-versus-host disease: pathogenesis and clinical management. *Drugs*. 2006;66(8):1041–1057. doi:10.2165/00003495-200666080-00002

62. Carpenter PA, Johnston L, Fernandez HF, et al. Posttransplant feasibility study of nilotinib prophylaxis for high-risk Philadelphia chromosome positive leukemia. *Blood*. 2017;130(9):1170–1172. doi:10.1182/blood-2017-03-771121

63. Olavarria E, Siddique S, Griffiths MJ, et al. Posttransplantation imatinib as a strategy to postpone the requirement for immunotherapy in patients undergoing reduced-intensity allografts for chronic myeloid leukemia. *Blood*. 2007;110(13):4614–4617. doi:10.1182/blood-2007-04-082990

64. DeFilipp Z, Langston AA, Chen Z, et al. Does post-transplant maintenance therapy with tyrosine kinase inhibitors improve outcomes of patients with high-risk Philadelphia chromosome-positive leukemia? *Clin Lymphoma Myeloma Leuk*. 2016;16(8):466–471.e461. doi:10.1016/j.clml.2016.04.017

65. Kolb H-J, Schattenberg A, Goldman JM, et al. Graft-versus-leukemia effect of donor lymphocyte transfusions in marrow grafted patients. *Blood*. 1995;86(5):2041–2050. doi:10.1182/blood.V86.5.2041.bloodjournal8652041

66. Dazzi F, Szydlo RM, Cross NC, et al. Durability of responses following donor lymphocyte infusions for patients who relapse after allogeneic stem cell transplantation for chronic myeloid leukemia. *Blood*. 2000;96(8):2712–2716. doi:10.1182/blood.V96.8.2712

67. Luznik L, Fuchs EJ. Donor lymphocyte infusions to treat hematologic malignancies in relapse after allogeneic blood or marrow transplantation. *Cancer Control*. 2002;9(2):123–137. doi:10.1177/107327480200900205

68. Michallet AS, Nicolini F, Fürst S, et al. Outcome and long-term follow-up of alloreactive donor lymphocyte infusions given for relapse after myeloablative allogeneic hematopoietic stem cell transplantations (HSCT). *Bone Marrow Transplant*. 2005;35(6):601–608. doi:10.1038/sj.bmt.1704807

69. Weisser M, Tischer J, Schnittger S, Schoch C, Ledderose G, Kolb HJ. A comparison of donor lymphocyte infusions or imatinib mesylate for patients with chronic myelogenous leukemia who have relapsed after allogeneic stem cell transplantation. *Haematologica*. 2006;91(5):663–666. https://haematologica.org/article/view/3960

70. Chalandon Y, Passweg JR, Guglielmi C, et al. Early administration of donor lymphocyte infusions upon molecular relapse after allogeneic hematopoietic stem cell transplantation for chronic myeloid leukemia: a study by the chronic malignancies working party of the EBMT. *Haematologica*. 2014;99(9):1492–1498. doi:10.3324/haematol.2013.100198

71. Schmidt S, Liu Y, Hu Z-H, et al. The role of donor lymphocyte infusion (DLI) in post-hematopoietic cell transplant (HCT) relapse for chronic myeloid leukemia (CML) in the tyrosine kinase inhibitor (TKI) era. *Biol Blood Marrow Transplant*. 2020;26(6):1137–1143. doi:10.1016/j.bbmt.2020.02.006

72. Nuwal P, Dixit R, Dargar P, George J. Pleural effusion as the initial manifestation of chronic myeloid leukemia: report of a case with clinical and cytologic correlation. *J Cytol*. 2012;29(2):152–154. doi:10.4103/0970-9371.97165

CHAPTER 32

Chronic Lymphocytic Leukemia

Tamer Othman and Brian A. Jonas

INTRODUCTION

Chronic lymphocytic leukemia (CLL) is a lymphoproliferative disorder referring to the accumulation of monoclonal, small, and mature CD5+ B-lymphocytes in the peripheral blood, bone marrow, and lymphoid tissues.[1] CLL is the most common adult leukemia in the Western world, with an incidence of 4.9 per 100,000 individuals and represents 1.1% of all new cancer cases in the United States.[2] In 2022, it is estimated that 20,160 new cases will be diagnosed, and that 4,410 individuals will die from the disease.[2] The disease is most commonly diagnosed in people 65 years old and older, at a median age of 70 years. In more recent decades, CLL is diagnosed incidentally on routine labs in 80% or more of cases,[3] although symptomatic manifestations can include unexplained fevers, drenching night sweats, unintentional weight loss, severe fatigue, lymphadenopathy (LAD), hepatosplenomegaly, cytopenias, recurrent infections, and autoimmune complications.[1,4,5] Small lymphocytic lymphoma (SLL) is a different presentation of the same disease process as CLL, with the difference being that the disease is found mostly in bone marrow, lymph nodes (LNs), and other lymphoid tissues, with very little to none circulating in the peripheral blood.[6]

The precise mechanism of CLL development involves a complex interaction between CLL cells and the tissue microenvironment (that is, T-cell, macrophages, and stromal cells) in a manner similar to normal B-lymphocytes expanding in germinal centers during an adaptive immune response.[1] These processes activate B-cell receptors (BCRs), causing downstream signaling via spleen tyrosine kinase (SYK), Bruton tyrosine kinase (BTK), and phosphatidylinositol 3-kinase (PI3K), ultimately promoting expansion and proliferation of CLL cells. The emergence of new agents targeting pathways that drive CLL pathogenesis, as discussed in detail in this chapter, have extended the life expectancy of older adult CLL patients to match the general population.[7]

CASE SUMMARIES

Case 32.1: Newly Diagnosed Chronic Lymphocytic Leukemia

A 71-year-old male with a past medical history (PMH) of hypertension and hyperlipidemia was found to have a white blood cell (WBC) count of 28.6 × 10⁸/L on routine labs with 85% lymphocytes on the cell differential. His complete blood count (CBC) was also notable for a hemoglobin (Hgb) of 12.6 g/dL and a platelet count of 321 × 10⁸/L. He returns 1 week later for follow-up, at which time he denies fevers, night sweats, and unintentional weight loss. Physical exam at a subsequent appointment was notable for a 2-cm left cervical LN and 1.5-cm left axillary LN. No splenomegaly was appreciated.

How Is a Diagnosis Established?

- In cases of suspected CLL, a bone marrow biopsy is not required, and the diagnosis can be made off a CBC with cell differential, blood smear, and flow cytometry.[8]
- Although a bone marrow biopsy is not required for the diagnosis, it may help to distinguish cytopenias secondary to disease-burden in the marrow versus an immune-related process.
- CLL requires a monoclonal B-lymphocyte population greater than 5×10^8/L in the peripheral blood for 3 months or more. Clonality can be confirmed with immunophenotyping by flow cytometry. Characteristic surface markers seen on CLL cells include CD5, CD19, CD20 (although weakly), and CD23. Smudge cells on peripheral blood smear are classic. SLL is diagnosed by lymphadenopathy (LAD) without cytopenias as a direct result of the disease and a monoclonal B-cell population less than 5×10^8/L. Typically, the SLL diagnosis is made histopathologically by a LN biopsy. Also of note, CLL is a disease of B-lymphocytes, whereas a neoplastic mature T-cell disorder would be termed T-prolymphocytic leukemia.[9]
- When CLL is suspected, other similar diagnoses, such as mantle cell lymphoma (MCL) and monoclonal B-cell lymphocytosis (MBL) should be ruled out.[4] MCL and CLL are both B-lymphoproliferative disorders expressing CD5, but MCL typically expresses CD20 strongly and is negative for CD23, while CLL is generally weakly CD20 positive and is CD23 positive.[10] MBL is defined by a monoclonal B-cell population less than 5×10^8/L in the peripheral blood for 3 months or more without cytopenias, LAD, or organomegaly.[11] MBL with a monoclonal lymphocytosis greater than 0.5×10^8/L progresses to CLL necessitating treatment at a rate of 1% to 2%/year.[12,13]
- It should also be noted that while CLL commonly presents with very high WBC counts, even above 200×10^8/L, they generally do not cause symptomatic hyperleukocytosis.[14]

Patient's Diagnosis

- *Repeat CBC shows a WBC of 27×10^8/L with 80% lymphocytes. Flow cytometry shows 19×10^8 lambda-restricted B-cells expressing CD5, CD23, and weak expression of CD20. A diagnosis of CLL is made.*

How Is This Tumor Staged?

- Several staging and prognostic scoring systems exist for CLL:
  - Rai staging accounts for CBC and the presence of LAD and/or hepato- or splenomegaly (H/SM; Table 32.1A).[5]
  - The Binet staging system also accounts for the same criteria (Table 32.1B).[15,16]
  - CLL international prognostic index (IPI) awards 1 point for age 65 or older and Rai stage 1 to 4 or Binet B to C, and 2 points for serum β2-microglobulin greater than 3.5 mg/L, *IGHV* unmutated, and del(17p) and/or *TP53* alteration (Table 32.1C).[17]

Patient's Clinical Stage

- *Serum β2-microglobulin is 1.3 mg/L.*
- *Patient is Rai stage 1, Binet stage A, CLL IPI score 2, overall intermediate-risk disease.*

Table 32.1 Staging and Prognostication Systems for CLL

(A) Rai

Low-Risk	Intermediate-Risk		High-Risk	
Stage 0	Stage 1	Stage 2	Stage 3	Stage 4
Lymphocytosis alone	Lymphocytosis + LAD	Lymphocytosis + H/SM ± LAD	Lymphocytosis + Hgb <11 g/dL ± LAD ± H/SM	Lymphocytosis + platelets <100 × 10⁸/L ± Hgb <11 g/dL ± LAD ± H/SM

(B) Binet

Stage A	Stage B	Stage C
<3 lymphoid sites involved[†]	≥3 lymphoid sites involved[†]	Hgb <10 g/dL or platelets <100 × 10⁸/L

(C) CLL IPI

	0–1 Point	2–3 Points	4–6 Points	7–10 Points
Risk-stratification	Low	Intermediate	High	Very high
5-year overall survival (%)	93.2	79.3	63.3	23.3

[†]Refers to cervical LNs (unilateral or bilateral would count as 1), axillary LNs (unilateral or bilateral would count as 1), inguinal LNs (unilateral or bilateral would count as 1), spleen, and liver.

CLL, chronic lymphocytic leukemia; Hgb, hemoglobin; H/SM, hepato- or splenomegaly; LAD, lymphadenopathy; LN, lymph node.

What Are Appropriate Treatment Options?

- Not all patients with CLL require treatment. The international workshop on CLL (iwCLL) has provided guidance on when treatment is indicated (Table 32.2).[4] Generally, patients with Rai stage 0 and Binet stage A do not require treatment.

Recommended Treatment Plan for This Patient
- *Therapy is withheld, and the patient is monitored with a history, physical exam, and CBC with differential every 3 months initially and is gradually spaced out.*
- *Patient remains stable over the following 8 years.*

Table 32.2 Indications for Treatment by the iwCLL

Progressive cytopenias due to CLL (Hgb <10 g/dL or platelets <100 × 10⁸/L, although may monitor if below these cutoffs and stable over long period of time)

Progressive or symptomatic splenomegaly (that is, ≥6 cm below the costal margin)

Progressive LAD (that is, longest diameter ≥10 cm)

≥50% increase in lymphocytosis over 2 months or lymphocyte doubling time <6 months

Autoimmune phenomenon related to CLL refractory to steroids

Structural or functional impairment of other organs due to extranodal involvement

CLL-related B-symptoms: unintentional weight loss ≥10% within 6 months, fatigue causing significant functional impairment, fevers ≥38.0°C (100.4°F) for ≥2 weeks, and night sweats for ≤1 month

CLL, chronic lymphocytic leukemia; Hgb, hemoglobin; CLL, International Workshop on Chronic Lymphocytic Leukemia; LAD, lymphadenopathy.

Case 32.2: Chronic Lymphocytic Leukemia Requiring Treatment

A 74-year-old female with a PMH of asthma presents with a 3-month history of progressive fatigue, rendering her with an Eastern Cooperative Oncology Group (ECOG) 3. Routine physical exam shows cervical and axillary LAD bilaterally, with the largest diameter measuring 4 cm. CBC with differential is obtained, revealing a WBC 210 × 10⁸/L with 91% lymphocytes, Hgb 7.1 g/dL, and platelets 111 × 10⁸/L. Peripheral blood smear shows numerous smudge cells. Subsequent flow cytometry reveals a monoclonal B-cell population with restricted kappa expression, CD5+, CD19+, CD20 (dim positive), and CD23+. Fluorescent in situ hybridization (FISH) reveals del(17p), and IGHV is unmutated.

What Further Molecular or Genomic Testing Is Required?

- Once the decision to begin treatment for CLL by the physician has been made, FISH should be obtained on the peripheral blood prior to treatment to assess for del(13q), del(11q), del(17p), +12. *TP53* mutation and *IGHV* mutation analyses should also be obtained on the peripheral blood. Cytogenetic analysis assessing for the presence of a complex karyotype can be considered.[6]
- Patients with del(13q) without other cytogenetic abnormalities, mutated *IGHV*, and no *TP53* alterations tend to have a favorable prognosis. Patients with del(11q), del(17p), unmutated *IGHV*, or *TP53* alterations have a worse prognosis. Patients with normal cytogenetics or +12 have intermediate-risk disease.
- *TP53* mutations, del(17p), and/or unmutated *IGHV* predict a poor response to chemoimmunotherapy.[6] Therefore, patients possessing these genetic alterations should be treated with small molecule inhibitor-based treatments, such as a BTK inhibitor (ibrutinib or acalabrutinib) or BCL2 antagonist (venetoclax)-based regimen, rather than chemoimmunotherapy.

What Are Appropriate Treatment Options?

- In the modern era, first-line treatment with ibrutinib, acalabrutinib ± obinutuzumab, or venetoclax,[18-23] regardless of age, comorbidities, cytogenetics, *TP53*, and *IGHV* mutational status, is preferred over chemoimmunotherapy according to National Comprehensive Cancer Network (NCCN) guidelines.[6]
- It should be noted, however, that ibrutinib is known to induce mostly partial but durable remissions (in the upfront setting, 7-year progression-free survival [PFS] 83%, and in the relapsed/refractory setting, 34%).[24] Thus, this requires long-term therapy, which can lead to complications such as toxicity and the emergence and expansion of resistant clones.[1] Therefore, in younger patients able to tolerate chemoimmunotherapy and without *TP53* mutations or del(17p) and have a mutated *IGHV*, fludarabine, cyclophosphamide, and rituximab (FCR) may be a reasonable alternative as it can induce remissions exceeding 10 years in these low-risk patients.[25] However, the National Clinical Trials Network E1912 trial, which consisted predominantly of patients younger than 60 years, demonstrated superior PFS and overall survival (OS) with ibrutinib over FCR.[21]
- Venetoclax plus obinutuzumab is given for a finite duration and is able to produce deep remissions. Unlike ibrutinib, the disease-free interval depends on the depth of response with venetoclax plus obinutuzumab, with complete remissions with undetectable measurable residual disease (MRD) producing the longest duration of response. However, resistance and relapses post-venetoclax therapy still occur.[1]
- Autoimmune complications, such as autoimmune hemolytic anemia (AIHA), immune thrombocytopenic purpura (ITP), and pure red cell aplasia (PRCA), may occur with CLL.[6] In this case, if there are no treatment indications per the iwCLL criteria, management is similar to what is used in the absence of malignancy, starting with steroids

first-line, and rituximab, intravenous immunoglobulin (IVIg), splenectomy, or immunosuppressive therapy in later lines.[26] If treatment is indicated, fludarabine should be avoided due to the increased incidence of AIHA noted with it.

Recommended Treatment Plan for This Patient
- *Any of the small molecular inhibitors would be a reasonable choice for this patient given her age. Thus, she is started on ibrutinib 420 mg once daily.*

What Are the Toxicities Associated With Bruton Tyrosine Kinase Inhibitors?
- Cytopenias, gastrointestinal disturbances, rash, headaches, and musculoskeletal pain are common adverse events (AEs) with ibrutinib and acalabrutinib.[6]
- AEs of special interest include hypertension, atrial fibrillation, and hemorrhage, and should be accounted for when selecting a treatment regimen. Fatal and non-fatal infections, such as fungal (like aspergillus), viral, and bacterial, including *Pneumocystis jiroveci* pneumonia (PJP), have been reported.
- BTK inhibitors induce a well-described lymphocytosis upon initiation and even re-initiation of therapy, which should not be confused for disease progression. This phenomenon is thought to be due to disruption of adhesion factors by BCR signaling inhibition in the bone marrow and LNs, leading to lymphocyte mobilization. This generally resolves within 8 months. In some patients it may persist more than 12 months, but it does not correlate with overall prognosis.[27]

What Are Other Treatment Considerations?

Monitoring Response
- The iwCLL created a list of criteria for assessing response to therapy, based on reduction of tumor load (A) and restoration of hematopoietic function (B; Table 32.3).[4]
- MRD status post-definite duration therapies, such as chemoimmunotherapy and venetoclax-based regimens as previously discussed, are emerging as an important prognosticator.[28-31]
- There are different techniques to measure MRD:[32]
  - Six-color/multiparameter flow cytometry (MRD flow)
  - Allele-specific oligonucleotide PCR (ASO-PCR)
  - High-throughput sequencing using the ClonoSEQ assay, a method that relies on amplifying and sequencing of the immunoglobulin heavy (IGH) locus to characterize CLL-specific VDJ recombination[32,33]
- The timing of response assessment should be after at least 2 months upon completion of finite treatment, such as with chemoimmunotherapy, and after at least 2 months from maximal response attained for indefinite treatments (Table 32.3).
- For patients undergoing fludarabine- or bendamustine-based chemoimmunotherapy, anti-infective prophylaxis with acyclovir and an antibiotic targeting PJP is recommended.[6] In high-risk patients, prophylaxis against and monitoring of hepatitis B (HBV) and cytomegalovirus (CMV) is also recommended. Prophylaxis against opportunistic infections for patients on a BTK inhibitor who are at an increased risk should be considered.[34,35] Patients should be screened for HBV before starting anti-CD20 monoclonal antibodies due to the high risk of HBV reactivation.[36]

Patient's Response
- *After 4 months of ibrutinib, the patient's ECOG returns to 0, and her Hgb rises to 12.1 g/dL, but lymphocytes remain elevated at 222×10^8/L.*
- *After 6 months of therapy, lymphocytes decrease to 90×10^8/L.*
- *After 9 months of therapy, lymphocytes decrease further to 70×10^8/L.*

Table 32.3   Response Assessment as per the iwCLL

	CR	PR	PD	SD
Group A				
LNs	All <1.5 cm	≥50% ↓ from baseline	≥50% ↑ from baseline or from response	Δ –49% to +49%
Liver and spleen size	Spleen <13 cm, normal liver size	≥50% ↓ from baseline	≥50% ↑ from baseline or from response	Δ –49% to +49%
Constitutional symptoms	None	Present	Present	Present
Circulating lymphocyte count	Within normal limits	≥50% ↓ from baseline	≥50% ↑ from baseline	Δ –49% to +49%
Group B				
Platelets	≥100 × 10⁸/L	≥100 × 10⁸/L or ≥ 50% ↑ from baseline	≥50% ↓ from baseline due to CLL	Δ –49% to +49%
Hgb	≥11 g/dL without transfusion or erythropoietin support	≥11 g/dL or ≥50% ↑ from baseline	2 g/dL ↓ from baseline due to CLL	↑ <11.0 g/dL or <50% from baseline, or ↓ < 2 g/dL
Neutrophils	Absolute neutrophil count >1500/ μL without growth factor support	Absolute neutrophil count >1500/ μL or ≥ 50% ↑ from baseline without growth factor support		
Bone marrow	Normocellular without CLL involvement	CLL present or not done	≥50% ↑ in CLL cells on successive biopsies	No Δ in marrow involvement

CLL, chronic lymphocytic leukemia; CR, complete remission (requires all criteria to be met); Hgb, hemoglobin; iwCLL, International Workshop on Chronic Lymphocytic Leukemia; LN, lymph node; PD, progressive disease (requires at least 1 criteria from group A or B); PR, partial remission (requires 2 parameters from group A and 1 from B if previously abnormal, but if only 1 parameter from both groups is abnormal prior to therapy, only 1 improvement is required); SD, stable disease (requires all criteria to be met, and is not defined by constitutional symptoms alone).

Special Considerations During Monitoring

- Patients with CLL, especially those previously treated, are generally at risk for infectious complications due to low immunoglobulin (Ig) levels.[37]
- This is better described in patients treated with chemoimmunotherapy, but patients treated with ibrutinib appear to experience improvements in IgA levels, reducing infectious complications.[38] Decreasing IgG levels in patients treated with ibrutinib has been reported with prolonged treatment, but does not correlate with an increased infection rate.
- In patients experiencing recurrent sinopulmonary infections requiring hospitalization and Ig levels lower than 500 mg/dL, monthly IVIg targeting a nadir of 500 mg/dL can reduce infection rates, but does not increase OS.[39–41]

Patient's Outcome

- *After 28 months of therapy, the patient's lymphocytes remain elevated at 50 × 10⁸/L but her Hgb and platelets remain within normal limits.*

Case 32.3: Chronic Lymphocytic Leukemia Undergoing Richter's Transformation

A 66-year-old male with a recurrent history of diverticular bleeding and atrial fibrillation presents to the ED for bright red blood per rectum. On CBC with differential, he is noted to have a WBC of 100.4×10^8/L with 77% lymphocytes, an Hgb of 9.4 g/dL, and a platelet count of 33×10^8/L. Flow cytometry confirms CLL. Further workup shows an IGHV unmutated state and del(17p). He is stabilized from a bleeding perspective and establishes care with a hematologist 1 week after discharge. Repeat CBC shows an improvement in Hgb to 11.2 g/dL, but stable leukocytosis and thrombocytopenia.

What Are Appropriate Treatment Options?

- As previously discussed, small molecule inhibitors are preferred in patients with *TP53* mutations, del(17p), and/or unmutated *IGHV*.
- Special attention to comorbidities can help guide the choice of first-line therapy. BTK inhibitors such as ibrutinib and acalabrutinib should be avoided in patients on antiplatelet therapy or anticoagulation at increased risk of hemorrhage, or in those who have uncontrollable hypertension or atrial fibrillation.[6]
- Venetoclax and obinutuzumab is a category 1 recommendation for older adult patients with comorbidities that prevent the use of BTK inhibitors.[6,22]

Recommended Treatment Plan for This Patient
- *The patient is started on venetoclax and obinutuzumab.*

What Are Important Considerations With BCL2 Inhibitors?

- Venetoclax is ramped up over a 5-week period, starting at 20 mg daily during week 1, then increased weekly to 50 mg daily, 100 mg daily, 200 mg daily, and finally to 400 mg daily week 5. It is then continued at 400 mg daily for every 28-day cycle for a total of 12 cycles of venetoclax plus 6 cycles of obinutuzumab.
- Venetoclax leads to an increased risk of tumor lysis syndrome (TLS) when used for CLL treatment. Careful assessment of tumor burden by LN size and absolute lymphocyte count can guide management. Specifically, patients should receive intravenous hydration and allopurinol at minimum prior to initiating venetoclax with close monitoring of TLS labs. Patients should undergo radiographical assessment of LNs for proper TLS risk stratification. Patients at high risk of TLS (that is, any LN size 10 cm or greater or those who have an absolute lymphocyte count of 25×10^8/L or greater with an LN of 5 cm or greater) should be admitted for their first 20 mg and 50 mg dose, and can receive subsequent ramp-ups outpatient.[42]

The Patient's Treatment Course
- *The patient successfully completes 6 cycles of obinutuzumab and 12 cycles of venetoclax.*
- *After 3 months post-treatment, the patient undergoes full response evaluation and is in complete remission and MRD-negative by flow.*
- *The patient, 4 years after achieving CR, reports to his hematologist that he has noticed a "lump growing in his left armpit" over the past 3 weeks with intermittent fevers and drenching night sweats.*

What Diagnostic Tests Should Be Considered for This Patient?

- The patient's CLL has been quiescent for several years, so the acuity of his new symptoms should raise concerns for a serious complication of CLL known as Richter's transformation (RT).[43,44] RT is a histological transformation into a more aggressive lymphoma, more commonly diffuse large B-cell lymphoma (DLBCL) but occasionally Hodgkin lymphoma (HL) as well. RT occurs in 2% to 10% of cases.

- Examples of risk factors for the development of RT include an unmutated *IGHV*, the presence of del(17p) or a complex karyotype, and abnormalities in *c-MYC*, *NOTCH1*, *CDKN2A/B*, or *TP53*.[45–50]
- A biopsy is required to establish the diagnosis of RT. When RT is suspected, a PET/CT should be obtained to identify the ideal biopsy site (that is, the lesion with the highest standardized uptake value [SUV]).[51–53]
- Molecular analysis can help determine if the RT is clonally related to CLL. *IGHV* gene sequencing or clonal *IGHV* rearrangements can also be used. Generally, clonally related CLL is associated with unmutated *IGHV* and *TP53* mutations, and a worse prognosis.[50,54]

The Patient's Diagnosis

- *PET/CT is obtained and reveals high fluorodeoxyglucose (FDG)-uptake in the left axillary LNs, with an SUV of 33.*
- *Subsequent biopsy is obtained, showing sheets of large, atypical B-cell consistent with DLBCL.*

What Are the Treatment Options for Richter's Transformation?

- Clonally unrelated DLBCL can be managed similarly to de novo DLBCL.[6]
- In the absence of a clinical trial, which is especially encouraged in clonally related transformed lymphoma, RT with HL histology should be treated with HL-type regimens, while RT with DLBCL histology should be treated with DLBCL-type regimens.[55,56] Autologous and allogeneic hematopoietic stem cell transplantation (allo-HSCT) can be considered in RT with DLBCL histology in those demonstrating chemosensitive disease, as retrospective data suggests these patients may benefit from a consolidative transplant approach.[57]
- Unfortunately, RT is associated with an extremely poor prognosis, and patients with DLBCL histology in particular tend to have resistant disease.[55,58,59]

REVIEW QUESTIONS

1. A 71-year-old male with a past medical history (PMH) remarkable for chronic lympho-cytic leukemia (CLL) treated with fludarabine, cyclophosphamide, and rituximab (FCR) 11 years ago presents to his hematologist with debilitating fatigue and anorexia over the past 2 weeks. Physical exam is notable for a 3-cm right cervical lymph node (LN) that was not present on his last exam 3 months ago. Complete blood count (CBC) shows a white blood cell (WBC) count of 31.4×10^8/L and an absolute lymphocyte count of 24,000/μL, compared to 28.0×10^8/L and 22,000/μL, respectively, 3 months ago. Hemoglobin (Hgb) and platelets are within normal limits. What is the most appropriate next step in manag-ing this patient?
   A. Bone marrow biopsy
   B. Excisional biopsy of right cervical LN
   C. PET/CT
   D. Start ibrutinib
   E. Repeat CBC in 2 weeks

2. A 57-year-old female is found to have a WBC of 77.4×10^8/L and a normal hemoglobin (Hgb) and platelet count on routine labs. Cell differential shows an absolute lymphocyte count of 67,000/μL. Subsequent flow cytometry reveals a monoclonal B-cell population with restricted kappa expression, CD5+, CD19+, CD20 (dim positive), and CD23+, con-firming the diagnosis of chronic lymphocytic leukemia (CLL). The patient denies any symptoms, and physical exam is unremarkable. Which of the following is the next best step in managing this patient?
   A. Start ibrutinib
   B. Observation
   C. CT of the chest, abdomen, and pelvis
   D. Bone marrow biopsy
   E. Start dexamethasone

3. A 64-year-old woman who was diagnosed with chronic lymphocytic leukemia (CLL) 4 years ago and has not required any treatment to date presents to the ED for significant dizziness and dyspnea with minimal exertion, without any other symptoms. Complete blood count (CBC) reveals a white blood cell (WBC) count of 38.0×10^8/L with 88% lym-phocytes, a hemoglobin (Hgb) of 7.5 g/dL, with a mean corpuscular volume (MCV) of 88 fL, and a platelet of 330×10^8/L. Additional labs demonstrate no nutritional deficiencies, but direct antiglobulin test, haptoglobin, reticulocyte count, and lactate dehydrogenase support autoimmune hemolytic anemia (AIHA). Bone marrow biopsy shows 15% involve-ment of her CLL, and erythroid precursors are present and increased. What is the next appropriate step in management?
   A. Start ibrutinib
   B. Fluorescent in situ hybridization (FISH) to assess for del(13q), del(11q), del(17p), +12, and *TP53* mutation and *IGHV* mutation analyses
   C. Fludarabine, cyclophosphamide, and rituximab (FCR)
   D. Prednisone 1 mg/kg daily
   E. Rituximab monotherapy

4. A 62-year-old male with a past medical history (PMH) of hypertension on lisinopril presents due to "lumps" along his right neck and significant progressive fatigue over the past 6 months. Physical exam reveals right cervical, supraclavicular, and axillary

lymphadenopathy (LAD). Complete blood count (CBC) shows a white blood cell (WBC) count of 101×10^8/L with 81% lymphocytes, a platelet of 77×10^8/L, and a normal hemoglobin (Hgb). Flow cytometry confirms chronic lymphocytic leukemia (CLL), and fluorescent in situ hybridization (FISH) is remarkable for del(17p). *IGHV* is unmutated. What is the next appropriate step in managing this patient?

A. Chemoimmunotherapy
B. Venetoclax ± obinutuzumab
C. Ibrutinib
D. High-dose chemotherapy followed by autologous hematopoietic stem cell transplantation
E. B or C

5. Which of the following is false regarding chronic lymphocytic leukemia (CLL) and its management?

A. CLL most commonly presents asymptomatically
B. CLL undergoing Richter's transformation (RT) resembling diffuse large B-cell lymphoma (DLBCL) should always be considered for a clinical trial upfront
C. Ibrutinib is generally given indefinitely until disease progression or unacceptable toxicity
D. Ibrutinib has high complete remission (CR) and measurable residual disease (MRD)-negativity rates
E. Small molecular inhibitor-based regimens, such as ibrutinib, acalabrutinib ± obinutuzumab, or venetoclax ± obinutuzumab, are the preferred first-line treatments irrespective of age, performance status (PS), and comorbidities

6. A 66-year-old female who was recently diagnosed with chronic lymphocytic leukemia (CLL) and started on ibrutinib 1 week ago calls in as she noted her white blood cell (WBC) count increased from 135×10^8/L to 205×10^8/L. She denies any fevers or localizing infectious symptoms or any new symptoms since starting ibrutinib. Which of the following is the most appropriate step in managing this patient?

A. Assure her that this is secondary to ibrutinib and continue to monitor
B. Recommend that she present to the ED to rule out an occult infectious cause of rapid rise in WBC count
C. Recommend that she present to the ED for leukapheresis as she is at high risk for leukostasis
D. Schedule urgent follow-up with her as her disease is progressing
E. Increase dose of ibrutinib

7. A 68-year-old male underwent percutaneous coronary intervention with placement of two coronary stents 4 months ago. He is currently on dual anti-platelet therapy and presents to the ED with increasing abdominal pain over the past 2 months that has rendered him unable to perform activities of daily living (ADLs). Abdominal exam is notable for splenomegaly 10 cm below the left costal margin. A complete blood count (CBC) at this time shows white blood cell (WBC) count of 76×10^8/L with 81% lymphocytes, a hemoglobin (Hgb) of 9.2 g/dL, and platelets of 77×10^8/L. A full diagnostic workup is performed and he is ultimately diagnosed with chronic lymphocytic leukemia (CLL). *IGHV* is unmutated, but no *TP53* mutation is detected and fluorescent in situ hybridization (FISH) is unremarkable. His hematologist determines that treatment is necessary given his symptomatic disease interfering with his performance status (PS; Eastern Cooperative Oncology Group

[ECOG] 3) and cytopenias. Which of the following would be the most ideal treatment option for this patient?

A. Ibrutinib

B. Venetoclax ± obinutuzumab

C. Acalabrutinib ± obinutuzumab

D. Dexamethasone

E. Fludarabine, cyclophosphamide, and rituximab (FCR)

8. A 45-year-old male is diagnosed with chronic lymphocytic leukemia (CLL) after presenting with early satiety and 35 lbs weight loss over the past 3 months. Fluorescent in situ hybridization (FISH) shows a del(13q), and further analysis reveals a mutated *IGHV* and an unmutated *TP53*. His Eastern Cooperative Oncology Group (ECOG) is 0 and he has no other comorbidities. Given his anorexia, his hematologist decides to treat him and reviews his treatment options. The patient is interested in treatment, but prefers the shortest regimen possible, whether he has to present for an IV infusion or not. Which of the following is an acceptable first-line treatment in this patient?

A. Fludarabine, cyclophosphamide, and rituximab (FCR)

B. Obinutuzumab monotherapy

C. Rituximab plus dexamethasone

D. Allogeneic hematopoietic stem cell transplantation (allo-HSCT)

E. Advise the patient that given the cytogenetic profile, small molecular inhibitor therapy is the most reasonable option

9. The patient from question 8 is successfully treated with 6 cycles of fludarabine, cyclophosphamide, and rituximab (FCR) and achieved complete remission (CR) and measurable residual disease (MRD) negativity by flow. However, since completion of treatment, he has required three hospitalizations over the past 8 months for pneumonia. His complete blood count (CBC) is within normal limits. In addition to continuing trimethoprim/sulfamethoxazole prophylaxis, which of the following is appropriate?

A. Granulocyte colony-stimulating factor (G-CSF) support at scheduled intervals until the patient remains infection-free for 6 months or more

B. Prophylaxis with levofloxacin

C. Bone marrow biopsy to rule out persistent chronic lymphocytic leukemia (CLL)

D. Routine intravenous immunoglobulin (IVIg) to maintain a nadir of 500 mg/dL

10. Which of the following regarding chronic lymphocytic leukemia (CLL) and its treatment is true?

A. Patients starting ibrutinib should be hospitalized for the first few days of treatment to watch for signs of leukostasis

B. Patients starting venetoclax-based regimens should undergo CT assessment of lymphadenopathy (LAD)

C. Patients with CLL treated with ibrutinib are not at risk for fungal infections

D. Persistent lymphocytosis after 6 months of ibrutinib indicates treatment failure

E. Cytopenias are not a typical complication of Bruton tyrosine kinase (BTK) inhibitors

ANSWERS AND RATIONALES

1. **C. PET/CT.** This patient with rapid development of B-symptoms and lymphadenopathy (LAD) is concerning for Richter's transformation (RT). Although excisional biopsy is the preferred method of obtaining tissue, this should be targeted toward the lesion on PET/CT with the highest fluorodeoxyglucose (FDG)-avidity if feasible. Ibrutinib would be appropriate if biopsy confirms CLL progression rather than histological transformation.

2. **B. Observation.** The patient does not meet any of the international workshop on chronic lymphocytic leukemia (iwCLL) criteria to begin treatment and should thus be carefully monitored. A bone marrow biopsy is not required to establish the diagnosis of CLL, and CT scans are not routinely a part of the initial evaluation, unless clinically indicated.

3. **D. Prednisone 1 mg/kg daily.** In the absence of indications for CLL-directed therapy as per the international workshop on chronic lymphocytic leukemia (iwCLL) criteria, autoimmune hemolytic anemia (AIHA) should be treated the same as any other patient without CLL, starting with steroids. Rituximab is generally used in steroid-refractory AIHA. Cytogenetic and mutational analyses would be appropriate if the patient met the criteria for CLL treatment. Fludarabine is associated with an increased risk of AIHA and should be avoided if treatment for CLL was indicated.

4. **E. B or C.** With a del(17p) and unmutated *IGHV*, this patient will have a poor response to chemoimmunotherapy, and thus, a small molecule inhibitor should be considered. Therefore, either ibrutinib or venetoclax-based therapy is appropriate. Autologous hematopoietic cell transplantation is not indicated in frontline CLL management.

5. **D. Ibrutinib has high complete remission (CR) and measurable residual disease (MRD) negativity rates.** Ibrutinib induces mostly partial but very durable responses.

6. **A. Assure her that this is secondary to ibrutinib and continue to monitor.** Bruton tyrosine kinase (BTK) inhibitors induce a well-described lymphocytosis upon initiation and even re-initiation of therapy, which should not be confused for disease progression. This generally resolves within 8 months. In some patients it may persist more than 12 months, but it does not correlate with overall prognosis. CLL does not typically cause leukostasis.

7. **B. Venetoclax ± obinutuzumab.** It is best to avoid Bruton tyrosine kinase (BTK) inhibitors in patients with a risk for a major or life-threatening hemorrhage, either from an irreversible cause or because the patient is on dual antiplatelet therapy or long-term anticoagulation. FCR should not be used in a patient with an unmutated *IGHV*.

8. **A. Fludarabine, cyclophosphamide, and rituximab (FCR).** Chemoimmunotherapy has become less routinely used in the era of small molecular inhibitors for CLL. However, for a young and fit patient with a mutated *IGHV* and no *TP53* mutations/del(17p), FCR is a reasonable option as it can lead to disease-free intervals greater than 10 years in these patients.[1] While small molecular inhibitors are the preferred agents now regardless of age, fitness, and cytogenetics, their duration is longer than that of chemoimmunotherapy, so given his preferences, FCR is acceptable in this particular patient. Obinutuzumab monotherapy may be appropriate in a patient unable to tolerate other therapies due to age or comorbidities, but would not apply to this particular patient. Allo-HSCT is not indicated as first-line treatment for CLL.

9. **D. Routine intravenous immunoglobulin (IVIg) to maintain a nadir of 500 mg/dL.** Patients with CLL, especially those previously treated with chemoimmunotherapy, are generally at risk for infectious complications due to low immunoglobulin (Ig) levels.[37] In patients

experiencing recurrent sinopulmonary infections requiring hospitalization and Ig levels less than 500 mg/dL, monthly IVIg targeting a nadir of 500 mg/dL can reduce infection rates, but does not increase overall survival (OS). Prophylaxis with levofloxacin or routine use of G-CSF post-treatment for CLL is not commonly done, and the infection risk in CLL patients is due to hypogammaglobulinemia as opposed to neutropenia.

10. **B. Patients starting venetoclax-based regimens should undergo CT assessment of lymphade-nopathy (LAD).** Venetoclax leads to an increased risk of tumor lysis syndrome (TLS) when used for CLL treatment. Careful assessment of tumor burden by lymph node (LN) size and absolute lymphocyte count can guide management. Specifically, patients should receive intra-venous (IV) hydration and allopurinol at minimum prior to initiating venetoclax with close monitoring of TLS labs. Patients should undergo radiographical assessment of LNs for proper TLS risk stratification. Patients at high risk of TLS (that is, any LN size of 10 cm or greater or have an absolute lymphocyte count of 25×10^8/L or greater with an LN of 5 cm or greater) should be admitted for their first 20-mg and 50-mg dose, and can receive subsequent ramp-ups outpatient. The lymphocytosis seen with ibrutinib is expected; it can persist past 6 months and would not indicate treatment failure. Furthermore, ibrutinib more commonly induces partial remission (PR) rather than complete remission (CR), so lymphocytosis may persist indefinitely while on ibrutinib. Leukocytosis seen with CLL in general does not cause leukostasis. Fungal infections can be seen in patients treated with ibrutinib. Cytopenias are seen with ibrutinib.

REFERENCES

1. Burger JA. Treatment of chronic lymphocytic leukemia. *N Engl J Med.* 2020;383(5):460-473. doi:10.1056/NEJMra1908213
2. Surveillance, Epidemiology, and End Results Program. Cancer stat facts: leukemia—chronic lymphocytic leu-kemia (CLL). National Cancer Institute. Accessed June 8, 2022. https://seer.cancer.gov/statfacts/html/clyl.html
3. Catovsky D, Else M, Oscier D. The clinical presentation of CLL. In: Hallek M, Eichhorst B, Catovsky D, eds. *Chronic Lymphocytic Leukemia.* Springer International Publishing; 2019:39–50.
4. Hallek M, Cheson BD, Catovsky D, et al. iwCLL guidelines for diagnosis, indications for treatment, response assessment, and supportive management of CLL. *Blood.* 2018;131(25):2745–2760. doi:10.1182/blood-2017-09-806398
5. Rai KR, Sawitsky A, Cronkite EP, Chanana AD, Levy RN, Pasternack BS. Clinical staging of chronic lympho-cytic leukemia. *Blood.* 1975;46(2):219–234. doi:10.1182/blood.V46.2.219.219
6. Wierda WG, Byrd JC, Abramson JS, et al. Chronic lymphocytic leukemia/small lymphocytic lymphoma, ver-sion 4.2020, NCCN clinical practice guidelines in oncology. *J Natl Compr Canc Netw.* 2020;18(2):185–217. doi:10.6004/jnccn.2020.0006
7. Furman RR, Allan JN, Howes AJ, Mahler M, Wildgust MA. Comparing overall survival (OS) outcomes in patients with newly diagnosed chronic lymphocytic leukemia (CLL) with normal life expectancy. *J Clin Oncol.* 2016;34(3_suppl):7. doi:10.1200/jco.2016.34.3_suppl.7
8. Hallek M. Chronic lymphocytic leukemia: 2020 update on diagnosis, risk stratification and treatment. *Am J Hematol.* 2019;94(11):1266–1287. doi:10.1002/ajh.25595
9. Catovsky D, Muller-Hermelink HK, Ralfkiaer E, eds. T-cell prolymphocytic leukaemia. In: Swerdlow SH, Campo E, Harris NL, et al., eds. *WHO Classification of Tumours or Haematopoietic and Lymphoid Tissues.* 4th ed. Lyon; 2008:346–347.
10. Puente XS, Jares P, Campo E. Chronic lymphocytic leukemia and mantle cell lymphoma: crossroads of genetic and microenvironment interactions. *Blood.* 2018;131(21):2283–2296. doi:10.1182/blood-2017-10-764373
11. Marti GE, Rawstron AC, Ghia P, et al. Diagnostic criteria for monoclonal B-cell lymphocytosis. *Br J Haematol.* 2005;130(3):325–332. doi:10.1111/j.1365-2141.2005.05550.x
12. Rawstron AC, Shanafelt T, Lanasa MC, et al. Different biology and clinical outcome according to the absolute numbers of clonal B-cells in monoclonal B-cell lymphocytosis (MBL). *Cytometry B Clin Cytom.* 2010;78(suppl 1):S19–S23. doi:10.1002/cyto.b.20533
13. Swerdlow SH, Campo E, Pileri SA, et al. The 2016 revision of the World Health Organization classification of lymphoid neoplasms. *Blood.* 2016;127(20):2375–2390. doi:10.1182/blood-2016-01-643569
14. Singh N, Singh Lubana S, Dabrowski L, Sidhu G. Leukostasis in chronic lymphocytic leukemia. *Am J Case Rep.* 2020;21:e924798. doi:10.12659/AJCR.924798

15. Binet JL, Leporrier M, Dighiero G, et al. A clinical staging system for chronic lymphocytic leukemia: prognostic significance. *Cancer*. 1977;40(2):855–864. doi:10.1002/1097-0142(197708)40:2<855::aid-cncr2820400239>3.0.co;2-1

16. Binet JL, Auquier A, Dighiero G, et al. A new prognostic classification of chronic lymphocytic leukemia derived from a multivariate survival analysis. *Cancer*. 1981;48(1):198–206. doi:10.1002/1097-0142(19810701)48:1<198::aid-cncr2820480131>3.0.co;2-v

17. Pflug N, Bahlo J, Shanafelt TD, et al. Development of a comprehensive prognostic index for patients with chronic lymphocytic leukemia. *Blood*. 2014;124(1):49–62. doi:10.1182/blood-2014-02-556399

18. Burger JA, Tedeschi A, Barr PM, et al. Ibrutinib as initial therapy for patients with chronic lymphocytic leukemia. *N Engl J Med*. 2015;373(25):2425–2437. doi:10.1056/NEJMoa1509388

19. Burger JA, Barr PM, Robak T, et al. Long-term efficacy and safety of first-line ibrutinib treatment for patients with CLL/SLL: 5 years of follow-up from the phase 3 RESONATE-2 study. *Leuk*. 2020;34(3):787–798. doi:10.1038/s41375-019-0602-x

20. Woyach JA, Ruppert AS, Heerema NA, et al. Ibrutinib regimens versus chemoimmunotherapy in older patients with untreated CLL. *N Engl J Med*. 2018;379(26):2517–2528. doi:10.1056/NEJMoa1812836

21. Shanafelt TD, Wang XV, Kay NE, et al. Ibrutinib–rituximab or chemoimmunotherapy for chronic lymphocytic leukemia. *N Engl J Med*. 2019;381(5):432–443. doi:10.1056/NEJMoa1817073

22. Fischer K, Al-Sawaf O, Bahlo J, et al. Venetoclax and obinutuzumab in patients with CLL and coexisting conditions. *N Engl J Med*. 2019;380(23):2225–2236. doi:10.1056/NEJMoa1815281

23. Sharman JP, Egyed M, Jurczak W, et al. Acalabrutinib with or without obinutuzmab versus chlorambucil and obinutuzmab for treatment-naive chronic lymphocytic leukaemia (ELEVATE TN): a randomised, controlled, phase 3 trial. *Lancet*. 2020;395(10232):1278–1291. doi:10.1016/S0140-6736(20)30262-2

24. Byrd JC, Furman RR, Coutre SE, et al. Ibrutinib treatment for first-line and relapsed/refractory chronic lymphocytic leukemia: final analysis of the pivotal phase Ib/II PCYC-1102 study. *Clin Cancer Res*. 2020;26(15):3918–3927. doi:10.1158/1078-0432.CCR-19-2856

25. Thompson PA, Tam CS, O'Brien SM, et al. Fludarabine, cyclophosphamide, and rituximab treatment achieves long-term disease-free survival in IGHV-mutated chronic lymphocytic leukemia. *Blood*. 2016;127(3):303–309. doi:10.1182/blood-2015-09-667675

26. Go RS, Winters JL, Kay NE. How I treat autoimmune hemolytic anemia. *Blood*. 2017;129(22):2971–2979. doi:10.1182/blood-2016-11-693689

27. Woyach JA, Smucker K, Smith LL, et al. Prolonged lymphocytosis during ibrutinib therapy is associated with distinct molecular characteristics and does not indicate a suboptimal response to therapy. *Blood*. 2014;123(12):1810–1817. doi:10.1182/blood-2013-09-527853

28. Kovacs G, Robrecht S, Fink AM, et al. Minimal residual disease assessment improves prediction of outcome in patients with chronic lymphocytic leukemia (CLL) who achieve partial response: comprehensive analysis of two phase III studies of the German CLL Study Group. *J Clin Oncol*. 2016;34(31):3758–3765. doi:10.1200/JCO.2016.67.1305

29. Molica S, Giannarelli D, Montserrat E. Minimal residual disease and survival outcomes in patients with chronic lymphocytic leukemia: a systematic review and meta-analysis. *Clin Lymphoma Myeloma Leuk*. 2019;19(7):423–430. doi:10.1016/j.clml.2019.03.014

30. Kater AP, Seymour JF, Hillmen P, et al. Fixed duration of venetoclax-rituximab in relapsed/refractory chronic lymphocytic leukemia eradicates minimal residual disease and prolongs survival: post-treatment follow-up of the MURANO phase III study. *J Clin Oncol*. 2019;37(4):269–277. doi:10.1200/JCO.18.01580

31. Kater AP, Kipps TJ, Eichhorst B, et al. Five-year analysis of murano study demonstrates enduring undetectable minimal residual disease (uMRD) in a subset of relapsed/refractory chronic lymphocytic leukemia (R/R CLL) patients (Pts) following fixed-duration venetoclax-rituximab (VenR) therapy (Tx). *Blood*. 2020;136(suppl 1):19–21. doi:10.1182/blood-2020-136109

32. Rawstron AC, Fazi C, Agathangelidis A, et al. A complementary role of multiparameter flow cytometry and high-throughput sequencing for minimal residual disease detection in chronic lymphocytic leukemia: an European Research Initiative on CLL study. *Leukemia*. 2016;30(4):929–936. doi:10.1038/leu.2015.313

33. Gimondi S, Cavanè A, Vendramin A, et al. Identification of clonal IGH gene rearrangements by high-throughput sequencing of cell free DNA in multiple myeloma patients. *Blood*. 2015;126(23):2987. doi:10.1182/blood.V126.23.2987.2987

34. Pharmacyclics. Imbruvica prescribing information. Revised February 2018. https://www.accessdata.fda.gov/drugsatfda_docs/label/2018/210563s000lbl.pdf

35. AstraZeneca Pharmaceuticals. Calquence prescribing information. Revised October 2017. https://www.accessdata.fda.gov/drugsatfda_docs/label/2017/210259s000lbl.pdf

36. Hwang JP, Somerfield MR, Alston-Johnson DE, et al. Hepatitis B virus screening for patients with cancer before therapy: American Society of Clinical Oncology provisional clinical opinion update. *J Clin Oncol*. 2015;33(19):2212–2220. doi:10.1200/JCO.2015.61.3745

37. Tsai H-T, Caporaso NE, Kyle RA, et al. Evidence of serum immunoglobulin abnormalities up to 9.8 years before diagnosis of chronic lymphocytic leukemia: a prospective study. *Blood*. 2009;114(24):4928–4932. doi:10.1182/blood-2009-08-237651

38. Sun C, Tian X, Lee YS, et al. Partial reconstitution of humoral immunity and fewer infections in patients with chronic lymphocytic leukemia treated with ibrutinib. *Blood*. 2015;126(19):2213–2219. doi:10.1182/blood-2015-04-639203

39. Chapel H, Dicato M, Gamm H, et al. Immunoglobulin replacement in patients with chronic lymphocytic leukaemia: a comparison of two dose regimes. *Br J Haematol*. 1994;88(1):209–212. doi:10.1111/j.1365-2141.1994.tb05002.x

40. Boughton BJ, Jackson N, Lim S, Smith N. Randomized trial of intravenous immunoglobulin prophylaxis for patients with chronic lymphocytic leukaemia and secondary hypogammaglobulinaemia. *Clin Lab Haematol*. 1995;17(1):75–80. doi:10.1111/j.1365-2257.1995.tb00322.x

41. Molica S, Musto P, Chiurazzi F, et al. Prophylaxis against infections with low-dose intravenous immunoglobulins (IVIG) in chronic lymphocytic leukemia. Results of a crossover study. *Haematologica*. 1996;81(2):121–126. https://haematologica.org/article/view/759

42. AbbVie, Genentech USA. Venclexta prescribing information. Revised April 2016. https://www.accessdata.fda.gov/drugsatfda_docs/label/2016/208573s000lbl.pdf

43. Tsimberidou A-M, O'Brien S, Kantarjian HM, et al. Hodgkin transformation of chronic lymphocytic leukemia: the M. D. Anderson Cancer Center experience. *Cancer*. 2006;107(6):1294–1302. doi:10.1002/cncr.22121

44. Bockorny B, Codreanu I, Dasanu CA. Hodgkin lymphoma as Richter transformation in chronic lymphocytic leukaemia: a retrospective analysis of world literature. *Br J Haematol*. 2012;156(1):50–66. doi:10.1111/j.1365-2141.2011.08907.x

45. Scandurra M, Rossi D, Deambrogi C, et al. Genomic profiling of Richter's syndrome: recurrent lesions and differences with de novo diffuse large B-cell lymphomas. *Hematol Oncol*. 2010;28(2):62–67. doi:10.1002/hon.932

46. Rossi D, Rasi S, Spina V, et al. Different impact of NOTCH1 and SF3B1 mutations on the risk of chronic lymphocytic leukemia transformation to Richter syndrome. *Br J Haematol*. 2012;158(3):426–429. doi:10.1111/j.1365-2141.2012.09155.x

47. Villamor N, Conde L, Martínez-Trillos A, et al. NOTCH1 mutations identify a genetic subgroup of chronic lymphocytic leukemia patients with high risk of transformation and poor outcome. *Leukemia*. 2013;27(5):1100–1106. doi:10.1038/leu.2012.357

48. Chigrinova E, Rinaldi A, Kwee I, et al. Two main genetic pathways lead to the transformation of chronic lymphocytic leukemia to Richter syndrome. *Blood*. 2013;122(15):2673–2682. doi:10.1182/blood-2013-03-489518

49. Fabbri G, Khiabanian H, Holmes AB, et al. Genetic lesions associated with chronic lymphocytic leukemia transformation to Richter syndrome. *J Exp Med*. 2013;210(11):2273–2288. doi:10.1084/jem.20131448

50. Rossi D, Spina V, Deambrogi C, et al. The genetics of Richter syndrome reveals disease heterogeneity and predicts survival after transformation. *Blood*. 2011;117(12):3391–3401. doi:10.1182/blood-2010-09-302174

51. Bruzzi JF, Macapinlac H, Tsimberidou AM, et al. Detection of Richter's transformation of chronic lymphocytic leukemia by PET/CT. *J Nucl Med*. 2006;47(8):1267–1273. https://jnm.snmjournals.org/content/47/8/1267

52. Noy A, Schöder H, Gönen M, et al. The majority of transformed lymphomas have high standardized uptake values (SUVs) on positron emission tomography (PET) scanning similar to diffuse large B-cell lymphoma (DLBCL). *Ann Oncol*. 2009;20(3):508–512. doi:10.1093/annonc/mdn657

53. Papajík T, Myslíveček M, Urbanová R, et al. 2-[18F]fluoro-2-deoxy-D-glucose positron emission tomography/computed tomography examination in patients with chronic lymphocytic leukemia may reveal Richter transformation. *Leuk Lymphoma*. 2014;55(2):314–319. doi:10.3109/10428194.2013.802313

54. Mao Z, Quintanilla-Martinez L, Raffeld M, et al. IgVH mutational status and clonality analysis of Richter's transformation: diffuse large B-cell lymphoma and Hodgkin lymphoma in association with B-cell chronic lymphocytic leukemia (B-CLL) represent 2 different pathways of disease evolution. *Am J Surg Pathol*. 2007;31(10):1605–1614. doi:10.1097/PAS.0b013e31804bdaf8

55. Tsimberidou A-M, O'Brien S, Khouri I, et al. Clinical outcomes and prognostic factors in patients with Richter's syndrome treated with chemotherapy or chemoimmunotherapy with or without stem-cell transplantation. *J Clin Oncol*. 2006;24(15):2343–2351. doi:10.1200/JCO.2005.05.0187

56. Parikh SA, Habermann TM, Chaffee KG, et al. Hodgkin transformation of chronic lymphocytic leukemia: incidence, outcomes, and comparison to de novo Hodgkin lymphoma. *Am J Hematol*. 2015;90(4):334–338. doi:10.1002/ajh.23939

57. Cwynarski K, van Biezen A, de Wreede L, et al. Autologous and allogeneic stem-cell transplantation for transformed chronic lymphocytic leukemia (Richter's syndrome): a retrospective analysis from the chronic lymphocytic leukemia subcommittee of the chronic leukemia working party and lymphoma working party of the European Group for Blood and Marrow Transplantation. *J Clin Oncol*. 2012;30(18):2211–2217. doi:10.1200/JCO.2011.37.4108. Epub 2012 Apr 3

58. Al-Sawaf O, Robrecht S, Bahlo J, et al. Richter transformation in chronic lymphocytic leukemia (CLL)—a pooled analysis of German CLL Study Group (GCLLSG) front line treatment trials. *Leukemia*. 2021;35(1):169–176. doi:10.1038/s41375-020-0797-x

59. Wang Y, Tschautscher MA, Rabe KG, et al. Clinical characteristics and outcomes of Richter transformation: experience of 204 patients from a single center. *Haematologica*. 2020;105(3):765–773. doi:10.3324/haematol.2019.224121

CHAPTER 33

Myelodysplastic Syndrome

Tamer Othman and Brian A. Jonas

INTRODUCTION

Myelodysplastic syndrome (MDS) refers to a spectrum of myeloid neoplasms describing clonal proliferation of hematopoietic stem cells, ineffective hematopoiesis, cytopenias, and a tendency to progress to acute myeloid leukemia (AML).[1] The incidence of MDS in the general population is 4.5 per 100,000 individuals per year,[2] but increases to 26.9 per 100,000 in those between the ages of 70 to 79 years of age, and 55.4 per 100,000 in those 80 years of age and older. The median age of diagnosis is 71 years.[3]

MDS is thought to arise from the expansion of a somatically mutated clone of hematopoietic stem cells.[1] First, an initial driver mutation conferring a survival advantage occurs within a normal hematopoietic stem cell capable of self-renewal, forming a clonal population of aberrant hematopoietic progenitor and precursor cells. The next step involves migration and propagation of these abnormal stem cells through the peripheral blood and other bone marrow compartments, forming local clones in distinct bone marrow reservoirs throughout the body (that is, sternum, ilium, femur, and so on). Clonal hematopoiesis continues to increase, usually with the acquisition of more somatic mutations that also help to block differentiation, until it becomes significant in the bone marrow. Ultimately, clonal selection and proliferation occurs, leading to leukemic transformation, often with the assistance of additional driver mutations.[1]

Despite an improved understanding of MDS biology, therapeutic advances have been limited. Managing MDS is difficult given that the majority of patients are diagnosed at older ages, and often have several comorbidities and limited performance status (PS), prohibiting curative treatments like allogeneic hematopoietic cell transplantation (allo-HCT).[4] Management of MDS requires proper classification and risk stratification, along with careful assessment of comorbidities and attention to goals of care.

CASE SUMMARIES

Case 33.1: Myelodysplastic Syndrome With Excess Blasts-1

A 47-year-old female with previously diagnosed stage 3 hormone receptor-positive, human epidermal growth factor receptor 2 (HER2)-negative breast cancer is found to have a platelet count of 87 × 10⁹/L. Six years ago, she underwent lumpectomy and axillary lymph node (LN) dissection and received adjuvant dose-dense doxorubicin plus cyclophosphamide, followed by paclitaxel. She was placed on tamoxifen. Currently, her hemoglobin (Hgb) is 10.6 g/dL, and white blood cell (WBC) count is 3.7 × 10⁹/L with an absolute neutrophil count (ANC) of 2100/

μL. *Peripheral blood smear is significant for reduced hypogranular and large platelets. Three months ago, her platelets were 222 × 10⁹/L. She denies a history of alcohol use, and workup investigating nutritional deficiencies, viral infections, new medications, and liver pathology all return unremarkable.*

How Is a Diagnosis Established?

- MDS is a malignancy of the bone marrow leading to disrupted hematopoiesis.[5,6] This manifests as peripheral blood cytopenia(s), which is required for the diagnosis. Cytopenia(s) are defined by the World Health Organization (WHO) as Hgb less than 10 g/dL, ANC less than 1800/μL, and/or platelets less than 100,000 × 10⁹/L, for 4 to 6 months.[5] The remaining diagnostic criteria by the WHO 2016 criteria are summarized in Table 33.1. Thus, bone marrow examination is required to diagnose MDS.
- MDS also requires the exclusion of other causes of pancytopenia, such as medications, viral infections, and nutritional deficiencies.
- Of note, 20% or greater myeloblasts in the peripheral blood or bone marrow, or the presence of t(15;17), inv(16), or t(8;21) regardless of blast count, would be considered AML and not MDS.
- MDS should also be separated from other related indolent clonal hematopoietic disorders.[7]
  ○ Clonal hematopoiesis of indeterminant potential (CHIP): 1 somatic myeloid mutation without persistent cytopenia(s).
  ○ Idiopathic cytopenia of undetermined significance (ICUS): Cytopenia(s) for 6 months or greater without other causes, lacks somatic myeloid mutations, and does not fulfill diagnostic criteria of myeloid neoplasms/MDS.
  ○ Clonal cytopenia of undetermined significance (CCUS): 1 or more somatic myeloid mutation(s) with an allele frequency of 2% or greater plus cytopenia(s) for 4 months or more without other causes and does not fulfill diagnostic criteria of myeloid neoplasms/MDS.
  ○ Of note, CHIP and CCUS lack cytogenetic lesions.[7]
  ○ Those with these conditions have a low probability of developing a hematologic malignancy in their lifetime but are at a higher risk compared to those without such clonal disorders.[8] Thus, monitoring with complete blood counts (CBCs), at least every 6 months, is recommended (Table 33.1).[4]

The Patient's Diagnosis
- *The patient undergoes a bone marrow biopsy and is found to have greater than 10% dysplastic cells in the erythroid and megakaryocyte lineages and 5% blasts, giving her the diagnosis of MDS-EB-1.*

What Further Molecular or Genomic Testing Is Required?

- Cytogenetic and molecular characterization can help to determine diagnosis, prognosis, and management.

Patient's Molecular and Genomic Testing
- *Karyotyping reveals complex cytogenetics with greater than three abnormalities.*
- *Molecular panel reveals a TP53 mutation.*

How Is This Tumor Staged?

- MDS does not have a staging system, but risk stratification by the Revised International Prognostic Scoring System (IPSS-R) is used to help determine treatment goals and approaches (Table 33.2).[10] Lower-risk patients may be designated as patients scoring 3.5 or less, while higher-risk would be greater than 3.5.[4]

Table 33.1   Diagnostic Criteria for MDS in Adults by WHO 2016 Criteria[5]

Entity	# of Dysplastic Lineages	# of Cytopenias	% of RBCs With RS	BM/PB Blasts (No Auer Rods Present)	Cytogenetics
MDS with single lineage dysplasia (MDS-SLD)	1	1–2	<15%, or <5% + *SF3B1* mutation	BM <5%, PB <1%	Any if it doesn't fulfill criteria for MDS with isolated del(5q)
MDS with multi-lineage dysplasia (MDS-MLD)	2 or 3	1–3	<15%, or <5% + *SF3B1* mutation	BM <5%, PB <1%	Any if it doesn't fulfill criteria for MDS with isolated del(5q)
MDS-RS					
MDS-RS with single lineage dysplasia (MDS-RS-SLD)	1	1–2	<15%, or <5% + *SF3B1* mutation	BM <5%, PB <1%	Any if it doesn't fulfill criteria for MDS with isolated del(5q)
MDS-RS with multilineage dysplasia (MDS-RS-MLD)	2–3	1–3	<15%, or <5% + *SF3B1* mutation	BM <5%, PB <1%	Any if it doesn't fulfill criteria for MDS with isolated del(5q)
MDS with isolated del(5q)	1–3	1–2	Not accounted for	BM <5%, PB <1%	del(5q) alone or with 1 additional abnormality except –7 or del(7q)
MDS With Excess Blasts (MDS-EB)					
MDS-EB-1	0–3	1–3	Not accounted for	BM 5%–9% or PB 2%–4%	Any
MDS-EB-2	0–3	1–3	Not accounted for	BM 10%–19% or PB 5%–19%	Any
MDS, Unclassifiable (MDS-U)					
With 1% blood blasts	1–3	1–3	Not accounted for	BM <5%, PB = 1% on two assays	Any
With single lineage dysplasia and pancytopenia	1	3	Not accounted for	BM <5%, PB <1%	Any

(continued)

Table 33.1   Diagnostic Criteria for MDS in Adults by WHO 2016 Criteria[5] *(continued)*

Entity	# of Dysplastic Lineages	# of Cytopenias	% of RBCs With RS	BM/PB Blasts (No Auer Rods Present)	Cytogenetics
Based on defining cytogenetic abnormality[†]	0	1–3	<15% (≥15% RS are classified as MDS-RS-SLD)	BM <5%, PB <1%	MDS-defining abnormality
Refractory cytopenia of childhood	1–3	1–3	None	BM <5%, PB <2%	Any

[†] The WHO lists specific unbalanced, such as -7/del(7q), -5/del(5q), i(17q)/t(17p), -13/del(13q), del(11q), del(12p)/r(12p), del(9q), or idic(X)(q13), and balanced abnormalities, such as t(11;16)(q23;p13.3), t(3;21)(q26.2;q22.1), t(1;3)(p36.3;q21.1), t(2;11)(p21;q23), inv(3)(q21q26.2), or t(6;9)(p23;q34), that meet this criteria.[9]

BM, bone marrow; MDS, myelodysplastic syndrome; PB, peripheral blood; RBC, red blood cells; RS, ring sideroblasts; WHO, World Health Organization.

Source: Arber DA, Orazi A, Hasserjian R, et al. The 2016 revision to the World Health Organization classification of myeloid neoplasms and acute leukemia. *Blood.* 2016;127(20):2391–2405. doi:10.1182/blood-2016-03-643544

Table 33.2   IPSS-R

A) Variables considered for IPSS-R

Variable	Status	Point(s)
Cytogenetics	Very good: del(11q), -Y	0
	Good: normal karyotype, del(5q), del(12p), del(20q), double including del(5q)	1
	Intermediate: +8, del(7q), i(17q), + 19 or any other single or double independent clones	2
	Poor: -7, inv(3)/t(3q)/del(3q), double including -7/del(7q) or complex (3 abnormalities)	3
	Very poor: complex >3 abnormalities	4
Bone marrow blasts (%)	≤2	0
	>2 to <5	1
	5–10	2
	>10	3
Hgb (g/dL)	≥10	0
	8 to <10	1
	<8	1.5
Platelets (x 10^9/L)	≥100	0
	50 to <100	0.5
	<50	1

(continued)

Table 33.2   IPSS-R (continued)

A) Variables considered for IPSS-R

Variable	Status	Point(s)
ANC (10^9/L)	≥0.8	0
	<0.8	0.5

B) Variables translated into risk category

IPSS-R Risk Stratification	Total Score
Very low	≤1.5
Low	>1.5 to ≤3.0
Intermediate	>3.0 to ≤4.5
High	>4.5 to ≤6.0
Very high	>6.0

ANC, absolute neutrophil count; Hgb, hemoglobin; ISPP-R, Revised International Prognostic Scoring System.

Patient's Clinical Stage

- Her IPSS-R score is 6.5, placing her in the high-risk category for mortality and transformation to AML.

What Are Appropriate Treatment Options?

- Not all MDS requires treatment. In some instances, close observation ± supportive care is appropriate.[4]
- However, patients with higher-risk MDS are more likely to progress to AML; thus, treatment to modify the natural history of this disease and improve survival is indicated.
- Patients with higher-risk MDS (some cases of intermediate, high, or very high risk) should always be evaluated for allo-HCT, a potentially curative treatment for MDS.[11–13] Patients deemed eligible for allo-HCT may receive low or high intensity chemotherapy as a bridge to transplant during the donor search, although the true benefit of receiving chemotherapy prior to allo-HCT versus directly proceeding to transplant is not known at this time.[14]
- Low intensity options include the hypomethylating agents (HMAs), decitabine and azacitidine. Azacitidine demonstrated superior efficacy to conventional care, which was defined as best supportive care, low-dose cytarabine, or intensive chemotherapy, in the AZA-001 trial.[15] HMAs induce responses, although they are not durable, across high-risk biological subsets of MDS, such as those with *TP53* mutations.[16] In general, poor-risk cytogenetics, detectable peripheral blasts, high transfusion requirements, and a poor PS predict worse outcomes with MDS.[17] Neither HMA has demonstrated greater efficacy over the other in a prospective trial, so either choice is acceptable based on institutional availability and provider experience or preference.[18]
- More recently, the U.S. Food and Drug Administration (FDA) approved the combination of oral decitabine and cedazuridine, a cytidine deaminase inhibitor that allows for increased bioavailability of decitabine, based on a Phase 2 randomized crossover study that showed equal efficacy and safety to that of intravenous decitabine.[19]
- Higher intensity chemotherapy may lead to remissions but they are generally not durable; thus, they should be used only in patients planned for allo-HCT and need reduction in their disease burden prior to transplant.[4,20,21]

Table 33.3   Brief Summary of Response Criteria (Responses Need to Last 4 or More Weeks)

Response	Criteria
Complete remission	≤5% blasts in the bone marrow with normal maturation of all cell lines restored
	Persistent dysplasia must be within normal limits of dysplasia
	Hgb ≥11 g/dL
	Platelets ≥100 × 10⁹/L
	ANC ≥1.0 × 10⁹/L
	0% blasts in peripheral blood
Partial remission	All CR criteria if abnormal pretreatment, with the exception of:
	↓Bone marrow blasts by ≥50% over pretreatment but >5%
	Cellularity and morphology not relevant
Marrow complete remission	≤5% myeloblasts in bone marrow and ↓ ≥50% from pretreatment
Complete cytogenetic response	Complete disappearance of any chromosomal abnormalities
Partial cytogenetic response	≥50% reduction of the chromosomal abnormality
Hematologic Improvement	
Hgb response if <11 g/dL pretreatment	↑ Hgb by ≥1.5 g/dL
pRBC transfusion response	↓ # of units transfused by 4 units over 8 weeks compared to pretreatment. Only pRBC transfusions given for Hgb ≤9.0 g/dL count
Platelet response if <100 × 10⁹/L pretreatment	↑ by ≥30 × 10⁹/L if pretreatment platelets >20 × 10⁹/L
	↑ >20 × 10⁹/L and by 100% if <20 × 109/L
ANC	↑ by 100% and >500/μL

ANC, absolute neutrophil count; CR, complete response; Hgb, hemoglobin; pRBC, packed red blood cell.

Recommended Treatment Plan for This Patient

- *Given her young age, excellent PS, and seemingly cured breast cancer, she is selected for an allo-HCT, and begins oral decitabine-cedazuridine as the matched unrelated donor search takes place.*

What Are the Toxicities Associated With Hypomethylating Agents?

- The primary toxicities of HMAs are myelosuppression and related issues, nausea, and constipation.[22,23]
- Oral decitabine-cedazuridine induces cytopenias at a similar rate to intravenous decitabine.[24]

What Are Other Treatment Considerations?

Monitoring Response

- An International Working Group (IWG) developed criteria for assessing responses to therapy for MDS, including to alter the natural history of the disease (that is, increase

overall survival [OS] and time to AML transformation) and improve blood cell counts. Table 33.3 provides a brief summary of the IWG response criteria.[25]
- Two categories of HMA failure have been suggested.[26] Primary resistance is defined as progression to AML while on HMA therapy without ever achieving hematologic improvement; progression to a higher-risk MDS; or stable disease after 4 to 6 cycles (that is, never achieved complete or partial remission, a marrow complete remission, or no hematologic improvement) by the IWG criteria (Table 33.3).[25] Secondary resistance is defined as the emergence of any of the conditions of primary resistance after an initial response has been maintained for any number of cycles without having experienced HMA interruption or a delay greater than 5 weeks (Table 33.3).

The Patient's Outcome
- *She receives 4 cycles of decitabine-cedazuridine and undergoes a bone marrow biopsy.*
- *She achieves a complete remission and subsequently undergoes reduced-intensity conditioning and allo-HCT.*
- *She remains disease free 2 years post-HCT.*

Case 33.2: Myelodysplastic Syndrome With Ring Sideroblasts

A 75-year-old man with a history of chronic obstructive pulmonary disease (COPD) presents to his primary care provider (PCP) for 2 weeks of dizziness, fatigue, and near syncope after rising from a seated position earlier in the week. Physical exam is significant for conjunctival pallor, but no other remarkable findings. CBC returns showing a WBC of 5.5×10^9/L with an ANC of 3400/\mu L, an Hgb of 7.3 g/dL with a mean corpuscular volume (MCV) of 103 fL, and a platelet count of 175×10^9/L. Comprehensive metabolic panel (CMP) is unremarkable. Bone marrow biopsy shows greater than 10% dysplastic red blood cells (RBCs) with 6% ring sideroblasts (RS), with 2% blasts.

What Other Tests Are Required to Complete the Diagnostic Workup?

- A full molecular panel should be obtained, as that could help determine his subtype and, in some instances, may be predictive of response to specific therapies and prognosis.

The Patient's Final Diagnosis
- *He is noted to have a mutated SF3B1. Cytogenetics show 46,XY.*
- *His final diagnosis is MDS with ring sideroblasts with single lineage dysplasia (MDS-RS-SLD).*
- *By IPSS-R, he has very-low risk disease.*

What Are Treatment Options for Lower-Risk Myelodysplastic Syndrome?

- In contrast to higher-risk MDS, where the goal of treatment is to alter the natural course of MDS, the goal of managing lower-risk MDS is to improve blood counts in order to reduce complications and transfusion requirements, and improve quality of life.[14]
- Given the lower risk of disease-related mortality, a watch and wait approach is reasonable for many patients with lower-risk MDS, particularly in those with cytopenias with very mild symptoms, no increased blasts, or poor cytogenetics or molecular mutations, such as *ASXL1, RUNX1, TP53, EZH2,* and *ETV6*.[27]
- In patients with predominantly anemia and anemia-related symptoms, in the absence of del(5q), the next step would be to check an erythropoietin (EPO) level. Figure 33.1 summarizes an approach to treatment and supportive care tactics in lower-risk MDS. Notable from this figure are the following:

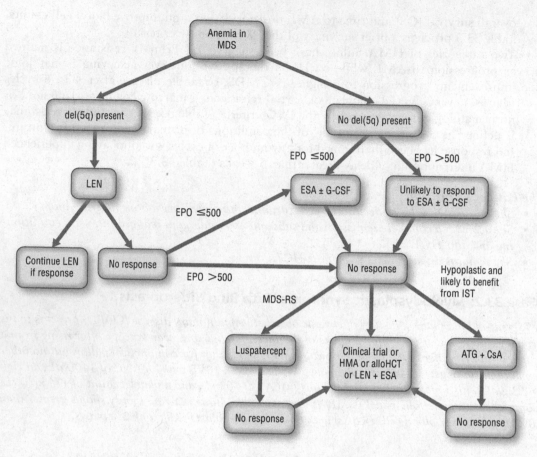

Figure 33.1 A proposed treatment and supportive care algorithm for anemia in lower-risk MDS

alloHCT, allogeneic hematopoietic cell transplantation; ATG, anti-thyocyte globulin; CsA, cyclosporine; EPO, erythropoictin; ESA, erythropoiesis-stimulating agent; G-CSF, granulocyte-colony stimulating factor; HMA, hypomethylating agent; IST, immunosuppressive therapy; LEN, lenalidomide; MDS, myelodysplastic syndrome; MDS-RS, MDS with ring sideroblasts.

- ○ Randomized data has demonstrated a synergistic effect with an erythropoiesis-stimulating agent (ESA) and granulocyte-colony stimulating factor (G-CSF) in patients with a low EPO level.[28] Moreover, a survival benefit has been reported with this combination, primarily in those requiring less than 2 transfusions per month.[29] This synergy is especially evident in patients with MDS-RS; thus, for this particular subset, starting with the combination of ESAs and G-CSF is recommended, while starting with EPO alone in lower-risk MDS without RS is acceptable.[4,25,30,31]
- ○ Responses with ESA generally occur within 3 months and have a median duration of response of 15 to 18 months.[32] If no response is seen by 12 weeks, G-CSF can be added to ESA.
- ○ Immunosuppressive therapy (IST) with anti-thymocyte globulin (ATG) and cyclosporine (CsA) has been reported to be primarily beneficial in patients 60 years of age or younger plus 5% or less bone marrow blasts, or patients with hypocellular bone marrows, a detectable paroxysmal nocturnal hemoglobinuria (PNH) clone, or signal transducer and activator of transcription 3 (STAT-3) mutant cytotoxic T-cell clones.[4]
- ○ Lenalidomide plus EPO has been shown to significantly improve erythroid response compared to lenalidomide alone in lower-risk MDS patients without del(5q) with ESA-refractory disease.[33]

- Patients with predominantly a clinically significant thrombocytopenia or neutropenia should be treated in the context of a clinical trial if available; otherwise, they should receive an HMA or ATG + CsA in select cases as previously discussed. In lower-risk patients with refractory or significant thrombocytopenia, thrombopoietin-stimulating agonists, such as eltrombopag or romiplostim, can be used.[34,35] Routine platelet transfusions in the absence of bleeding is not recommended if the platelet count is greater than 10×10^9/L. G-CSF support should be considered in neutropenic patients with MDS experiencing recurrent infections, although their use over an extended period of time has not been shown to increase survival (Figure 33.1).[4,36]

The Patient's Treatment Course
- *His EPO level is found to be 150 mU/mL, and he is started on EPO + filgastrim.*
- *His Hgb initially increases to 8.9 g/dL maximally off transfusions after 3 months of therapy; however, 7 months later his Hgb drops to 7.1 g/dL.*
- *He is next started on luspatercept.*

What Are the Toxicities Associated With Erythropoietin, Granulocyte Colony-Stimulating Factor, and Luspatercept?

- A very rare and serious complication of G-CSF is splenic rupture.[37]
- Utilization of ESAs in order to target an Hgb greater than 11 g/dL increases the risk of serious adverse cardiovascular events.[38] Other toxicities include hypertension, increased risk of seizures, and rarely pure red cell aplasia.[39]
- Common side effects with luspatercept include fatigue, GI intolerance, and hypertension.[40,41]

What Are Other Treatment Considerations?

- Prophylactic antibiotics are only recommended for recurrent infections.[4]
- If a patient has received 20 to 30 pRBC transfusions, iron chelation can be considered. In the event that serum ferritin levels exceed 2500 ng/mL, targeting a level less than 1000 ng/mL is reasonable.
- Consider treatment failure if no response to ESA ± G-CSF. Of note, if EPO is used as the first ESA, then one can consider switching to darbepoetin ± G-CSF for second-line treatment.
- Of note, patients with MDS-RS have a shorter median duration of response to ESAs than patients without RS, but still have synergy with G-CSF and respond well to the combination.[28-31,40]
- Luspatercept is an *SMAD2 to SMAD3* pathway inhibitor that enables RBC maturation and differentiation, and is indicated in patients with very-low to intermediate-risk MDS-RS with anemia, failing or not a candidate for (e.g., high EPO level) ESA therapy, and requiring 2 or more packed red blood cell (pRBC) transfusions over 8 weeks.[40,41]
- The key endpoint in the MEDALIST trial with luspatercept was transfusion independence for 8 or more weeks, which was seen in 38% of patients.[40]
- Luspatercept failure is defined as lack of a 1.5 g/dL increase in Hgb or lack of a pRBC transfusion requirement decrease at 3 to 6 months.
- If a patient is not pRBC transfusion-free after at least 2 consecutive doses (6 weeks) at the 1 mg/kg starting dose, the dose should be increased to 1.33 mg/kg.

The Patient's Outcome
- *The patient remains transfusion independent for 12 weeks on luspatercept.*

Case 33.3: Myelodysplastic Syndrome With Isolated Del(5q)

A 61-year-old man with a past medical history of basal cell carcinoma of the scalp, status post-surgical resection without chemotherapy or radiation 15 years ago, presents due to a 3-month history of progressive fatigue. Physical exam is notable for generalized pallor. CBC is obtained and shows an Hgb of 6.6 g/dL, an MCV of 105 fL, a WBC of 4.5 ×10⁹/L with an ANC of 3000/μL, and a platelet count of 202 × 10⁹/L. No blasts are seen on the differential or smear. A bone marrow biopsy is obtained which shows 1% blasts, greater than 10% dysplastic RBCs. Cytogenetics reveal a del(5q) with no other chromosomal abnormalities, and no mutations were seen on molecular profiling.

What Further Tests for Diagnosis and Therapy Planning Are Required at This Point?

- None: the bone marrow biopsy, as well as cytogenetic and molecular workup, should be performed in all cases of new MDS and have been completed here.

The Patient's Diagnosis and Risk Stratification

- *The patient meets the morphological criteria for MDS with a cytopenia, and shows an isolated del(5q) without a –7 or del(7q), meeting the criteria for MDS with isolated del(5q) as per Table 33.1.*
- *IPSS-R score stratifies his disease as low risk.*

What Are the Treatment Options and Considerations for MDS With Del(5q)?

- MDS with an isolated del(5q) may be treated with lenalidomide at 10 mg/day for 21 days out of every 28-day cycle or 28 days monthly, followed by a response assessment at the 2 to 4 month mark.[4,42,43] The efficacy of lenalidomide in MDS with del(5q) was seen in an international multicenter trial, where 112 of 148 patients (76%) had a decreased transfusion requirement, and 99 patients (67%) required no more transfusions.[44] The median duration of transfusion independence was not reached after a median follow-up of 104 weeks. Sixty-two of 85 evaluable patients (73%) had a cytogenetic improvement, 38 (45%) of whom had a complete cytogenetic remission.
- Lenalidomide failure is defined as a lack of a 1.5 g/dL increase in Hgb or lack of a pRBC transfusion decrease at 3 to 6 months.
- Lenalidomide is thought to induce a direct cytotoxic effect on the del(5q) clone, leading to a decrease in transfusion needs.
- Patients failing lenalidomide should follow the treatment pathway similar to those without del(5q), as depicted in Figure 33.1.
- Patients with a -7 or del(7q) should be treated as a higher-risk MDS.[4]

What Are the Toxicities Associated With Lenalidomide?

- Lenalidomide frequently induces thrombocytopenia and neutropenia in patients with MDS, and may require a dose reduction.[42]

The Patient's Outcome

- *The patient's Hgb improves to 9 to 10 g/dL after 2 months and begins to require a transfusion once every 8 weeks.*
- *Eight months after his response, he is immediately admitted from the hematology clinic after CBC shows 16% blasts in his peripheral blood with an Hgb of 7.0 g/dL.*
- *A bone marrow biopsy is obtained, and shows 26% blasts consistent with AML.*
- *The patient is started on CPX-351 and is referred for allo-HCT.*

1. Which of the following regarding myelodysplastic syndrome (MDS) and its treatment is false?
   A. Allogeneic hematopoietic cell transplantation (allo-HCT) is the only curative option
   B. MDS requires urgent treatment upon diagnosis to prevent leukemic transformation
   C. Cytopenia(s) are a diagnostic feature of all MDS subtypes per the World Health Organization (WHO) criteria
   D. Patients with high erythropoietin (EPO) levels are unlikely to respond to erythropoiesis-stimulating agent (ESA) ± granulocyte colony-stimulating factor (G-CSF)

2. A 69-year-old male presents to his primary care provider (PCP) with 3 weeks of progressive fatigue and dyspnea on exertion. Complete blood count (CBC) shows a white blood cell (WBC) count of 5.2×10^9/L (absolute neutrophil count [ANC] 3,100/μL), hemoglobin (Hgb) 8.1 g/dL (mean corpuscular volume [MCV] 101 fL), and platelets 255×10^9/L. The only medications the patient is on are lisinopril for hypertension and metformin for diabetes. Which of the following is the next appropriate step in managing this patient?
   A. Bone marrow biopsy with cytogenetic analysis and molecular profiling
   B. Nutritional deficiency and viral workup
   C. Repeat CBC in 6 weeks
   D. Erythropoietin (EPO)

3. The patient in question 2 is found to have normal folate, vitamin B12, and copper levels, and viral workup is negative. He undergoes a bone marrow biopsy and is diagnosed with myelodysplastic syndrome with ring sideroblasts (MDS-RS). Karyotype is normal. He has 1% blasts on his bone marrow biopsy and none in his peripheral blood. An erythropoietin (EPO) level returns at 196 mU/mL. What is the next best step in management?
   A. 7+3 followed by allogeneic hematopoietic cell transplantation (allo-HCT)
   B. Azacitidine
   C. Luspatercept
   D. Epoetin alfa plus granulocyte colony-stimulating factor (G-CSF)
   E. Supportive packed red blood cell (pRBC) transfusions alone

4. A 75-year-old male presented to his primary care provider (PCP) for dizziness over the past 2 weeks, and was found to have pancytopenia with a white blood cell (WBC) count of 2.9×10^9/L, hemoglobin (Hgb) of 7.5 g/dL, and platelets of 88×10^9/L. A bone marrow biopsy is performed, revealing 6% myeloblasts and overall consistent with myelodysplastic syndrome with excess blasts-1 (MDS-EB-1). Which of the following is the next best step in managing this patient?
   A. Clinical trial if available
   B. CPX-351 induction
   C. Azacitidine
   D. Epoetin alfa ± granulocyte colony-stimulating factor (G-CSF)

5. A patient who presented with progressive fatigue underwent a bone marrow biopsy after basic blood work failed to find a cause for a hempglobin (Hgb) of 7.0 g/dL, revealing myelodysplastic syndrome with ring sideroblasts (MDS-RS). He was initially trialed on epoetin alfa plus granulocyte colony-stimulating factor (G-CSF) given his erythropoietin (EPO) of 202 mU/mL, but after 3 months he still required weekly packed red blood cell (pRBC) transfusions. He was switched over to luspatercept 1 mg/kg, but after 2 doses, he is still requiring

weekly pRBC transfusions. His latest complete blood count (CBC) shows no change in his other counts, and no blasts. Which of the following is the best next step in management?

A. Repeat bone marrow biopsy to rule out leukemic transformation
B. Obtain parvovirus B19 serologies
C. Increase the dose of luspatercept to 1.33 mg/kg
D. Start azacitidine
E. Keep the luspatercept dose the same and continue for now

6. Which of the following regarding myelodysplastic syndrome (MDS) and its treatment is false?

A. Prophylactic antibiotics are only recommended for recurrent infections
B. In lower-risk patients with significant thrombocytopenia, thrombopoietin-stimulating agonists can be considered
C. Use of granulocyte colony-stimulating factor (G-CSF) has not been shown to improve overall survival (OS) in MDS
D. The only role for lenalidomide in treating MDS is in the presence of del(5q)
E. Acute myeloid leukemia (AML) is the final stage of the pathway leading to the pathogenesis of MDS

7. A 51-year-old male with no prior past medical history was in his usual state of health until he contracted an upper respiratory infection that persisted after 2 weeks. He presents to his local ED, where on complete blood count (CBC) he is found to have a white blood cell (WBC) count of $1.1 \times 10^9/L$ with an absolute neutrophil count (ANC) of 400/μL and 4% blasts. Hemoglobin (Hgb) is 9.1 g/dL and platelets are $111 \times 10^9/L$. The patient undergoes a bone marrow biopsy and is found to have 8% blasts. Cytogenetics reveal t(8;21), and molecular studies are still pending. Which of the following is the most appropriate next step in managing this patient?

A. 7 + 3 induction (add gemtuzumab ozogamicin if CD33+)
B. Azacitidine
C. Azithromycin
D. Begin donor search and plan for allogeneic hematopoietic cell transplantation (allo-HCT)
E. Supportive care

8. A 60-year-old female with a past medical history (PMH) of hyperthyroidism presents after developing shortness of breath, dizziness, and near syncope after walking up a flight of stairs. She reports previously having no limitations in her daily living. Physical examination was remarkable for pallor and scattered ecchymosis. Complete blood count (CBC) showed a white blood cell (WBC) count of $2.0 \times 10^9/L$ with an absolute neutrophil count (ANC) of 300/μL and 1% immature mononuclear cells, hemoglobin (Hgb) of 6.8 g/dL (mean corpuscular volume [MCV] 99 fL), and platelets of $15 \times 10^9/L$. Nutritional and viral workup is unremarkable. Her bone marrow aspirate and biopsy demonstrated an overall cellularity of 40% with trilineage dysplasia with 7% blasts. Karyotype revealed del(7). Which of the following is the most appropriate initial treatment for this patient?

A. Oral decitabine-cedazuridine
B. Referral for allogeneic hematopoietic cell transplantation (allo-HCT)
C. Lenalidomide
D. Anti-thymocyte globulin (ATG) + cyclosporine
E. A and B

9. Which of the following regarding hypomethylating agents (HMAs) is false?
   A. HMAs induce responses in high-risk biological subsets of myelodysplastic syndrome (MDS), such as those with *TP53* mutations
   B. Neither HMA has demonstrated greater efficacy over the other in a prospective trial
   C. Oral decitabine and cedazuridine has equal efficacy and safety to that of intravenous (IV) decitabine
   D. HMA responses are not durable, and thus should only be used if allogeneic hematopoietic cell transplantation (allo-HCT) is planned
   E. Cytopenias are a well-recognized complication of HMAs

10. A 62-year-old female with no prior past medical history (PMH) is noted to have a platelet of 99 × 10⁹/L, with an otherwise remarkable complete blood count (CBC). She denies alcohol use and does not take any medications or herbal agents. She denies arthralgias and other constitutional symptoms. Nutritional and viral workup and chemistry labs at that time are unrevealing. Abdominal ultrasound is also unremarkable. She is eventually referred to hematology, and repeat labs 5 months after her thrombocytopenia was discovered show a platelet count of 92 × 10⁹/L and an otherwise unremarkable CBC. She undergoes a bone marrow biopsy that shows a normocellular marrow without blasts or lineage dysplasia. Cytogenetics show 46,XX, and a *TET2* mutation with a variant allele frequency of 8% is noted on molecular profiling. Which of the following is her diagnosis?
    A. Clonal hematopoiesis of indeterminant potential (CHIP)
    B. Clonal cytopenia of undetermined significance (CCUS)
    C. Idiopathic cytopenia of undetermined significance (ICUS)
    D. Myelodysplastic syndrome (MDS)
    E. Acute myeloid leukemia (AML)

ANSWERS AND RATIONALES

1. **B. MDS requires urgent treatment upon diagnosis to prevent leukemic transformation.** Not all MDS requires treatment. In some instances, such as lower-risk MDS, close observation ± supportive care is appropriate.

2. **B. Nutritional deficiency and viral workup.** A diagnosis of myelodysplastic syndrome (MDS) requires exclusion of other causes of cytopenias that resemble MDS. A bone marrow biopsy will eventually be indicated if the rest of the anemia workup is unremarkable. Repeating the CBC without any further diagnostic workup would not be appropriate as his anemia would not correct itself without addressing the underlying cause. EPO may be useful depending on the etiology of his anemia, but addressing the underlying cause should be the priority.

3. **D. Epoetin alfa plus granulocyte colony-stimulating factor (G-CSF).** The patient has lower-risk MDS, and thus can just be managed with supportive care. Supportive pRBC transfusions alone will over time lead to iron overload, so therapy directed toward reducing transfusion burden is preferred, and the synergy of erythropoiesis-stimulating agent (ESA) + G-CSF in MDS-RS is well described.

4. **A. Clinical trial if available.** Patients with MDS, or in general any patient with cancer, should always be encouraged to enroll in a clinical trial when available. If none are available, azacitidine would be appropriate. CPX-351 is used for acute myeloid leukemia (AML) with myelodysplastic-related changes and therapy-related AML, not MDS. Supportive care alone would not be sufficient for higher-risk MDS.

5. **C. Increase the dose of luspatercept to 1.33 mg/kg.** Luspatercept failure is defined as a lack of a 1.5 g/dL increase in Hgb or lack of a pRBC transfusion decrease at 3 to 6 months. As the patient has only received 6 weeks of therapy, luspatercept should be continued rather than switching therapies. However, if the patient is still pRBC transfusion dependent after 2 doses, then the dose should be increased from 1.0 mg/kg to 1.33 mg/kg.

6. **D. The only role for lenalidomide in treating MDS is in the presence of del(5q).** Lenalidomide can be combined with erythropoiesis-stimulating agent (ESA) in patients with del(5q) who have failed ESA ± G-CSF.

7. **A. 7 + 3 induction (add gemtuzumab ozogamicin if CD33+).** Although his presentation may appear to be consistent with myelodysplastic syndrome with excess blasts-1 (MDS-EB-1), the presence of t(15;17), inv(16), or t(8;21) regardless of blast count would be considered acute myeloid leukemia (AML) and not myelodysplastic syndrome (MDS). Thus, he should be treated with intensive chemotherapy given his overall good state of health, performance status (PS), and core-binding factor AML. With the information available, he would be considered favorable-risk and may not need allo-HCT in first complete remission if his molecular profile doesn't elevate his risk status.

8. **E. A and B.** The patient has high-risk myelodysplastic syndrome (MDS) and, thus, should be treated with a hypomethylating agent (HMA). This patient is still in the age range of allo-HCT, and she appears to have limited comorbidities and good performance status (PS), so referral for transplant evaluation is appropriate. Immunosuppressive therapy (IST) is generally used for hypoplastic marrows. Lenalidomide is used to treat anemia in patients with del(5q) or non-del(5q) failing erythropoiesis-stimulating agent (ESA)-therapy.

9. **D. HMA responses are not durable, and thus should only be used if allogeneic hematopoietic cell transplantation (allo-HCT) is planned.** Although it is true that HMA responses are transient, they still may be used for palliative purposes in patients with high-risk MDS ineligible for allo-HCT to prolong overall survival (OS) and time to acute myeloid leukemia (AML) transformation.

10. **B. Clonal cytopenia of undetermined significance (CCUS).** The diagnostic criteria for CCUS is 1 or more somatic myeloid mutation with an allele frequency of 2% or greater plus cytopenia(s) for 4 or more months without other causes and does not fulfill diagnostic criteria of myeloid neoplasms/MDS. CHIP refers to 1 somatic myeloid mutation without persistent cytopenia(s). ICUS refers to cytopenia(s) for 6 or more months without other causes, lacks somatic myeloid mutations, and does not fulfill diagnostic criteria of myeloid neoplasms/MDS. The patient does not meet criteria for MDS based on the World Health Organization (WHO) criteria (Table 33.1), nor AML on the basis of less than 20% blasts in her bone marrow and no AML-defining cytogenetic lesion.

REFERENCES

1. Cazzola M. Myelodysplastic syndromes. *N Engl J Med*. 2020;383(14):1358–1374. doi:10.1056/NEJMra1904794
2. National Cancer Institute. Browse the SEER Cancer Statistics Review (CSR) 1975–2016. https://seer.cancer.gov/archive/csr/1975_2016/browse_csr.php?sectionSEL=30&pageSEL=sect_30_intro.01
3. Sallman DA, Padron E. Myelodysplasia in younger adults: outlier or unique molecular entity? *Haematologica*. 2017;102(6):967–968. doi:10.3324/haematol.2017.165993
4. Greenberg PL, Stone RM, Al-Kali A, et al. NCCN Guidelines® Insights: Myelodysplastic syndromes, version 3.2022. *J Natl Compr Canc Netw*. 2022 Feb;20(2):106–117. doi:10.6004/jnccn.2022.0009
5. Arber DA, Orazi A, Hasserjian R, et al. The 2016 revision to the World Health Organization classification of myeloid neoplasms and acute leukemia. *Blood*. 2016;127(20):2391–2405. doi:10.1182/blood-2016-03-643544
6. Della Porta MG, Travaglino E, Boveri E, et al. Minimal morphological criteria for defining bone marrow dysplasia: a basis for clinical implementation of WHO classification of myelodysplastic syndromes. *Leukemia*. 2015;29(1):66–75. doi:10.1038/leu.2014.161
7. DeZern AE, Malcovati L, Ebert BL. CHIP, CCUS, and other acronyms: definition, implications, and impact on practice. *Am Soc Clin Oncol Educ Book*. 2019;(39):400–410. doi:10.1200/EDBK_239083
8. Jaiswal S, Fontanillas P, Flannick J, et al. Age-related clonal hematopoiesis associated with adverse outcomes. *N Engl J Med*. 2014;371(26):2488–2498. doi:10.1056/NEJMoa1408617
9. Vardiman JW, Thiele J, Arber DA, et al. The 2008 revision of the World Health Organization (WHO) classification of myeloid neoplasms and acute leukemia: rationale and important changes. *Blood*. 2009;114(5):937–951. doi:10.1182/blood-2009-03-209262
10. Greenberg PL, Tuechler H, Schanz J, et al. Revised International Prognostic Scoring System for myelodysplastic syndromes. *Blood*. 2012;120(12):2454–2465. doi:10.1182/blood-2012-03-420489
11. de Witte T, Bowen D, Robin M, et al. Allogeneic hematopoietic stem cell transplantation for MDS and CMML: recommendations from an international expert panel. *Blood*. 2017;129(13):1753–1762. doi:10.1182/blood-2016-06-724500
12. Robin M, Porcher R, Zinke-Cerwenka W, et al. Allogeneic haematopoietic stem cell transplant in patients with lower risk myelodysplastic syndrome: a retrospective analysis on behalf of the Chronic Malignancy Working Party of the EBMT. *Bone Marrow Transplant*. 2017;52(2):209–215. doi:10.1038/bmt.2016.266
13. Platzbecker U, Mufti G. Allogeneic stem cell transplantation in MDS: How? When? *Best Pract & Res Clin Haematol*. 2013;26(4):421–429. doi:10.1016/j.beha.2013.09.008
14. Platzbecker U. Treatment of MDS. *Blood*. 2019;133(10):1096–1107. doi:10.1182/blood-2018-10-844696
15. Fenaux P, Mufti GJ, Hellstrom-Lindberg E, et al. Efficacy of azacitidine compared with that of conventional care regimens in the treatment of higher-risk myelodysplastic syndromes: a randomised, open-label, phase III study. *Lancet Oncol*. 2009;10(3):223–232. doi:10.1016/S1470-2045(09)70003-8
16. Welch JS, Petti AA, Miller CA, et al. TP53 and decitabine in acute myeloid leukemia and myelodysplastic syndromes. *N Engl J Med*. 2016;375(21):2023–2036. doi:10.1056/NEJMoa1605949
17. Itzykson R, Thépot S, Quesnel B, et al. Prognostic factors for response and overall survival in 282 patients with higher-risk myelodysplastic syndromes treated with azacitidine. *Blood*. 2011;117(2):403–411. doi:10.1182/blood-2010-06-289280

18. Lee Y-G, Kim I, Yoon S-S, et al. Comparative analysis between azacitidine and decitabine for the treatment of myelodysplastic syndromes. *Br J Haematol*. 2013;161(3):339–347. doi:10.1111/bjh.12256

19. Garcia-Manero G, Griffiths EA, Steensma DP, et al. Oral cedazuridine/decitabine for MDS and CMML: a phase 2 pharmacokinetic/pharmacodynamic randomized crossover study. *Blood*. 2020;136(6):674–683. doi:10.1182/blood.2019004143

20. Beran M, Shen Y, Kantarjian H, et al. High-dose chemotherapy in high-risk myelodysplastic syndrome: covariate-adjusted comparison of five regimens. *Cancer*. 2001;92(8):1999–2015. doi:10.1002/1097-0142(20011015)92:8<1999::aid-cncr1538>3.0.co;2-b

21. Tricot G, Boogaerts MA. The role of aggressive chemotherapy in the treatment of the myelodysplastic syndromes. *Br J Haematol*. 1986;63(3):477–483. doi:10.1111/j.1365-2141.1986.tb07524.x

22. Gao C, Wang J, Li Y, et al. Incidence and risk of hematologic toxicities with hypomethylating agents in the treatment of myelodysplastic syndromes and acute myeloid leukopenia: a systematic review and meta-analysis. *Medicine*. 2018;97(34):e11860. doi:10.1097/MD.0000000000011860

23. Celgene Corporation. Vidaza prescribing information. Revised August 2018. https://www.accessdata.fda.gov/drugsatfda_docs/label/2008/050794s011lbl.pdf

24. Otsuka Pharmaceutical Company. Inqovi prescribing information. Revised July 2020. https://www.accessdata.fda.gov/drugsatfda_docs/label/2020/212576s000lbl.pdf

25. Cheson BD, Greenberg PL, Bennett JM, et al. Clinical application and proposal for modification of the International Working Group (IWG) response criteria in myelodysplasia. *Blood*. 2006;108(2):419–425. doi:10.1182/blood-2005-10-4149

26. Santini V. How I treat MDS after hypomethylating agent failure. *Blood*. 2019;133(6):521–529. doi:10.1182/blood-2018-03-785915

27. Bejar R, Stevenson K, Abdel-Wahab O, et al. Clinical effect of point mutations in myelodysplastic syndromes. *N Engl J Med*. 2011;364(26):2496–2506. doi:10.1056/NEJMoa1013343

28. Balleari E, Rossi E, Clavio M, et al. Erythropoietin plus granulocyte colony-stimulating factor is better than erythropoietin alone to treat anemia in low-risk myelodysplastic syndromes: results from a randomized single-centre study. *Ann Hematol*. 2006;85(3):174–180. doi:10.1007/s00277-005-0044-6

29. Jädersten M, Malcovati L, Dybedal I, et al. Erythropoietin and granulocyte-colony stimulating factor treatment associated with improved survival in myelodysplastic syndrome. *J Clin Oncol*. 2008;26(21):3607–3613. doi:10.1200/JCO.2007.15.4906

30. Hellström-Lindberg E, Ahlgren T, Beguin Y, et al. Treatment of anemia in myelodysplastic syndromes with granulocyte colony-stimulating factor plus erythropoietin: results from a randomized phase II study and long-term follow-up of 71 patients. *Blood*. 1998;92(1):68–75. doi:10.1182/blood.V92.1.68.413k23_68_75

31. Hellström-Lindberg E, Negrin R, Stein R, et al. Erythroid response to treatment with G-CSF plus erythropoietin for the anaemia of patients with myelodysplastic syndromes: proposal for a predictive model. *Br J Haematol*. 1997;99(2):344–351. doi:10.1046/j.1365-2141.1997.4013211.x

32. Park S, Hamel J-F, Toma A, et al. Outcome of lower-risk patients with myelodysplastic syndromes without 5q deletion after failure of erythropoiesis-stimulating agents. *J Clin Oncol*. 2017;35(14):1591–1597. doi:10.1200/JCO.2016.71.3271

33. Toma A, Kosmider O, Chevret S, et al. Lenalidomide with or without erythropoietin in transfusion-dependent erythropoiesis-stimulating agent-refractory lower-risk MDS without 5q deletion. *Leukemia*. 2016;30(4):897–905. doi:10.1038/leu.2015.296

34. Platzbecker U, Wong RS, Verma A, et al. Safety and tolerability of eltrombopag versus placebo for treatment of thrombocytopenia in patients with advanced myelodysplastic syndromes or acute myeloid leukaemia: a multicentre, randomised, placebo-controlled, double-blind, phase 1/2 trial. *Lancet Haematol*. 2015;2(10):e417–e426. doi:10.1016/S2352-3026(15)00149-0

35. Fenaux P, Muus P, Kantarjian H, et al. Romiplostim monotherapy in thrombocytopenic patients with myelodysplastic syndromes: long-term safety and efficacy. *Br J Haematol*. 2017;178(6):906–913. doi:10.1111/bjh.14792

36. Fenaux P, Adès L. How we treat lower-risk myelodysplastic syndromes. *Blood*. 2013;121(21):4280–4286. doi:10.1182/blood-2013-02-453068

37. Amgen. Neupogen prescribing information. Revised February 2015. https://www.accessdata.fda.gov/drugsatfda_docs/label/2015/103353s5184lbl.pdf

38. Janssen Pharmaceutical. Epogen prescribing information. Revised September 2017. https://www.accessdata.fda.gov/drugsatfda_docs/label/2017/103234s5363s5366lbl.pdf

39. Schellekens H. Immunologic mechanisms of EPO-associated pure red cell aplasia. *Best Pract Res Clin Haematol*. 2005;18(3):473–480. doi:10.1016/j.beha.2005.01.016

40. Fenaux P, Platzbecker U, Mufti GJ, et al. Luspatercept in patients with lower-risk myelodysplastic syndromes. *N Engl J Med*. 2020;382(2):140–151. doi:10.1056/NEJMoa1908892

41. Celgene Corporation. Reblozyl prescribing information. Revised April 202. https://www.accessdata.fda.gov/drugsatfda_docs/label/2020/761136orig2lbl.pdf

42. Sekeres MA, Maciejewski JP, Giagounidis AA, et al. Relationship of treatment-related cytopenias and response to lenalidomide in patients with lower-risk myelodysplastic syndromes. *J Clin Oncol.* 2008;26(36):5943–5949. doi:10.1200/JCO.2007.15.5770

43. Revicki DA, Brandenburg NA, Muus P, Yu R, Knight R, Fenaux P. Health-related quality of life outcomes of lenalidomide in transfusion-dependent patients with low- or intermediate-1-risk myelodysplastic syndromes with a chromosome 5q deletion: results from a randomized clinical trial. *Leuk Res.* 2013;37(3):259–265. doi:10.1016/j.leukres.2012.11.017

44. List A, Dewald G, Bennett J, et al. Lenalidomide in the myelodysplastic syndrome with chromosome 5q deletion. *N Engl J Med.* 2006;355(14):1456–1465. doi:10.1056/NEJMoa061292

Index

abraxane, metastatic non-small cell
lung cancer, 46
ABVD. *See* adriamycin, bleomycin, vinblastine,
and dacarbazine
ACC. *See* adenoid cystic carcinoma
accelerated phase chronic myeloid leukemia
(AP-CML), 506
acute lymphoblastic leukemia (ALL)
adolescent and young adult, 461–465
classification, 461
clinical features, 461
complete response criteria, 462
Philadelphia chromosome positive, 465–467
pre-B cell, 467–469
T-cell, 469–470
treatment, 461–462
acute myeloid leukemia (AML)
acute promyelocytic leukemia, 477–482
complications, 477
drug approvals, 479
European LeukemiaNet Genetic Risk
Stratification, 478
older adults, 484–486
risk factors, 477
younger adults, 482–484
acute promyelocytic leukemia (APL)
case study, 477–478
central nervous system prophylaxis, 482
diagnosis, 478, 480
hypergranular, 479
microgranular variant, 479
relapsed, 481–482
treatment, 480–481
adenocarcinoma
locally advanced rectal, 196–197
lung, 42, 46
metastatic gastric, 125–130
unknown primary, 394–397
adenoid cystic carcinoma (ACC), metastatic
adjuvant therapy, 8
case study, 7
diagnosis, 7
recommended follow-up, 8
treatment, 7–8

adolescent and young adult acute lymphoblastic
leukemia
case study, 462
diagnosis, 462–463
initial treatment, 464
intrathecal chemotherapy, 463
lumbar puncture, 463
post-induction therapy, 464–465
surveillance, 465
treatment options, 465
workup, 463
adriamycin, bleomycin, vinblastine, and
dacarbazine (ABVD), 407–408
AHCT. *See* autologous hematopoietic cell
transplantation
AI. *See* aromatase inhibitors
AIHA. *See* autoimmune hemolytic anemia
AJCC eighth edition staging system. *See* American
Joint Committee on Cancer eighth edition
staging system
alcohol consumption, esophageal SCC, 115
ALL. *See* acute lymphoblastic leukemia
alpelisib, toxicities, 79
alpha-thalassemia/intellectual disability syndrome
X-linked (ATRX), 161, 367
alveolar rhabdomyosarcoma (ARMS), 352
American Joint Committee on Cancer (AJCC)
eighth edition staging system
anal cancer, 208
breast cancer, 69
differentiated thyroid cancer, 25–26
localized prostate cancer, 218–219
localized testicular cancer, 232
localized triple-negative breast cancer, 88
locally advanced cholangiocarcinoma, 185
locally advanced colon adenocarcinoma, 194
locally advanced triple-negative breast
cancer, 90
metastatic cholangiocarcinoma, 186
metastatic colon adenocarcinoma, 198
metastatic gastric adenocarcinoma, 127
metastatic hepatocellular carcinoma, 182
metastatic hormone-sensitive prostate
cancer, 223

American Joint Committee on Cancer (AJCC)
eighth edition staging system (*cont.*)
metastatic triple-negative breast cancer, 93
nasopharyngeal cancer, 5–6
oropharyngeal cancer, 2, 3
resectable gastric cancer, 121
resectable pancreatic cancer (PC), 141
AML. *See* acute myeloid leukemia
amyloid light chain amyloidosis, 451–452
anal canal, 207–208
anal cancer
human papilloma virus infection, 207
locally advanced, 208–210
metastatic, 211
staging system, 208
very early-stage, 210
anaplastic large-cell lymphoma, 406
anaplastic thyroid cancer
locally advanced, 21–22
mutations, 20
anemia, 284
Ann Arbor staging system, Hodgkin
lymphoma, 407
anthracyclines
locally advanced anaplastic thyroid cancer, 22
toxicities, 89, 95
anti-angiogenesis tyrosine kinase inhibitors, 250
antrectomy, 159
AP-CML. *See* accelerated phase chronic myeloid
leukemia
APL. *See* acute promyelocytic leukemia
appendiceal duodenal neuroendocrine
tumor, 166
ARMS. *See* alveolar rhabdomyosarcoma
aromatase inhibitors (AI), 71, 83
adverse effects, 72–73
selection, 73
ARTIST 1 trial, 121–122
ARTIST 2 trial, 122
astrocytoma, *IDH* mutant
case study, 366
diagnosis, 366–367
follow-up and survivorship, 371
grade 2, 368
grade 3, 368
grade 4, 369
staging, 367–368
treatment considerations, 371
treatment toxicities, 370
atezolizumab
lung adenocarcinoma, 42
metastatic hepatocellular carcinoma, 182
SCC, lung, 43
toxicities, 183
ATRX. *See* alpha-thalassemia/intellectual
disability syndrome X-linked
autoimmune hemolytic anemia (AIHA), 522

autologous hematopoietic cell transplantation
(AHCT), 448
avapritinib, rhabdomyosarcoma, 357
avelumab, metastatic bladder cancer, 265
azacitidine, 490

Barcelona Clinic Liver Cancer (BCLC) staging
system, 182
Barrett's esophagus, 101, 116
BC. *See* breast cancer
BCLC staging system. *See* Barcelona Clinic Liver
Cancer staging system
BEP. *See* bleomycin, etoposide, and cisplatin
bevacizumab
metastatic cervical cancer, 279
metastatic colon adenocarcinoma, 199
midgut neuroendocrine tumor, 167
toxicities, 183, 199
biliary tract cancers (BTC), 184, 185, 186
biochemically recurrent prostate cancer
case study, 220
diagnosis, 220–221
staging, 221
treatment options, 221–222
bladder cancer
incidence, 259
metastatic, 263–265
muscle invasive, 259–263
bleomycin, etoposide, and cisplatin (BEP)
malignant germ cell tumors, 312, 317
metastatic germ cell tumor, 244
stage IIB seminoma, 243
stage IIIA seminoma, 243
blinatumomab, adolescent and young adult acute
lymphoblastic leukemia, 465
bone marrow examination, lymphoma
involvement, 437
bone metastases, 95
bone sarcoma
benign bone lesions, 339
chondrosarcoma, 343–344
Ewing sarcoma, 341–343
osteosarcoma, 339–341
borderline ovarian tumors (BOTs)
extraovarian spread, 306
fertility-sparing surgery, 307
histologies, 306
invasive implants, 307
prognosis, 307–308
staging, 307
borderline resectable pancreatic cancer (BRPC)
diagnosis, 143
staging, 144
treatment options, 144–145
bosutinib, side effects, 496
BOTs. *See* borderline ovarian tumors
brachytherapy, cervical cancer, 285

BRAF mutation
  locally advanced anaplastic thyroid cancer, 22
  melanoma, 321, 335
BRAF V600 mutation-positive disease,
    melanoma, 327–329
brain magnetic resonance imaging
  localized testicular cancer, 232
  melanoma, 335
  metastatic bladder cancer, 264
  oligodendroglioma, *IDH*-mutant, 378
brain tumors, primary
  astrocytoma, *IDH* mutant, 366–371
  glioblastoma, *IDH* wildtype, 361–366
  oligodendroglioma, *IDH* mutant, 1p/19q
    co-deleted, 371–375
BRCA mutation
  locally advanced breast cancer, 74–75
  triple-negative breast cancer (TNBC), 94
breast cancer (BC)
  early stage, 67–71
  hormone receptor positive, 67–80
  human epidermal growth factor receptor 2
    (HER2) positive, 68, 69, 83
  locally advanced, 73–75
  stage IV, 75–78
  subtypes, 68–69
  triple negative, 87–95
brentuximab vedotin, Hodgkin lymphoma, 411
BRPC. *See* borderline resectable pancreatic cancer
BTC. *See* biliary tract cancers
Burkitt lymphoma
  case study, 431
  central nervous system prophylaxis, 433
  diagnosis, 431
  front-line treatment, 432–433
  lumbar puncture, 433
  prognostic system, 432
  relapsed/refractory, 433
  staging, 432
  subtypes, 431–432
  surveillance, 433

CA-125, ovarian cancer, 304
CA 19-9, resectable pancreatic cancer (PC), 140
cabozantinib
  intermediate-risk RCC, 256
  for medullary thyroid carcinoma, 23
  metastatic hepatocellular carcinoma, 183
  metastatic RAI-refractory differentiated
    thyroid cancer, 31
CAeLYx in Platinum Sensitive Ovarian Patients
    (CALYPSO) trial, 311
calcitonin, medullary thyroid carcinoma, 31, 31
CALYPSO trial. *See* CAeLYx in Platinum
    Sensitive Ovarian Patients trial
cancers of unknown primary (CUPs)
  adenocarcinoma, 394–397

  clinical presentation, 381
  cytokeratin markers, 382
  histological subtypes, 381
  immunohistochemistry (IHC) markers, 381–383
  molecular gene expression profiling, 382
  neuroendocrine cancer, 390–394
  poorly differentiated, 387–390
  squamous cell carcinoma of the head and
    neck, 384–387
  staging, 381
  subtypes, 383
capecitabine
  locally advanced cholangiocarcinoma, 185
  locally advanced colon adenocarcinoma, 195
  toxicity, 186, 195
capecitabine and temozolomide (CAPTEM)
  pancreatic neuroendocrine tumors, 163, 176
  toxicities, 164
capecitabine/oxaliplatin, poorly differentiated
    carcinoma of unknown primary, 389
CAPTEM. *See* capecitabine and temozolomide
carboplatin, side effects, 233
carboplatin and paclitaxel
  average lifetime risk, 306
  metastatic anal cancer, 211
  metastatic cervical cancer, 279
  poorly differentiated carcinoma of unknown
    primary, 389
  toxicity, 294
carcinoid syndrome, 166
cardia gastric cancer, 120
cardiac toxicities, 280
CARMENA trial, 251
CCUS. *See* clonal cytopenia of undetermined
    significance
CELESTIAL Phase III trial, 183
cemiplimab monotherapy
  lung adenocarcinoma, 42
  SCC, lung, 43
Central Nervous System International Prognostic
    Index (CNS-IPI) model, 427
central nervous system prophylaxis
  acute promyelocytic leukemia, 482
  Burkitt lymphoma, 433
  peripheral T-cell lymphoma, 430
  surveillance, 430
cervical cancer
  distant metastatic and recurrent, 278–280
  early, 274–277
  eidemiology, 273
  FIGO surgical staging, 275
  incidence, 273
  locally advanced, 277–278
  natural history and prognosis, 273
  pathology, 273
  risk factors, 273
  symptoms and signs, 273

cervical esophageal squamous cell carcinoma, 106–107

cetuximab, colorectal cancer, 204

CHAARTED criteria, 223

checkpoint inhibitor immunotherapies immune-related adverse events, 250

chemoradiation (CRT)
gastrointestinal symptoms, bladder cancer, 263
locally advanced anal cancer, 209
locally advanced rectal cancer, 196
locally advanced unresectable lung cancer, 39
nasopharyngeal cancer, 6
oropharyngeal cancer, 2–3
toxicities, 3

chemoradiotherapy toxicities
Hodgkin lymphoma, 408
locally advanced unresectable lung cancer, 40

chemotherapy
endometrial cancer, 300
localized soft-tissue sarcoma, 350
metastatic esophageal adenocarcinoma, 108
metastatic soft-tissue sarcoma, 351
osteosarcoma, 340
poorly differentiated carcinoma of unknown primary, 389–390
side effects, advanced seminoma treatment, 234

chemotherapy toxicity
advanced seminoma, 234
advanced type 2 endometrial cancer, 294
early-stage resectable lung cancer, 37
locally advanced cholangiocarcinoma, 186
locally advanced colon adenocarcinoma, 195
malignant germ cell tumor, 312
metastatic cholangiocarcinoma, 187
metastatic colon adenocarcinoma, 199
metastatic hepatocellular carcinoma, 183
metastatic pancreatic cancer, 147

CHIP. *See* clonal hematopoiesis of indeterminant potential

cHL. *See* classical Hodgkin lymphoma

cholangiocarcinoma
extrahepatic, 184
intrahepatic, 184
locally advanced, 184–186
metastatic, 186–187
risk factors, 184

chondrosarcoma, 343–344

chromosomal instability (CIN)
colorectal cancer (CRC), 193
DNA mismatch repair (MMR) process, 193

chronic lymphocytic leukemia (CLL)
incidence, 511
mechanism, 511
newly diagnosed, 511–513
requiring treatment, 514–516

Richter's transformation, 517–518
staging and prognostication systems, 513

chronic myeloid leukemia (CML)
incidence, 493
lymphoid blast crisis, 500–502
newly diagnosed, 493–498
T315I mutation, 498–500

CIN. *See* chromosomal instability

cisplatin, toxicities, 187

cisplatin/gemcitabine, poorly differentiated carcinoma of unknown primary, 389

CLARINET study, 162, 167

CLASSIC trial, 122

classical Hodgkin lymphoma (cHL), 406, 411

CLL. *See* chronic lymphocytic leukemia

clonal cytopenia of undetermined significance (CCUS), 528, 541

clonal hematopoiesis of indeterminant potential (CHIP), 528

CML. *See* chronic myeloid leukemia

CNS-IPI model. *See* Central Nervous System International Prognostic Index model

coagulopathy, 480

Codman's triangle, 340

colon adenocarcinoma
locally advanced, 194–194
unresectable metastatic, 197–199

colonoscopy, 203

colorectal cancer (CRC)
chromosomal instability (CIN), 193
incidence and death rate, 193
locally advanced colon adenocarcinoma, 194–194
locally advanced rectal cancer, 196–197
microsatellite instability (MSI), 193
risk factors, 193

computed tomography (CT)
adenocarcinoma of unknown primary, 395
advanced type 2 endometrial cancer, 292
early stage renal cell carcinoma, 246
early-stage resectable lung cancer, 36
esophageal adenocarcinoma, 103
leiomyosarcoma, 300
localized prostate cancer, 218
localized testicular cancer, 232
locally advanced anal cancer, 208
metastatic bladder cancer, 264
metastatic colon adenocarcinoma, 198
muscle invasive bladder cancer, 260
neuroendocrine cancer of unknown primary, 391

computed tomography (CT) urography, muscle invasive bladder cancer, 260

concurrent chemoradiotherapy (CRT)
cervical esophageal SCC, 115
limited-stage small cell lung cancer, 58
locally advanced unresectable lung cancer, 39

concurrent chemoradiotherapy (CRT) (*cont.*)
    metastatic bladder cancer, 270
    nasopharyngeal carcinoma, 15
    oropharyngeal cancer, 15
conization, 285
craniotomy, 378
CRC. *See* colorectal cancer
CREATE-X trial, 91–92
CRITICS trial, 122
CRT. *See* chemoradiation
CT. *See* computed tomography
CUPs. *See* cancers of unknown primary
cyclin-dependent kinase 4/6 inhibitors,
        toxicities, 77–78
cystoscopy, muscle invasive bladder
        cancer, 260
cytoreductive nephrectomy, 256
cytoreductive surgery
    neuroendocrine tumor, 164
    ovarian cancer, 308
cytotoxic chemotherapy, toxicities, 89, 95

dabrafenib, *BRAF* V600E-positive metastatic
        differentiated thyroid cancer, 27
DA-EPOCH-R. *See* dose-adjusted etoposide,
        prednisone, vincristine, cyclophosphamide,
        doxorubicin, and rituximab
daratumumab, relapsed/refractory multiple
        myeloma (RRMM), 450
dasatinib, toxicity, 495, 506
DAXX. *See* death-domain associated protein
dd-MVAC. *See* dose dense methotrexate,
        vinblastine, doxorubicin, and cisplatin
death-domain associated protein
        (DAXX), 161
dermatologic toxicity, CTLA-4/PD-1/PD-L1
        blockade, 43
diagnostic laparoscopy, resectable gastric
        cancer, 120
differentiated thyroid cancer
    anaplastic thyroid cancer, 20
    follicular thyroid cancer, 19
    Hürthle cell carcinoma, 20
    medullary thyroid carcinoma, 20
    metastatic radioactive iodine
        refractory, 25–28
    papillary thyroid cancer, 19
    treatment overview, 20
differentiation syndrome (DS), 480
diffuse large B-cell lymphoma (DLBCL)
    case study, 424–425
    central nervous system prophylaxis, 427
    diagnosis, 425
    first relapse, 427–428
    genetic testing, 425–426
    lumbar puncture, 427

multiply-relapsed disease, 428
    prognostic stratification system, 426
    staging, 426
    surveillance, 427
    treatment options, 426
diffusion capacity of the lung for carbon
        monoxide (DLCO), 312
distant relapse-free survival, locally advanced
        breast cancer, 74
DLBCL. *See* diffuse large B-cell lymphoma
DLCO. *See* diffusion capacity of the lung for
        carbon monoxide
DNA mismatch repair (MMR) process, 193
docetaxel
    metastatic non-small cell lung cancer, 46
    side effects, 224
dose-adjusted etoposide, prednisone, vincristine,
        cyclophos phamide, doxorubicin, and
        rituximab (DA-EPOCH-R), 427
dose dense methotrexate, vinblastine,
        doxorubicin, and cisplatin
        (dd-MVAC), 270
DS. *See* differentiation syndrome
ductal and lobular carcinoma, breast, 68
duloxetine, 128
durvalumab, locally advanced unresectable lung
        cancer, 39
Dutch D1D2 trial, 123
dysgerminoma, 312

early stage cancer
    breast cancer, 68, 69, 70, 72
    cervical cancer, 274–277
    ovarian cancer, 304–306
    renal cell carcinoma, 245, 246, 248
    resectable lung cancer, 36–38
EBRT. *See* external beam radiation therapy
EBUS–TBNA. *See* endobronchial ultrasound
        transbronchial needle aspiration
EGD. *See* esophagogastroduodenoscopy
EGFR inhibitor toxicities, metastatic colon
        adenocarcinoma, 199
EGFR mutations, lung adenocarcinoma, 45
embryonal rhabdomyosarcoma (ERMS), 352
enasidenib, 486
endemic Burkitt lymphoma, 431
endobronchial ultrasound transbronchial needle
        aspiration (EBUS–TBNA), 38
endometrial biopsy, advanced type 2 endometrial
        cancer, 292
endometrial cancer
    advanced type 2, 292–294
    risk factors, 289
    type 1, 289–292
endoscopic retrograde cholangiopancreatography,
        resectable pancreatic cancer, 140

endoscopic ultrasound (EUS)
    gastric neuroendocrine neoplasms
      (g-NETs), 157
    locally advanced pancreatic cancer
      (LAPC), 145
    metastatic gastric adenocarcinoma, 127
    resectable gastric cancer, 120
    resectable pancreatic cancer, 140
enfortumab vedotin, adverse events, 266
eribulin, 98
ERMS. *See* embryonal rhabdomyosarcoma
esophageal adenocarcinoma
    diagnosis, 103–104
    locally advanced and resectable, 103–106
    metastatic, 107–110
    staging, 104
    surveillance, 106
    treatment modality, 105–106
esophageal cancer
    adenocarcinoma, 103–106
    clinical presentation, 102
    histological subtypes, 101
    human epidermal growth factor receptor 2
      positive metastatic, 110–111
    risk factors, 101
    squamous cell carcinoma, 106–107
    staging, 102–103
esophagogastric junction (EGJ), 102
esophagogastroduodenoscopy, 190
    gastric neuroendocrine neoplasms (g-NETs), 157
    metastatic gastric adenocarcinoma, 127
esophagus, 101, 102
etoposide/cisplatin, stage IIB nonseminoma germ
    cell tumor, 243
EUS. *See* endoscopic ultrasound
everolimus
    midgut neuroendocrine tumors, 167
    pancreatic neuroendocrine tumors, 176
    toxicities, 164
Ewing sarcoma
    case study, 341
    metastatic disease, 342
    surveillance, 342
    treatment course, 342
    treatment toxicities, 342
excess blasts-1, myelodysplastic syndrome
    case study, 527–528
    diagnosis, 528
    diagnostic criteria, 529
    staging, 529
    treatment options, 532–533
extensive-stage small cell lung cancer
    clinical presentation, 54
    diagnosis, 54
    molecular biomarker analysis, 55
    prognosis, 56

    staging, 54–55
    surveillance, 55–56
    treatment, 55
external beam radiation therapy (EBRT)
    advanced type 2 endometrial cancer, 293
    cervical cancer, 284
    medullary thyroid carcinoma, 24
extrahepatic cholangiocarcinoma, 184

FCR. *See* fludarabine, cyclophosphamide, and
    rituximab
FDG PET/CT scan. *See* fluorodeoxyglucose PET/
    CT scan
    fertility preservation, locally advanced triple-
      negative breast cancer, 92
fertility sparing surgery
    borderline ovarian tumors (BOTs), 307
    cervical cancer, 277
    ovarian cancer, 304–305
fine needle aspiration (FNA) biopsy
    metastatic colon adenocarcinoma, 198
    oropharyngeal cancer, 2
    FLIPI-1. *See* Follicular Lymphoma
      International Prognostic Index
fludarabine, cyclophosphamide, and rituximab
    (FCR), 522
fluorodeoxyglucose (FDG) PET/CT scan
    early-stage resectable lung cancer, 36
    metastatic lung cancer, 41, 44
    pancreatic neuroendocrine neoplasms
      (PNENs), 161
    poorly differentiated carcinoma of unknown
      primary, 388
fluoropyrimidine toxicity, 109
5-fluorouracil, cervical cancer, 284
5-fluorouracil, oxaliplatin, irinotecan, and
    leucovorin (FOLFOXIRI), 198, 199
5-fluorouracil and irinotecan (FOLFIRI), 198
5-fluorouracil and oxaliplatin (FOLFOX)
    locally advanced colon adenocarcinoma, 195
    metastatic cholangiocarcinoma, 187
    metastatic colon adenocarcinoma, 198, 203, 204
5-flurauracil, leucovorin, oxilaplatin, and
    doxetaxel (FLOT4/AIO) trial, 134
FNA biopsy. *See* fine needle aspiration biopsy
follicular lymphoma
    case study, 422
    diagnosis, 422–423
    relapse, 424
    risk stratification, 423
    staging, 423
    surveillance, 424
    treatment strategies, 423–424
Follicular Lymphoma International Prognostic
    Index (FLIPI-1), 423
follicular thyroid cancer, 19

gallbladder adenocarcinoma, 184
gastrectomy, 159
gastric cancer
  incidence, 119
  metastatic adenocarcinoma, 125–130
  resectable, 119–123
  unresectable locally advanced, 123–125
gastric neuroendocrine neoplasms (g-NETs)
  biochemical testing, 158
  case studies, 156
  diagnosis, 157
  follow-up, 159
  molecular/genetic markers, 158
  staging, 157
  subtypes, 156–157
  treatment options, 158–159
  types, 158
gastric outlet obstruction (GOO), 124
gastrointestinal stromal tumor (GIST)
  adjuvant therapy, 354
  diagnosis, 353
  staging, 353–354
  treatment options and toxicities, 354
gastrointestinal tract neuroendocrine
    neoplasms, 155
gemcitabine, metastatic non-small cell lung
    cancer, 46, 46
gemcitabine/cisplatin, metastatic
    cholangiocarcinoma, 186, 190
genetic syndromes, endometrial cancer, 289
genitourinary problems, bladder cancer
    radiation, 263
germ cell tumor, malignant, 311–312
germinal center B cell type (GCB) DLBCL, 425
germline mutations
  pancreatic neuroendocrine neoplasms
      (PNENs), 161
  poorly differentiated neuroendocrine
      carcinoma, 171
GIST. See gastrointestinal stromal tumor
glioblastoma, IDH wildtype
  case study, 361
  diagnosis, 363
  follow-up and survivorship, 366
  MR imaging, 362
  staging, 363–364
  treatment options, 364
  treatment toxicities, 365
g-NETs. See gastric neuroendocrine
    neoplasms
GOO. See gastric outlet obstruction

HCC. See hepatocellular carcinomas
head and neck cancers
  adenoid cystic carcinoma, 7–8
  metastatic squamous cell carcinoma, 9–11

oropharyngeal cancer, 1–4
  risk factors, 1
head and neck squamous cell carcinoma
    (HNSCC)
  diagnosis, 384
  recurrent/persistent disease, 387
  regional lymph node involvement, 384–385
  treatment recommendations, 386
hematological toxicity
  carboplatin, 55
  cisplatin-based chemotherapy regimens, 265
hepatocellular carcinomas (HCC)
  cholangiocarcinoma, 184–187
  hepatitis B, 181
  incidence, 181
  metastatic, 181–184
  risk factors, 181
  surveillance plan, 181
hereditary renal cell carcinoma syndromes, 247
HER2. See human epidermal growth factor
    receptor
HL. See Hodgkin lymphoma
HMAs. See hypomethylating agents
HNSCC. See head and neck squamous cell
    carcinoma
Hodgkin lymphoma (HL)
  advanced stage, 410–412
  classical, 406
  early stage, favorable risk, 405–408
  early stage, unfavorable risk, 408–410
  familial predisposition, 405
  mantle cell lymphoma, 420–422
  relapsed/refractory, 412
  subtypes, 406
hormone-positive breast cancer, early-stage, 71–73
hormone receptor-positive breast cancer, 67–80
human epidermal growth factor receptor 2
    (HER2), 115
  gastric cancer, 120, 124, 127
  HER2-positive breast cancer, 68, 69, 83
  hormone receptor-positive breast cancer, 68,
      69, 76, 83
  positive metastatic esophageal cancer, 110–111
  triple-negative breast cancer, 87
Hürthle cell carcinoma, 20
hypercalcemia, squamous cell lung cancer, 64
hyperglycemia, 80, 84
hypergranular acute promyelocytic
    leukemia, 479
hyperleukocytosis, 482
hypodiploidy, B-cell acute lymphoblastic
    leukemia, 474
hypomethylating agents (HMAs)
  excess blasts-1, myelodysplastic syndrome, 531
  toxicities, 532
hypophysitis, 335

ibrutinib, 522
ICUS. *See* idiopathic cytopenia of undetermined
    significance
IDH 1/2 mutation, chondrosarcoma, 347
idiopathic cytopenia of undetermined significance
    (ICUS), 528
IHC. *See* immunohistochemist
imatinib
    for GIST, 354
    side effects, 354
IMbrave 150 trial, 182
IMDC criteria. *See* International Metastatic
    Renal Cell Carcinoma Database Consortium
    criteria
immune-related adverse events (irAEs)
    melanoma, 327
    platinum-refractory metastatic bladder
        cancer, 266
immunodeficient B Burkitt lymphoma, 432
immunohistochemistry (IHC)
    breast, 68
    human epidermal growth factor receptor 2
        (HER2), 115
    metastatic esophageal adenocarcinoma, 107
immunotherapy
    human epidermal growth factor receptor
        2-positive metastatic esophageal cancer, 110
    locally advanced unresectable lung cancer, 39
    metastatic cervical cancer, 280
    metastatic cholangiocarcinoma, 187
    metastatic esophageal adenocarcinoma,
        108–109
    metastatic hepatocellular carcinoma, 183
    metastatic lung cancer, 45
    metastatic renal cell carcinoma, 250
    neuroendocrine cancer of unknown
        primary, 393
    toxicities, 95
immunotherapy toxicities
    anti-PD-1/PD-L1 therapies, 280
    IMpower-133 and CASPIAN, 55
    melanoma, 327
    metastatic lung cancer, 43, 45
iMODEL score, 311
IMpower010 Phase III trial, 37
IMRT. *See* intensity modulated radiotherapy
induction therapy
    acute promyelocytic leukemia, 480–481
    favorable-risk acute myeloid leukemia, 483
    intermediate and unfavorable risk acute
        myeloid leukemia, 484
inotuzumab ozogamicin, 474
intensity modulated radiotherapy (IMRT)
    medullary thyroid carcinoma, 24
    nasopharyngeal cancer, 6
interferon, midgut neuroendocrine tumor, 167

International Metastatic Renal Cell Carcinoma
    Database Consortium (IMDC) criteria, 249
International Prognostic Index (IPI), 426
intrahepatic cholangiocarcinoma, 184
intramuscular epinephrine, 474
intrathecal chemotherapy, adolescent and young
    adult acute lymphoblastic leukemia, 463
intravenous cytarabine, 490
invasive disease-free survival, locally advanced
    breast cancer, 74
invasive ductal carcinoma, breast, 72
involved-field radiation therapy, early-stage
    favorable risk classical Hodgkin lymphoma,
    407–408
IPI. *See* International Prognostic Index
IPSS-R. *See* Revised International Prognostic
    Scoring System
irAEs. *See* immune-related adverse events
irinotecan toxicity, 199
ivosidenib, 187, 485

Karnofsky Performance Status (KPS), 125,
    249, 261
Ki-67 proliferation index
    hormone receptor-positive breast cancer, 69
    neuroendocrine tumors (NETs), 155
    pancreatic neuroendocrine neoplasms
        (PNENs), 160
KPS. *See* Karnofsky Performance Status
Krenning scale, 172

Lambert-Eaton myasthenic syndrome, 64
lanreotide toxicity, 164
LAPC. *See* locally advanced pancreatic cancer
larotrectinib, metastatic cholangiocarcinoma, 187
LATITUDE criteria, 223
LBC. *See* lymphoid blast crisis
leiomyosarcoma
    case study, 294
    diagnosis, 295
    follow-up and survivorship, 297
    preoperative evaluations, 295
    staging, 296
    treatment options, 296
lenvatinib
    metastatic hepatocellular carcinoma, 182
    radioactive iodine refractory metastatic
        differentiated thyroid cancer, 27
    toxicities, 183
leukapheresis, 490
leukostasis, 490
limited-stage small cell lung cancer
    prognosis, 58
    prophylactic cranial irradiation, 59
    staging, 58
    treatment, 58

LI-RADS. *See* liver imaging reporting and data systems

liver imaging reporting and data systems (LI-RADS), 182

liver metastasis, 243

LNETs. *See* lung neuroendocrine tumors

localized cancer
 adenocarcinoma of unknown primary, 396
 prostate cancer, 217–219
 soft-tissue sarcoma, 349–351
 testicular cancer, 231–233

locally advanced cancer
 anaplastic thyroid cancer, 21–22
 breast, 73–74
 breast cancer, 73–75
 cholangiocarcinoma, 184–186
 nasopharyngeal cancer, 4–7
 oropharynx, 1–4
 pancreatic cancer, 145–146
 rectal cancer, 196–197
 triple-negative breast cancer, 90–92
 unresectable lung cancer, 38–40

locally advanced pancreatic cancer (LAPC)
 case study, 145
 diagnosis, 145
 staging, 145–146
 treatment options, 146

lumbar puncture
 adolescent and young adult acute lymphoblastic leukemia, 463
 Burkitt lymphoma, 433
 peripheral T-cell lymphoma, 430

lung cancer
 early-stage resectable, 36–38
 locally advanced unresectable, 38–40
 metastatic, 35–46
 non-small cell, 35–46
 risk factors, 35
 small cell, 53–60
 systemic therapy, 35
 5-year overall survival, 35

lung neuroendocrine tumors (LNETs), 176

luspatercept, 535

Lutathera radioisotope
 midgut neuroendocrine tumor, 167
 pancreatic neuroendocrine neoplasms (PNENs), 163

lymphoid blast crisis (LBC), 500–502

Lynch syndrome, 303

MAGIC study trial, 121

magnetic resonanace imaging (MRI)
 early cervical cancer, 274
 early stage renal cell carcinoma, 246
 leiomyosarcoma, 295
 locally advanced triple-negative breast cancer, 90

metastatic lung cancer, 44
 nasopharyngeal cancer, 5

maintenance therapy
 acute promyelocytic leukemia, 481
 intermediate and unfavorable risk acute myeloid leukemia, 484
 ovarian cancer, 309–310

malignant mixed mullerian tumors (MMMTs), 317

mantle cell lymphoma
 case study, 420
 diagnosis, 421
 follow-up and relapsed disease, 422
 staging, 421
 treatment options, 421–422

Mayo MGUS model, 443

MBL. *See* monoclonal B-cell lymphocytosis

mCRPC. *See* metastatic castration-resistant prostate cancer

MDS. *See* myelodysplastic syndrome

medullary thyroid carcinoma, 20
 calcitonin levels, 31, 31
 diagnosis, 22
 metastatic, 22–24
 pheochromocytoma, 32, 32
 treatment options, 23

melanoma
 early-stage, 321
 histological subtypes, 321
 merkel cell carcinoma, 329–331
 metastatic *BRAF* V600 mutation-positive disease, 327–329
 stage I to II disease, 322–324
 stage III, 324–327
 systemic treatment, 321

Memorial Sloan Kettering Cancer Center (MSKCC) PSADT calculator tool, 221

Memorial Sloan Kettering Cancer Center (MSKCC) prognostic model, 249

MEN. *See* multiple endocrine neoplasia

MEN1 germline mutation. *See* multiple endocrine neoplasia type 1 germline mutation

merkel cell carcinoma
 case study, 329
 diagnosis, 330
 locoregional, 330
 management, 330
 staging workup, 330
 treatment options, 331

metastatectomy, 159

metastatic adenocarcinoma
 esophageal, 107–100
 gastric, 125–130

metastatic cancer
 anal cancer, 211
 bladder cancer, 263–266
 hepatocellular carcinoma, 181–184

metastatic cancer (*cont.*)
  lung cancer, 35–46
  nonseminoma testicular cancer, 237–239
  pancreatic, 146–148
  soft-tissue sarcoma, 351–352
metastatic castration-resistant prostate cancer
  (mCRPC), 228
metastatic hormone-sensitive prostate cancer,
  222–224
MGUS. *See* monoclonal gammopathy of
  undetermined significance
microsatellite instability (MSI)
  metastatic cholangiocarcinoma, 187
  metastatic esophageal adenocarcinoma, 107
midgut neuroendocrine tumor
  carcinoid syndrome, 166
  diagnosis, 165
  pathological features, 165
  prognosis, 169
  treatment options, 166–167
midostaurin, 490
minimally invasive versus open surgery, localized
  prostate cancer, 220
mitomycin C (MMC)
  locally advanced anal cancer, 209
  microangiopathic hemolytic anemia, 214
mitotane treatment, adenoid cystic carcinoma
  (ACC) resection, 177
mitotic index, pancreatic neuroendocrine
  neoplasms (PNENs), 160
MM. *See* multiple myeloma
MMC. *See* mitomycin C
MMMTs. *See* malignant mixed mullerian tumors
MMR process. *See* DNA mismatch repair process
molecular and genomic testing
  adenocarcinoma of unknown primary,
    394–395
  advanced type 2 endometrial cancer, 292
  astrocytoma, *IDH* mutant, 367
  chronic myeloid leukemia (CML), 494
  early-stage resectable lung cancer, 37
  excess blasts-1, myelodysplastic syndrome, 528
  glioblastoma, *IDH* wildtype, 363
  leiomyosarcoma, 296
  localized prostate cancer, 218
  locally advanced anaplastic thyroid cancer,
    21–22
  locally advanced breast cancer, 74
  locally advanced colon adenocarcinoma, 194
  locally advanced pancreatic cancer (LAPC), 145
  locally advanced unresectable lung cancer,
    38–39
  metastatic bladder cancer, 264
  metastatic colon adenocarcinoma, 198
  metastatic esophageal adenocarcinoma, 107
  metastatic gastric adenocarcinoma, 127

metastatic hormone-sensitive prostate
  cancer, 223
metastatic lung cancer, 41, 44–45
metastatic SCC, head and neck, 9
metastatic triple-negative breast cancer, 93
muscle invasive bladder cancer, 262
nasopharyngeal cancer, 2
oligodendroglioma, *IDH* mutant, 1p/19q
  co-deleted, 372
oropharyngeal cancer, 2
poorly differentiated carcinoma of unknown
  primary, 388–389
recurrent stage IV breast cancer, 78–79
resectable gastric cancer, 120
resectable pancreatic cancer, 140
stage IV breast cancer, 76
unresectable locally advanced gastric
  cancer, 124
MONALEESA-2 trial, 77
MONALEESA-7 trial, 77
Monarch-3 trial, 77
monoclonal B-cell lymphocytosis (MBL), 512
monoclonal gammopathy of undetermined
  significance (MGUS)
  case study, 441–442
  diagnostic criteria, 442–443
  risk stratification, 443
MOSAIC trial, 195
MRI. *See* magnetic resonanace imaging
MSI. *See* microsatellite instability
MSKCC prognostic model. *See* Memorial Sloan
  Kettering Cancer Center prognostic model
MSKCC prostate-specific antigen doubling
  time calculator tool. *See* Memorial Sloan
  Kettering Cancer Center PSADT calculator
  tool
MSLT-I. *See* Multicenter Selective
  Lymphadenectomy Trial-I
mSMART 3.0 Model, 447
Multicenter Selective Lymphadenectomy Trial-I
  (MSLT-I), 321
multiple endocrine neoplasia (MEN), 32
multiple endocrine neoplasia type 1 (MEN1)
  germline mutation, 176, 177
multiple myeloma (MM)
  amyloid light chain amyloidosis, 451–452
  MGUS, 441–446
  newly diagnosed, transplant-eligible, 446–448
  newly diagnosed, transplant-ineligible,
    448–449
  relapsed/refractory, 449–451
  risk factors, 441
  smoldering, 441–446
muscle invasive bladder cancer
  in nonsurgical candidate, 262–263
  in surgical candidate, 259–262

myasthenia gravis, 64
myelodysplastic syndrome (MDS)
　excess blasts-1, 527–533
　incidence, 527
　with isolated Del(5q), 536
　ring sideroblasts, 533–535

nasopharyngeal cancer
　case study, 4
　diagnosis, 4–5
　histological subclassifications, 5
　staging, 5–6
　surveillance recommendations, 7
　treatment options, 6
necrosis, leiomyosarcoma, 300
nelarabine
　T-cell acute lymphoblastic leukemia, 470
　T-cell ALL, 475
NENs. See neuroendocrine neoplasms
neoadjuvant chemotherapy
　early stage breast cancer, 70
　ovarian cancer, 308–309
neoadjuvant endocrine therapy
　early stage breast cancer, 70–71
nerve sparing retroperitoneal lymph node
　　dissection
　stage IB seminoma, 243
neuroendocrine cancer of unknown primary
　case study, 390
　diagnosis, 390–391
　histological differentiation, 391
　imaging, 391
　laboratory testing, 391–392
　localized, 392
　management, 393
　metastatic, 392
　surveillance, 393–394
neuroendocrine neoplasms (NENs)
　gastric, 155–159
　gastrointestinal (GI) tract, 155
　incidence, 155
　pancreatic, 159–165
　WHO classification, 156
neuroendocrine tumors (NETs)
　appendiceal duodenal NETs, 166
　cytoreductive surgery, 164
　gastric NETs (g-NETs), 157
　lung NETs (LNETs), 176
　midgut NETs, 165–169
　nonmetastatic duodenal NETs, 166
　pancreatic NETs, 163, 176
　rectal duodenal NETs, 166
next-generation sequencing (NGS)
　Burkitt lymphoma, 431
　locally advanced anaplastic thyroid cancer, 21
　metastatic bladder cancer, 264

metastatic cholangiocarcinoma, 186
metastatic esophageal adenocarcinoma, 110
metastatic lung cancer, 44
poorly differentiated carcinoma of unknown
　　primary, 387
radioactive iodine refractory metastatic
　　differentiated thyroid cancer, 25
NGS. See next-generation sequencing
NHL. See non-Hodgkin lymphomas
nilotinib, side effects, 496
nivolumab
　platinum-refractory metastatic bladder
　　cancer, 265
　platinum-refractory recurrent/metastatic
　　HNSCC, 10, 16
　toxicities, 109
nivolumab plus cabozantinib, metastatic
　　RCC, 256
nonfunctional pancreatic neuroendocrine
　　neoplasms, 161
non-Hodgkin lymphomas (NHL)
　Burkitt lymphoma, 431–433
　clinical manifestations, 417
　diagnosis, 417, 420
　diffuse large B-cell lymphoma, 424–428
　follicular lymphoma, 422–424
　mantle cell lymphoma, 420–422
　pathogenesis, 417
　peripheral T-cell lymphoma, 428–431
　risk factors, 417
　staging, 420
nonmetastatic duodenal neuroendocrine
　　tumor, 166
nonseminoma testicular cancer
　locally advanced, 236–237
　metastatic, 237–238
　stage I, 236–237
　stage II, 237
　subtypes, 236
non-small cell lung cancer (NSCLC)
　algorithmic/decision-tree model, 35
　early-stage resectable lung cancer, 36–38
　locally advanced unresectable lung cancer,
　　38–40
　metastatic lung cancer, 35–46
　NSCLC. See non-small cell lung cancer
NTRK inhibitors
　for papillary thyroid cancer, 27
　radioactive iodine refractory metastatic
　　differentiated thyroid cancer, 27–28
nuclear medicine bone scan
　gastric cancer, 134
　metastatic bladder cancer, 264
　muscle invasive bladder cancer, 260
nucleoside diphosphate-linked moiety X motif 15
　　(NUDT15), 475

NUDT15. *See* nucleoside diphosphate-linked
    moiety X motif 15
numb chin syndrome, 475

obesity, endometrial cancer, 289
olaparib, 98
    metastatic castration-resistant prostate cancer
        (mCRPC), 228
    side effects, 95
oligodendroglioma, *IDH* mutant, 1p/19q
        co-deleted
    case study, 371–372
    diagnosis, 372
    follow-up and survivorship, 375
    grade 2, 373
    grade 3, 373–374
    treatment considerations, 375
    treatment toxicities, 374
    tumor grading, 372–373
oligometastatic disease
    case study, 251
    diagnosis, 251
    treatment options, 251–252
OlympiA trial, 92
omental biopsy, endometrial cancer, 300
oropharyngeal cancer
    case study, 1
    diagnosis, 2
    staging, 2
    surveillance recommendations, 4
    treatment options, 2–4
osteosarcoma
    case study, 339
    diagnosis, 340
    recommended treatment, 340
    staging system, 340
    surveillance, 341
    treatment toxicities, 341
osteosclerotic bone metastases, 222
ovarian cancer
    average lifetime risk, 303
    borderline, 306–308
    cytoreductive surgery, 308
    early, 304–306
    epithelial, 304
    family history, 303
    maintenance therapy, 309–310
    malignant germ cell tumor, 311–312
    neoadjuvant chemotherapy, 309
    nonepithelial, 304
    recurrent, 310–311
    symptoms, 304
oxaliplatin
    locally advanced colon adenocarcinoma, 195
    metastatic esophageal adenocarcinoma, 108
    toxicities, 109, 199

oxaliplatin-fluoropyrimidine-based therapy,
    neuroendocrine cancer of unknown
    primary, 393

packed red blood cell transfusion, cervical
    cancer, 284
PALOMA-2 trial, 77
pancreatic cancer (PC)
    five-year survival rate, 139
    incidence, 139
    locally advanced, 145–146
    metastatic, 146–148
    resectable, 139–145
    risk factors, 139
pancreatic neuroendocrine neoplasms
        (PNENs)
    advanced unresectable/metastatic well-
        differentiated G3, 163–164
    biochemical hormone testing, 161
    case study, 159–160
    classification, 160
    diagnosis, 160–161
    follow up, 165
    functional, 161
    germline mutation, 161
    hormonal syndromes, 162
    molecular markers, 161
    nonfunctional, 161
    pathology report, 160
    prognostic markers, 164–165
    systemic therapy toxicities, 164
    treatment options, 162–163
papillary thyroid cancer, 19
para-aortic lymph node metastases, 278
paraneoplastic phenomena, renal cell
    carcinoma, 245
paraneoplastic syndromes, 54
PARP inhibitor. *See* poly adenosine diphosphate-
    ribose polymerase inhibitor
pazopanib
    midgut neuroendocrine tumor, 167
    pulmonary complications, 256
PC. *See* pancreatic cancer
PCI. *See* prophylactic cranial irradiation
pembrolizumab
    colorectal cancer (CRC), 203–204
    early stage renal cell carcinoma, 248
    locally advanced anaplastic thyroid
        cancer, 22
    lung adenocarcinoma, 42
    metastatic cervical cancer, 280
    metastatic esophageal adenocarcinoma, 109
    nonplatinum-refractory disease, 16
    oligometastatic disease, 252, 256
    platinum-refractory metastatic bladder
        cancer, 265

pembrolizumab (*cont.*)
  platinum-refractory recurrent/metastatic
    HNSCC, 10, 15
  plus lenvatinib, metastatic RCC, 256
  SCC, lung, 43
  stage III RCC, clear cell type, 256
pemigatinib, metastatic cholangiocarcinoma, 187
PEPI score. *See* preoperative endocrine prognostic
    index score
peptide receptor radionucleotide
    therapy (PRRT)
  pancreatic neuroendocrine neoplasms
    (PNENs), 163
  toxicities, 164
percutaneous image-guided biopsy, metastatic
    lung cancer, 41
peripheral neuropathy, 128
peripheral T-cell lymphoma
  case study, 428
  central nervous system prophylaxis, 430
  diagnosis, 428
  first-line treatment options, 429–430
  genetic testing, 428–429
  lumbar puncture, 430
  prognostic stratification system, 429
PET/CT scan. *See* positron emission tomography/
    computed tomography scan
PFTs. *See* pulmonary function tests
pheochromocytoma, medullary thyroid
    carcinoma, 32, 32
Philadelphia chromosome-positive acute
    lymphoblastic leukemia (ALL)
  case study, 465–466
  induction strategies, 466
  post-induction therapy, 467
  significance, 466
  surveillance, 467
  treatment options, 467
phosphoinositide 3 kinase (PI3K), 79
PI3K. *See* phosphoinositide 3 kinase
platinum-based chemotherapy regimens,
    neuroendocrine cancer of unknown
    primary, 393
platinum-based doublet chemotherapy, extensive-
    stage small cell lung cancer, 64
platinum-refractory disease, head and neck
    squamous cell carcinoma, 9–10
platinum-refractory metastatic bladder cancer,
    265–266
platinum-resistant ovarian cancer, 310, 316
platinum-sensitive cancer, 310
PNENs. *See* pancreatic neuroendocrine
    neoplasms
poly adenosine diphosphate-ribose polymerase
    (PARP) inhibitor, 316
ponatinib

chronic myeloid leukemia, 499, 506
  Philadelphia chromosome-positive acute
    lymphoblastic leukemia (ALL), 467, 474
  toxicities, 500
poorly differentiated carcinoma of unknown
    primary
  case study, 387
  chemotherapy, 389–390
  molecular gene expression profiling, 388–389
  prognosis, 389
  systemic therapy, 389
  treatment recommendations, 389
  workup, 387–388
poorly differentiated neuroendocrine carcinoma
  diagnosis, 170
  germline mutations, 171
  molecular markers, 171
  pathology, 170
  treatment options, 171–172
poorly differentiated neuroendocrine
    tumor, 401
positron emission tomography/computed
    tomography (PET/CT) scan
  advanced stage Hodgkin lymphoma, 412
  biochemically recurrent prostate cancer, 221
  Burkitt lymphoma, 432
  early cervical cancer, 274
  limited-stage small cell lung cancer, 65
  locally advanced anal cancer, 208
  locally advanced cervical cancer, 278
  muscle invasive bladder cancer, 260
  nasopharyngeal cancer, 5
  non-Hodgkin lymphomas (NHL), 417
  oropharyngeal cancer, 2
  resectable gastric cancer, 120
postmenopausal bleeding, endometrial
    cancer, 300
pralsetinib, RET-mutated medullary thyroid
    cancer, 24, 31
pre-B cell acute lymphoblastic leukemia (ALL)
  case study, 467
  diagnosis, 467–468
  high-risk features, 468
  prognostic and risk assessment
    variables, 468
  treatment, 468–469
preoperative endocrine prognostic index (PEPI)
    score, 70, 71
procarbazine, lomustine, and vincristine
  astrocytoma, *IDH*-mutant, 371
  oligodendroglioma, *IDH* mutant, 1p/19q
    co-deleted, 374, 375
  toxicities, 365
PRODIGE 23 trial, 197
prophylactic cranial irradiation (PCI), limited-
    stage small cell lung cancer, 59, 65

prostate cancer
  biochemically recurrent, 220–222
  localized, 217–220
  metastatic hormone-sensitive, 222–224
PRRT. *See* peptide receptor radionucleotide
    therapy
pulmonary function tests (PFTs), early-stage
    resectable lung cancer, 37

radiation therapy (RT)
  advanced stage Hodgkin lymphoma, 412
  astrocytoma, *IDH* mutant, 370
  genitourinary problems, bladder cancer
    treatment, 263
  leiomyosarcoma, 296
radical prostatectomy (RP)
  localized prostate cancer, 219
  toxicities, 220
radioactive iodine refractory metastatic
    differentiated thyroid cancer
  case study, 24–25
  next-generation sequencing (NGS), 25
  staging, 25
  treatment options, 26–28
ramucirumab, metastatic esophageal
    adenocarcinoma, 109
RAPIDO trial, 197
RCC. *See* renal cell carcinoma
REACH-2 Phase III trial, 183
rectal cancer, locally advanced, 196–197
rectal duodenal neuroendocrine tumor, 166
refractory disease, 56
relapsed small cell lung cancer, 56–57
relapsed/refractory multiple myeloma (RRMM),
    449–451
renal cell carcinoma (RCC)
  clinical presentation, 245
  early stage, 245–248
  incidence, 245
  metastatic, 248–250
  oligometastatic disease, 251–252
  paraneoplastic phenomena, 245
resectable gastric cancer
  diagnosis, 120
  follow-up and survivorship, 123
  staging, 121
  surgical resection, SCLC, 122–123
  treatment options, 121–122, 141–143
resectable pancreatic cancer (PC)
  borderline, 143–145
  case study, 139
  diagnosis, 140
  follow-up and survivorship, 143
  staging, 141
resistant relapse, 56
RESORCE trial, 183

RET inhibitors, radioactive iodine refractory
    metastatic differentiated thyroid cancer, 27
retroperitoneal soft-tissue sarcoma, 350
Revised International Prognostic Scoring System
    (IPSS-R), 529–531
rhabdomyosarcoma, 352–353
Richter's transformation, 517–518
ring sideroblasts, myelodysplastic syndrome,
    533–535
RP. *See* radical prostatectomy
RRMM. *See* relapsed/refractory multiple myeloma
RT. *See* radiation therapy

sacituzumab govitecan, 94–95
salvage radiation therapy
  biochemically recurrent prostate cancer, 222
  toxicities, 222
SCC. *See* squamous cell carcinoma
SCLC. *See* small cell lung cancer
SCORPION trial, 308
selective estrogen receptor degrader (SERD), 71
selective estrogen receptor modulators (SERM), 71
  adverse effects, 72–73
  selection, 73
selpercatinib, 23–24, 27
seminoma
  risk stratification, 232
  second-line therapy, 235
  stage I, 233
  stage II, 234
  stage III, 234
  third-line options, 235
sensitive relapse, SCLC, 56
SERD. *See* selective estrogen receptor degrader
SERM. *See* selective estrogen receptor modulators
serum protein electrophoresis (SPEP), 347
SHARP trial, 182
SIADH. *See* syndrome of inappropriate diuretic
    hormone
skeletal-related events (SREs), 448
skin rash, alpelisib toxicity management, 80
small cell lung cancer (SCLC)
  extensive-stage, 53–56
  limited-stage, 57–59
  recent trials, 60
  relapsed, 56–57
SMM. *See* smoldering multiple myeloma
smoking
  esophageal adenocarcinoma, 101
  esophageal SCC, 115
smoldering multiple myeloma (SMM)
  case study, 441–442
  diagnosis, 442
  risk group categorization, 444
  risk stratification, 443–444
  treatment plan, 445–446

soft-tissue sarcoma
gastrointestinal stromal tumor (GIST), 353–354
localized, 349–351
metastatic, 351–352
rhabdomyosarcoma, 352–353
somatostatin analogues (SSAs), midgut
neuroendocrine tumor, 167
somatostatin receptor analogue (SSRA)
functional imaging
gastric neuroendocrine neoplasms (g-NETs), 157
pancreatic neuroendocrine neoplasms
(PNENs), 160
sorafenib, radioactive iodine refractory metastatic
differentiated thyroid cancer, 26
SPEP. *See* serum protein electrophoresis
sporadic Burkitt lymphoma, 431
sporadic pancreatic neuroendocrine neoplasms
(PNENs), 162
squamous cell carcinoma (SCC)
of the anus, 207–208
cervical esophageal, 106–107
esophageal cancer, 106–107
head and neck, 384–387
head and neck cancers, 9–11
metastatic lung cancer, 42–43
SREs. *See* skeletal-related events
SSAs. *See* somatostatin analogues
SSRA. *See* somatostatin receptor analogue
stage IV breast cancer
diagnosis, 75–76
recurrent, 78–80
staging, 76
treatment options, 76–78
sunitinib
early stage renal cell carcinoma, 248
toxicities, 164
superior vena cava (SVC) syndrome, 54
supportive care
acute promyelocytic leukemia, 480
favorable-risk acute myeloid leukemia, 482
SVC syndrome. *See* superior vena cava syndrome
syndrome of inappropriate diuretic hormone
(SIADH), 54
systemic therapy
locally advanced triple-negative breast
cancer, 91
medullary thyroid carcinoma, 23
oligometastatic disease, 251
stage I to II melanoma, 324
unresectable recurrent/metastatic HNSCC, 11

talazoparib, 95, 98
tamoxifen, side effects, 73
taxanes
locally advanced anaplastic thyroid cancer, 22
toxicities, 89, 95

T-cell acute lymphoblastic leukemia, 469–470
telotristat, bowel movement, 177
temozolomide
astrocytoma, *IDH* mutant, 370
glioblastoma, *IDH* wildtype, 364
oligodendroglioma, *IDH* mutant, 1p/19q
co-deleted, 364, 378, 379
toxicities, 365, 370
testicular cancer
advanced, 233–235
germ cell tumors, 230
localized, 231–233
locally advanced nonseminoma, 236–237
thyroid cancer
anaplastic, 20
differentiated, 19–20
follicular, 19
histology categories, 19
incidence, 19
5-year survival rate, 19
thyroid-stimulating hormone (TSH) suppression,
differentiated thyroid cancer, 31
TKIs. *See* tyrosine kinase inhibitors
TLS. *See* tumor lysis syndrome
TNBC. *See* triple-negative breast cancer
TNM staging system. *See* tumor, lymph node,
metastasis staging system
total neoadjuvant therapy, locally advanced rectal
cancer, 196–197
transurethral resection of bladder tumor
(TURBT), 260
trastuzumab
human epidermal growth factor receptor 2
(HER2)-positive metastatic esophageal cancer,
110, 111
toxicity, 294
treatment toxicities
chondrosarcoma, 344
Ewing sarcoma, 342
metastatic gastric adenocarcinoma, 128
osteosarcoma, 341
TREAT study. *See* Trial to Reduce Cardiovascular
Events With Aranesp Therapy study
Trial on Radical Upfront Surgical Therapy in
Advanced Ovarian Cancer (TRUST) trial, 308
Trial to Reduce Cardiovascular Events With
Aranesp Therapy (TREAT) study, 37
triple-negative breast cancer (TNBC), 69
localized, 87–89
locally advanced, 89–92
metastatic, 92–95
TRUST trial. *See* Trial on Radical Upfront
Surgical Therapy in Advanced Ovarian
Cancer trial
TSH suppression. *See* thyroid-stimulating
hormone suppression

TTFields. *See* tumor treating fields
tumor, lymph node, metastasis (TNM) staging
    system
    extensive-stage small cell lung cancer, 54
    metastatic gastric adenocarcinoma, 127
    resectable gastric cancer, 121
    resectable pancreatic cancer (PC), 141
    stage IV breast cancer, 76
tumor lysis syndrome (TLS), 55, 517, 523
tumor markers
    ovarian cancer, 304
    poorly differentiated carcinoma of unknown
      primary, 388
tumor pseudoprogression, glioblastoma, 365
tumor treating fields (TTFields), 364
TURBT. *See* transurethral resection of bladder
    tumor
tyrosine kinase inhibitors (TKIs)
    chronic myeloid leukemia (CML), 495
    mechanisms of resistance, 499
    medullary thyroid carcinoma, 23
    toxicities, 495–496

unresectable locally advanced gastric cancer
    case study, 123
    diagnosis, 124
    gastric outlet obstruction, 124
    staging, 124
    treatment options, 125
unresectable metastatic colon adenocarcinoma,
    197–199
UPEP. *See* urine protein electrophoresis

urine cytology, adenocarcinoma of unknown
    primary, 395
urine protein electrophoresis (UPEP), bone lesion, 347
uterine cancer
    endometrial cancer, 289–294
    leiomyosarcoma, 294–297

vaginal cuff brachytherapy, complications, 291
vaginal cuff radiation, endometrial cancer, 300
vandetanib, medullary thyroid carcinoma, 23
vemurafenib, metastatic *BRAF*-mutated RAI-
    refractory differentiated thyroid cancer, 27
venetoclax, 517, 523
venous thromboembolism (VTE), metastatic
    pancreatic cancer, 148
VTE. *See* venous thromboembolism

WBRT. *See* whole breast radiation therapy
well-differentiated neuroendocrine tumor, 401
WHO classification. *See* World Health
    Organization classification
whole breast radiation therapy (WBRT), localized
    triple-negative breast cancer, 88–89
World Health Organization (WHO) classification
    adenocarcinoma, 41
    mature lymphoid neoplasms, 418–420
    neuroendocrine neoplasms, 156

zoledronic acid, 456
    skeletal-related events, lytic bone disease,
      multiple myeloma, 448, 456, 457
    stage IV breast cancer, 78

Printed in the United States
by Baker & Taylor Publisher Services

Printed in the United States
by Baker & Taylor Publisher Services